Geriatric Medicine and Elderly Care
Lecture Notes

Geriatric Medicine and Elderly Care

Lecture Notes

Claire G. Nicholl

MB FRCP
Consultant Geriatrician (Emerita)

K. Jane Wilson

MB FRCP
Consultant Geriatrician

Shaun D'Souza

MB MRCP
Consultant Geriatrician

All of:
Department of Medicine for the Elderly
Addenbrooke's Hospital
Cambridge University Hospitals NHS Foundation Trust
Cambridge, UK

Ninth Edition

WILEY Blackwell

This ninth edition first published in 2025

© 2025 John Wiley & Sons Ltd.

Edition History

[8e, 2012, by Wiley-Blackwell]

All rights reserved, including rights for text and data mining and training of artificial technologies or similar technologies. No part of this publication may be reproduced, stored in a retrieval system, or transmitted in any form or by any means, electronic, mechanical, photocopying, recording or otherwise, except as permitted by law. Advice on how to obtain permission to reuse material from this title is available at http://www.wiley.com/go/permissions.

The right of Claire G. Nicholl, K. Jane Wilson, and Shaun D'Souza to be identified as the authors of this work has been asserted in accordance with the law.

Registered Offices

John Wiley & Sons, Inc., 111 River Street, Hoboken, NJ 07030, USA

New Era House, 8 Oldlands Way, Bognor Regis, West Sussex, PO22 9NQ, UK

For details of our global editorial offices, customer services, and more information about Wiley products, visit us at www.wiley.com.

Wiley also publishes its books in a variety of electronic formats and print-on-demand. Some content that appears in standard print versions of this book may not be available in other formats.

Trademarks: Wiley and the Wiley logo are trademarks or registered trademarks of John Wiley & Sons, Inc. and/or its affiliates in the United States and other countries and may not be used without written permission. All other trademarks are the property of their respective owners. John Wiley & Sons, Inc. is not associated with any product or vendor mentioned in this book.

Limit of Liability/Disclaimer of Warranty

The contents of this work are intended to further general scientific research, understanding, and discussion only and are not intended and should not be relied upon as recommending or promoting scientific methods, diagnoses, or treatments by physicians for any particular patient. In view of ongoing research, equipment modifications, changes in governmental regulations, and the constant flow of information relating to the use of medicines, equipment, and devices, the reader is urged to review and evaluate the information provided in the package insert or instructions for each medicine, equipment, or device for, among other things, any changes in the instructions or indication of usage and for added warnings and precautions. While the publisher and authors have used their best efforts in preparing this work, they make no representations or warranties with respect to the accuracy or completeness of the contents of this work and specifically disclaim all warranties, including without limitation any implied warranties of merchantability or fitness for a particular purpose. No warranty may be created or extended by sales representatives, written sales materials or promotional statements for this work. This work is sold with the understanding that the publisher is not engaged in rendering professional services. The advice and strategies contained herein may not be suitable for your situation. You should consult with a specialist where appropriate. The fact that an organisation, website, or product is referred to in this work as a citation and/or potential source of further information does not mean that the publisher and authors endorse the information or services the organisation, website, or product may provide or recommendations it may make. Further, readers should be aware that the websites listed in this work may have changed or disappeared between when this work was written and when it is read. Neither the publisher nor the authors shall be liable for any loss of profit or any other commercial damages, including but not limited to special, incidental, consequential, or other damages.

Library of Congress Cataloguing-in-Publication Data applied for

Paperback ISBN: 9781119627593

Cover Design: Wiley

Cover Image: © Francesca DB Photography

Set in 8.5/11pt Utopia by Straive, Pondicherry, India

Printed and bound by CPI Group (UK) Ltd, Croydon, CR0 4YY

C9781119627593_310725

The manufacturer's authorized representative according to the EU General Product Safety Regulation is Wiley-VCH GmbH, Boschstr. 12, 69469 Weinheim, Germany, e-mail: Product_Safety@wiley.com.

Contents

Preface

The ninth edition was commissioned before COVID-19, but the pandemic and its aftermath diverted attention from book writing, and the landscape of medicine has changed since the previous edition in 2012. Much of the text has been completely rewritten to reflect this.

Whatever branch of medicine you are studying or working in, with a few exceptions such as obstetrics or paediatrics, most of your patients will be older, or very old. Apart from Africa, this is now true across the world. Geriatricians have always promoted treating a person's 'biological age' rather than their 'chronological age', but this was difficult to define. The concept of frailty and simple ways to assess it are making this a reality. Outcomes across a range of specialties are linked to frailty rather than age, and older people who are likely to benefit are getting better access to new drugs and surgical procedures. All 21st century doctors need a solid grounding in geriatric medicine to be comfortable treating the majority of the patients they will see.

The biggest change for UK undergraduates is the upcoming Medical Licensing Assessment. Some medical schools still teach a 'geriatrics-light' version of the medical curriculum, but the General Medical Council content map focuses on topics that doctors are likely to encounter during the UK Foundation Programme. This obviously includes medicine that is relevant to older people, the biggest users of the health service.

The British Geriatrics Society published an updated curriculum for undergraduates in 2023, and this book covers this as well as the current European version. Global aspects of ageing are explained, and there is some detail on the organisation and delivery of health care in the UK. This can be difficult for students to grasp and will be particularly helpful for overseas-trained doctors taking the Professional and Linguistic Assessments Board (PLAB) examinations to work here. With increasing differences across the four nations, most detail is given about England, but the main differences are highlighted. The content will also provide a useful starting point for trainees revising for their Specialty Certificate Examination.

When so much information is instantly available online, is there still a place for textbooks? We believe so! The clue is the amount of information. Consider a well-defined topic such as 'Parkinson's disease' (PD). The National Institute for Health and Care Excellence (NICE) website currently lists 18 'products' about PD, with hundreds of pages, dating back to 2003. NICE Clinical Knowledge Summaries are shorter but also run to tens of pages, require multiple clicks to navigate, and sometimes give different advice to NICE guidelines. Then there are multiple 'best practice' sites, specialist society guidelines and finally the vast resource of primary literature. The advantage of a book is that we have provided a synthesis of the most important points that are relevant to our clinical practice and highlighted areas of controversy. Once you have a basic grasp of an area, exploring it online will be more rewarding.

This book, like the population, is a little fatter than its predecessors. This is the result of both more advances in medicine being offered to older people (there is a new chapter on geriatric oncology) and a decision to include more explanation in the text. For example, there is enough detail about bone metabolism to understand, rather than just memorise, the drugs for osteoporosis. Our approach to medicine that empowers patients, and values working with the multidisciplinary team is relevant to patients of any age with chronic disease. For simplicity, when describing the prevalence of disease, female sex is used when referring to those assigned female at birth.

A typical older patient is more complex than a younger patient because of the interaction between their unique long-life experience and various comorbidities. Therefore, geriatric medicine is the medicine of complexity – interesting, varied, and challenging. If you enjoy using clinical acumen, leading and working in a team, and thinking about what really matters to an individual patient rather than following guidelines, consider a career in geriatric medicine. In addition to their core inpatient and community work, geriatricians are in demand across a wide and expanding range of clinical areas, for example in orthopaedics, surgical liaison, acute assessment, falls and syncope and movement disorders.

Geriatricians provide a large proportion of the examiners for PACES, the Practical Assessment of Clinical Examination Skills examination for the Royal College of Physicians. They are often excellent teachers, successful as medical managers and there are numerous opportunities for basic, epidemiological, and clinical research. There are many options for working overseas. After retiring from full-time work, CN had an enjoyable and satisfying time working and teaching in Botswana and teaching the European geriatrics curriculum as a visiting professor at the University of Pavia in Italy.

For years, geriatricians may have felt a little overshadowed by their single-organ specialty colleagues. In a world where patients are told they must present a single problem in a consultation with their GP and guideline medicine prevails in hospitals, the value of a comprehensive but individualised approach is increasingly recognised by patients, families, and colleagues. This edition has reverted to its original name, Lecture Notes in Geriatric Medicine.

Claire G. Nicholl
K. Jane Wilson
Shaun D'Souza
Cambridge, October 2024

Note about the cover

Cover image by Francesca DB Photography.

Isabella Mastantuono with her first great-granddaughter, Sofia.

Isabella had a very prolonged hospital stay. Her medical team began to wonder if they should keep on with burdensome rounds of treatment, striving to try to get her better. Isabella and her family had a very different perspective. Four months after her discharge, they sent the team this photograph of Isabella, who was doing well and especially enjoying spending time with Sofia.

Published with permission from Isabella, Sofia's parents, and Francesca.

Note about doses

We have given doses of common drugs to help with familiarity and have tried to ensure that there are no errors, but please always check with a primary source such as the BNF or product literature before prescribing.

Acknowledgments

Thanks to Dr Matthew Butler for his input to the cardiology chapter, Prof. Liz Warburton for her contribution to the stroke chapter and Dr James Tanner for providing images.

We would also like to thank Nigel, Jo, and Hettie for their patience and support.

Abbreviations

5-HT	5 hydroxytryptamine (serotonin)
5-HT$_{2A}$	5-HT2A receptor
A&E	accident and emergency, usually now known as the emergency department
AA	alcoholics anonymous
AA	attendance allowance
AAA	abdominal aortic aneurysm
AADC	aromatic amino acid decarboxylase
AAFB	acid and alcohol fast bacilli
AaPO$_2$	alveolar-arterial oxygen tension difference
AAV	adeno-associated virus
Aβ	amyloid beta-peptide
ABCDE	approach for resuscitation: airway, breathing, circulation, disability, exposure
ABG	arterial blood gas
ABL-1	tyrosine protein kinase proto-oncogene
ABPI	arterial brachial pressure index
ACA	anterior cerebral artery
ACB	anticholinergic burden
ACE	angiotensin-converting enzyme
ACEi	ACE inhibitor
AChE	acetylcholinesterase
AChEi	acetylcholinesterase inhibitor
AChR	acetylcholine receptor
ACiS	anterior circulation ischaemic stroke
ACP	advanced care planning
ACR	albumin : creatinine ratio
ACS	acute coronary syndrome
ACS	anterior circulation stroke (context essential)
ACS NSQIP	American College of Surgeons national surgical quality improvement program
ACTH	adrenocorticotrophic hormone
AD	advance decision
AD	Alzheimer's disease
ADH	antidiuretic hormone
ADL	activities of daily living
ADORE	drug trial of edaravone in ALS
ADR	adverse drug reaction
ADRT	advance decision to refuse treatment
ADT	androgen deprivation therapy
AEDs	anti-epileptic drugs, now known as ASMs, see below
AF	atrial fibrillation
AFO	ankle-foot orthosis
AIDP	acute inflammatory demyelinating polyradiculoneuropathy
AIDS	acquired immune deficiency syndrome
AIHA	autoimmune haemolytic anaemia
AIP	acute interstitial pneumonia
AJGP	Australian Journal of General Practice
AKI	acute kidney injury
AKT	a serine/threonine protein kinase, also known as protein kinase B, PKB
ALD	alcoholic liver disease
ALL	acute lymphoblastic leukaemia
ALP	alkaline phosphatase
ALS	amyotrophic lateral sclerosis
AMD	age-related macular degeneration
AMHP	approved mental health practitioner
AML	acute myeloid leukaemia
AMP/ADP/ATP	adenosine mono di and triphosphate
AMPA	α-amino-3-hydroxy-5-methyl-4-isoxazolepropionic acid, a receptor for glutamate
AMP-K	adenosine monophosphate activated protein kinase
AMTS	abbreviated mental test score
ANH	artificial nutrition and hydration
ANS	autonomic nervous system
anti-CCP/ACPA	anticitrullinated peptide antibody
AP	antero-posteriorly
APOE	apolipoprotein E
APP	amyloid precursor protein
ARB	angiotensin receptor blocker
ARDS	acute respiratory distress syndrome
ARIA	amyloid-related imaging abnormalities
ARNI	ARB/ neprilysin inhibitor combination e.g. valsartan/ sacubitril
AS	Alzheimer's society
AS	aortic stenosis
ASA	American Society of Anesthesiology
ASM	anti-seizure medication, previously anti-epileptic drugs
ATN	acute tubular necrosis
AV	atrioventricular
AVP	arginine vasopressin
AXR	abdominal X-ray
BACE	β-secretase enzyme that cleaves transmembrane APP
BAFTA	Birmingham atrial fibrillation treatment of the aged study
BAME	Black, Asian and ethnic minorities
BC	breast cancer
BCC	basal-cell carcinoma
BCE	before common era
BCG	bacille Calmette Guérin
BD	twice a day
BiTEs	bispecific T cell engagers
BMA	British Medical Association
BMD	bone mineral density
BMI	body mass index
BMJ	British Medical Journal
BNF	British National Formulary
BNP	brain natriuretic peptide
BOO	bladder outflow obstruction
BOOP	bronchiolitis obliterans organizing pneumonia
BP	blood pressure
BPH	benign prostatic hyperplasia
BPI	bactericidal/permeability-increasing protein fold gene
BPL	below the poverty line (households in India)
BPPV	benign paroxysmal positional vertigo
BPSD	behavioural and psychological symptoms of dementia
BRAF	a serine/threonine protein kinase proto-oncogene with a critical role in MAPK cell signalling pathway.
BRAN	questions to ask about a new drug - benefits, risks, alternatives, do nothing?
BRCA	breast cancer genes 1 and 2 (also increase risk of other cancers including ovary, pancreas, prostate)
BTS	British Thoracic Society
BZD	benzodiazepine
CAA	cerebral amyloid angiopathy
CABG	coronary artery bypass graft

CAD	coronary artery disease
CADASIL	cerebral autosomal dominant arteriopathy with subcortical infarcts and leukoencephalopathy
CAG	cytosine, adenine, guanine triplet repeats found in high numbers in Huntington's
CAGE	screen for problem alcohol use
CAM	confusion assessment method
CAP	community acquired pneumonia
CAPD	continuous ambulatory peritoneal dialysis
CAR	chimeric antigen receptor
CASSR	council with adult social services responsibility
CAT	COPD assessment test
CAUTI	catheter-associated UTI
CBD	corticobasal degeneration
CBT	cognitive behavioural therapy
CBTI	cognitive behavioural therapy for insomnia
CCK	cholecystokinin
CCL5	chemokine ligand 5
CCP	cyclic citrullinated peptide
CCU	coronary care unit
CDAD	Clostridioides difficile-associated diarrhoea
CDK	cyclin dependent kinase
CFH	complement factor H
CFS	clinical frailty score (Rockwood)
CGA	comprehensive geriatric assessment
CGM	continuous glucose monitoring
CHA_2DS_2VASc	score for risk of stroke in atrial fibrillation
CHARM	candesartan in heart failure assessment of reduction in morbidity and mortality study
CHART	continuous hyperfractionated accelerated radtiotherapy
CHC	continuing healthcare funding
CHF	chronic heart failure
CI	confidence interval
CIDP	chronic inflammatory demyelinating polyradiculoneuropathy
CIWA	clinical institute withdrawal assessment - alcohol
CK	creatine kinase
CKD	chronic kidney disease
CKM	conservative kidney management
CK-MB	creatine kinase with muscle and brain subunits
CKS	clinical knowledge summary
CLL	chronic lymphocytic leukaemia
CMA	chaperone-mediated autophagy
CMC	carpometocarpal
CML	chronic myeloid leukaemia
CNS	central nervous system
CO	carbon monoxide
CO_2	carbon dioxide
COHb	carboxyhaemoglobin
COMT	catechol-O-methyltransferase
COP	cryptogenic organizing pneumonia
COPD	chronic obstructive pulmonary disease
COX-2	cyclo-oxygenase-2
CPAP	continuous positive airways pressure
CPN	community psychiatric nurse
CPPD	calcium pyrophosphate deposition disease
CPR	cardiopulmonary resuscitation
CQC	Care Quality Commission
CREST	acronym for calcinosis, Raynaud phenomenon, esophageal dysmotility, sclerodactyly, and telangiectasia
CRHT	crisis resolution and home treatment team
CRP	C-reactive protein
CRT	conformal radiotherapy
CRT-P	cardiac resynchronisation therapy - pacemaker
CSF	cerebrospinal fluid
CSM	carotid sinus massage

CSS	carotid sinus syndrome
CT	computerized tomography
CTPA	computerized tomography pulmonary angiogram
CTZ	chemoreceptor trigger zone
CUH	Cambridge University Hospitals (Addenbrooke's)
CVA	cerebrovascular accident
CVP	central venous pressure
CVS	cardiovascular system
CVT	central venous thrombosis
CXR	chest X-ray
DA	dopamine
DAA	direct acting antiviral
DAME	acronym for causes of falls (drugs, ageing, medical and environmental causes - female preponderance)
DAMPs	damage-associated molecular patterns
DAN	diabetic autonomic neuropathy
DAPT	dual antiplatelet therapy
DAT	dopamine transporter
DBS	deep brain stimulation
DBS	disclosure and barring service
DC	direct current
DE	dementia (elderly) - in the context of care home provision
DESH	disproportionately enlarged subarachnoid space hydrocephalus
DFLE	disability-free life expectancy
DGH	district general hospital
DHSC	Department of Health and Social Care
DI	diabetes insipidus
DIC	disseminated intravascular coagulation
DIP	distal interphalangeal
DLB	dementia with Lewy bodies
DLCO	diffusing capacity for carbon monoxide
DLUHC	Department for Levelling Up, Housing and Communities
DM	dermatomyositis
DM	diabetes mellitus
DMARD	disease-modifying anti-rheumatic drug
DMT1	divalent metal transporter1
DNA	deoxyribonucleic acid
DNACPR	do not attempt cardiopulmonary resuscitation
DOAC	direct oral anticoagulant
DOLS	deprivation of liberty safeguards
DORA	dual orexin receptor antagonists
DPLD	diffuse parenchymal lung disease
DPP	dipeptidyl peptidase
DRD	Daratumumab + Revlimid (lenalidomide) + dexamethasone, an immunotherapy regimen for myeloma
DRE	digital rectal examination, sometimes abbreviated as PR (per rectum) which is also a route for drug administration
DSPN	diabetic sensorimotor polyneuropathy
DVLA	Driver and Vehicle Licensing Authority
DVT	deep vein thrombosis
DWI	diffusion weighted imaging (MRI)
DXA	dual-energy X-ray absorptiometry
E&W	England and Wales
ECG	electrocardiogram
ECMO	extracorporeal membrane oxygenation
ECOG	Eastern Cooperative Oncology Group
ECT	electroconvulsive therapy
ED	emergency department
EEG	electroencephalogram/graphy
eGFR	estimated glomerular filtration rate
EGFR	epidermal growth factor receptor
EuGMS	European Geriatric Medicine Society
EIBC	early invasive breast cancer

ELISA	enzyme-linked immunosorbent assay
EMA	endomysial antibodies
EMG	electromyogram/electromyography
ENT	ear, nose and throat
EOFAD	early-onset familial Alzheimer's disease
EPO	erythropoietin
ER	(o)estrogen receptor
ER	endoplasmic reticulum
ERAD	endoplasmic reticulum-associated degradation
ERCP	endoscopic retrograde cholangiopancreatography
ESC	European Society of Cardiology
ESKD	end stage kidney disease
ESR	erythrocyte sedimentation rate
ET	essential tremor
ET	essential thrombocythaemia
EU	European Union
EVAR	endovascular aneurysm repair
EWGSOP2	European Working Group on Sarcopenia in Older People 2
FaME programme	fitness and mobility exercise programme
FAST	face, arms, speech, time, score for stroke
FBC	full blood count
FDA	Food and Drug Administration (US)
FDG	fluorodeoxyglucose
FEV1	forced expiratory volume in 1 s
FGFR	fibroblast growth factor receptor
FIMDT	feeding issues multidisciplinary team
FIT	faecal immunochemical test
FLAIR	fluid-attenuated inversion recovery, MRI sequence that shows grey matter as bright and CSF as dark
FNC	NHS funded nursing care
FOCUS	fluoxetine on functional outcomes after acute stroke trial
FOXO	forkhead box O: transcription factors with key roles in insulin signalling and ageing
FRAX	fracture risk tool advocated by NOGG and NICE
FRIDS	falls-risk increasing drugs
FRS	family research survey
FSH	follicle stimulating hormone
FTD	frontotemporal dementia
FTLD	frontotemporal lobar degeneration
FUS	focused ultrasound
FVC	forced vital capacity
GABA	gamma-aminobutyric acid
GARS	glycyl-tRNA synthetase
GBS	Guillain–Barré syndrome
GCA	giant-cell arteritis
GCS	Glasgow coma score
G-CSF	granulocyte colony stimulating factor
GDNF	glial cell-line derived nerve growth factor
GDP	gross domestic product
GDS	geriatric depression score
GFR	glomerular filtration rate
GH	growth hormone
GI	gastrointestinal
GIP	glucose-dependent insulinotropic polypeptide
GLP-1	glucagon-like peptide 1
GLUT4	glucose transporter - a rate-limiting step in insulin-stimulated glucose uptake in muscle and adipocytes
GMC	General Medical Council
GnRH	gonadotrophin releasing hormone
GORD	gastro-oesophageal reflux disease
GP	general practitioner
GPCOG	general practice cognitive screening test for dementia
GRACE	global registry of acute coronary events
GSF	gold standards framework

GSK	a pharma company, previously GlaxoSmith Kline
GSM	genitourinary syndrome of menopause (new term for vulvovaginal atrophy)
GTN	glyceryl trinitrate
GU	genitourinary tract
GWAS	genome-wide association study
h	hour
HALE	health-adjusted life expectancy
HASBLED	score for predicting bleeding risk of anticoagulation for AF, superseded by ORBIT
HCM	hypertrophic cardiomyopathy
HDU	high dependency unit
HPC	haemoprogenitor cell
HSC	haemopoietic stem cell
HER2	human epidermal growth factor receptor 2
HERMES	outcomes of thrombectomy : highly effective reperfusion evaluated in multiple endovascular stroke trials
HFE	high iron (Fe)/ human homeostatic iron regulator protein/ gene (mutations cause haemochromatosis)
HFmrEF	heart failure with mildly reduced ejection fraction
HFpEF	heart failure with preserved ejection fraction
HFrEF	heart failure with reduced ejection fraction
HHS	hyperosmolar hyperglycaemic syndrome
HINTS test	head impulse, nystagmus, test of skew test in vertigo
HIV	human immunodeficiency virus
HL	Hodgkin's lymphoma
HLA	human leucocyte antigen
HLE	healthy life expectancy
HLY	health-adjusted life expectancy
HMRN	Haematological Malignancy Research Network
HOOF	home oxygen order form
HPC	haematoprogenitor cell
HPV	human papilloma virus
HRCT	high resolution computerized tomography scan
HRT	hormone replacement therapy
HSC	haematopoietic stem cells
HSMN	hereditary motor and sensory neuropathy
HSV	Herpes simplex virus
HUT	head-up tilt
HWB	health and wellbeing board
I131	iodine-131
IA	intraarticular
IADL	instrumental activities of daily living
IBD	inflammatory bowel disease
IBM	inclusion body myositis
IBS	irritable bowel syndrome
IC	intermediate care
ICA	internal carotid artery
ICB	integrated care board
ICD	implantable cardioverter-defibrillator
ICH	intracerebral haemorrhage
ICP	intracranial pressure
ICP	integrated care partnership
ICS	inhaled corticosteroids
ICS	integrated care system
ICU	intensive care unit
IDA	iron deficiency anaemia
IE	infective endocarditis
Ig G, M, A, D and E	immunoglobulin classes
IGF-1	insulin-like growth factor 1
IHD	ischaemic heart disease
IL	interleukin
ILD	interstitial lung disease
IM	intramuscular
IMCA	independent mental capacity advocate
INR	international normalized ratio
IOP	intraocular pressure

IPF	idiopathic pulmonary fibrosis
IS	ischaemic stroke
ISC	intermittent self-catheterisation
IU	international units
IV	intravenous
IVT	intravenous thrombolysis
IVU	intravenous urogram
JAK	Janus kinases, cytoplasmic tyrosine kinases and their genes
JVP	jugular venous pressure
KRT	kidney replacement therapy
LA	local authority
LAA	left atrial appendage
LABA	long-acting beta$_2$ agonist
LACI	lacunar infarct
LAMA	long-acting muscarinic antagonist
LASI	longitudinal aging study in India
LBBB	left bundle branch block
LBD	Lewy body disease, an umbrella term including DLB and PDD
LCP	Liverpool care pathway for the dying patient
LDH	lactate dehydrogenase
LDL-C	low density lipoprotein cholesterol
LE	life expectancy
LED	levodopa equivalent dose
LFT	liver function test
LGBTQ+	lesbian, gay, bisexual, transgender, queer plus other emerging gender and sexual identities
LH	luteinizing hormone
LHRH	luteinizing hormone-releasing hormone
LMIC	low or middle income country
LMN	lower motor neuron
LMWH	low molecular weight heparin
LOAD	late-onset Alzheimer's disease
LOC	loss of consciousness
LP	lumbar puncture
LPA	lasting power of attorney
LPL	lymphoplasmacytic lymphoma
LPS	liberty protection safeguards
LTOT	long-term oxygen therapy
LUTS	lower urinary tract symptoms
LV	left ventricular
LVEF	left ventricular ejection fraction
LVF	left ventricular failure
LVH	left ventricular hypertrophy
LVO	large vessel occlusion
M$_{1-5}$	muscarinic receptors
M band	monoclonal band
Mab	monoclonal antibody
MAO-A or B	monoamine oxidase A or B
MAP	mean arterial pressure
MAP-K	mitogen-activated protein kinases: serine/threonine-specific protein kinases that relay signals from the cell surface to the nucleus
MAR	medicines administration record
MASD	moisture-associated skin damage
MASLD	metabolic dysfunction-associated steatotic liver disease (replacing the term NAFLD)
MBBS	Bachelor of Medicine, Bachelor of Surgery (UK professional medical qualification)
MCA	Mental Capacity Act
MCA	middle cerebral artery
MCCD	Medical Certificate of Cause of Death
MCI	mild cognitive impairment
MCV	mean corpuscular volume
MDRD	modification of diet in renal disease
MDS	myelodysplastic syndrome
MDT	multidisciplinary team

MEK	mitogen-activated protein kinase, also known as MAP2K
MFRA	multifactorial falls risk assessment
MG	myasthenia gravis
MGUS	monoclonal gammopathy of unknown significance
MHA	Mental Health Act
MHC	major histocompatibility complex
MHRA	Medicines and Healthcare Products Regulatory Agency (UK)
MI	myocardial infarction
min	minute
MIND	a mental health charity in England and Wales
MMSE	mini-mental state examination
MNA	mini-nutritional assessment
MND	motor neuron disease
MoCA	Montreal cognitive assessment
MOVES	Trial of chondroitin and glucosamine for knee pain in osteoarthritis
MPTP	1-methyl-4-phenyl-1,2,3,4-tetrahydropyridine
MRA	magnetic resonance angiography
MRC	Medical Research Council
MRCP	magnetic resonance cholangiopancreatography
MRCP	Membership of the Royal College of Physicians
MRgFUS	MRI-guided focused ultrasound
MRI	magnetic resonance imaging
mRNA	messenger RNA
MRSA	methicillin-resistant Staphylococcus aureus
MS	multiple sclerosis
MSA	multiple system atrophy
MSU	midstream urine
MT	mechanical thrombectomy
mtDNA	mitochondrial DNA
mTOR	mammalian target of rapamycin: a serine/threonine protein kinase regulating cell growth and proliferation
MTP	metatarso-phalangeal
MuSK	muscle specific tyrosine kinase
MUST	malnutrition universal screening tool
NA	noradrenaline
NABCOP	national audit of breast cancer in older patients
NAD +	nicotinamide adenine dinucleotide
NAFLD	non-alcoholic fatty liver disease, now known as MASLD
NAIF	national audit of inpatient falls
NaSSa	serotonin noradrenaline reuptake inhibitor
NBM	nil by mouth
NCEPOD	National Confidential Enquiry into Patient Outcomes and Death
NCS	nerve conduction studies
NCSE	non-convulsive status epilepticus
NELA	national emergency laparotomy audit
NF-kB	nuclear factor kappa light chain enhancer of activated B cells
NG	nasogastric
NGO	non-governmental organisation
NHS	National Health Service
NHS CC	NHS continuing care
NIA-AA	National Institute on Aging and the Alzheimer's Association (new criteria for diagnosis of AD)
NICE	National Institute for Health and Care Excellence
NICs	national insurance contributions
NIH	National Institutes of Health (Agency of the US Dept. of Health)
NIHSS	National Institutes of Health stroke scale
NIV	non-invasive ventilation
NKT	natural killer T cells
NMDA	N-methyl-D-aspartate, a receptor for glutamate
NMJ	neuromuscular-junction

NMS	neurally-mediated syncope		PMF	primary myelofibrosis
NNT	number needed to treat		PMR	polymyalgia rheumatica
NOF	neck of femur		POADR	prospective old age dependency ratio
NOGG	National Osteoporosis Guidelines Group		POAG	primary open angle glaucoma
NPH	normal pressure hydrocephalus		POCI	posterior circulation infarct
NSAID	non-steroidal anti-inflammatory drug		POP	plaster of Paris
NSCLC	non-small-cell lung cancer		POPS	perioperative medicine for older people having surgery
NSIP	non-specific interstitial pneumonia			
NSTE-ACS	non-ST elevation acute coronary syndromes		PP	pulse pressure
NSTEMI	non-ST elevation myocardial infarction		PPARγ	peroxisome-proliferator-activated receptor gamma
NT-proBNP	N-terminal pro-B-type natriuretic peptide		PPCs	postoperative pulmonary complications
NVH	non-visible haematuria		PPI	proton pump inhibitor
NYHA	New York Heart Association		PPI	patient and public involvement
O2	oxygen		PPO	potential prescribing omissions
OA	osteoarthritis		PPS	post-polio syndrome
OADR	old age dependency ratio		PRISMA	a self-reported questionnaire for frailty
OD	once a day		PRISMS	potential of rtPA for ischemic strokes with mild symptoms trial
OECD	Organization for Economic Cooperation and Development			
OGD	oesophago gastro duodenoscopy		PSA	prostate specific antigen
ONS	Office of National Statistics		PSP	progressive supranuclear palsy
OPG	osteoprotegerin		PSR	potential support ratio
ORBIT	acronym for a risk score for bleeding on anticoagulants for AF (older, renal impairment, bled before, iron low, taking antiplatelet drugs)		PT (or physio.)	physiotherapy/ physiotherapist
			PTCA	percutaneous transluminal coronary angioplasty
			PTH	parathyroid hormone
			PTHrP	parathyroid hormone-related protein
OSA/HS	obstructive sleep apnoea/hyponoea syndrome		PUVA	psoralen + UVA treatment
OT	occupational therapy/ therapist		PV	polycythaemia vera
OTC	over-the-counter (medicines)		PVD	peripheral vascular disease
P2Y12	purinergic receptors on platelets (bind clopidogrel family)		PVS	persistent vegetative state
			QDS	four times a day
PA	pernicious anaemia		Qfracture	fracture risk tool advocated by SIGN and NICE
PACG	primary angle closure glaucoma		QOF	quality and outcomes framework
PACI	partial anterior circulation infarct		QRISK3	UK cardiovascular risk calculator
PAF	paroxysmal atrial fibrillation		QT	the time between the start of the Q wave and end of the T wave on an ECG
PaO2	partial pressure of oxygen			
PARP	poly ADP-ribose polymerase		RA	rheumatoid arthritis
PBC	primary biliary cirrhosis		RA	right atrium
PCI	percutaneous coronary intervention		RAAS	renin angiotensin aldosterone system
PCiS	posterior circulation ischaemic stroke		RAGE/AGE	receptor for advanced glycation endproducts
PCR	polymerase chain reaction		RANKL	receptor activator of nuclear factor kappa-B ligand
PCS	posterior circulation stroke		RAS	renal artery stenosis
PCT	primary care trust		Ras	ras proto-oncogenes: GTPases that act as molecular switches in pathways for cell proliferation and survival
PD	Parkinson's disease			
PD-1 inhibitor	programmed cell death protein 1 inhibitor (an immune checkpoint inhibitor)			
			RBBB	right bundle branch block
PDB	Paget's disease of the bone		RBC	red blood cell
PDD	Parkinson's disease dementia		RCC	renal cell cancer
PDE	phosphodiesterase		RCGP	Royal College of General Practitioners
PDK1	phosphoinositide-dependent kinase 1		RCP	Royal College of Physicians
PD-LI inhibitor	programmed cell death ligand inhibitor		RCT	randomized controlled trial
PE	pulmonary embolism		RDW	red cell distribution width
PEC	percutaneous endoscopic colopexy		Rehab.	rehabilitation
PEFR	peak expiratory flow rate		REM	rapid eye movement
PEG	percutaneous endoscopic gastrostomy		RGSC	Registrar General's socio-economic class
PEG-J	percutaneous endoscopic gastrostomy with a jejunal extension		RLS	restless legs syndrome
			RNA	ribonucleic acid
PEJ	percutaneous endoscopic jejunostomy		RNIB	Royal National Institute for Blind people
PET	positron-emission tomography		ROS	reactive oxygen species
PHC	primary health centre (India)		ROSIER	recognition of stroke in the emergency room scale
PICC	peripherally inserted central catheter		RoSPA	Royal Society for the Prevention of Accidents
PICH	primary intracranial haemorrhage		RPE	retinal pigment epithelium
PIM	potentially inappropriate medication		RS3PE	remitting seronegative symmetrical synovitis with pitting (o)edema
PIP	proximal interphalangeal			
PIP2/3	phosphatidylinositol 4,5-bisphosphate and 3,4,5-trisphosphate (cell membrane phospholipids)		RSPCA	Royal Society for Prevention of Cruelty to Animals
			RTA	road traffic accident
PJ	slang for pyjama, as in pj paralysis		rt-PA	recombinant tissue-type plasminogen activator
PLMS	periodic limb movements in sleep		RUQ	right upper quadrant
PM	polymyositis		SA	sino-atrial

SABA	short-acting beta$_2$ agonist
SABR	stereotactic ablative radiotherapy
SAE	serious adverse event (with a medical product)
SAH	subarachnoid haemorrhage
SAMA	short-acting muscarinic antagonist
SaO2	arterial oxygen saturation
SARI	serotonin antagonist-reuptake inhibitor
SARS-CoV-2	severe acute respiratory syndrome coronavirus 2
SASP	senescence-associated secretory phenotype
SBOT	short-burst oxygen therapy
SBP	systolic blood pressure
SC	subcutaneous
SCC	squamous-cell carcinoma
SCLC	small-cell lung cancer
SCN	suprachiasmatic nucleus
SD	standard deviation
SDH	subdural haematoma
SE	status epilepticus
sec	second
SERM	selective estrogen modulator
Sestamibi or 'mibi' scan	technetium 99m methoxy isobutyl isonitrile scan
sFLC	serum free light chain
SGLT2i	sodium-glucose co-transporter-2 inhibitor
SIADH	syndrome of inappropriate antidiuretic hormone
SIGN	Scottish intercollegiate guidelines network
SIRT	sirtuins: nicotine adenine dinucleotide-dependent histone deacetylases regulating critical signalling pathways
SITS-MOST	safe implementation of treatments in stroke monitoring study
SIVD	subcortical ischaemic vascular disease
SLE	systemic lupus erythematosus
SLT	selective laser trabeculoplasty
SLT	speech and language therapist/ therapy
SN	substantia nigra
SNP	single nucleotide polymorphism (pronounced snip)
SNRI	serotonin and norepinephrine reuptake inhibitor
SNS	sympathetic nervous system
SOD	superoxide dismutase, an enzymatic antioxidant, which catalyses the dismutation of superoxide ions into oxygen and hydrogen peroxide
SOL	space-occupying lesion
SPA	state pension age
SPECT	single-photon emission computerized tomography
SPF	sun protection factor
SPLATT	acronym for falls assessment (symptoms, previous falls, location, activity, time, and trauma)
SSNAP	sentinel stroke national audit programme
SSRI	selective serotonin reuptake inhibitor
Stat.	usually a one-off dose, given immediately, from the Latin statim
STEMI	ST-elevation myocardial infarction
STOPP/START	screening tool of older persons prescriptions and screening tool to alert doctors to right treatment
SVC	superior vena cava
T1/T2 DM	type 1/type 2 diabetes mellitus
T3	triiodothyronine
T4	thyroxine
TACI	total anterior circulation infarct
TAVI	transcatheter aortic valve insertion
TB	tuberculosis
TCC	transitional cell carcinoma
tDCS	transcranial direct current stimulation
TDP	transactive response DNA-binding protein
TDS	three times a day
TEDS	thromboembolic deterrent stockings

TENS	transcutaneous electrical nerve stimulation
T$_{FH}$	T follicular helper cells
TFTs	thyroid function tests
TGA	transient global amnesia
TH	tyrosine hydroxylase
T$_H$	subset of T helper cells
TIA	transient ischaemic attack
TIBC	total iron binding capacity
TLOC	transient loss of consciousness
TMJ	temporomandibular joint
Tn	troponin
TNFα	tumour necrosis factor alpha
TOE	transoesophageal echocardiography
tPA	tissue plasminogen activator
TPN	total parenteral nutrition
T$_{reg}$	regulatory T cells, a T helper subset with role in immune tolerance
TSH	thyroid stimulating hormone
tTG-IgA	tissue transglutaminase antibodies
TTT	tilt-table testing
TUG	timed up and go test
TUIP	transurethral incision of the prostate
TUMT	transurethral microwave therapy
TUNA	transurethral needle ablation
TURBT	transurethral resection of bladder tumour
TURP	transurethral resection of the prostate
TVN	tissue viability nurse
TVT	tension-free vaginal tape
U&Es	urea and electrolytes
UA	unstable angina
UC	ulcerative colitis
UCL	University College, London
UI	urinary incontinence
UIP	usual interstitial pneumonia
UK	United Kingdom
UKHSA	UK Health Security Agency
UKPDS	UK prospective diabetes study
UMN	upper motor neuron
UN	United Nations
UNHCR	UN High Commissioner for refugees
UPR	unfolded protein response
URTI	upper respiratory tract infection
US	United States
US$	US dollar
UTI	urinary-tract infection
UV A and B	ultra violet light: A - longer wavelength associated with tanning and ageing, B - causes more sunburn
V/Q	ventilation/perfusion
VA	visual acuity
VAC	vacuum-assisted wound closure
VaD	vascular dementia
VAT	value added tax
VATS	video-assisted thoracoscopic surgery
VCSE	voluntary, community and social enterprise sector
VE	vaginal examination
VEGF	vascular endothelial growth factor
VGCC	voltage-gated calcium channels
VO$_2$max	the maximum rate of oxygen the body can use during exercise
VTE	venous thromboembolism
WBC	white blood cell
WCC	white cell count
WHO	World Health Organisation
YAG	yttrium aluminium garnet laser
Z drugs	hypnotics in the zopiclone family
ZIO	tradename of a biosensor to detect cardiac arrythmias

About the companion website

This book is accompanied by a companion website:

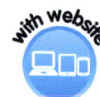

www.wiley.com/go/lecturenotesgeriatricmedicine9e

The website includes:

- Key revision points for each chapter
- Appendix
- Extended content for specialty trainees
- Further reading

Global ageing

Introduction

The Western world turned grey in the 20th century, and the rest of the world is following this century at a more rapid pace.

In response to population ageing, the United Nations General Assembly declared 2021–2030 the Decade of Healthy Ageing and asked the WHO to lead on implementation, but the Coronavirus disease 2019 (COVID-19) pandemic has diverted attention.

The common afflictions of old age are now accepted, not as a cause for shame but as serious diseases. Films and novels portray various aspects of ageing. There is increasing discussion in mainstream media about dementia and its effects on individuals from all levels of society, including former heads of state, sporting, and literary figures. However, ageism is still an issue. In the developed world, experience of death is often limited to the deaths of very elderly parents, and there is a loss of familiarity with death as a natural process.

Changes in the global population

The world is affected by the four global demographic 'megatrends', all of which have implications for older people:

1 Population **growth**
2 Population **ageing**
3 International **migration**
4 **Urbanisation** (local migration)

Population growth

From antiquity, the world population increased gradually, with fluctuations due to factors including famine and pandemics, reaching one billion around 1800. Since then, the growth rate has been remarkable (see Figure 1.1).

Population growth is determined by the balance of birth and death rates.

In outline:

- Once childhood death rates start to fall, life expectancy (LE) increases.
- More people reach reproductive age, high birth rates continue, the median age of the population stays low, and the population grows rapidly.
- Birth rates then start to fall; the population continues to increase, but ages.
- Eventually, older people outnumber the young, and the population begins to fall.

This process is called demographic transition (see Figure 1.2).

Major drivers of the transition include improvements in food security, nutrition, housing, clean water and sanitation, income, education (especially for women), and public health measures such as immunisation and contraception. Medical interventions such as the management of cardiovascular risk factors and earlier detection and management of cancer have extended LE in later life.

World stages of transition in 2019 (Wang, Lancet 2020)

1 **Pre-transition:** no countries
2 **Early transition:** no countries (1970, 17 countries)
3 **Intermediate:** 35 countries
4 **Late transition:** 131 countries
5 **Post-demographic:** 38 countries, 18 with net emigration, and 20 with net immigration.

Population pyramids usually show the population divided into males and females in 5-year age bands. The shape shows the stage of transition, moving from expansive, a wide-based triangle where young children predominate, to a more rectangular shape as the population ages, constrictive as the base shrinks, and finally a rocket shape as there is little death until old age. The changing shape can be seen in the world population pyramids 70 years apart (see Figure 1.3).

The world population reached eight billion in 2022. The rate of world population growth has been slowing since the 1960s. Until recently, the UN estimated that the world population would peak at 11 billion in 2100, but the rapidity of the decline in fertility has exceeded predictions.

- Many women wish or need to work.
- Widespread television, mobile phones, and internet access have brought a quantum leap in access to information, education, and awareness of how others live.
- Aspirations for a higher standard of living and better opportunities for children may be factors driving the rapidity of change.

The latest modelling suggests that peak world population will occur sooner and will be falling by 2100 to 10.4 billion (UN 2022), a peak of 9.7 billion in 2065 with a fall to 8.8 billion by 2100 (Lancet 2020), or more optimistically, a peak of 8.6 billion in 2050 with a fall to 7 billion by 2100 (New Scientist 2023). See Figure 1.4.

Geriatric Medicine and Elderly Care: Lecture Notes, Ninth Edition. Claire G. Nicholl, K. Jane Wilson, and Shaun D'Souza.
© 2025 John Wiley & Sons Ltd. Published 2025 by John Wiley & Sons Ltd.
Companion website: www.wiley.com/go/lecturenotesgeriatricmedicine9e

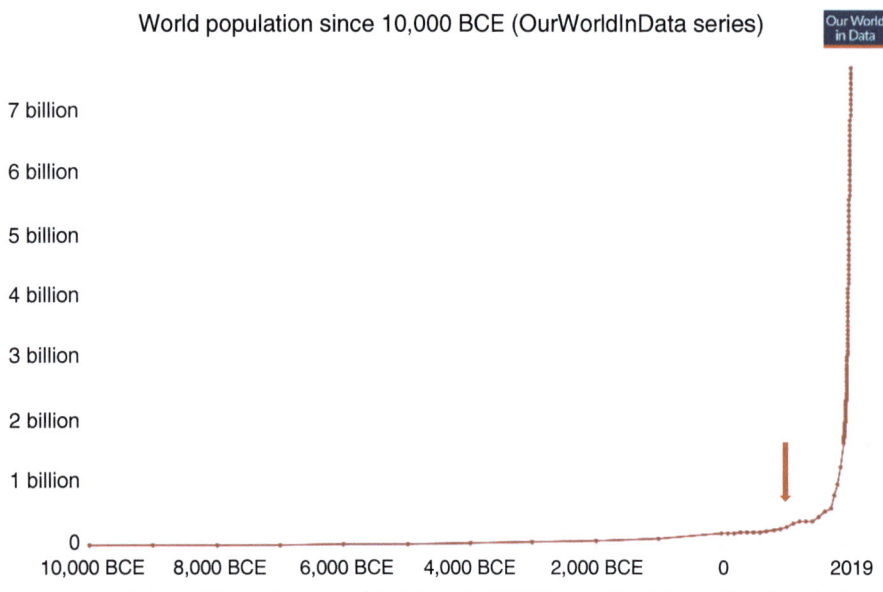

Figure 1.1 World population from 10,000 BCE to 2019 (BCE is before the common era, CE is the common era, previously AD or anno domini). The arrow shows the impact of the Black Death. *Source*: Adapted from Our World in Data.

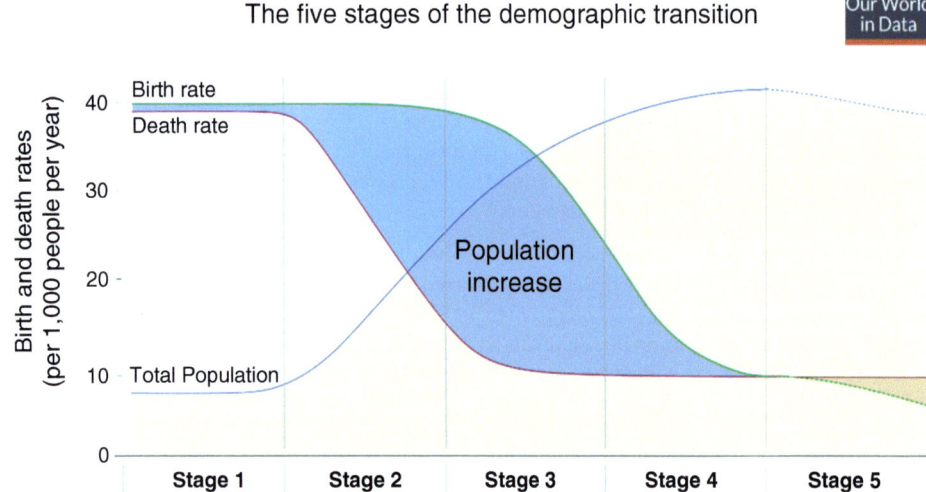

Figure 1.2 Demographic transition. *Source*: Our World in Data / CC BY - 4.0.

Population ageing

As discussed earlier, populations tend to age as they grow.

Population ageing has four key characteristics (UN 2009). It is:

1 **Unprecedented**, without parallel in the history of humanity.
2 **Pervasive,** affecting nearly all the countries in the world. Better treatment for HIV has enabled LE in sub-Saharan Africa to increase following a dip. Civil wars still have an impact on affected areas. It is too early to assess the overall effect of the COVID pandemic, but LE dipped for the first time in decades in many countries.
3 **Profound**, with major consequences and implications for all aspects of life.
4 **Enduring**, as short of a worldwide disaster, the trend will not be reversed.

Ways of expressing the age of a population
Median age

- Age at which half of the population is older and half is younger.
- It enables a single figure to compare countries and measure change.

World median age: 22.6 years in 1960, 30.9 in 2020, projected 36.2 in 2050.

Population over a specified age

- The age at which populations are considered 'elderly' is over 65 years in many statistics.
- Some data sets categorise people of 60+ as older and people of 80+ as the 'oldest old.'

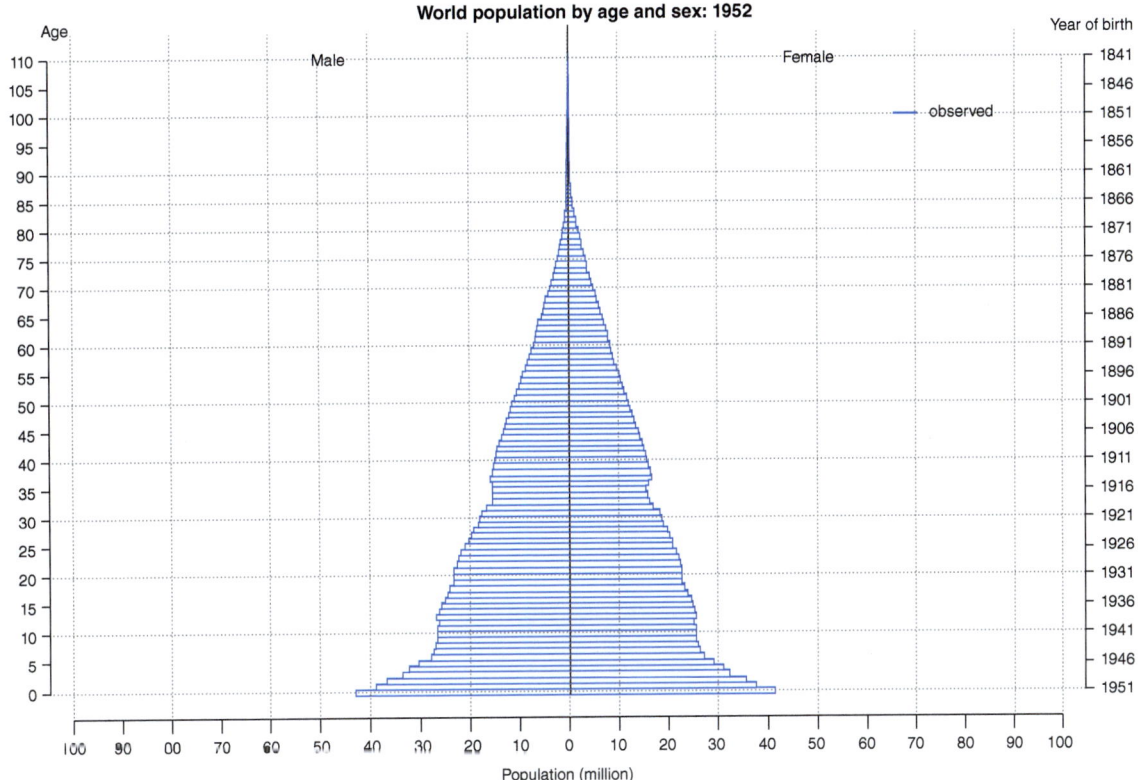

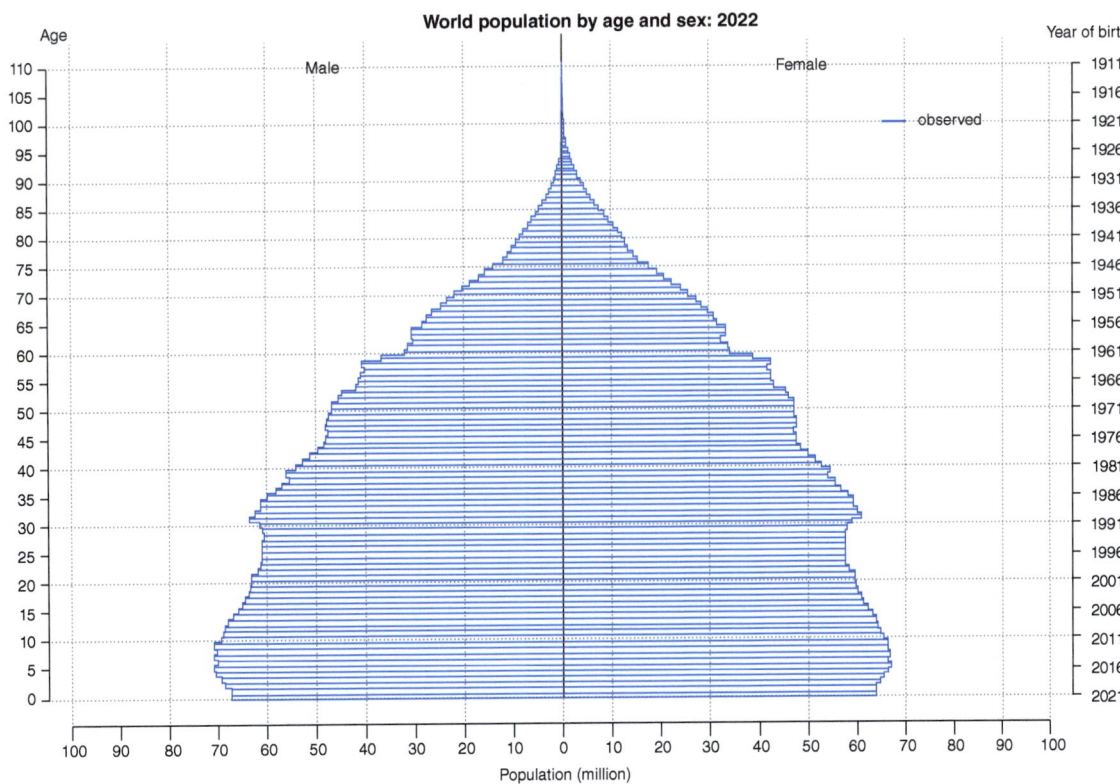

Figure 1.3 World population pyramids for 1952 and 2022. *Source*: United Nations (UN) World population prospects 2024 / CC BY 3.0.

Global population size: estimates, 1950–2022, and medium scenario with 95 per cent prediction intervals and high- and low-fertility scenarios, 2022–2100

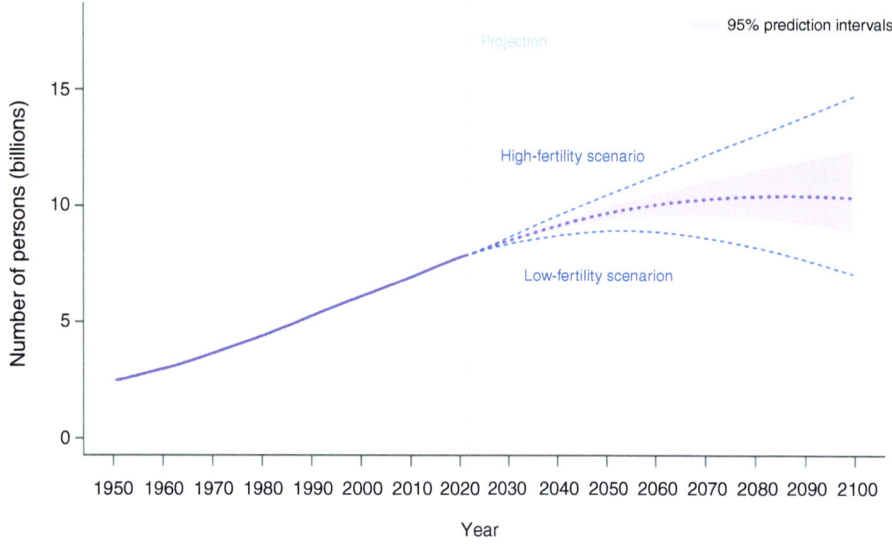

Figure 1.4 Global population and projections *Source*: UN World population prospects summary, 2022 / CC BY 3.0.

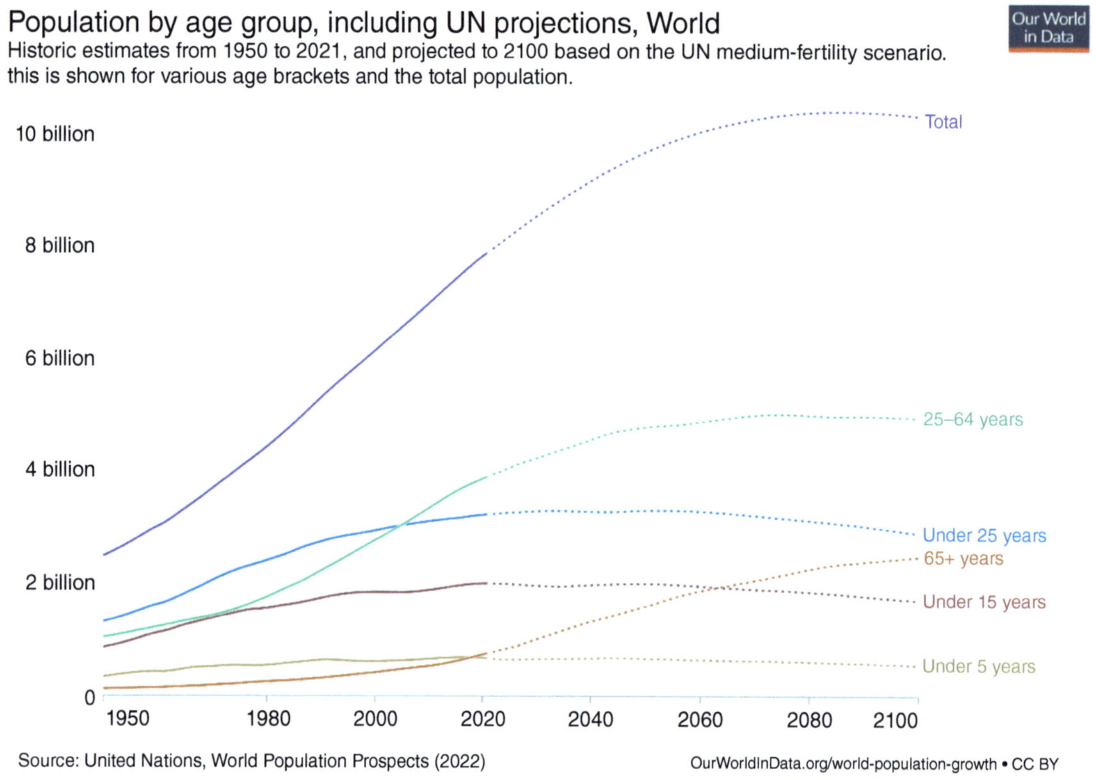

Population by age group, including UN projections, World
Historic estimates from 1950 to 2021, and projected to 2100 based on the UN medium-fertility scenario. this is shown for various age brackets and the total population.

Source: United Nations, World Population Prospects (2022)

OurWorldInData.org/world-population-growth • CC BY

Figure 1.5 The changing proportions of different age bands within the global population. *Source*: Modified from Our World in Data / CC BY 4.0.

The proportion of the world population aged 65+ was 5% in 1960, 10% in 2022, and predicted to rise to 16% in 2050. For the first time in world history, in 2018, people aged 65+ outnumbered children under 5 (see Figure 1.5).

Within the older population, the number of people aged 80+ will increase markedly (see Figure 1.6). This has implications for health and social services, as this age group has more needs. This will occur in middle-income countries as well as high-income countries.

Life expectancy at birth

Prior to 1800, global LE at birth is estimated to have been between 20 and 30. Extremely high infant and child mortality was the major factor, but people have always lived into middle and older age, just a much smaller proportion than today. In the absence of data, inferences about ageing can be made from artistic artefacts, e.g. figurines, drawings, and contemporary texts. In the 7th century BCE, the Greek poet Hesiod wrote

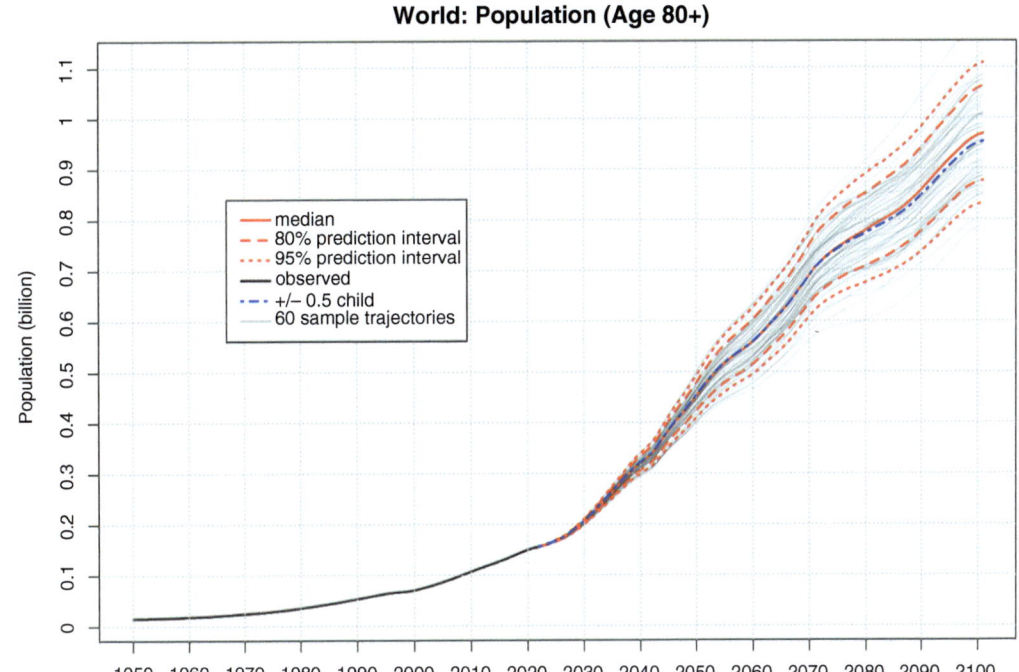

Figure 1.6 Projected world population aged 80 and over. *Source*: UN World population prospects 2024 / CC BY 3.0.

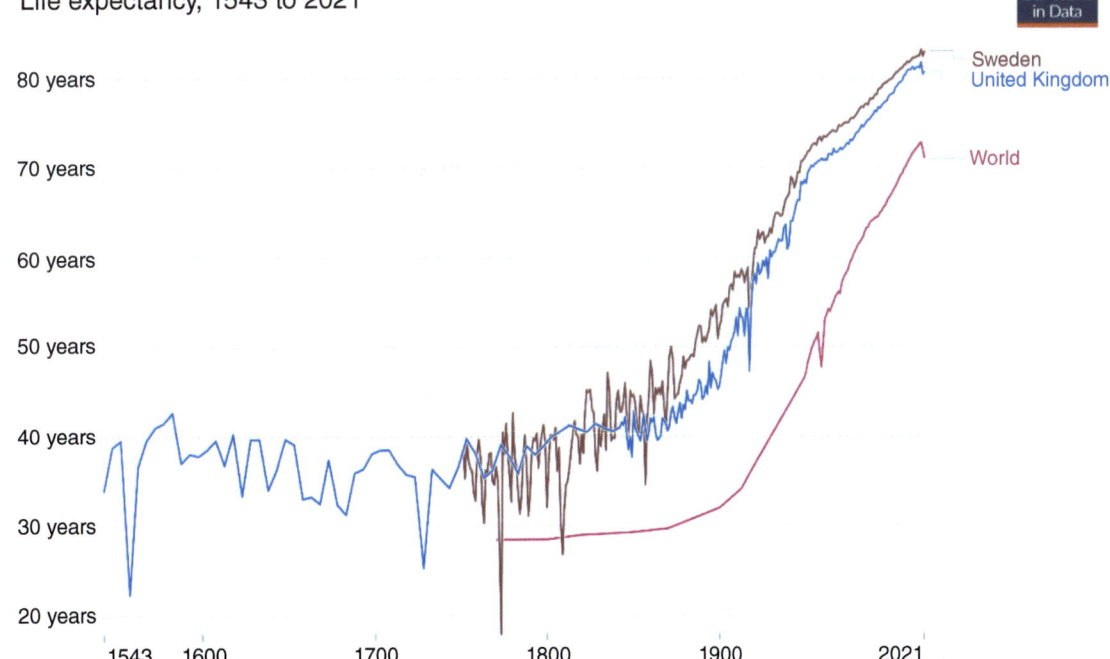

Source: UN WPP (2022); Zijdeman et al. (2015); Riley (2005)   OurWorldInData.org/life-expectancy • CC BY
Note: Shown is the 'period life expectancy'. This is the average number of years a newborn would live if age-specific mortality rates in the current year were to stay the same throughout its life.

Figure 1.7 The changing life expectancy at birth in the UK and Sweden over several centuries. *Source*: Modified from Our World in Data / CC BY 4.0.

that a man should marry at 'not much less than 30, and not much more'. To be a consul in ancient Rome, you had to be 43 – 8 years older than the minimum age of 35 to hold the presidency of the US. In the 1st century, Pliny records a few individuals with well-documented life spans of over 100 years, including Cicero's wife Terentia (103 years).

- Data about LE in populations is available for the UK from 1543 and Sweden from 1750.

- In 1800, more countries began collecting data, but global data, compiled by the UN, has only been available since 1948 (see Figure 1.7).
- Before 1800, no country had a sustained LE at birth over 40 years.
- Global inequality increased after 1850 as LE began to increase in parts of Europe and widened in 1900 as LE also increased in Australia and the US. By 1950, Norway had a LE of 72 years; the mean across Africa was 36 years, and in Mali, only 26 years.

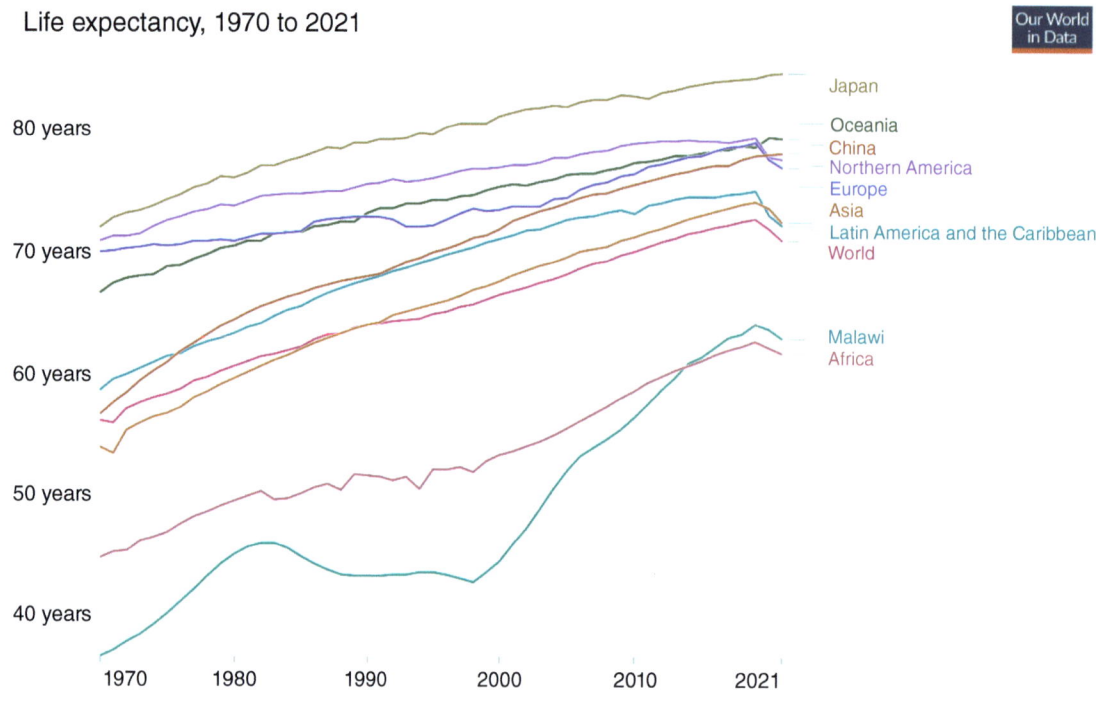

Life expectancy, 1970 to 2021

Source: UN WPP (2022); Zijdeman et al. (2015); Riley (2005)   OurWorldInData.org/life-expectancy • CC BY
Note: Shown is the 'period life expectancy'. This is the average number of years a newborn would live if age-specific mortality rates in the current year were to stay the same throughout its life.

Figure 1.8 Life expectancy in a wider range of countries showing convergence. *Source*: Modified from Our World in Data / CC BY 4.0.

- From the 1950s, LE in most regions increased at a comparable rate until the HIV epidemic, which peaked in sub-Saharan Africa in the 1980s–1990s, caused a marked fall there.
- Since 2000, LE has again increased in all regions, with a faster trajectory in Africa, so the global gap is narrowing (see Figure 1.8).
- The average world citizen born in 1950 could expect to live to 46 years, to 66 by 2000, and to 73 in 2019, with a projection of 77 years by 2050.
- Since 2020, COVID has caused LE to fall. Data on the extent is incomplete, but there has been a fall of almost 3 years in the US, and the dip is now visible in world data.

To visualise the increase in LE since records became available, look at the interactive site in Our World in Data: life expectancy-increased-in-all-countries-of-the-world.

Life expectancy at age 65

Life expectancy at age 65 is the average number of additional years of life a 65-year-old person would live if subjected to the age-specific mortality risks of a given period for the rest of their life.

- Worldwide, a person reaching 65 years old in 2020 can expect to live an additional 17 years, increasing to 19 years by 2050.
- Australia and New Zealand currently have the highest LE at age 65 (21 years), followed by Europe and Northern America (19 years).
- Life expectancy at age 65 is projected to increase in all regions, but with the smallest gain in sub-Saharan Africa.

Estimating years spent in health

There is now more focus on whether the extra years of life are spent in health. There are several similar metrics with different definitions, so to compare data, e.g. across countries, use the same metric.

Health-adjusted life expectancy (HALE), used by the WHO, is the expected number of remaining years of life spent in good health, i.e. without irreversible limitations in activities of daily living, from birth or age 65, assuming current rates of mortality and morbidity. Health status is derived from health statistics. In the EU, the Healthy Life Years indicator (HLY) is also known as disability-free life expectancy (DFLE) and uses self-reported data on disability. The UK metric of Healthy Life Expectancy (HLE) is not synonymous with DFLE, as it asks about the perception of health rather than disability.

Across the world, people live longer and live more years in good health. Between 2000 and 2019:

- LE at birth increased from 66.8 to 73.3 years.
- HALE increased from 58.3 to 63.7 years.
- LE and HALE are consistently higher for females.

Within individual countries, there are socio-economic gradients for LE and HALE.

Old-age dependency ratio

The old-age dependency ratio (OADR), the number of old-age dependents (people aged 65+) per 100 persons of working age (aged 20 to 64 years), is used to compare the economic prospects of countries related to their ageing population (see Figure 1.9).

In 2020:

- Japan tops the list and will continue to do so in 2050.
- Most countries with high OADRs are European; more Asian countries will be among this group by 2050.

Some data still uses 15–64 as 'working age', but the age of 20 reflects longer education and later entry into the work force. The use of 'age 64' will also become outdated as older people choose or need to defer retirement.

Whatever age bands are used, a more intuitive way of expressing the number of working people available to support older people is the Potential Support Ratio (PSR), i.e. the inverse of OADR. Using data for people aged 25–64 per person aged 65+; in 2019, Japan had a ratio of 1.8,

Economic old-age dependency ratios, world and regions, estimates for 1990–2021 and projections for 2022–2050

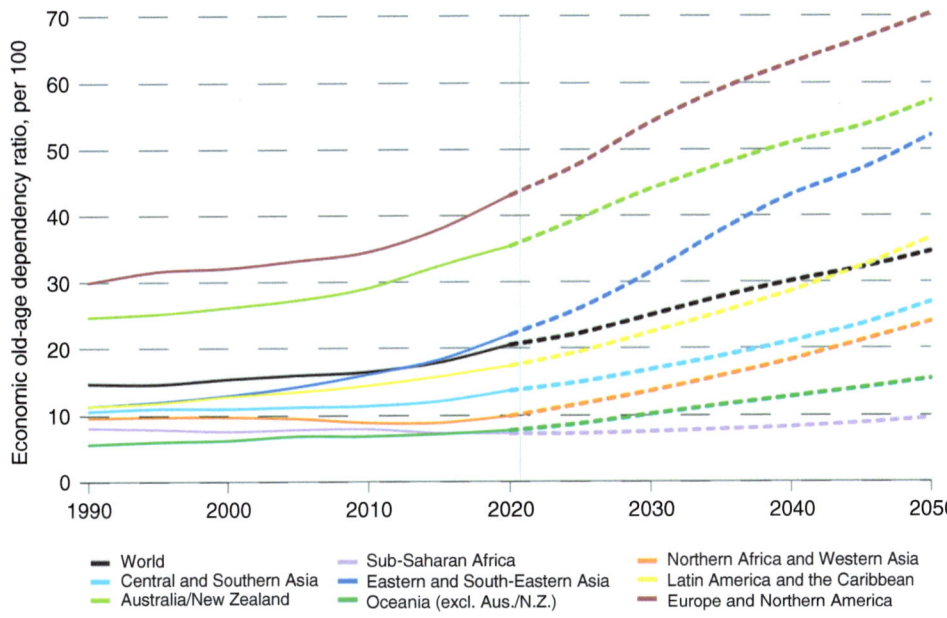

Figure 1.9 OADRs calculated from numbers of people aged 65+ per 100 persons aged 20–64. *Source*: UN World social report 2023 / CC BY 3.0.

the lowest in the world. A further 29 countries, mostly in Europe and the Caribbean, already have PSRs below 3.

Prospective old-age dependency ratio

As LE increases and older people stay economically active, rather than defining people as 'old' at an arbitrary age, newer metrics are being used. The prospective old-age dependency ratio (POADR) is calculated as the number of persons above the age closest to a remaining LE of 15 years compared to the number of persons between age 20 and that age.

Sex ratios and the age-sex gap

Unless there is intervention, more male infants are born than females in all populations (105:100). However, boy babies have higher perinatal and infant mortality. For data and discussion on sex ratios in different countries, see Our World in Data.

In antiquity, men were said to outlive women. This may have been true, but it may be a reporting phenomenon as most cultures recorded more information about men. Once comprehensive data became available, it was clear that, on average, women outlived men. The difference results from a complex interaction between biological, behavioural, and socio-economic factors that is uneven throughout the lifespan (e.g. due to the risks of childbirth, attitude to risk, military service and dangerous jobs, and cardiovascular disease). The size of the difference has varied historically.

- By 2020, it was universal that women live longer than men, although the difference ranges from less than a year in Nigeria to over 10 years in Russia (the global average is 4.8 years).
- 90% of supercentenarians (people reaching 110 years of age or older) are women.
- Thus, in many countries, particularly those with older populations, women outnumber men.

Countries where most older people live

India overtook China as the world's most populous country in April 2023. It is likely that between 2060 and 2070, sub-Saharan Africa will become the most populous region in the world.

The proportion of older people varies greatly from country to country, but as countries undergo demographic transition, the differences are diminishing. Globally, there were 703 million people aged 65+ in 2019. The region of Eastern and South-Eastern Asia was home to the largest number of older people (261 million), followed by Europe and Northern America (over 200 million).

Data from a range of countries are shown in Table 1.1.

Japan's population is the oldest in the world; most European countries have median ages around 43 years, but population ageing is not restricted to the developed world. In 2019:

- Nearly one in four people aged 65+ lived in China.
- Five countries (China, India, the US, Japan, and the Russian Federation) accounted for half of the world's population aged 65+.
- Five countries (China, the US, India, Japan, and Germany) were home to half of people aged 80+.

Table 1.1 Percentage of people aged 65+ and median age in 2019 (Our World in Data).

	% aged 65+	Median age years	World population ranking	Number of people aged 65+ (million)
Japan	28	46.7	11	35.6
Italy	23	45.7	23	14.0
UK	19	40.1	21	12.5
US	16	37.7	3	53.3
Russian Fed	15	39.4	9	22.0
China	12	37.0	1 (2 from 2023)	164.5
Brazil	9	33.5	6	19.3
Mexico	7	29.2	10	9.5
India	6	28.4	2 (1 from 2023)	87.1
Indonesia	6	29.7	4	16.3
Nigeria	3	18.1	7	5.5
WORLD	9	30.7	7.7 billion	702.9

Over the next three decades, the number of people aged 65+ is projected to more than double, reaching more than 1.6 billion people in 2050.

All regions will see an increase in the 65+ population between 2019 and 2050.

- The largest increase (312 million) is projected to occur in Eastern and South-Eastern Asia.
- The fastest increase (226%) is expected in Northern Africa and Western Asia.
- The second fastest increase (218%) is projected for sub-Saharan Africa.
- The increase is expected to be relatively small in Australia and New Zealand (84%) and in Europe and Northern America (48%), where the population is already older.

An excellent resource to look at demographic changes in individual countries is Our World in Data – the trends with time, effects of war (e.g. France 1918, 1944; Japan 1945), earlier flu pandemics, and HIV (e.g. Eswatini) are readily seen.

The pace of population ageing

The pace of population ageing is accelerating. It took 115 years (1865–1980) for the proportion of older people to double in France (from 7 to 14%), whilst in China the proportion will have doubled between 2000 and 2026. This gives countries very little time to adjust.

International migration

International migration is increasingly important.

- The number of people living outside their country of birth or citizenship reached 281 million in 2020, up from 173 million in 2000.
- The rate is continuing to increase due to economic migration and people fleeing war and persecution.

Most economic migrants are of working age and move to developed countries with older populations, so the countries they leave 'age' and the age in the destination country falls (e.g. Sweden). Immigration has an immediate impact on population age and growth in countries where natural population growth has fallen; in half of these 38 countries, immigration has ensured stable or rising populations.

However, emigration may worsen natural population decline, such as in Romania, where waves of immigration and emigration have caused marked fluctuations (see Figure 1.10).

The effect on populations of rapid, massive migration due to war depends on the situation, but typically more women and children are displaced. It is too early to evaluate the effect of the Russian invasion of Ukraine in 2022, but over 2 million refugees fled the fighting in the first 2 weeks. For context, United Nations High Commissioner for Refugees (UNHCR) estimates that there were 43.4 million refugees globally in 2023.

Urbanisation

The other major change affecting populations is urbanisation. The UN estimates that in 2007, for the first time in human history, the number of people in urban areas overtook the number in rural settings (see Figure 1.11). As with international migration, it is mainly younger people who leave the countryside, fragmenting families and altering the age distribution of areas within a country. Conflicts also cause massive internal displacements in countries.

Typical patterns of health and social care

More developed countries

Demographic changes

- Death, which was common in infancy and usual before 65 years, is now rare in infancy and unusual before 65 years.
- Life expectancy has generally continued to rise, but the rate of increase has flattened since 2010 in the US, Canada, Australia, the UK, and several European countries. By contrast, in Japan, a period of low gains in LE was followed by a return to faster improvement.
- Life expectancies have dipped because of the direct and indirect effects of COVID, but it is still too soon to be sure of the size and duration of this effect.
- The dramatic rise in the older population over the past 100 years is now slowing.
- The number of 'very old', i.e. those ≥80 years of age, is still increasing rapidly.
- Ageing populations are associated with slower economic growth due to lower productivity, less innovation and a risk of 'ageing recessions' due to labour shortages plus increased demands for care. In 2010, China overtook Japan as the world's second-largest economy, due in part to the ageing and shrinking population of Japan.

Medical services

- Sophisticated health systems are set up with specialised services for elderly people.
- An older person costs health services nine times as much as a young person.
- Population ageing requires increased health funding, estimated in the EU at 0.6% per year between 2015 and 2050, so price growth and technological advancements will be the main contributors to future growth in health care expenditure.
- Most deaths are due to cardiovascular disease, dementia, and cancer (see Figure 1.12).
- Time-to-death, particularly the final year of life, rather than age, is a stronger driver of healthcare expenditure, and there is an inverse relationship between age and the cost of end-of-life care.
- Rising expectations of older people and their carers also fuel rising health costs.
- Ethical dilemmas will become more pressing, e.g. the prolongation of death by technological intervention and the debate about access to euthanasia.
- Medical training continues to value increasing specialisation, so practitioners struggle to deal with complex aetiologies (sociological, psychological, and medical), multiple pathology and the frailty and atypical presentations common in older patients. This can result in a mismatch between the aspirations of young medics and the needs of their older patients.

Community services

- The provision of community care is more varied than for acute care. Inter-country comparisons are complex because of political, socio-economic, and demographic differences. The most straightforward comparison is the proportion of people in care homes; there used to be marked variation, but figures are converging to 4–7% of those aged 65+.

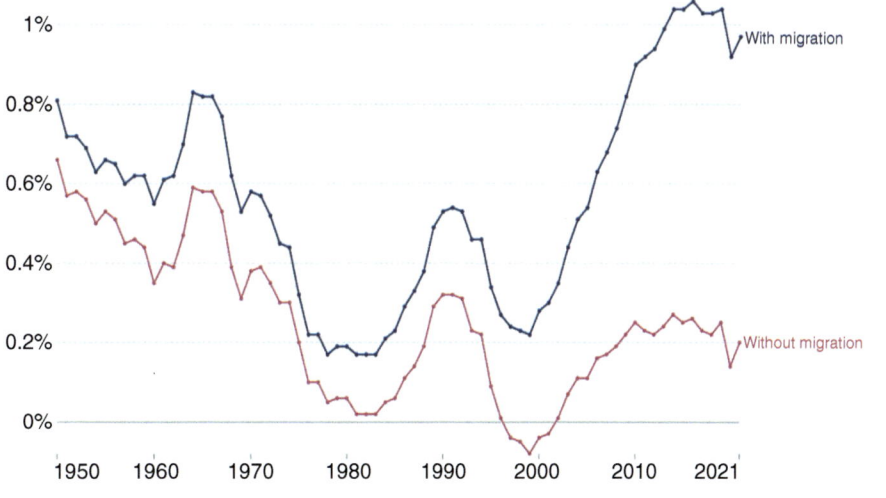

Population growth rate with and without migration, Sweden
The annual change in population with migration included, versus the change if there was zero migration (neither emigration or immigration). The latter therefore represents the change in population based solely on domestic births and deaths.

Source: United Nations, World Population Prospects (2022)   OurWorldInData.org/world-population-growth • CC BY

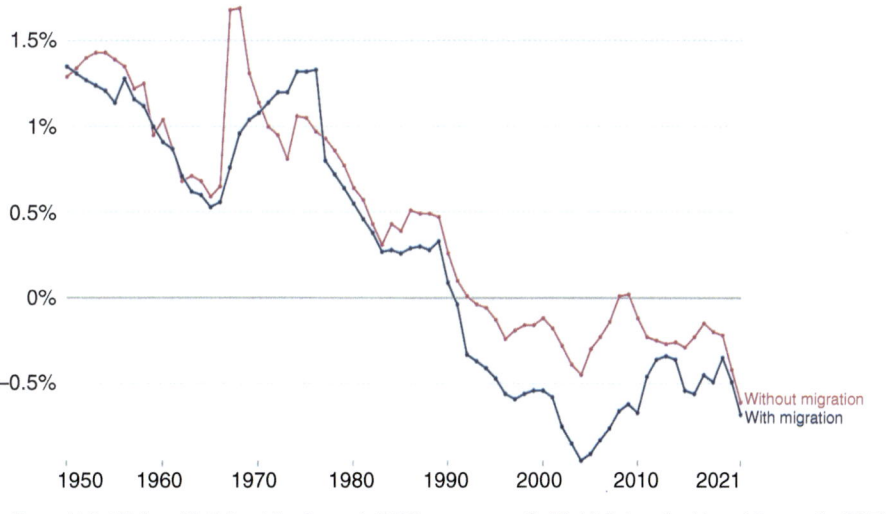

Population growth rate with and without migration, Romania
The annual change in population with migration included, versus the change if there was zero migration (neither emigration or immigration). The latter therefore represents the change in population based solely on domestic births and deaths.

Source: United Nations, World Population Prospects (2022)   OurWorldInData.org/world-population-growth • CC BY

Figure 1.10 Population growth with and without migration: in Sweden, where migration is increasing the population, and in Romania, where it has decreased the population. *Source*: Our World in Data / CC BY 4.0.

- The development of patterns of care is similar. Historically, there was a heavy reliance on self-sufficiency and family care. The healthy and wealthy elderly have always fared the best. The more disadvantaged have always needed support from others.
- In the 'Old World', non-family support was provided by the church or by occupationally related charities or guilds. In England, the state began to take a more active role after the dissolution of the monasteries with the first Poor Law Act of 1601, which provided workhouse care and 'outdoor relief'. This continued until the end of the 19th century. The 20th century saw the beginning of the welfare state – gradually growing in the first half of the century, reaching a peak mid-century, and then declining towards the end of the 1980s. State provision of services was replaced by state regulation of services provided by other organisations. This regulation was gradually devolved and often weakened.
- From the 1980s on, nursing homes in the US, Europe, and Australia were increasingly run for profit, now mainly by multinational companies.
- Detailed case studies (2021) describe the provision and financing of long-term care (facility-based health care, home-based care, residential care, and personal care) in Australia, several European countries, Japan, the Republic of Korea, and the US. Common themes are issues with eligibility, equity, quality, affordability, and funding streams.
- Care for people with dementia is a major issue.

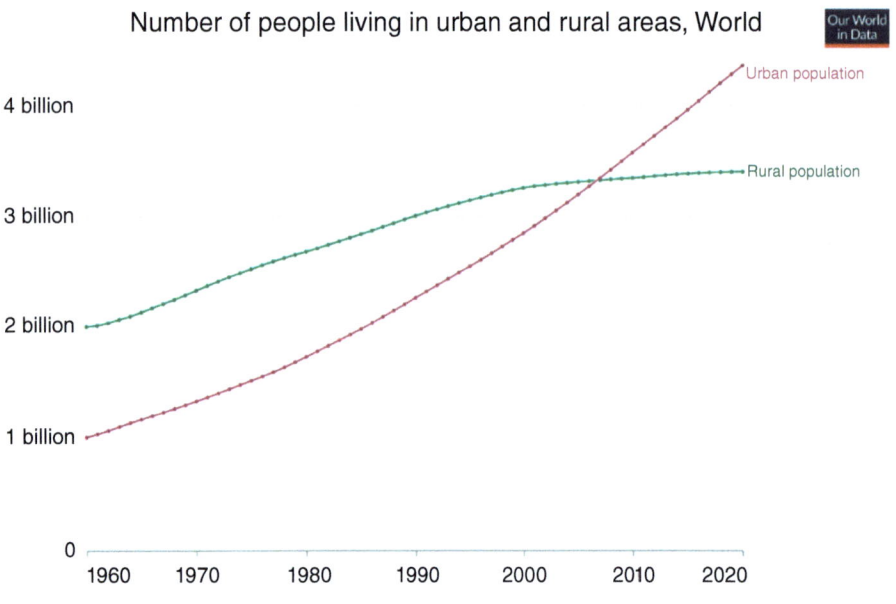

Number of people living in urban and rural areas, World

Source: World Bank based on data from the UN Population Division   OurWorldInData.org/urbanization • CC BY
Note: Urban populations are defined based on the definition of urban areas by national statistical offices.

Figure 1.11 Most people now live in urban areas. *Source*: Our World in Data / CC BY 4.0.

Leading causes of death in high-income countries

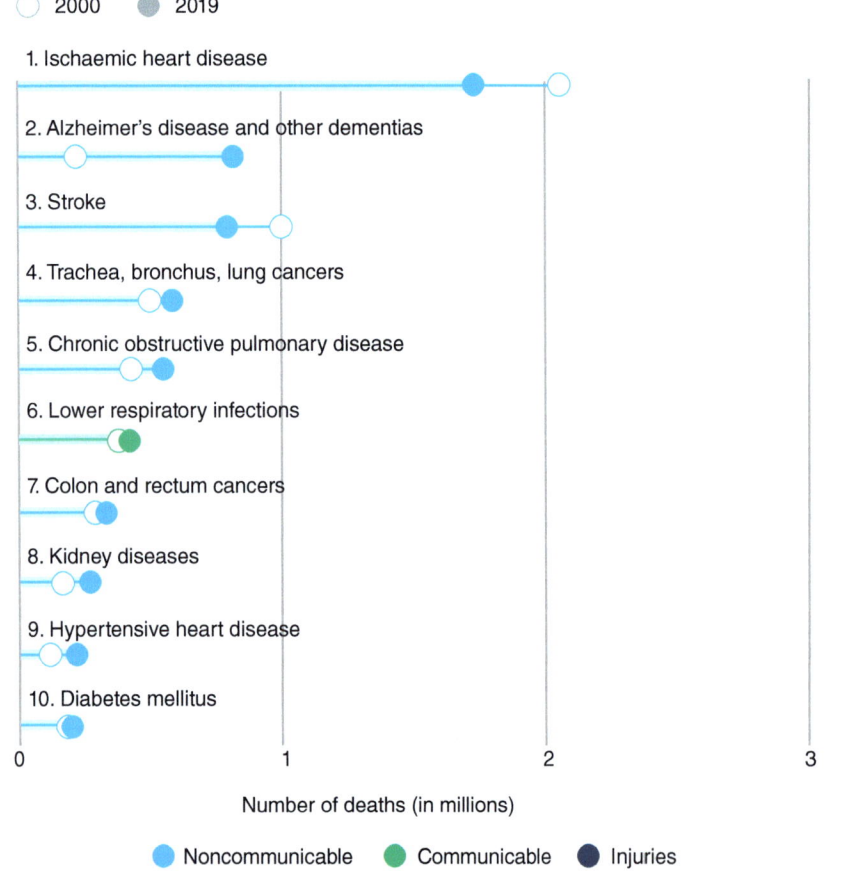

○ 2000   ● 2019

1. Ischaemic heart disease
2. Alzheimer's disease and other dementias
3. Stroke
4. Trachea, bronchus, lung cancers
5. Chronic obstructive pulmonary disease
6. Lower respiratory infections
7. Colon and rectum cancers
8. Kidney diseases
9. Hypertensive heart disease
10. Diabetes mellitus

Number of deaths (in millions)

● Noncommunicable   ● Communicable   ● Injuries

Source: WHO Global Health Estimates. Note: World Bank 2020 income classification.

Figure 1.12 Top ten causes of death in high-income countries. *Source*: WHO Global Health Estimates.

Less developed countries

Demographic changes

- Once people reach old age in developing countries, their LE is not much lower than in the developed world (Table 1.2).
- Until recently, the proportion of older people was low, but as countries such as China and India are so populous, over 60% of the world's elderly population already lives in these countries.
- These countries' population structures are changing rapidly with falling birth rates as contraceptive policies become effective (or are imposed), infant mortality is reduced, and survival in adult life improves.
- European studies show that babies with low birth weight and reduced growth in the first year have poor adult health, e.g. with hypertension and hyperglycaemia. This is likely to have significant consequences in India and Southeast Asia.
- Potentially preventable congenital and childhood disabilities will complicate old age.
- Poor people will be unable to get sufficient wealth to provide for themselves in old age, so the total burden will either fall on the state or older people will be neglected.
- Governments have many competing financial demands, e.g. education, housing, and the development of infrastructure.
- Many countries struggle with debt, and political instability is common.
- Population patterns are at risk of distortion by epidemics, e.g. HIV/AIDS, civil war, and migration, e.g. sub-Saharan Africa.

Medical services

- Communicable diseases still claim most lives, but cardiovascular disease is increasing (see Figure 1.13).
- Health services are often primitive, patchy, and inappropriate for needs with huge urban/rural divides.
- There may be conflict between traditional healers and scientific approaches.
- The state may pursue 'high-tech' for the few over public health measures that would help many.
- Private health care clinics grow rapidly in cities, regulation may be limited, and people may shop around until they get an opinion that they like.

Table 1.2 Mean life expectancy at different ages (UN 2019).

Country	At birth	At 60 years	At 80 years
World	73.3	21.1	8.2
Low-income	65.1	17.4	5.9
Lower-middle income	69.4	18.6	6.8
Higher-middle income	76.3	21.2	7.7
High income	80.9	24.3	9.8

Leading causes of death in low-income countries

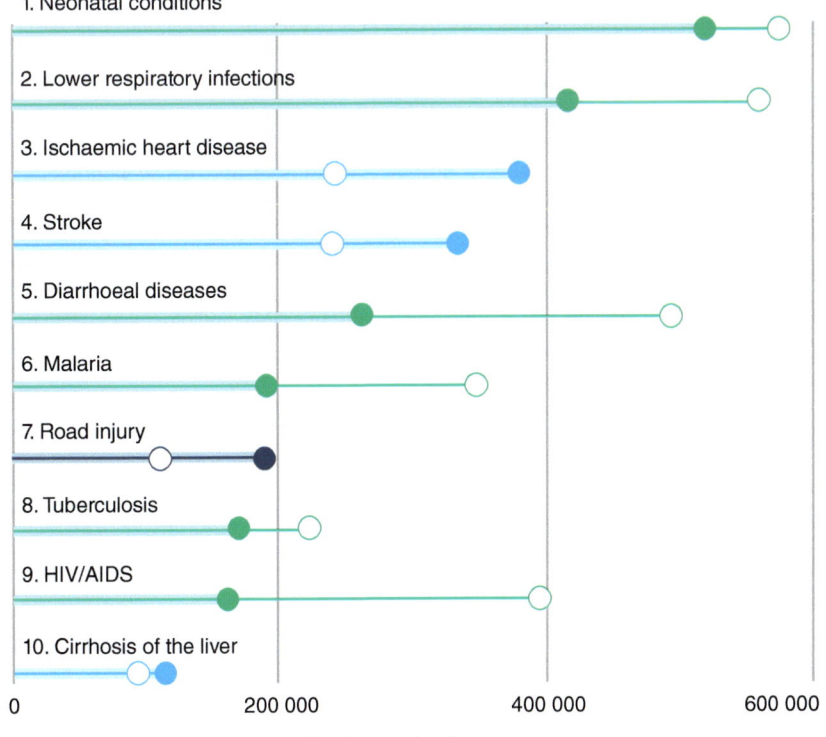

Source: WHO Global Health Estimates. Note: World Bank 2020 income classification.

Figure 1.13 Top ten causes of death in low-income countries. *Source*: WHO Global Health Estimates.

- There is often limited access to therapies and equipment for rehabilitation.
- Doctors and nurses need training in geriatrics because of worldwide demographic change.
- Development may be restricted by the tight macro-economic practices enforced by the International Monetary Fund, which encourage privatisation and limit a government's ability to invest in public health.
- Globalisation via the World Trade Organisation has resulted in conflict over the cost of drugs. Unaffordable prices for patented drugs ensure financial profits for Pharma, enabling the development of new drugs, but developing countries need access to cheap generic drugs, e.g. for hypertension, diabetes, and HIV. Efforts to distribute COVID vaccines worldwide and limited countries of manufacture highlighted the difficulties.
- World trade tends to promote bad health habits, e.g. smoking, high sugar intake, excess alcohol, and recreational drug abuse.

Community services

- Most of the population continues to work for as long as they are able, and when they cannot, they must rely on family support; retirement, at least for most people, is a concept of the developed world.

Ageing in India in 2023

Demographic changes

India is in a rapid phase of transition. Life expectancy at birth has been increasing since the 1950s, with a recent dip due to COVID (see Figure 1.14). Of note, male LE was longer than that of females until 1980. As the birth rate is higher in India than in China, India became the most populous country in 2023.

- The population of India is around 1.5 billion people (UN data).
- India has 17.8% of the world's population.
- The median age in India is 28.7 years.
- Fertility has fallen from 5.9 children per woman in 1965 to 2.1 in 2020.
- The number of children under the age of five peaked in 2007.
- The population growth rate has been falling since 1983.
- Urbanisation has increased from 20% in 1970 to 35% in 2020.
- About half a million people emigrate every year.

The fall in the numbers of children means that the base of the population pyramid is becoming progressively constricted (see Figure 1.15) and young adults are the largest group.

Life expectancy at the age of 65 and older in India has also increased for both men and women since 1955, and as a result, India's elderly population is growing rapidly (Table 1.3).

Between 1970 and 2020, the number of children aged 0–14 increased, plateaued and has been falling since 2010. The population age 15–64 has increased steadily by threefold; the over-65s have gone up over fourfold; and the over-80s, sevenfold, although they still make up only 7% and 1% of the population, respectively (see Figure 1.16).

Causes of death and disability

Indian states are in different phases of epidemiological transition, and there are large variations in disease burden across the states. People are living longer, but in 2019, only a fifth of registered deaths in India had a medically certified cause of death, so causes of death are based on extrapolation.

India generates considerable data on health aspects, but the data are fragmented and non-standardised, and there is little quality control. The Ayushman Bharat Digital Mission developed a system to generate a unique health identification number for every individual for use across a range of healthcare providers (to document cases of COVID and vaccinations), but the use of this number is still optional.

- Communicable diseases have fallen.
  - Polio has been eliminated, but malaria, tuberculosis, leprosy, AIDS, and a swathe of 'neglected tropical diseases' are still significant (see Figure 1.17).
  - Mortality from TB has halved since 1990 to 23 per 100,000, but India still has a quarter of the world's cases, an estimated 28 million new cases in 2018.
  - 1.47 million of these are drug-resistant TB, a situation local sources believe has arisen because of 'unregulated treatment by private providers'.
- The prevalence of noncommunicable diseases is rising steadily as the population ages.
  - Tobacco and alcohol use, a lack of exercise, and a poor diet have resulted in a high prevalence of metabolic syndrome and hypertension. Death rates from ischaemic heart disease (IHD), stroke, diabetes, and cancer are increasing.
  - Although domestic air pollution has fallen with cleaner cooking, poor air quality contributes to chronic obstructive pulmonary disease (COPD).
  - Malnutrition is still widespread. The 2019 Global Hunger Index ranks India at 102 out of 117 countries assessed and accounts for over two-thirds of deaths under 5 years old. The sequelae in the survivors will include poor health in middle and older age.
  - Injuries are another significant cause of mortality and morbidity.

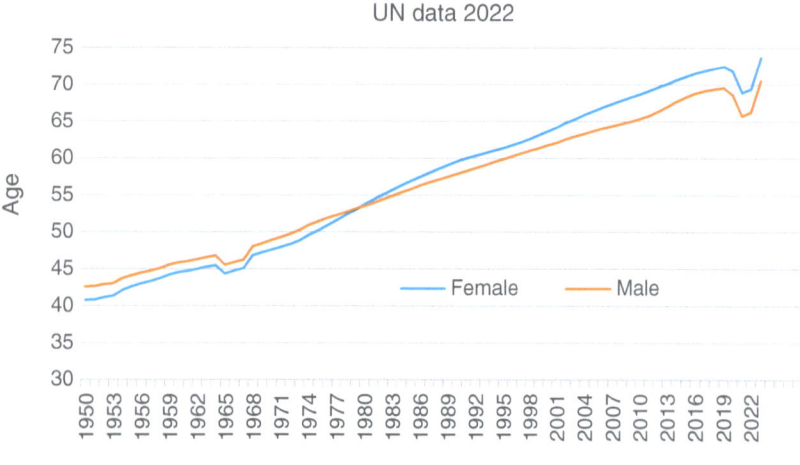

Figure 1.14 Life expectancy in India is now higher in women than men. The dip after 2019 was due to COVID. *Source*: UN World population prospects 2024 / CC BY 3.0.

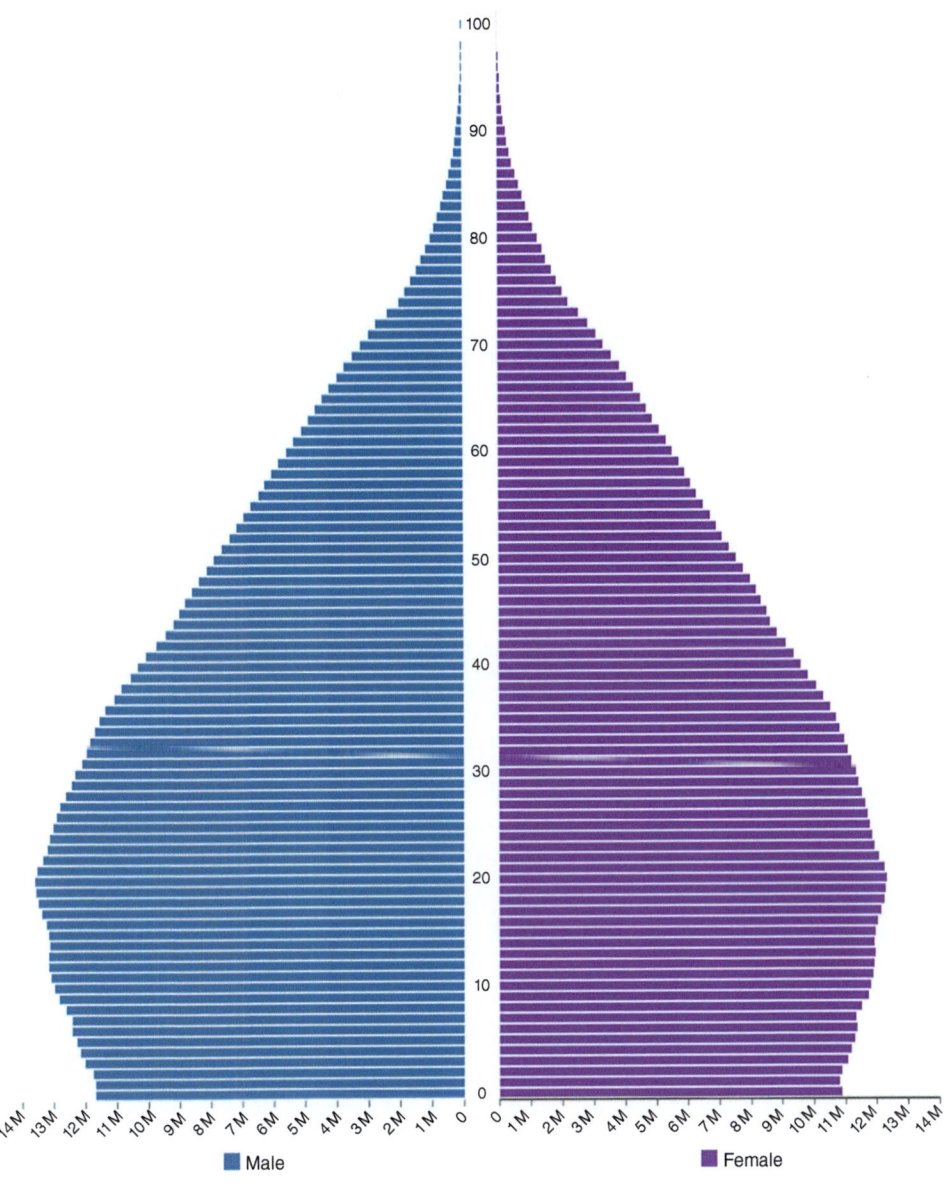

Figure 1.15 India population pyramid 2023. *Source*: UN World population prospects 2024 / CC BY 3.0. M, a million.

Table 1.3 Life expectancy for older people in India (UN 2019).

Age	1950–1955		1980–1985		2010–2015		2045–2050 projected	
	Males	**Females**	**Males**	**Females**	**Males**	**Females**	**Males**	**Females**
65	9.4	10.2	11.4	12.4	13.8	14.8	15.5	17.2
80	4.1	5.1	5.1	6.0	6.5	6.9	7.2	7.9

More detail about the diseases within these broad classifications is given in Figure 1.18 and IHD, COPD and stroke are now the three top causes of death.

Reliable data on the prevalence of disabilities is limited, with estimates ranging from 2.2% (2011 census) to much higher figures. In the census, the main types of disability were impaired mobility, hearing, and vision. Long-term disability from congenital disorders, perinatal problems, poor nutrition, polio, injury from road traffic and industrial accidents, breathlessness from cardiorespiratory problems, and problems of older age, including stroke, arthritis, cataracts, macular degeneration and presbycusis, are all common.

Better data are now available from the Longitudinal Ageing Study in India (LASI), a nationally representative survey of 72,250 adults aged 45 and older across all states of India. Data collection for wave 1 was carried out from 2017 to 2018.

Some of the social data emphasises the challenges India faces in modernising:

All ages in rural areas:

- Households practicing open defecation: 38%
- Households without electricity: 11%.

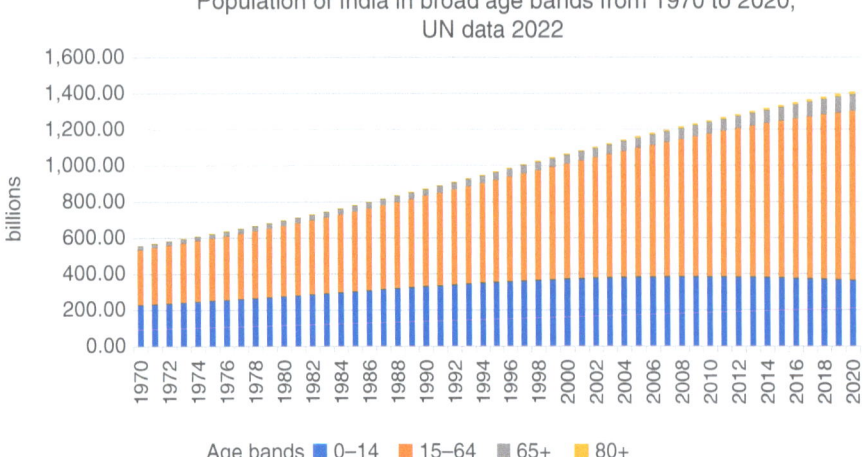

Figure 1.16 The increasing proportion of older and very old people in India. *Source*: UN data 2022.

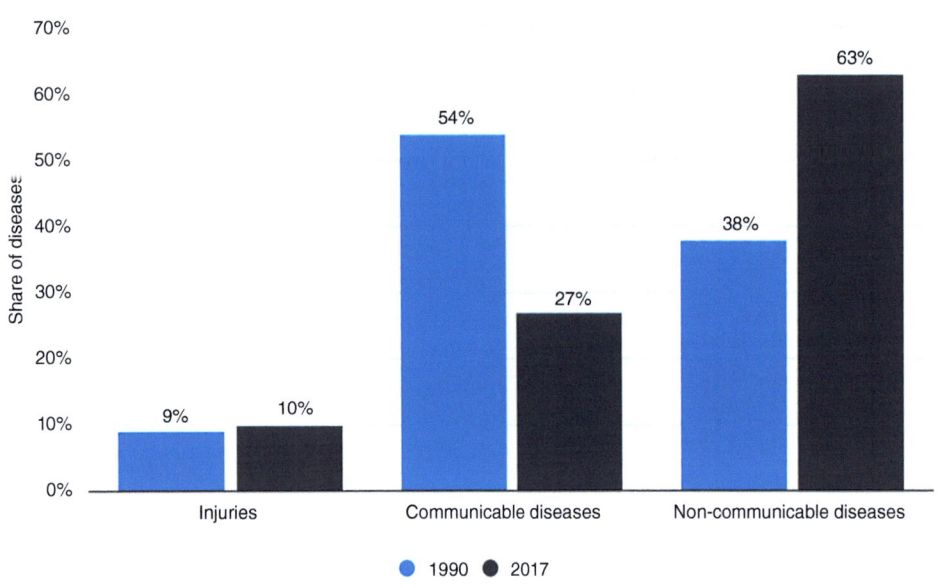

Figure 1.17 Distribution of disease burden across India in 1990 and 2017, by type. *Source*: Statista https://www.statista.com/statistics/1180661/india-distribution-of-disease-burden-by-type.

What causes the most deaths?

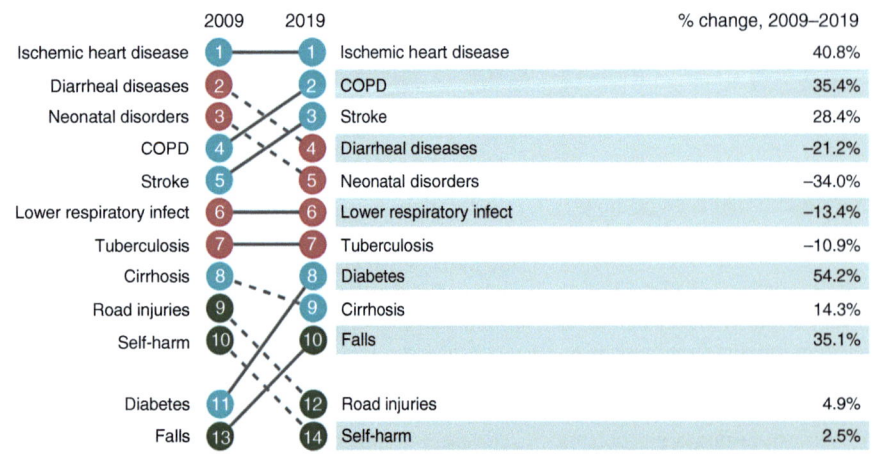

Top 10 causes of total number of deaths in 2019 and percent change 2009–2019, all ages combined

Figure 1.18 Top 10 causes of death in India. COPD, chronic obstructive pulmonary disease. *Source*: The Institute for Health Metrics and Evaluation.

People aged 60+ in all areas:

- No schooling: 57%;
- Currently receiving a retirement pension: 6%;
- Living alone: 6%;
- Poor or very poor self-rated health: 24%;
- Any activities of daily living (ADL) limitation: 24%;
- Any instrumental activities of daily living (IADL) limitation: 48%;
- Persons who need help with ADL/IADL limitations: 25%;
- Low vision: 37% (measured, better eye, with own glasses).

There is a lot of data on self-reported medical conditions, and some conditions were measured directly. Eye problems and hypertension reported by participants were similar to the levels found on examination. However, self-reported neurological and psychiatric problems were extremely low, at 2% at all ages and 3% in people aged 60 and over. This probably reflects a marked underdiagnosis and reluctance to disclose mental health problems because of the associated stigma.

- In LASI, a depression screening questionnaire gave a rate of 8% for all ages.
- Pilania found that depression may affect 34% of the older population.
- Dementia will be underdiagnosed (lack of recognition and lack of schooling make standard tests difficult), but an add-on study to LASI estimates the prevalence of dementia in the over-60s at 7%.
- In childhood, neurodevelopmental disorders are common (14% of children aged 6–9 years in one study), and these disorders will persist into adulthood.

Provision of health care

Within India, there is huge variation in health care. There are high standards in large centres, but much of the country still lacks basic provision. India has one of the lowest public healthcare budgets in the world, at 1.26% of Gross Domestic Product (GDP) in 2020. The private sector accounts for over 70% of healthcare spending. The extremes are exemplified by cardiac centres, which offer coronary surgery to health tourists and are feted by Western politicians, contrasting with 10% of Primary Health Centres (PHCs), which have no MBBS doctor (2019).

Health care is decentralised, and each state organises its own health services. In principle, all Indian citizens can get free outpatient and inpatient care at government facilities. However, due to limited availability and shortages of staff and supplies, many households pay for private care, even though they incur debt to do so.

In 2018, the Indian Government announced the Ayushman Bharat Programme with two components:

- Health and Wellness Centres, to deliver comprehensive primary health care to the entire population. This was aimed at upgrading 150,000 government PHCs by the end of 2022.
- Pradhan Mantri Jan Arogya Yojana for improving access to secondary and tertiary hospital services for the bottom 40% of the population.

Training in medicine

Medicine is a sought-after, competitive career in India, and there are many medical graduates every year. Others travel abroad to study, particularly to Eastern Europe. Many qualify with high debts and specialist aspirations, so a career in rural India is not attractive. State schemes to mandate a period of rural medicine are very unpopular.

In 1999, the Government of India Ministry of Social Justice and Empowerment developed the 'National Policy on Older Persons'. This stressed the importance of setting up geriatric services and proper training, but implementation has been limited. Professional organisations include the Indian Academy of Geriatrics, which publishes a quarterly journal, the Geriatric Society of India, and the charity HelpAge India.

Higher degrees in geriatrics are available at an increasing number of universities, including the top state and private institutions, the All India Institute of Medical Sciences, and the Christian Medical College.

Provision of social care

Most older Indians live with family members, but as younger people move into cities or emigrate and women work, the proportion of older people living just with a spouse is increasing. Since the Maintenance and Welfare of Parents and Senior Citizens Act (2008), it has been a legal obligation for children to support their parents with a monthly allowance, but most older people are not aware of this. HelpAge India (2019) has documented that many careers of older relatives (usually a daughter-in-law) find care burdensome, and elder abuse occurs here as elsewhere. Wealthy families can fund private care at home or access luxury old-age communities and nursing homes. At the other end of the market, the Ministry of Social Justice and Empowerment supports 551 NGO-run old-age homes for 16,290 'destitute elderly' (2021). Data for private old-age homes is not kept by the government.

Small numbers of people have private or occupational pensions, as 90% of employment in India is in the informal sector. The benefits system is complicated. There are non-contributory pensions, the Indira Gandhi National Old-Age Pension Scheme, and a scheme for widows who live below the poverty line (BPL households) and have a BPL card to prove this. Pensions are claimed by about a third of rural older people from BPL households and a quarter of elderly widows. Many people are unaware of the scheme or find enrolment too cumbersome, and others make fraudulent claims. About a quarter of older people are aware of government concessions, e.g. for bus and train travel, telephone connections, special interest rates for bank accounts and loans, and income tax benefits; this proportion is lower amongst older rural inhabitants than their urban counterparts.

Ageing in Africa

Africa is the second-largest continent with the second-largest population, estimated at 1.4 billion people in 2020, and the youngest median age at 19.7. Demography in Africa has shown more perturbation than in the rest of the world due to HIV/AIDS, with a plateauing of the trend to improvement (marked falls in some countries) in both LE and childhood mortality between 1980 and 1995. The combination of HIV and conflicts resulted in skip generations where grandparents brought up children, but most of that older generation has died, and the 'missing' parents are now 'missing' grandparents.

Life expectancy has been increasing steadily again, since the management of HIV/AIDS improved, but the impact of the COVID pandemic is still to be determined. Overall, as age is the biggest risk factor for death from COVID, Africa, with its young population, had less early mortality than 'older' countries. However, sub-Saharan Africa is home to two-thirds of people living with HIV, which may increase the risk of death from COVID. Some governments denied the reality of COVID; there was little testing; ICU care is limited; and ascertainment of the cause of death is poor. COVID vaccination was slow. By July 2021, less than 3% of people in Africa had received a single dose of the vaccine. In developed countries, the pandemic disrupted cancer screening. In Africa, diagnostic and treatment programmes for HIV and TB were disrupted, and the effects of this may be delayed.

In 2021, Africa was still the continent with the highest number of ongoing wars (Uppsala definition), with 14–18 conflicts causing 1,000–10,000 direct, violent deaths in the year, but only 1–5 major wars (with 10,000 or more combat-related deaths in a year), including the conflict in Tigray. Most deaths due to direct violence are among those aged 15–45. Indirect factors, including the movement of refugees, rape, famine, poverty, and failure of infection control programmes, kill thousands more and limit sustainable economic development. A recent study across the entire continent found that the number of infant deaths related to armed conflicts from 1995 to 2015 was more than three times the number of direct deaths from these conflicts.

Ageing in Brazil

Brazilians' LE has shot up to near Western European levels from just 37 years in 1940, whilst the number of births per woman has fallen to 1.8 from nearly 6 in 1970. In 1990, it was predicted that AIDS would have a major impact, but strategies including widespread promotion of condom use, educating prostitutes, needle exchange programmes, and most controversially, the manufacture and provision of cheap generic antiretroviral drugs, were remarkably successful in limiting the threatened epidemic.

Income distribution is very unequal in Brazil, with concomitant inequalities in health status and quality of life. Disability rises with increasing age. Those with less education and wealth were almost twice as likely to suffer from disability compared with their peers. Urban dwellers were also more disabled than those in rural areas.

The climate emergency

According to the World Meteorological Organisation, 2022 continued the run of the world's hottest years with a temperature of 1.15°C above the average for the pre-industrial period (1850–1900). 2022 was the hottest summer on record in Europe, with the temperature topping 40°C in Britain for the first time, the worst drought in 500 years, and record wildfires and air pollution.

Climate change is a major threat to the world. It is already having a significant impact on human health by:

- **Direct effects:** changes in the normal temperature range with heatwaves and intense cold. Extreme weather events (floods, hurricanes, droughts, wildfires) and exposure to UV radiation.
- **Indirect effects:** changes in air quality (air pollution, pollen, and allergens), famine, unsafe food and water, and increased risk of transmission of vector-borne diseases.

Older people are more vulnerable to all these hazards and the chaos that follows disasters because of their physiology, medical problems, medication, and socio-economic factors. HelpAge International notes that humanitarian efforts often fail to provide adequate help for older people. An early example was the French experience in the 2-week summer heatwave of 2003, when most of the excess deaths occurred in people over 70, mainly due to the added stress on the cardiac and respiratory systems. After disasters like cyclones and floods, people with poor mobility and dementia are more challenging to rescue, and food- and water-borne diseases are more likely to be fatal.

Oxfam (2022) reports that:

- The number of climate-related disasters has tripled in the last 30 years.
- Between 2006 and 2016, the rate of global sea-level rise was two and half times faster than for almost all of the 20th century.
- More than 20 million people a year are forced from their homes by climate change.

Recent major events include cyclones Daniel in the eastern Mediterranean and Freddy in East Africa in 2023, the 2020 bushfires in Australia, ongoing droughts in the Horn of Africa, Southern Africa and Central America, and floods and landslides in India, Nepal, Bangladesh,

and Pakistan. The true toll of the floods in Pakistan in 2022 will not be known for years as the poverty resulting from destroyed livelihoods continues to claim lives.

Air pollution is the world's leading environmental cause of illness and premature death. Air pollutants and greenhouse gases often come from the same sources, and there is a complex interaction between pollutants and climate. Climate change is already increasing ozone levels, and the length of the wildfire season and number of large fires are contributing to increased particulate matter. $PM_{2.5}$ is the most hazardous particle and is cleared by rainfall, so the changes will vary in different localities.

Longer, hotter summers and rising CO_2 are increasing the length of pollen seasons and the quantity of pollen and fungal spores produced. Between 1995 and 2015, the season for ragweed pollen, a common allergen leading to asthma attacks, lengthened by around 3 weeks in the northern latitudes of North America, with later frosts in the autumn.

Mosquito-borne diseases are spreading. Mosquitoes that can carry the dengue fever virus were previously limited to elevations below 3,300 ft but are now found at over 7,000 ft in the Andes of Colombia. Malaria has been detected in new higher-elevation areas in Indonesia and Africa. Aedes mosquitoes, which transmit chikungunya, dengue fever, West Nile, and Zika viruses, are now found in much of Southern Europe. Lyme disease is becoming more widespread as the range of ticks increases.

Global poverty

Whilst the developed world confronts diseases of affluence, much of the world still struggles with poverty.

In 2019, half of the world's population (47%) lived in poverty defined, as living on less than US$ 6.85 a day.

The number of people living in extreme poverty, living on less than $2.15 a day, had been falling for three decades. The rate of decline slowed after 2015, partly because of conflict and climate change, but the trend was reversed in 2020, when poverty rose because of the disruption caused by the COVID pandemic. The effects of lockdowns and job losses were particularly hard on poor households everywhere, but in less economically developed regions there is less economic resilience, and older people who depended on family support fared badly. Global poverty resumed its pre-pandemic downward trajectory, but the ongoing effects of the pandemic and the war in Ukraine (from March 2022), with their inflationary effects on energy and food supply, are likely to have harmful effects for the next decade.

There is a clear positive correlation between the per capita income in a country and LE (see Figure 1.19), but there is a range of life expectancies across countries at all levels of income. Individual countries can be looked at dynamically on Gapminder. In many parts of the world, there is also marked variation within countries (see the discussion on the effect of social class in the UK in Chapter 2).

Inter-generational strife

This is a potential problem in both more and less economically developed countries. Strains and conflict could arise from:

- Decreasing numbers of working-age adults are trying to support and fund increasing numbers of retirees.
- Younger people in the economically developed world are not experiencing the ongoing increases in affluence that their parents and grandparents took for granted.

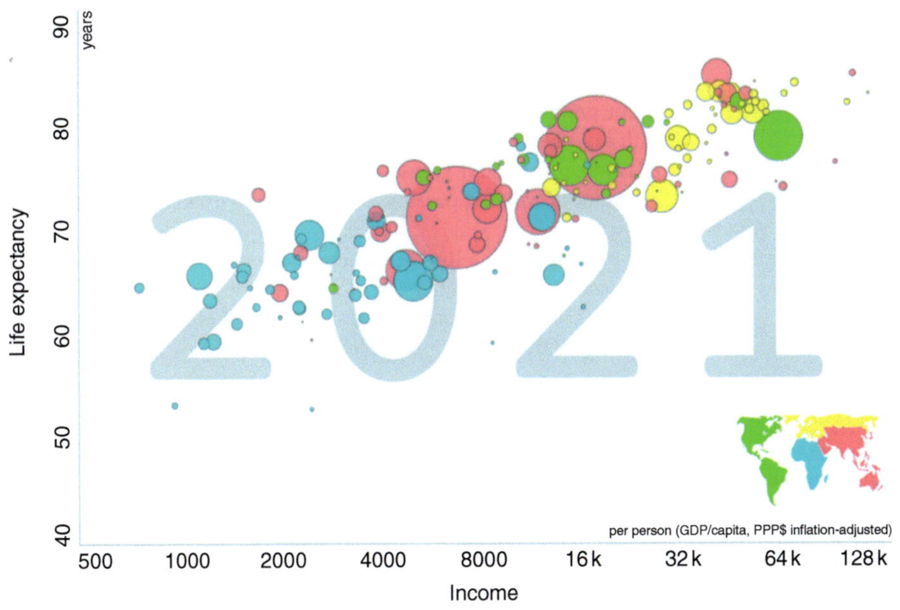

Figure 1.19 The relationship between gross domestic product and life expectancy. *Source*: Adapted from Gapminder.

- Increasing climate-change activism as those generations and parts of the world that gained from the consumption of resources are leaving a major challenge for the next generation and developing countries (several of which are at particular risk from rising sea levels).
- The prospect of relative poverty in old age for the current young due to increased LE but declining provision for pensions (compared with current retirees).
- High expectations of those growing old in the next two decades, e.g. aspiring to retire early with decreased disability but still expecting enhanced care services.
- In less economically developed countries, demographic change poses challenges for older people, services, and pensions.

Social aspects of ageing

Old age is a time of loss. The potential losses are varied but often inter-related. Some are inevitable; others depend on the socio-economic and cultural environment.

Losses in old age

- Health, due to declining homeostasis and increasing frailty and pathology.
- Independence, due to acquired disabilities.
- Wealth, as income falls on stopping work, and disabilities may result in added costs, e.g. for personal care, the need for a warmer environment, aids, and adaptations.
- Companionship after bereavement (spouse, siblings, and friends).
- Status following retirement, loss of independence, and ageism.
- Life.

The above changes and losses may expose people to the following consequences:

- Unhappiness, grief, depression, and suicide (see Chapter 8).
- Increased incidence of illness.
- Increased risk of accidents.
- Poverty.
- Dependence and abuse.
- Malnutrition (see Chapter 14).
- Hypothermia or risk of heat stroke (see Chapter 16).

Retirement

Retirement is an ancient concept dating back to 13 BCE when the Roman Emperor Augustus began paying pensions to legionnaires who had served 20 years. Pensions have always been contentious – in CE 14, an increase in the retirement age and a reduction in the pension resulted in a mutiny! From the 16th century, several European countries offered pensions to their troops, and after the American Civil War, disabled veterans received pensions. However, throughout the world, most people worked until they were no longer physically able. In 1880, the Baltimore and Ohio Railroad introduced the first retirement plan financed jointly by contributions from an employer and its workers. In 1889, the German chancellor, Bismarck, established government financial support for those aged 70+ who were 'disabled from work by age and invalidity'. State-funded pensions were gradually put in place by economically developed countries in the late 19th and early 20th centuries, usually with 65 as the retirement age. This was considered affordable, as the proportion of the population reaching this age was low.

In the 21st century, wealthy countries are increasing pension ages to try to maintain financial viability. However, even among the members of the Organisation for Economic Co-operation and Development (OECD), there is wide variation in pension structure, retirement age, and gender differences. In the least economically developed countries, retirement is for the privileged few, and most people still must work until they die or become unable to work and must rely on family support.

According to the International Labour Organisation (2019), at the global level, 68% of older people receive a pension, but only 20% in most low-income countries. Women are less likely than men to receive a pension, and if they do, benefits are often much lower.

Retirement is a major life transition. Even for those lucky enough to have the possibility of retirement, it is viewed as a mixed blessing. It may occupy one-third of life. In a 2018 survey in the UK, 38% looked forward to retiring, 11% did not, and 25% of retirees experienced difficulties with adverse psychosocial outcomes. Retirement is a potential period of loss of – income, companionship, status, and self-confidence.

To counteract the disadvantages, there are positive aspects of retirement:

- Many stay fit and healthy for most of this time.
- It is an opportunity to redesign one's lifestyle and promote good health.
- Time is available for new or renewed interests, activities, and relationships.

But retirement may bring social problems, and it is a time when some complex decisions will have to be made. Dilemmas encountered may include:

- Becoming a carer, e.g. of parents or grandchildren early in retirement or of a spouse or siblings later.
- Where to live – it is probably best to stay somewhere comfortable and well known. If a move is contemplated, earlier is better than later, as the retiree is likely to be fitter and one of a pair.
- What sort of accommodation? Somewhere enabling independence, despite acquired disabilities.
- Driving – may need to be given up at some stage, so beware of geographical isolation (see Chapter 21).
- Boredom affects 10% of the retired – another 20% (although not bored) would prefer to still be working. People who are poor, disabled, poorly educated and isolated are most likely to be dissatisfied with retirement.
- The economic consequences of an expanding number of retirees are causing widespread concern in the developed world. The retirement age has increased in many countries and may reach 70+ years. There will be a need to review the nature of paid employment in later years with consideration for manual workers and ways to enable partial or gradual retirement.
- Preparation for retirement is vital.
- The increasing vulnerability and unpredictability of the global financial markets also pose threats to pension provision. The pension aspirations of many current workers may not be met and may be considered a potential threat to world finance.

Some myths of ageing

- **It is a new problem.** No – there have always been elderly people; there are now more. In the past, most people were denied the opportunity of old age by dying young. Now, most babies born worldwide can expect to live into their 70s, and in developed countries, their 80s.
- **All older people are decrepit and confused.** No – most live independent lives in their own homes.
- **The chronic conditions of old age are untreatable**. No – medical treatment at all ages is primarily the management of chronic conditions. The course of disease can be slowed or modified, e.g. Parkinson's disease; symptoms can be alleviated, e.g. pain and breathlessness; and in deficiency diseases (pernicious anaemia, osteomalacia, and myxoedema), normal function can be restored.
- **Natural decline cannot be prevented.** No – regular physical activity can rejuvenate, and physical capacity can be improved by 10–15 years. Adopting a 'healthy lifestyle' in middle age (no smoking, minimal alcohol, avoidance of obesity, regular exercise and keeping social activity) can delay the onset and decrease the eventual severity and duration of disability towards the end of life.
- **Treating older patients is a waste of money.** No – not to treat is not only inhumane (see Human Rights Act 1998) but also often expensive, and neglected problems may lead to more expenditure in the long term (i.e. 'care' can be more expensive than 'cure').
- **All older people are depressed and lonely.** No – most elderly people are not depressed. Well-being and contentment may feature more in later life than during the ambitious and frustrated productive years. Although the general population thinks that 90% of elderly people are lonely, only 10% of the elderly consider themselves to be so.
- **Older people are just a burden.** No – they are a valuable resource with experience and, sometimes, wisdom. Most carers are older people, and these include grandparents caring for grandchildren because of absent or working parents. The old are the backbone of voluntary services.
- **Old patients have a limited future and a poor prognosis.** No – LE at 65 years is more than 17 years for a man and 20 years for a woman. To put this into context, survival for 5 years after many surgical and oncological treatments is recorded as a success.

📖 REFERENCES AND FURTHER READING

Our World in Data. *How has world population growth changed over time?* https://ourworldindata.org/world-population-growth.

Our World in Data. *Graph of demographic transition.* https://ourworldindata.org/demographic-transition.

Wang H, Abbas KM, Abbasifard M, et al. (2020) Global age-sex-specific fertility, mortality, healthy life expectancy (HALE), and population estimates in 204 countries and territories. *The Lancet* 396:1160–1203. doi: 10.1010/30140-6736(20)30977-6

UN Department of Economic and Social Affairs. Population Division. *World population prospects* 2022. *World population pyramids.* https://population.un.org/wpp/Graphs/DemographicProfiles/Pyramid/900

UN DESA PD *World population prospects; summary of results.* (2022) https://www.un.org/development/desa/pd/sites/www.un.org.development.desa.pd/files/wpp2022_summary_of_results.pdf

Vollset SE, Goren E, Yuan C-W, et al. (2020) Fertility, mortality, migration, and population scenarios for 195 countries and territories from 2017 to 2100: a forecasting analysis for the Global Burden of Disease Study. *The Lancet* 396:1285–1306. doi: 10.1016/S0140-6736(20)30677-2.

Our World in Data. *Population by age group.* https://ourworldindata.org/age-structure

UN DESA PD. *World population aged 80+.* https://population.un.org/wpp/Graphs/Probabilistic/POP/80plus/900

Our World in Data. *Life expectancy.* https://ourworldindata.org/life-expectancy

Tanne JH (2022) Life expectancy: US sees steepest decline in a century. *BMJ* 378:o2142. doi: 10.1136/bmj.o2142.

Our World in Data. *Life expectancy increase worldwide.* https://ourworldindata.org/life-expectancy#life-expectancy-increased-in-all-countries-of-the-world.

UN DESA World social report (2023) *Leaving no one behind in an ageing world* (shows OADR projections). https://www.un.org/development/desa/pd/sites/www.un.org.development.desa.pd/files/undesa_pd_2023_wsr-fullreport.pdf

Our World in Data. *Gender ratios.* https://ourworldindata.org/gender-ratio

Our World in Data. *Visualisation of demographic change in different countries.* https://ourworldindata.org/grapher/life-expectancy?country=~OWID_WRL

Our World in Data. *Migration.* https://ourworldindata.org/migration

Our World in Data. *Urbanization.* https://ourworldindata.org/urbanization#all-charts

WHO *Global health estimates.* https://www.who.int/news-room/fact-sheets/detail/the-top-10-causes-of-death

OECD *Data on care home provision.* https://stats.oecd.org/Index.aspx?QueryId=30142

Forster T, Kentikelenis AE, Stubbs TH, et al. (2020) The impact of structural adjustment programs on developing countries. *Social Science & Medicine* 267:112496. doi: 10.1016/j.socscimed.2019.112496.

UN DESA PD *Population Pyramid for India* (2023). https://population.un.org/wpp/Graphs/DemographicProfiles/Pyramid/356

World population review *India*. https://worldpopulationreview.com/countries/india-population?ModPagespeed=noscript

Dandona R (2022) Public health priorities for India. *The Lancet* 7e102–7e103. doi: 10.1016/S2468-2667(22)00008-1.

Desiraju K (2021) Issues in Public Health in India. *Journal of Public Health* 43(Suppl 2): ii3–ii9. doi: 10.1093/pubmed/fdab305

The Institute for Health Metrics and Evaluation *India*. https://www.healthdata.org/india

Bloom DE, Sekher TV, Lee J (2021) Longitudinal Aging Study in India (LASI): new data resources for addressing aging in India. *Nature Aging* 1:1070–1072. doi: 10.1038/s43587-021-00155-y.

Pilania M, Yadav V, Bairwa M, et al. (2019) Prevalence of depression among the elderly (60 years and above) population in India, 1997–2016: a systematic review and meta-analysis. *BMC Public Health* 19:832. doi: 10.1186/s12889-019-7136-z

Arora NK, Nair MKC, Gulati S, et al. (2018) Neurodevelopmental disorders in children aged 2-9 years: population-based burden estimates across five regions in India. *PLoS Medicine* 15(7):e1002615. doi: 10.1371/journal.pmed.1002615.

HelpAge India https://www.holpageindia.org

Akinrolie O, Iwuagwu AO, Kalu ME, et al. Emerging Researchers and Professionals in Ageing, African Networks (2024) Longitudinal studies of aging in sub-Saharan Africa: review, limitations, and recommendations in preparation of projected aging population. *Innovation in Aging* 8(4):igae002. https://academic.oup.com/innovateage/article/8/4/igae002/7585958.

Sawyer D. Getting Old Before Getting Rich – challenges of ageing in Brazil. https://revista.drclas.harvard.edu/challenges-of-aging-in-brazil

US Environmental Protection Agency. *Climate Change and the Health of Older Adults.* https://www.epa.gov/climateimpacts/climate-change-and-health-older-adults

US Environmental Protection Agency. *Climate change indicators: health and society (2024).* https://www.epa.gov/climate-indicators/health-society

International Institute for Population Sciences and United Nations Population Fund. *Caring for our Elders: institutional responses. India Ageing report 2023.* https://india.unfpa.org/sites/default/files/pub-pdf/20230926_india_ageing_report_2023_web_version_pdf

Oxfam 2020 *Five natural disasters that beg for climate action.* https://www.oxfam.org/en/5-natural-disasters-beg-climate-action

Colón-González FJ, Sewe MO, Tompkins AM, et al. (2021) Projecting the risk of mosquito-borne diseases in a warmer and more populated world: a multi-model, multi-scenario intercomparison modelling study. Lancet Planetary Health 5:e404–e414. https://www.thelancet.com/journals/lanplh/article/PIIS2542-5196(21)00132-7/fulltext

Gapminder. *The relationship between GDP and life expectancy.* https://www.gapminder.org/tag/life-expectancy/

Centre for Ageing Better. (2018) *The experience of the transition to retirement.* https://ageing-better.org.uk/sites/default/files/2018-12/Transition-to-retirement.pdf

WHO Health topics. *Ageing* https://www.who.int/health-topics/ageing#tab=tab_1

All websites were accessed in August 2024.

2

Health and social care in the UK

Population figures

The UK population topped 60 million in 2005 and was 68.3 million in 2023. The population in millions of the constituent nations is:

England	57.7
Scotland	5.5
Wales	3.2
Northern Ireland	1.9

When you look at any data, check which population it refers to, i.e. the UK/Great Britain/England and Wales. Not all of the 2021 census data has been processed, so you will find conflicting numbers as some are still estimates from 2011. Census data is for England and Wales. Also, check the age band and beware of 'pensionable age' as this keeps changing. The COVID-19 pandemic has caused perturbations in various data sets. The key source for data is the Office for National Statistics (ONS).

The population will continue to grow and age. See Figure 2.1.

- In mid-2020, there were more females than males, reflecting their higher life expectancy (LE).
- The spike at age 73 (in 2020) is the post-war baby boom.
- The bulge at age 55 is the 1960s baby boom.
- The deficit at around 20 reflects a drop in births around the millennium.
- By 2030, there will be more older people and fewer children, so the base narrows.

Nearly one-fifth of the UK population (19%) was aged 65+ in 2019, around 12.3 million people. The number of people in this age group increased by 23% between 2009 and 2019, at a time when the whole UK population only increased by 7%. By 2050, one in four people will be aged 65+.

The proportion of the population aged 75+ is projected to rise from 8% in 2018 to 13% in 2043, whilst the proportion aged 85+ is projected to double from 2 to 4%.

The number of centenarians in the UK rose to its highest-ever level in 2020, reaching 15,120, an increase of almost a fifth from 2019. This rapid growth is not due to LE but to the spike in births following World War I (numbers are too small to be visible on the population pyramid).

Life expectancy at birth

Life expectancy at birth increased steadily from 1970 to 2013, flatlined from 2013 (falling in deprived areas, leading to discussion about the impact of austerity), and has fallen overall since 2019 due to COVID (see King's Fund report). Life expectancy at birth in the UK in 2018–2020 was 79.0 years for males and 82.9 years for females. Amongst the four nations, England consistently has the highest LE and Scotland the lowest.

Life expectancy in old age

Life expectancy at extreme old age has always been longer than people think (see Figure 2.2). If a woman born in 1850 lived to be 80, her LE would be another 4 years. For a woman born in 1940, in 2020, this was estimated to be 9.7 years. This is important clinically – an 80-year-old newly diagnosed diabetic has time to develop complications! In 2018–2020, in the UK, a man of 65 can expect another 18.5 years of life and a woman another 21 years. However, only about half of these years are spent in good health (see later discussion).

Characteristics of the older population

Sex

In the population aged 65+, women outnumber men because of their LE. The difference has been decreasing for decades as LE has increased faster for men (changing smoking habits and safer working environments). The cohort effect of excess deaths of young men in World War II has passed.

At the age of 65+

- In 1984, there were 1.56 females for every male.
- In 2019, there were 1.29 females for every male.
- By 2034, there will be 1.18 females for every male (projected).

This ratio is greater in the very old, so at 90–94

- In 2002, there were 3.1 females for every male.
- In 2020, there were 1.9 females for every male.

Ethnicity

In the 2021 census, 18% of the population identified as having a Black, Asian and Minority Ethnic (BAME) background. Ethnic diversity is lower in older age groups but is increasing over time. 93.6% of the population aged 65 years and over living in England and Wales identified in the high-level White ethnic group, 3.8% identified in the Asian groups, 1.4% in the Black groups, and 1.2% of people in the Mixed or Other ethnic groups.

There is marked regional variation. London is the most ethnically diverse region, and Newham is the most diverse local authority.

Geriatric Medicine and Elderly Care: Lecture Notes, Ninth Edition. Claire G. Nicholl, K. Jane Wilson, and Shaun D'Souza.
© 2025 John Wiley & Sons Ltd. Published 2025 by John Wiley & Sons Ltd.
Companion website: www.wiley.com/go/lecturenotesgeriatricmedicine9e

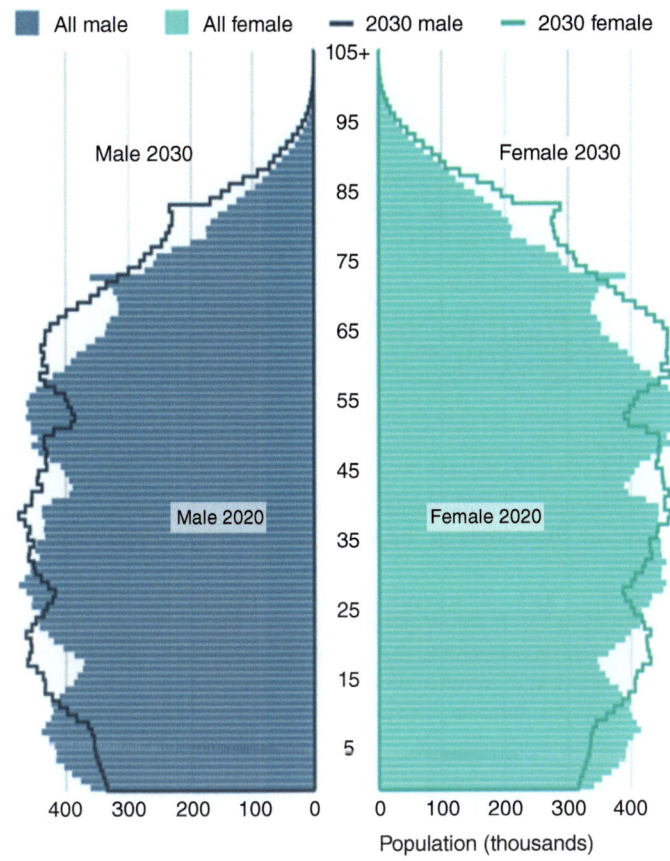

Figure 2.1 Age structure of the UK population in mid-2020 and mid-2030. *Source*: ONS / CC BY 3.0.

Table 2.1 Broad ethnic composition of the population in London by age.

Age	Number (thousands)	% population	Ethnic composition (%) White	Ethnic composition (%) BAME
0–15	1874	21	43	57
16–24	962	11	52	48
25–34	1689	19	60	40
35–49	2058	23	57	43
50–64	1446	16	61	39
65–79	777	9	71	29
80+	300	3	77	23
Total	9106	100	57	43

Source: Adapted from London datastore. BAME, Black, Asian and Minority Ethnic groups.

In Greater London, the proportion of White residents increases steadily above 50 years (Table 2.1), but even at 80+, nearly a quarter of residents are from a BAME background, so services need to be appropriate.

Within broad ethnic categories, in London (see Table 2.2),

- The White Irish population is the only group older than the White British.
- There are more Black Africans than Black Caribbeans, but the Black Caribbean population is older (earlier migration).
- Over 10% of the Indian population is also 65+.

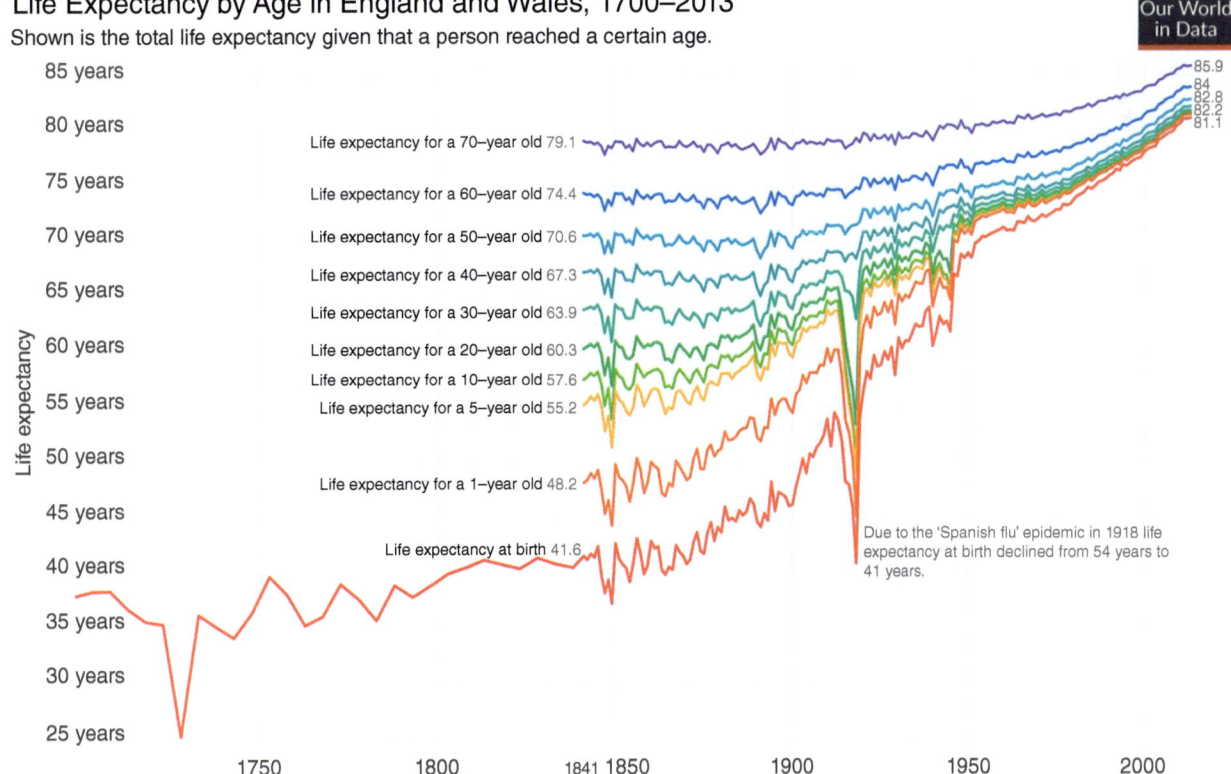

Figure 2.2 Changes in life expectancy at different ages in England and Wales since 1700. *Source*: Modified from Our World in Data / CC BY 4.0.

Table 2.2 Ethnic groups and their age structure in Greater London.

Ethnic group	Number (thousands)	% population	Age breakdown (%)		
			0–15	16–24	65+
White Irish	187	2	6	68	26
White British	3551	39	16	66	18
Black Caribbean	346	4	18	67	15
Indian	644	7	17	71	12
Chinese	156	2	10	82	8
Pakistani	277	3	27	66	7
Black African	660	7	30	65	5

Source: Adapted from London datastore.

Migration

Net migration has been the major contributor to the increase in population between 2001 and 2020, accounting for 60% of the population growth.

Geographical location

Older people migrate from towns to the country and seaside, so the age structure of the population is uneven (see Figure 2.3). London is a young city. In North Norfolk, over a third of the residents are over 65. If you look at the map, you can pick out university cities, because of their young populations.

Marital status

In 2021, amongst the over 11 million people aged 65+ in England and Wales (ONS 2023)

- 6% were single.
- 58% were married or in a civil partnership. Same-sex marriages/civil partnerships accounted for less than 0.25% of legal partnerships.
- 12% were divorced.
- 23% were widowed; this increases to 37% of men and 72% of women by 85+.

Living companions

About 3.3 million individuals aged 65+ live alone (see Figure 2.4). Older women are more likely to live alone than older men, particularly in their 80s.

The focus is on older people living alone, but there is a little data (mainly from the building industry) that multigenerational living is becoming more common in the UK (three generations – grandparents with children and grandchildren, or two generations – parents with adult children, or middle aged people with their elderly parents).

Health status

There are two common measures of health and LE. Women live longer but spend more time in poor health and with disabilities than men.

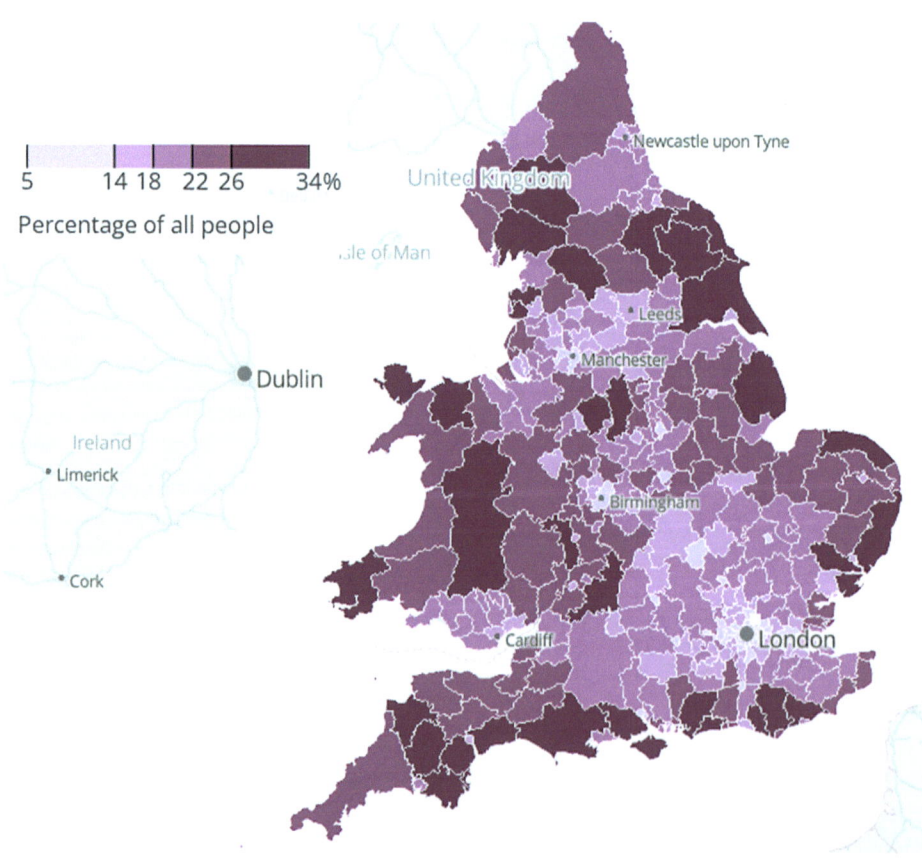

Percentage of all people
5 14 18 22 26 34%

Source: Office for National Statistics - Census 2021

Figure 2.3 Population aged 65 and over, 2021, local authorities in England and Wales. *Source*: ONS 2021 / CC BY3.0.

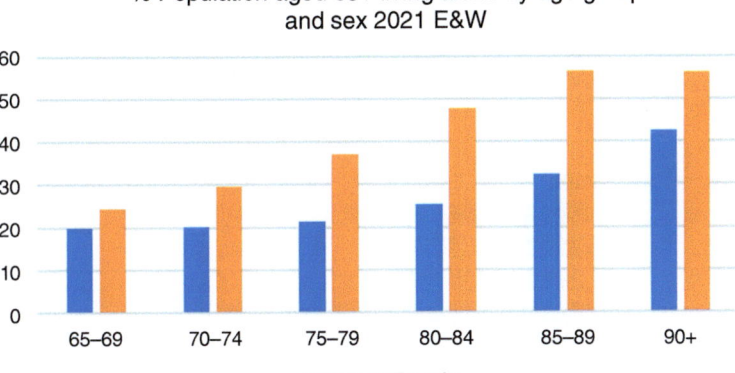

% Population aged 65+ living alone by age group and sex 2021 E&W

Figure 2.4 Percentage of the population aged 65+ who live alone by age groups and sex. *Source*: England and Wales 2021, ONS 2023 / CC BY 3.0

Table 2.3 Health state life expectancies for 2018–2020 at birth in the least and most deprived areas (deciles) of England. Note the health data is from the 2011 census.

Types of life expectancy	Females		Males	
	Least deprived	Most deprived	Least deprived	Most deprived
LE at birth	86.3	78.3	83.2	73.5
HLE at birth	70.7	51.9	70.5	52.3
DFLE at birth	66.4	50.3	69.0	51.4

Source: Adapted from ONS 2022. LE, life expectancy; HLE, healthy life expectancy; DFLE, disability-free life expectancy.

Table 2.4 Health state life expectancies in years at age 65 in England 2016–2018.

Types of life expectancy	Females	Males
LE at 65 years	21.2	18.9
HLE at 65 years	11.1	10.6
DFLE at 65 years	9.8	9.9

Source: Adapted from ONS 2019. LE, life expectancy; HLE, healthy life expectancy; DFLE, disability-free life expectancy.

Healthy life expectancy (HLE) is an estimate of the lifetime spent in 'very good' or 'good' health, based on how individuals perceive their general health.

Disability-free life expectancy (DFLE) is an estimate of the lifetime free from limiting long-term illness.

The effect of deprivation on life expectancy

People in deprived areas not only have shorter lives but spend a greater proportion of their lives in poor health. The difference is stark and worsening. The male-female difference in LE is greater in more deprived areas, but the effect of deprivation, measured by the index of multiple deprivation, is greater than the effect of sex (see Table 2.3).

A statistic that may surprise many is that despite higher levels of deprivation, male and female LE was higher in ethnic minority groups in England and Wales (2011–2014) than in White and Mixed groups (King's Fund). However, the pandemic had a disproportionate impact on ethnic minority communities, and more recent data is awaited.

By the age of 65, just over half of the remaining LE will be spent in good health (see Table 2.4). In deprived areas, this is less than half, but the effect of deprivation is less marked than at birth.

Disability

In England, 17.7% of people (18.7% of females and 16.5% of males) reported a disability in the 2021 census. People were asked if they had a long-term physical or mental health condition and, if so, how much it limited their day-to-day activities. (See Chapter 4 for more on impairments and disabilities and the resulting activity limitations).

Disability and age

The prevalence of disability increases with age, particularly after 70–74, with a marked increase in those whose activities were 'limited a lot' (see Figure 2.5).

The 2021 census data showed a small decrease in age-standardised disability compared with 2011, particularly in those 'limited a lot', and in older age, but the questions have changed and COVID may have had several effects.

Disability and deprivation

The prevalence of age-standardised disability varies across regions, following socioeconomic deprivation, so it is highest in Wales and Northeast England (both over 20%). In England, comparing the least deprived and most deprived deciles, disability is more common with deprivation from infancy to extreme old age, but the gulf is widest between 40 and 64 as increasing disability affects those living in deprivation in middle age. After the age of 64, the gap declines progressively and is minimal above the age of 85. Hence, councils in affluent areas, which get less central funding, struggle to fund care for very elderly people.

The data is similar to the Family Resources Survey 2021–2022, which found that 24% of people in the UK have a disability, up from 19% in 2010, with 44% of those aged 65+ and 58% aged 80+ reporting a disability.

Types of disability

Poor mobility is the most common, affecting two-thirds of older people who consider that they have a disability (see Figure 2.6).

The totals sum to over 100%, as respondents could report more than one impairment type. In 2020/2021, the State Pension Age (SPA) increased to 66 years.

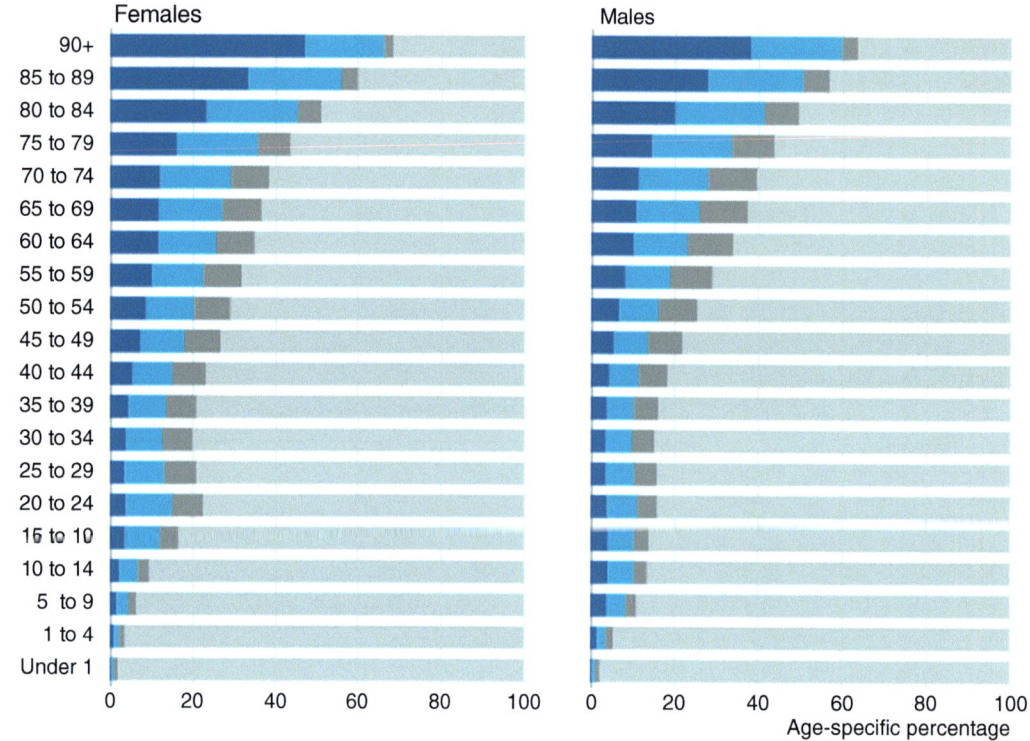

Figure 2.5 Percentage of the population reporting disability in England by age group and sex. *Source*: Adapted from ONS census data 2021.

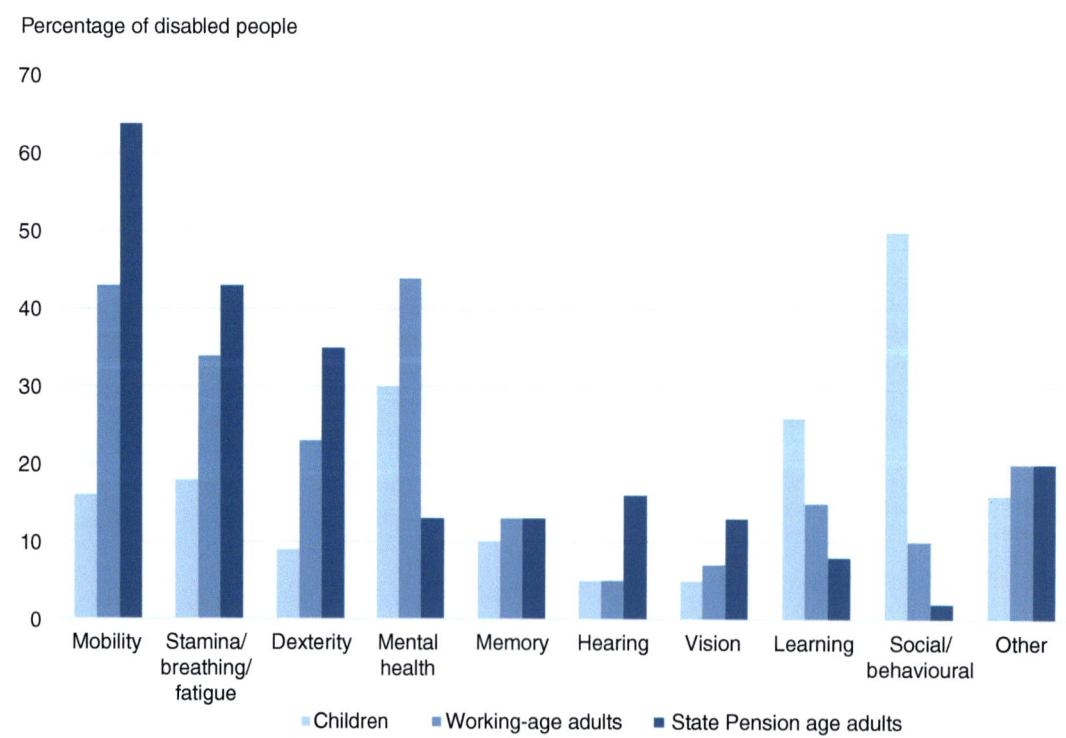

Figure 2.6 Impairment types reported by disabled people by age group, UK. *Source*: Family Resources Survey 2021 Crown Copyright / CC BY 3.0.

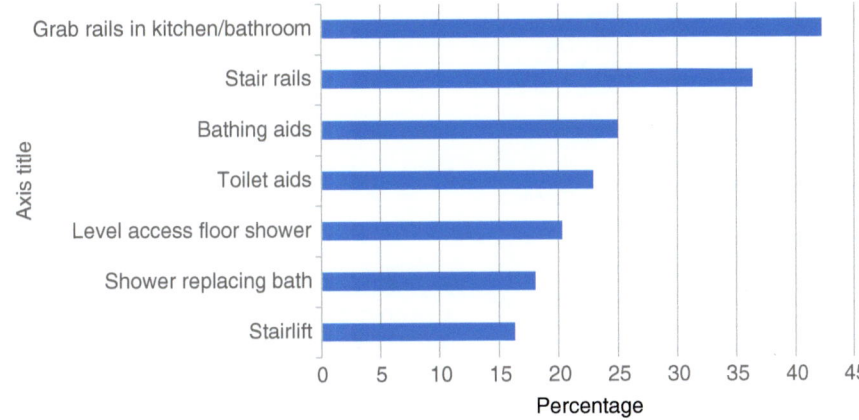

Figure 2.7 Indoor adaptations most often needed in 2019/20. *Source*: English Housing Survey / Public domain.

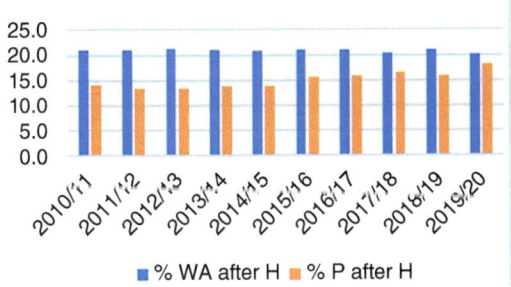

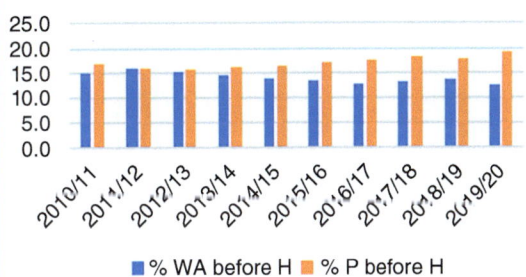

Figure 2.8 Percentage of working age (WA) and pensioner households (P) in poverty after and before consideration of housing costs (H). *Source*: DWP Households below average income 2019/2020.

Sensory impairment

- In the UK, more than 2 million people have sight loss that affects their daily lives (RNIB 2021). This is strongly related to age: 20% of this group are 65–74, 27% are 75–84, and 32% are 85+. Altogether, 340,000 people are registered as blind or visually impaired (but certification is very incomplete). Recent prevalence data is lacking, but around 1 in 8 over-75s and 1 in 3 over-90s have a serious visual impairment.
- Hearing loss is even more common, with 70% of the over-70-year-olds in the UK having some hearing loss, mild in 27%, moderate in 36%, and severe in 7%.

Home adaptations

Around 8% (1.9 million) of households in England included a person who needed adaptations to their home. 81% of households felt that their home itself was suitable, but the indoor adaptations needed are shown in Figure 2.7. The most common outdoor adaptations were ramps and rails for external steps. Care and Repair help organise building works, and a Disabled Facilities Grant may be available to help with costs.

Income

Over the last decade, pensioners as a group have faced less poverty than working-age adults. Three-quarters of pensioners own their homes, so after housing costs are considered, more working-age households are in relative poverty (defined as below 60% of contemporary median income). In 2021, half of pensioners were in the top half of the overall income distribution. However, there is considerable variation. If housing costs are not considered, the percentage of pensioner households in poverty has been rising gradually since 2013 (see Figure 2.8).

In 2019/20:

- 2.2 million of the 11.6 million pensioners lived in relative poverty.
- 6% of pensioners were defined as living with material deprivation.

Sources of income

Most income for pensioners comes from the state. 'Benefits' in Figure 2.9 include state pensions and any additional benefits. Over time, occupational and personal pensions and investment income have increased in importance. Female pensioners have lower incomes than men. Couples are less reliant on benefit income than single pensioners. Earnings make up a bigger proportion in the under 75s, but there is no marked difference in total income with age, except for couples where the head is under 75; the partner may still be working. Although pensioners have higher incomes than in 1995, the average pension income under 75 has been flat since 2010/2011 but has increased for the older group.

State benefits make up 86% of pensioner income in the lowest decile of income, but only 16% in the top decile. Ethnicity also has an impact; all White groups have a higher weekly income than Asians and Black groups (mainly due to lower occupational pensions).

Comparison between pensions in developed countries is complex, but the UK state pension is one of the lowest in Europe, providing just 58% of previous earnings from work – below the OECD average of 69% (2021). For discussion, see The Ferret 2022.

Housing

Ninety-seven per cent of people over 65 in the UK live in their own homes (including sheltered flats). This is termed living in 'the community', in contrast to institutional care, although care homes should be part of the community too!

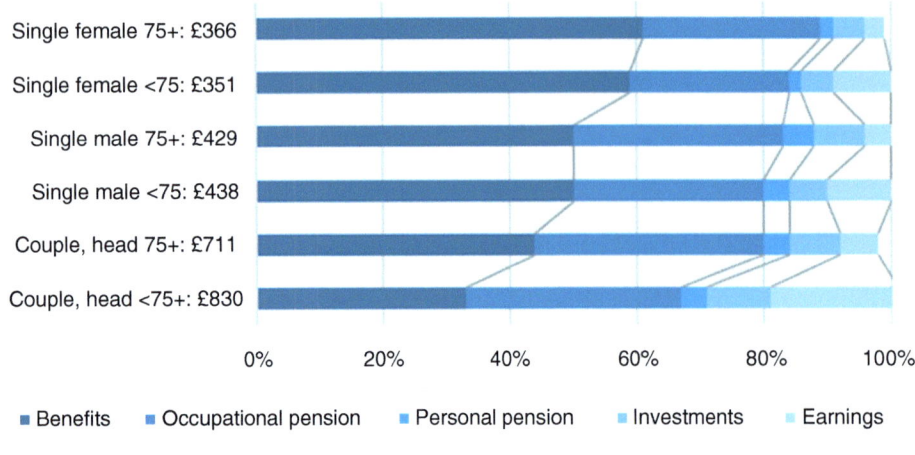

Figure 2.9 Average weekly gross income of pensioners by age, gender, and type of income, 2020/21. *Source*: DWP Pensioners' incomes series 2020 to 2021

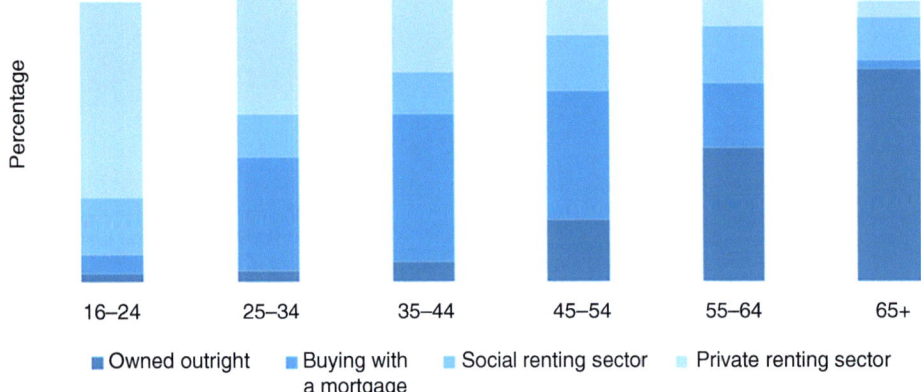

Figure 2.10 Households by tenure and age of head of household. *Source*: Adapted from English Housing Survey 2020/21/Public domain

Own home

From the English Housing Survey in 2020–2021 (see Figure 2.10) of the 6.9 million older households (led by someone aged 65 or older):

- 80% were owner-occupiers (5% had a mortgage).
- 15% were social renters.
- 6% were private renters (likely to increase).

In contrast with younger people, most older people live in a home they own outright, but issues for older households include:

- Overall, 15% lived in homes that did not meet the Decent Homes Standard; 30% in private renters (more damp and cold).
- 52% lived alone; of these, 12% felt lonely often or always and had lower life satisfaction scores.
- 45% had a household member with a long-term illness or disability.
- 13% did not have internet access at home.

Sheltered housing

In 2020/21, 439,000 households lived in sheltered accommodation (6% of older households). This is typically a group of small, self-contained flats (one or two bedrooms, a living room, a kitchenette, a bathroom, and a toilet) often around communal facilities for meals, services, and social activity.

- Provided by the local authority, housing associations, the voluntary sector, and increasingly the private sector for rent or purchase.
- Of most benefit to those with physical disabilities who lived in unsuitable housing.

- Scheme manager or 'warden' who may work office hours only.
- People with severe visual impairment struggle to adapt to new surroundings.
- Residents are generally able to wash, dress, transfer, and mobilise independently (including wheelchair users) and prepare their own food.
- Residents may have the usual help from social services.
- Assisted Living or Extra-Care housing is increasingly provided, with staff on-site 24-hr a day to provide 'extra care' (for washing, dressing, meals, etc.) and enabling much frailer residents with a degree of dementia to live there.
- Purpose-built developments may include components of 'assistive technology'.

Institutional care

Institutionalisation occurs when the person can no longer be supported at home within the resources available (see later discussion) because of:

- Severe physical disabilities.
- Immobility.
- Unpredictable and frequent care needs.
- Severe mental disability (usually dementia) requiring constant supervision. Providing care at home for a physically disabled but cognitively intact person is relatively straightforward – if problems arise between care visits, they can summon help. Dementia is the commonest reason for people to need institutional care.

Admission to a care home occurs sooner if the person does not get along well with home carers and there is no family support or even hostility towards the person remaining at home.

The complications of institutionalisation include:

- depersonalisation,
- marked restriction of choices, and
- accelerated dependence.

These can be minimised by the efforts of the staff, visitors, and sometimes the residents. Data is lacking, but restrictions on visiting and trips out during the COVID pandemic seemed to result in more rapid physical and mental decline, especially in residents with dementia.

Trends in care home provision

Historically, the NHS provided long-stay hospital beds, and the local authority provided residential homes. Since the 1980s, this pattern has changed radically. NHS long-stay beds for older people have all but disappeared, and almost everyone needing institutional care lives in:

- a care home providing personal care, a 'residential home' or
- a care home providing nursing care, a 'nursing home'.

There are about 17,000 care homes in the UK, about 70% of which are residential. Most provide care for older people; about 6,000 are registered to take people between 18 and 64, some exclusively, some with older people too. According to LaingBuisson 2024, the number of beds for people aged 65+ is around 467,000, about 45% of which are nursing beds (residential homes are typically smaller than nursing homes). The private sector provides most beds (83%), with 12% run by charities and 5% by the state. Provision is very fragmented with over 5,000 operators.

Trends in bed numbers over time show that:

- Beds have not kept pace with demographic change, so fewer people of a given age are in a care home. In E&W, the percentage of people aged 65+ in a care home was 3.5% in 2001, 3.2% in 2011, and 2.5% in 2021.
- Rates are higher with increasing age – around 14% of people aged 85+ are in a care home.
- Between 2012 and 2021, the number of both residential and nursing beds per 100 people aged 75+ fell (see Figure 2.11).
- The drop in age-adjusted demand for all beds is likely to be a combination of choice (preference for living at home), necessity (cost), and, since 2020, fear because of the risk of death and isolation experienced by care home residents due to COVID.

Residential homes

Residents need hotel services and help with personal hygiene. Most of the staff are care assistants. Twenty years ago, a new client would have been able to transfer and walk (with help as needed) to the communal dining and sitting areas. Now, the residents are often very frail and immobile. Nursing care, if needed for a brief period, is usually provided by a district nurse.

Nursing homes

A registered nurse must be on duty 24-hr a day. Most new residents are over 80, have multiple disabilities (both physical, usually being chair- or bed-bound, and mental), and need hotel services and help with personal hygiene, ***and*** nursing care. Medical cover is provided by the resident's general practitioner (GP). Residents may keep their GP if the home is local, but the move usually results in a change of GP at a very vulnerable time.

Specialist homes for people with dementia

An estimated 70% of care home residents have dementia (though not necessarily a formal diagnosis), so most care homes cope with a degree of dementia but must be registered for this. If dementia, with wandering or disruptive behaviour, is the main problem, a specialist Dementia (Elderly) or DE unit will be needed.

Moving to another type of home

All types of care homes are regulated by the Care Quality Commission (CQC), but the beds are registered for a specific client group. If a residential home resident becomes ill and is admitted to hospital, the home can refuse to take them back 'as it can no longer meet their needs'. The resident may have been deteriorating prior to the acute event, but the admission precipitates the statement that they need to move to nursing care. The wait for a nursing bed increases the length of the hospital stay. There may be less delay if the home has both nursing and care beds ('dual registered'). There is a lot of variation in the flexibility of both homes and commissioners. Many homes provide end-of-life care for their residents, and nursing homes may admit new residents for this (see Chapter 22).

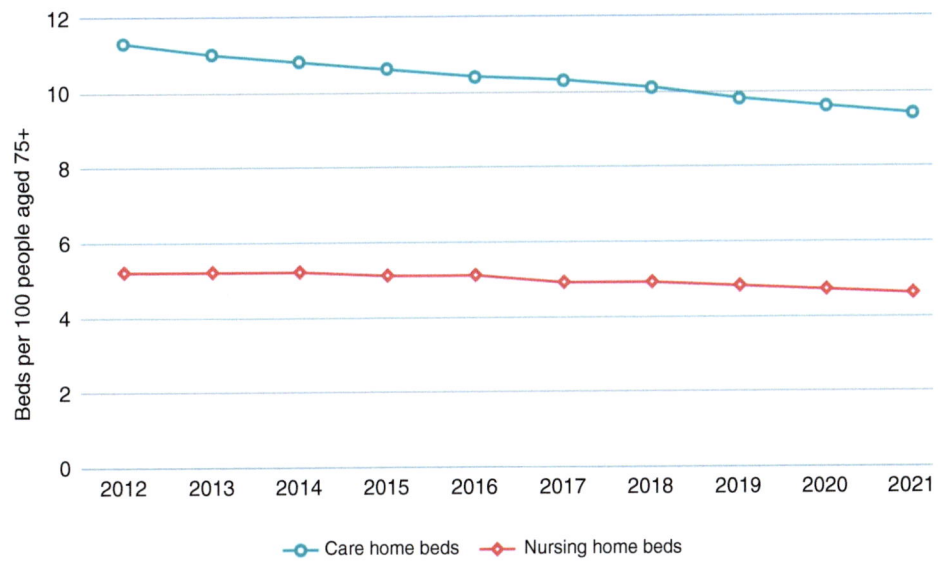

Figure 2.11 The change in the number of care home beds between 2012 and 2021, related to the population aged 75+, in England. *Source*: Nuffield Trust 2023 / Public domain.

Impact of COVID-19 on care homes

COVID destabilised what was already a difficult market, but none of the major providers closed. Of around 400,000 people living in care homes in England, during the two peak periods of COVID, April to September 2020 and October 2020 to March 2021, the CQC recorded 39,350 deaths in care homes attributed to COVID. This is the focus of an ongoing enquiry. The COVID legacy, the economic situation with rising wages and staffing difficulties are major challenges in 2024. As more people are supported at home, patients entering institutional care are frailer, and the costs outstrip the available funding.

Life expectancy in care homes

People underestimate care home costs (see later discussion) but overestimate the LE of residents. It is complex. If homes admit people specifically for end-of-life care, this will reduce average survival. Generally, death rates are high after people move in, but there is a tail of long survivors; a median may be a better guide than a mean.

The British Geriatrics Society (2020) states that the average LE in UK residential homes is 24 months and 12 months for nursing homes. Recent data gives longer LEs (see Figure 2.12). In the 2021 census, individuals aged 65+ made up 82% of the care home population (with and without nursing). LE is longer in females than males across all age groups, and all care home groups had a shorter LE than community dwellers.

Challenges for the UK care home sector

- Increasing numbers of very old people (i.e. >85 years).
- Increasing frailty of residents – especially dementia with behavioural problems.
- Rising public expectations.
- Demands of recent legislation about space.
- Financial consequences of increased staff numbers and training.
- National Living Wage, and increase in national insurance.

- Inadequate benchmark funding (self-funders subsidise state-funded clients).
- Staff recruitment and retention problems.
- Post-COVID legacy.
- Rapid rises in energy and food costs from 2022.

The organisation of care for older people

All agencies providing services have a responsibility to older people – town planning, housing, transport, law and order, even education – as all impact the quality of life for older people, but the big two are health and social care. Traditionally, health care was the responsibility of the NHS, and social care was the responsibility of the social services department of the local authority (LA). Over decades, the government departments responsible have been aggregated and disaggregated, regional and area planning has come and gone, and competition has vied with collaboration as the way forward.

NHS organisation

In 2018, the Department of Health became the Department of Health and Social Care (DHSC). The Department of Health already oversaw adult social care policy in England, but the change aims to promote closer working. DHSC sets the strategy and funds the health system in England. NHS England, the department's largest arm's-length body, sets the framework for commissioning (buying) healthcare services in England through seven regional teams.

The devolved administrations of Scotland, Wales, and Northern Ireland run their local NHS and social services.

The year 2022 saw yet another reorganisation of healthcare, recognising that the NHS needs to shift from treating single illnesses to managing

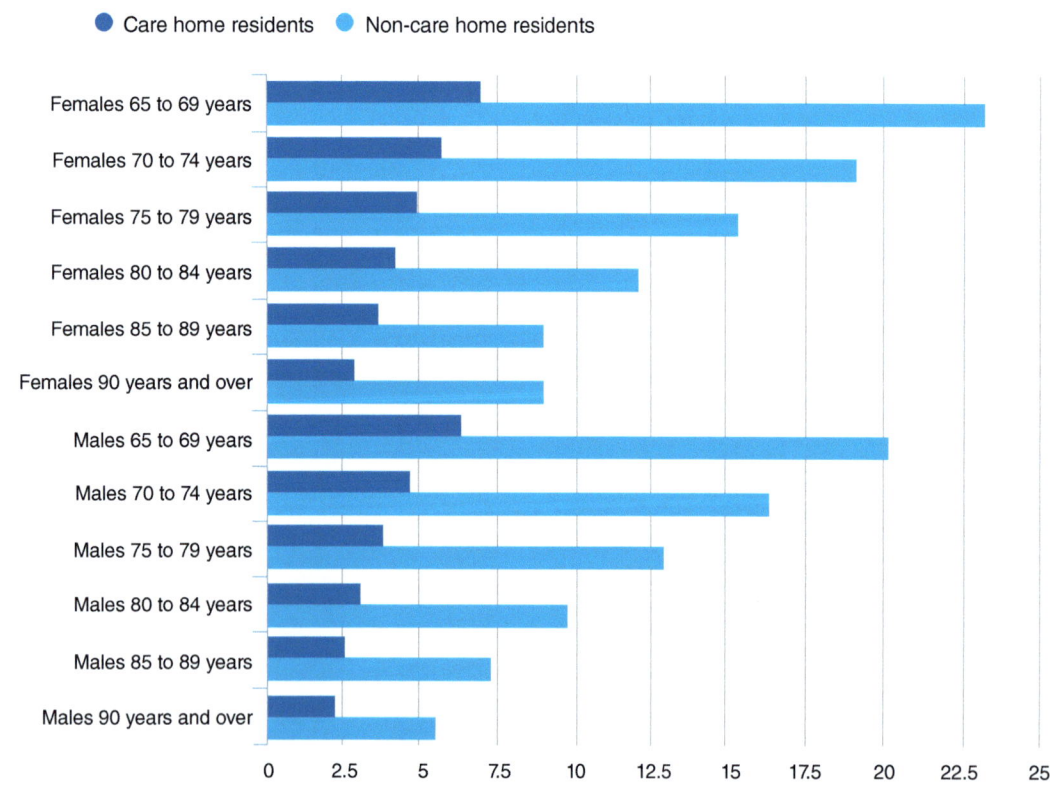

Figure 2.12 Life expectancy by age band and sex (England and Wales) 2021/22 in care home residents and community dwellers. *Source*: ONS / CC BY - 3.0.

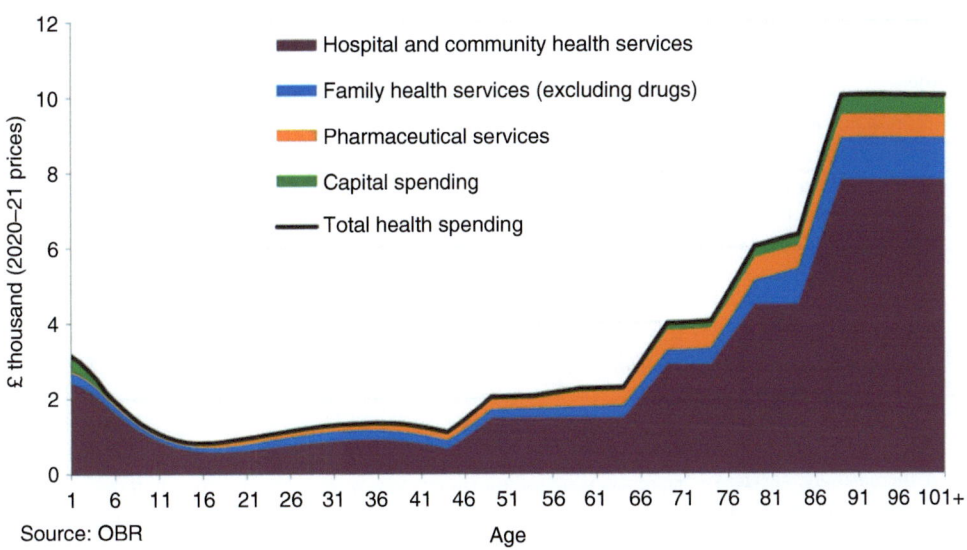

Figure 2.13 Representative profile for health spending with age in the UK. *Source*: Office for Budget Responsibility / Public domain.

multiple long-term conditions in an ageing population. This requires better integration between different parts of the health service and social care.

The Health and Care Act (2022) in England formalised the 42 Integrated Care Systems (ICSs), which have been developing for several years. They are partnerships between NHS organisations, LAs, and others to plan services and improve health based on LA boundaries.

An ICS (population of 0.5 to 3 million) has four aims:

1 Improve outcomes in health.
2 Tackle inequalities in access, experience, and outcomes.
3 Enhance productivity.
4 Support broader social and economic development.

Each ICS has two components:

1 An Integrated Care Board (ICB) to **plan and fund** most NHS services in its **area.**
2 An Integrated Care Partnership (ICP) to **develop an integrated health and care strategy** for its **area**.

The ICB has members from NHS trusts, general practice, and LAs. A member must have mental health expertise, and patients and communities must be involved.

The ICP is a statutory joint committee of the ICB, LAs, voluntary, community, and social enterprise sectors ('VCSE' organisations), and NHS organisations. The strategy should focus on the wider health care, public health, and social care needs of the population, building on the local joint strategic needs assessment. Inputs from local communities and Healthwatch are required.

Several partnerships and delivery structures with decreasing geographical footprints work within an ICS:
Provider collaboratives link across a **system** (population 1–2 million):
NHS trusts (specialist, acute, and mental health), VCSE organisations and the independent sector.
Place-based partnerships link across a **place** (population 250–500,000), often a single LA:
NHS trusts (acute, mental health, and community), VCSE organisations, Healthwatch, and primary care centres.
Health and Wellbeing Boards (HWBs) typically work in a **place**. These are formal local authority committees that bring together health and care partners to produce a Joint Strategic Needs Assessment and Joint Health and Wellbeing Strategy for their local population.
Primary care networks cover a **neighbourhood** (population 30–50,000):
General practice, opticians, dentistry, pharmacy

However, despite the rhetoric, the structure does not make integration easy; social care is still funded by a different ministry and commissioned by the local government. There is a very limited pooled budget – see later discussion.

Total healthcare expenditure in 2022 in the UK is estimated to have been £283 billion (11.3% of GDP), of which £230 billion was government spending (ONS). The DHSC spent £181.7 billion in England in 2022–2023 and has a budget of £190 billion for 2023–2024.

The cost of providing health care for older people increases with age (see Figure 2.13), but rather than age per se, it is proximity to death, particularly the last year of life, that is the stronger driver of healthcare expenditure.

Social services organisation

In England, there are 152 Councils with Adult Social Services Responsibilities or CASSRs. Most are now in groups in the 42 ICSs. It is not clear whether commissioning will be pooled between the CASSRs in an ICS.

Social care is funded through a combination of:

- a grant from the central government (Department for Levelling Up, Housing and Communities, DLUHC),
- local revenue from council tax and
- the social precept - an extra charge added to council tax.

ICBs must transfer a set amount of money to their LAs via the Better Care Fund. Social care funding is not ring-fenced, so councils can decide how much they spend on care. Hence, there is no national budget for adult social care in England! LAs spent £23.7 billion on adult social care in 2022–2023, less than 15% of government spending on health, even when cross-funding via the Better Care Fund is included.

Health care

The structure of the NHS is complex and confusing. At its simplest:

- Primary care is provided by teams in GP practices, opticians, dentists, and pharmacists.
- Secondary care is provided in the main local hospitals.
- Tertiary care is specialist hospital care provided at regional or national centres.
- Community health services are an increasing range of services provided outside the GP surgery or main hospitals and include

prevention, monitoring, chronic disease management, and urgent community response services to provide assessment in various settings, with the aim of keeping people at home.

Some of these provisions overlap with 'intermediate care', time-limited, short-term support to avoid unnecessary hospital or care home admission or to help people return to independence after a hospital stay. Mental health care is traditionally organised separately. Reforms aim to provide better integration between the different components of health and social care.

General practitioners

In the UK, every person should register with a GP. Almost all GPs work in group practices with a multidisciplinary team. The GP was the first point of contact for all NHS services, except the other components of primary care (opticians, dentists, and pharmacists), but increasingly, services can be accessed directly, e.g., self-referral to physiotherapy, minor illness, and injury centres, calling NHS 111 for advice. This increases patient choice but may fragment care. If multiagency care is to succeed, coordination is essential. A good GP needs:

- Wide knowledge of medicine and the skills of other team members and community services.
- Comprehensive records and a good summary of the patient's problems and treatment.
- An approachable manner so that neither older patients nor their carers are deterred from seeking help.
- Ready access to specialist advice and services.

Every consultation can be an opportunity to pick up on other health or social problems and look ahead. This is most likely to happen in a face-to-face consultation. The GP contract ensures that the practice is paid for specific QOF points (Quality and Outcomes Framework). GP practices have well-developed IT systems, and opportunities for paid prevention are flagged on screen for GPs as they consult. Practices must keep a frailty register, and this is done by using an electronic frailty index to find people over 65 who may be frail and then using clinical judgement.

Prevention and risk reduction for diseases in old age

- Seasonal influenza: annual vaccination.
- Pneumococcal pneumonia: a single vaccination at age 65.
- Severe COVID: vaccination has reduced the mortality from COVID – by winter 2024, a typical 65-year-old will have had 6 doses.
- Shingles: 2 Shingrix injections 6 months apart at 70, eventually, 65.
- Respiratory syncytial virus (RSV): a single vaccination for those aged 75–79 years. After a catchup programme, the vaccine will be offered as people turn 75.
- Stroke and possibly multi-infarct dementia: by treatment of high BP and anticoagulation for atrial fibrillation.
- Osteoporosis: by achieving good peak bone mass in adult life, continuing to exercise, vitamin D for all in winter, and bisphosphonates for primary prevention if at high risk.
- Ischaemic heart disease: by the avoidance of tobacco, the promotion of exercise, a 'Mediterranean' diet and prescription of statins.
- Consequences of alcohol: falls, alcoholic dementia, heart failure, pancreatitis, and cirrhosis, by safe drinking.
- Obesity with its effect on osteoarthritis and carbohydrate metabolism: by diet and exercise.
- Progression of prediabetes and Type 2 diabetes by maintaining an ideal body weight, regular walking and GLP-1 agonists.
- Falls, sarcopaenia, and frailty: by exercising for strength and balance.
- Diverticular disease: by increasing dietary fibre.

- Chronic obstructive pulmonary disease (COPD) bronchogenic carcinoma, and to a lesser extent, age-related macular degeneration are risks reduced by avoiding tobacco.
- A healthy lifestyle and social and cognitive activity reduce the likelihood of Alzheimer's disease.
- Dietary deficiency states.
- Iatrogenic disease.

GPs who wish to demonstrate their special expertise with older patients can take the Diploma of Geriatric Medicine examination of the Royal College of Physicians (RCP). They can take on extra responsibilities as a GP with a special interest in older people or care home medicine.

Opticians

NHS eye tests are free at 60 or over every 2 years (yearly if the optician recommends this) and can be conducted at home or in a care home if the person is unable to leave home unaccompanied. A contribution towards the cost of lenses is available for those on Pension Credit.

Dentists

Older people usually must pay NHS dental costs. Many areas of England are 'dental deserts' – it is impossible for adult patients to find an NHS dentist. Dental visits not only improve the health of the teeth and gums but also provide screening for oral cancers.

Pharmacists

Pharmacists dispense medicine and medical appliances, dispose of unwanted medicines, advise patients on self-care, and provide medicines support following hospital discharge. Some pharmacists provide other services, such as flu vaccination; support for patients on new long-term medication, such as for heart failure, COPD, osteoporosis, and Parkinson's disease; disease surveillance, such as BP checks; and private services, such as travel health. Patients can now get treatment for seven common conditions directly from their local pharmacy, without the need for a GP appointment or prescription. The conditions most relevant to older people are sinusitis, a sore throat, and shingles. Pharmacists are increasingly working in GP practices.

Community nursing staff

An increasing range of nurses work in the community. They are employed by GP practices, community trusts, or VCSEs. Examples include district nurses, disease- or system-specific specialist nurses, e.g. for heart failure, COPD/asthma, Parkinson's disease, continence, lymphoedema, stoma specialists, palliative care symptom control (Macmillan), and hands-on help (Marie Curie). Admiral nurses support the carers of people with dementia.

Many community nurses have prescribing rights, and much of their caseload is with older patients. They provide:

- Treatment, e.g. injections, dressings, enemas, syringe drivers for end-of-life.
- Monitoring, e.g. for heart failure and diabetes.
- Specialist care, e.g. stoma management and continence assessment.
- Liaison with other services.
- Hands-on nursing, mainly supervising health care assistants.
- Support for carers.

Community psychiatric nurses (CPNs) are registered mental health nurses based in the community mental health teams of the Old Age

Psychiatry service. They mainly work with patients with depression and dementia to:

- Support the patient and carers.
- Monitor progress.
- Liaise with other services.

Hospital care of older patients

This can take the following forms:

- Ambulatory care, i.e. emergency department attendance, outpatient clinics, and day assessments.
- Acute inpatient care.
- Intermediate care/rehabilitation.

Emergency department

Because of their liability to accidents and the effects of acute illness, older people are frequent users of the emergency department (ED). Their management in this setting may be suboptimal for several reasons:

- They may struggle to give an account of themselves owing to impaired consciousness, confusion or dementia, communication difficulties (speech or hearing impairment), anxiety, or fear.
- Their problems are frequently multiple and complex.
- They are often unaccompanied.
- Their accident or illness may be a consequence of long-term neglect or a lack of support.
- They may already have experienced considerable delays getting to the hospital and are more likely than most patients to require transport back home.

An overnight stay may allow time for an older person to regain their equilibrium and be assessed and discharged the next day with increased support, but the risk is that an overnight assessment will turn into a long admission. A rapid assessment by a senior geriatrician should be available at all hours, but in isolation, this achieves little; management requires diagnostic services, multidisciplinary assessment, and rapid access to social support to enable discharge.

Outpatient department

Appropriate patients have a right to be referred to any specialist clinic, regardless of age.

- Frail older patients are more likely to need help with transport to and within, the hospital.
- All clinics should be user-friendly, e.g. with appropriate seating (chairs with arms enable older people to get up independently), effective arrangements for deaf or partially sighted patients and wheelchair users in the waiting area, a working communicator in the clinic room, and variable height couches. Help with undressing and dressing is likely to be needed.
- Complex patients with multiple pathologies are best managed in specialist geriatric clinics, supported where necessary by organ-specific specialists.
- Routine follow-up should be avoided, but a good system is needed to track and send results, etc.

Day assessment

The day hospital was a part of a traditional service for older people. Transport was always problematic and most closed as it overlapped with 'social daycare'. However, many departments have opened day assessment units that offer diagnosis, investigation, procedures, e.g. blood transfusion, and multidisciplinary assessment.

Hospital inpatients

The number of hospital beds has been falling since the 1970s.

- Bed numbers in England have halved since 1990.
- Bed mix has changed with the closure of long stay beds and the creation of day-case beds.
- The rate of bed closure slowed after 2015 until the pandemic caused a rapid further reduction (infection control).
- Emergency admissions have continued to rise, especially in the 85+ group (more complex).
- The hospital system coped at first (just) by reducing the length of stay (increased pressure on GPs).
- Bed occupancy then started rising.
- Elective care is postponed.
- The number of delayed discharges has continued to increase despite huge efforts (a complex combination of low social care funding and hospital inefficiency due to high occupancy).

In January 2023, 14% of around 100,000 acute beds and around 50% of community beds were occupied by patients who were medically fit to leave; for all acute trusts, bed occupancy was 95%. More than 20,000 patients a year are 'warehoused' in community beds and care homes after hospital discharge without rehabilitation support (HSJ, 2024). A focus on care for older people is essential to resolving the health and social care crisis (Gordon, BMJ).

Most admissions (86%) are considered appropriate, but admissions may be avoidable for up to 20% of older patients and up to 40% of admissions from care homes. Rates of 'inappropriate' admission are very variable and depend on the quality of local general practice and the availability of alternative care. Older people have higher admission rates than younger people because of:

- More pathology, both acute and chronic.
- Living alone and social disadvantage.
- Polypharmacy.
- High accident/fall rates.
- Lower resilience to minor illnesses due to poor homeostasis.

Intensive case management of older patients with chronic disease in the community is designed to reduce admissions (e.g. by treating deteriorating cardiac failure before admission is necessary), and if admission is needed, faster discharge should be expedited by better, more flexible care in the community. The use of virtual wards is increasing – monitored care at home to prevent admission or speed up discharge – but this is always hardest to use in frail older patients. Admissions from care homes may be reduced if medical support and care planning are improved.

The acute hospital is a dangerous place for frail older people.

- Deconditioning occurs rapidly.
- Dependency may be encouraged by poor staff attitudes and practices (understaffing).
- Delirium is common.
- The nutrition of malnourished patients may deteriorate further due to poor catering and feeding.
- Sleep deprivation delays recovery.
- Nosocomial infections are more dangerous in old age. Rates of MRSA and *C. difficile* have fallen, but Gram-negative infections have been increasing (catheter-associated urine infections are a reason to avoid catheterization unless essential). Outbreaks of influenza and norovirus can be dangerous and debilitating for frail older patients, but since 2020, hospital-acquired COVID has been the most serious.
- Falls are common because of the impaired physical and cognitive function of the patient, hospital design, and inadequate supervision. The situation is often made worse by the inappropriate use of various

forms of restraint (both physical and pharmacological). In England, 3% of hip fractures are the result of an inpatient fall.

- Pressure ulcers may develop (2.5% of hip fracture patients).
- Older patients are not always given proper priority for investigations, and delays are detrimental. Sophisticated techniques may be needed, as older patients are less able to cope with demanding and invasive investigations than younger patients.
- Surgery is more dangerous, especially if it is delegated to junior surgeons and anaesthetists.
- Lack of attention to pre- and post-operative medical conditions compromises the success of essential surgery. Many hospitals involve geriatricians in perioperative assessment, and orthogeriatrics is a well-established subspecialty. See Chapter 10.
- Post-operative complications are more common and more serious.
- Bonds with preexisting carers may be broken.
- Lack of community services and/or accommodation may delay discharge, extending exposure to all these risks.

Medicine for older people

Frail older patients with multiple and complex problems are best managed in a specialist service for older people. A typical department has:

- acute beds in the hospital with the ED (the evidence base for Comprehensive Geriatric Assessment is strongest for speciality ward-based care),
- facilities for acute assessment,
- beds in community hospitals or intermediate care for rehabilitation,
- outpatient clinics,
- outreach provision to the community.

Inpatients should have rapid access to other specialist services, e.g. cardiology, and geriatricians offer a range of advice and support to older people under other hospital teams.

Geriatric medicine is the second-largest medical speciality. In addition to general geriatrics, most geriatricians take part in the general medical take and make up a major group of examiners for Membership of the Royal College of Physicians (MRCP).

Many geriatricians also have specialist roles, e.g. in orthogeriatrics, working with movement disorders, in the assessment and management of delirium and dementia, falls and syncope services, promotion of continence, rapid assessment of older people attending as emergencies, and providing pre-operative assessment for major gastrointestinal and vascular surgery. Stroke medicine is now a separate speciality, though many stroke physicians primarily train in geriatric medicine.

A third of geriatricians undertake some work in the community, but some specialise in community geriatrics, attached to the local acute service with outreach or based in a community trust, often in a community hospital. As well as working with inpatients and outpatients in community hospitals, many provide in-reach to care homes and work with GPs to assess patients in their own homes – domiciliary visits. See the BGS website for details of all the special interest groups.

There are not enough geriatricians. The scope of the speciality (as well as the number of very old people) is constantly expanding, with demand for geriatricians with expertise in cardiology and oncology limited only by the workforce. See the RCP report.

Academic geriatric medicine

Most medical schools have an academic department of geriatric medicine, but 90% of consultant geriatricians are employed by the NHS, and only 7% have academic posts (13% for physicians overall), so most teaching and training is carried out by NHS consultants. If the clinical workload is too onerous, this impacts educational provision, which may deter students from considering the speciality for their careers.

Older people, particularly those with multi-morbidity, frailty, and dementia, and those living in care homes, are underrepresented in clinical research and drug trials. This makes it hard to practice evidence-based medicine for an increasingly large group of people.

- The BGS website has a compilation of publications (2019) about research methodologies applicable to older people. It includes describing the participants in a study, cohort studies, recruiting for, running, and reporting clinical trials, test accuracy, statistics, qualitative studies, and systematic reviews.
- Everyone needs to be able to appraise research literature, and there is a useful paper on this.
- When deciding whether a research paper on 'older people' is relevant to your patients, look first at the mean or median age of the study population. An age range can be deceptive – the 'subjects aged between 60 and 85' may have a median age of 63!

There are practical challenges to including older people in research, and most geriatricians have a heavy clinical workload, but there are many questions that need addressing. Patient and public involvement (PPI) in study design helps to ensure that studies and outcome measures are relevant, more likely to be acceptable to participants, and improve patient information. Research opportunities include epidemiological studies (there are several large longitudinal studies of ageing) or laboratory-based work on the mechanisms of ageing (see Chapter 3).

The BGS offers grants and prizes for students and trainees, including funding to attend national meetings.

Mental health services for older people

Departments of old age psychiatry may be based in secondary care, often in a separate mental health facility, but do much of their work in the community. Traditionally, psychiatry has used an age cut-off; a patient with a psychiatric problem reaching a specific age – depending on the service, 65 to 75 years – 'graduates' from the adult service to the old age service, and new patients above that age go straight to old age psychiatry (see Chapter 8). The multidisciplinary team includes specialist nurses, therapists, psychologists, social workers, and case managers, in addition to the psychiatrist. In an acute hospital, there is often an Old Age Psychiatry Liaison Team. Patients are referred for advice but remain under the care of their medical team.

Intermediate care

Intermediate care comprises a range of therapeutic services that sit between primary and secondary care and overlap with community care. Services include:

- Prevention, e.g. fall clinics.
- Admissions avoidance by providing therapeutic intervention at home when needed, e.g. in a minor illness.
- Enabling earlier discharge by providing rehabilitation services in a community hospital or at home.
- Condition-specific programmes such as early discharge for stroke and hip fracture.
- Reablement is commonly provided after hospital discharge for a couple of weeks, with a maximum of 6 weeks. Whereas rehabilitation is therapy-led, reablement is usually provided by social care staff but also has specific goals, e.g. to get back confidence in preparing a meal and managing the stairs. Unlike other social care, it is not means-tested – there may be charges for ongoing care if it is needed after reablement.
- Direct admission to a community hospital, known as 'step-up care.'
- 'Step down care' from acute care; less intense, more user-friendly, less clinical, more domestic provision of inpatient services.
- End-of-life care when the community or family are unable to cope.

Community hospitals

There is a wide range of provision, both in terms of the number of beds, the facilities, and the medical and therapy input. Often, day-to-day care is provided by a local GP practice, with a consultant visiting twice a week. Community hospitals can be a fantastic resource, providing holistic, appropriate care and excellent nursing and therapy. However, they should not be used to deny older people access to the diagnostic facilities of the local acute hospital. 'Step-up care' has clinical risks unless there is a clear diagnosis.

Social care for older people

Most older people want to continue living at home. This aspiration is supported by the government, but good community services are not cheap. There is a significant unmet need for social care. Unmet need put pressure on unpaid carers. There is no UK-wide data set for domiciliary care. An overall picture is hard to obtain as many people arrange care from the private and voluntary sectors and pay for it themselves.

Support from social services

Since 2015, there has been a rise in requests for social support, 4 in 5 of which originate in the community. There was a dip during COVID, probably because people did not want carers coming into their homes, but demand is rising again. In November 2022, the Association of Directors of Adult Social Services estimated that there was a backlog of over 245,000 people waiting for assessments, a third for 6 months or longer.

The outcome of requests for support from social services is shown in Figure 2.14.

Of around 1.4 million requests (from a population of 10.5 million):

- A quarter received no service.
- A quarter were signposted to other services.
- Around 15% got reablement.
- 15% had ongoing low-level support.
- A small number had more intensive support.

There is wide variation in the hourly rate paid for home care by councils. In many areas, agencies that provide care struggle to recruit and retain carers. Three-quarters of councils reported that providers had closed, ceased trading, or handed back council contracts. Lack of home care is a major reason for delayed discharges.

Care at home

Over 95% of the older population live independently, but about 10% need domiciliary services to cope at home. Over the last decade, fewer clients have received home care as resources are focused on those most in need. More hours of home care are being delivered, but this is outstripped by the increasing demand. The trend is for short-term support to increase, but long-term support to fall. In 2019, Age UK estimated that 1.5 million older people, one in seven of the older population, had some unmet need for care. Not surprisingly, the percentage of people receiving care (formal, informal, or a combination) rises steeply around 75 years (see Figure 2.15).

Regular visits for care

Care may be organised privately, through the voluntary sector, or through social services.

- All agencies must carry out Disclosure and Barring Service (DBS) checks on staff, as the clients are vulnerable.
- Domestic tasks, e.g. shopping, cleaning, and laundry, must be paid for privately, so good-value 'home help' services, such as those run by AgeUK, are much in demand.
- In England and Wales, personal care is means-tested but it is free in Scotland.
- Care funded by social services involves assessment by a care manager, and a care package is drawn up. The care is commissioned, usually from the private sector through agencies.
- Private care is limited by the financial means of the individual and the local availability of suitable carers.
- However care is funded (see later discussion), it is provided by generic care assistants who will perform a range of tasks, e.g. a morning visit (30 min) to get the client up, toileted, washed, dressed, and breakfasted, a lunchtime visit (15 min) to heat the pre-delivered frozen meal, and an evening visit (20 min) to get the client back to bed. Carers may arrive at variable times and many clients find the evening call too early.
- Once the client can no longer use the toilet independently between visits or make themselves a hot drink, the situation becomes precarious, but many such individuals prefer to remain at home.

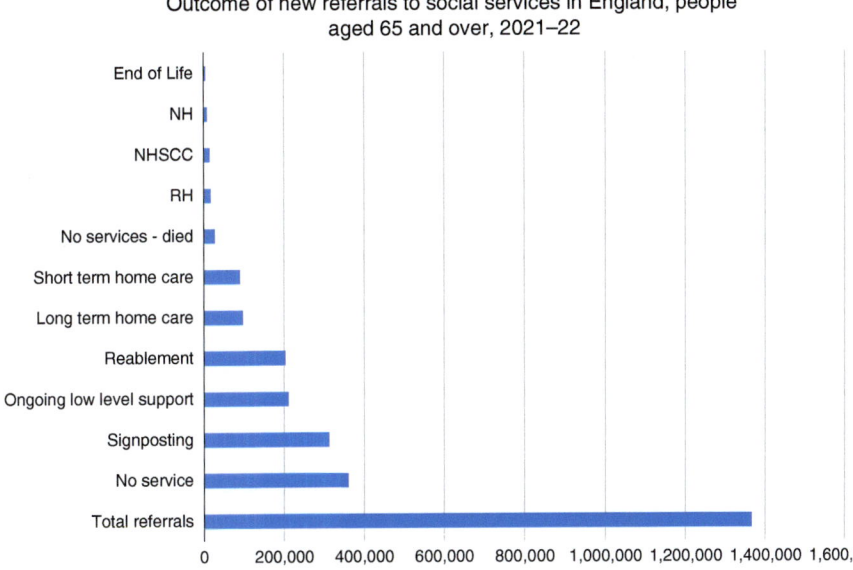

Outcome of new referrals to social services in England, people aged 65 and over, 2021–22

Figure 2.14 Requests for support from new clients aged 65 and over by what happened next. England, 2021–2022. *Source*: Adult Social Care Activity and Finance Report, England, 2021–22.

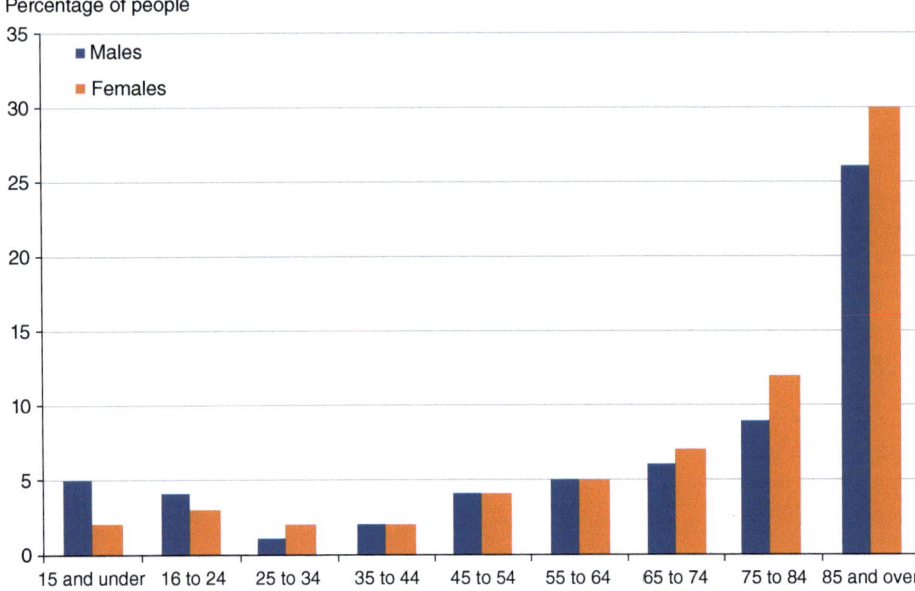

Percentage of people

Figure 2.15 Percentage of people receiving care by age and gender. *Source*: Family Resources Survey 2022 / Crown Copyright / CC BY 3.0.

- If the client cannot transfer with the help of one person, 'double-up' care may be needed (two carers), and such patients will usually be padded up (incontinence) and sit in their chairs until the next visit (risk of pressure sores). A hoist may be used to get the client from bed to chair.

Medicines support

People may be enabled to take their own medicines, e.g. with a blister pack or dosette box. Alternatively, carers may give medicines and will need a MAR chart (Medicine Administration Record).

Meals services

Historically, local authorities provided clients with a midday hot meal at home. Some clients loved them; others threw them away or were too muddled to eat them. Many areas moved to delivering frozen-ready meals. The client needs a freezer, microwave, and reasonable cognitive function to learn what may be a new method of heating food. However, hot meal services are reappearing, with the benefit of the daily human contact that this entails.

Specialist equipment

A range of traditional equipment can be provided, e.g. a pressure-relieving mattress, toilet frame, bath board, grab rails, bed rails, leg lifters, handling belts, a commode, and even a hospital bed, hoist, and wheelchair. Lifeline pendants or wrist alarms enable the wearer to summon help. More expensive equipment, such as stairlifts, can be fitted and modifications made to the house (see Figure 2.6), e.g. doorways widened for wheelchairs and the installation of a level access shower. There are often delays and wrangling over who pays.

Telecare

This is the use of electronic technology to monitor and help people to maintain independence in their own environment. A telecare service can monitor three components:

1 Safety and security,
2 Physiological parameters, and
3 Activity.

Devices include video-monitoring, falls detectors, sensors to monitor activity (a pressure mat activated as the person gets out of bed can turn on the light, detectors monitoring the fridge and front door can be used to check feeding and wandering, etc.), wet bed alerts can summon a night carer, automatic taps prevent floods, etc. Everyone should have smoke and carbon monoxide alarms.

Roving warden schemes

These are area-based and support a number of older people living in their original accommodation.

Twenty-four-hour care

This is expensive, costing from £800 to £1800 a week. At least two carers are needed to cover shifts and holidays. Individuals may pay for this privately, in addition to the expense of running the house, or it is very occasionally paid for by NHS CHC (see later).

Other community services

Luncheon clubs

These are centres where meals are provided, usually at subsidised prices, run by either the local authority or voluntary organisations. Luncheon clubs usually run just once or twice weekly but also offer companionship. Transport is often a limiting factor.

Day centres

These are very varied and may be run by the local authority, but more often now by voluntary groups. A charge for attendance is usual, and transport may be provided. About 5% of elderly people attend day centres.

The day centre aims to

- Combat loneliness.
- Provide diversional activity and recreation.
- Provide a meal and other comforts.
- Relieve carers.
- Disseminate health education, e.g. about falls risk.
- Encourage activity, e.g. regular exercise and balance groups.
- Introduce clients to other forms of care.

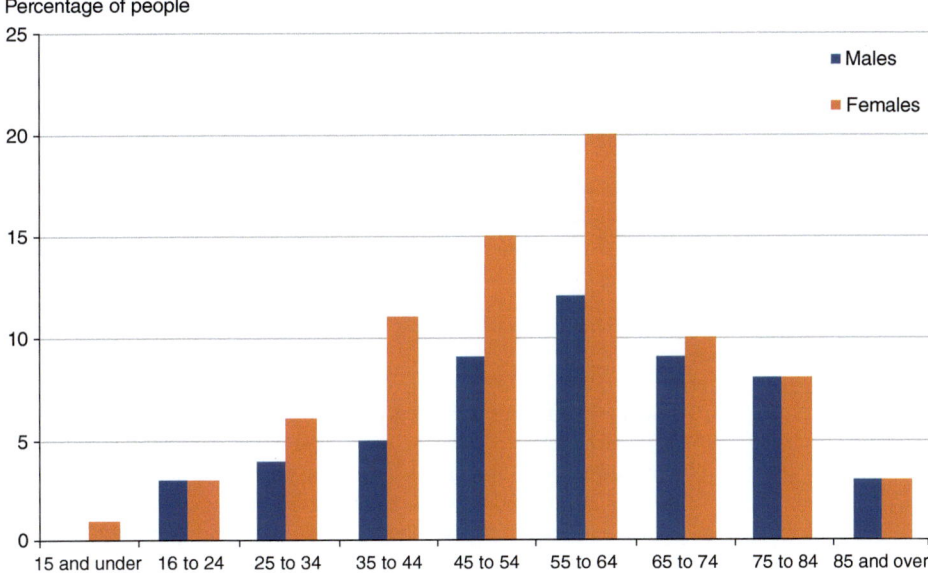

Figure 2.16 People providing informal care by age and gender. *Source*: Family Resources Survey 2022 / Crown Copyright / CC BY 3.0.

Respite care

This is the provision of a temporary bed, usually in a care home, for frail people with chronic irremediable diseases to give their informal carers a break. The service is organised by the LA and is means-tested. It may smooth the path to eventual permanent placement, e.g., for a person with dementia. However, respite care often has an adverse effect on the recipient – especially if they are unable to understand why it is needed. Respite care should not be confused with crisis intervention, i.e. when a supporting system collapses, nor is it top-up rehabilitation. Because of pressure to avoid hospital admission if a frail person suddenly deteriorates in a non-specific way (see Chapter 4), they may be put in a respite bed only to be admitted to the hospital several days later with a delayed diagnosis of severe pneumonia.

Regulation of health and social care

The CQC regulates all health and social care services in England. The regulatory bodies for the devolved nations are the Care Inspectorate (Scotland), the Health Inspectorate (Wales), and the Regulatory and Quality Improvement Authority (Northern Ireland).

Healthwatch England

This is a statutory body whose purpose is to understand the needs and experiences of people who use health and social care services and to speak out on their behalf. Local groups collaborate to share information, expertise, and learning to improve services. It reports to the CQC.

Informal carers

In the UK, informal carers, usually family and sometimes friends, provide most of the care for people at home. They are the key members of the care workforce. They are unpaid, untrained, usually devoted, and effective, but increasingly stressed with the decline in council services. In the UK, the total dependency ratio has been 50–60% since 1950; the fall in the number of children has balanced the rise in older people.

However, by 2030, the ratio will rise steadily, driven by the increase in older people. The range of options and support is much greater for children than for older people.

- Estimates of the number of carers vary widely (up to 13.6 million was quoted in Parliament in 2021). Carers often do not identify themselves in this role, and people move in and out of providing care.
- The 2021 census gave figures of 4.7 million carers in England (9% population); 310,000 in Wales (10.5%); 222,200 in North Ireland; and an estimated 700,000 in Scotland.
- Data from the annual Family Resources Survey (UK 2021–2022) gives a figure of 4.9 million, 7% of the *adult* population. There was no documented spike in the number of informal carers during the COVID pandemic, as described anecdotally, but if those already caring increased their support, this would not be apparent. From this survey:
  - Around 60% of carers are women (see Figure 2.16).
  - More women are carers than men up to age 74; above this, numbers are similar.
  - The modal age for caring is 55–64 when 20% of women and 12% of men provide care.
  - Most carers care for a parent.
  - Most carers provide 5–19 hr of care a week, but 16% provide more than 50 hr a week.
  - Around 25% of carers are retired.
  - 16% of carers are 'sandwich carers', caring for children and older relatives.
- Carers have the right to a LA assessment. If their needs arise from caring, their health is deteriorating, and their wellbeing is affected, there is a duty to meet those needs, but this is not achieved.
- In 2021–2022, only 380,700 carers were either supported or assessed by LAs, of whom 8.5% were aged 85+. Of these, 313,600 received 'direct support', but in over two-thirds of these, this was information and signposting. 18% got nothing. 8.7% received support for the cared-for person.
- Being a carer, particularly for many hours a week, affects:
  - **Physical health:** 28% report this is bad or very bad.
  - **Mental health:** 44% report this as bad or very bad.
  - **Access to the NHS**, e.g. difficulty getting to the dentist or optician.
  - **Feeling valued:** >90% felt ignored by the government. Of carers known to social services, >20% feel they have no encouragement or support.

- ○ **Social integration**: 90% are often/always lonely, and 50% have given up hobbies.
- ○ **Poverty**: 24% of carers live in relative poverty.

Estimates of the amount saved by informal care vary widely. The ONS estimate in 2014 was £57 billion, whilst Carers UK/University of Sheffield 2015 calculated more than twice this figure at £132 billion. Whatever the 'real' figure, compared with contemporaneous social services spending of £17 billion, the contribution is huge.

Needs of carers

Recognition

- By family and friends.
- By professionals.
- By the state.

Support

- Financial.
- Social.
- Psychological.
- Professional.
- Self-help groups.

Respite

- Short periods (e.g. day care).
- Extended periods: intermittent admission to care.
- Sitting services (e.g. Crossroads).
- Immediate in emergencies.

Information

- About the patient's illness.
- About available services.

Paying for care

If an older person has enough assets, they can arrange care at home or enter a home of their choice if they meet its admission criteria. In England and Wales, if a person may need care, the LA must carry out an assessment to decide whether they have 'eligible' needs for home care or meet criteria for care home admission, personal care, or nursing care. Then a financial assessment is done to determine whether the person will be a self-funder or get partial or full funding from the LA. The rules are complex. Recommend that patients/their families look at independent information, e.g. from AgeUK.

Paying for care at home

Eligibility for funding depends on income and capital, not including the person's home. In England, it is estimated that self-funders make up 30% of those using domiciliary care. (Nuffield Trust 2020). Care at home is expensive; at £25–30 per hr, 3-hr of daily home care costs around £30,000 per year.

Paying for a care home

The amount an individual must contribute to the cost of a care home ranges from losing their allowances to paying the full amount. The threshold for full self-funding in 2024 is >£23,250 (including income, assets, and savings). This is unchanged since 2010 and includes their house. Anyone with assets between £14,250 and £23,250 may be able to access some funding. Residents must be left with a personal expenses allowance of £28.25 per week.

According to LaingBuisson (2024) in England

- 46% of care home residents are completely self-funding.
- 11% pay a top-up.
- 35% are state-funded.
- 8% are NHS-funded (see later discussion).

Owner-occupiers must often sell their house to finance care unless a spouse or dependent relative continues to live in it; there is a '12-week disregard' that gives a brief window when the council must ignore the value of a house to allow the property to be sold. It may be possible to defer the sale of the house.

Local authority benchmarks

In each area, the commissioners (social services in discussion with their ICB) have benchmark prices for residential and nursing beds and a list of 'approved homes'. They may block purchase a number of beds in a home. Approval is intended to improve standards but reduces choice, as does block-purchasing. A social services client may need to pay a top-up if there is a gap between the cost of the home they choose and the benchmark.

Funding is constrained, and low benchmarks are set. Hard-to-place individuals with complex needs are managed by a broker. In 2023, English councils paid, on average, £828 for residential care and £1,146 for nursing care per week (LaingBuisson). There is wide geographic variation and a supplement for dementia.

Most LAs are coy about their benchmarks, but some are in the public domain, e.g. Hertfordshire 2023/2024, 'Long stay at a care home – what we pay per week'.

- Residential Care: £703.60
- Residential Care with Dementia and/or Mental Ill Health: £814.66
- Nursing Care (excludes FNC): £784.24
- Nursing Care with dementia and/or Mental Ill Health: £925

Costs for self-funders

Most people will not need a care home, but if they do and must fund it, the costs are huge.

- Fees paid by 'self-funders' are estimated to be up to 40% more than the LA pays for a place in the same home, so self-funders pay for themselves and subsidise council-funded residents.
- In 2023, average UK residential fees for self-funders were £1,136 per week, or £60,000 a year, and for nursing care, £1,409 per week, or £73,300 a year.

In 2021, the government announced reforms to the social care budget and a planned £86,000 cap on care costs from 2023, but this has been deferred.

In Scotland, in 2024, self-funders aged 65+ in care homes get £248.70 a week for personal care (they lose Attendance Allowance) and a further payment of £111.90 if they require nursing care; self-funders still pay for board and lodging.

The NHS's contributions to long-term care

Governments struggle with the NHS being 'free at the point of delivery', whilst care provided by social services is means-tested in England (free in Scotland). Forty years ago, many frail older people spent their last months in a geriatric long-stay hospital. This care had limitations but was free to the patient. Long-stay hospitals were closed to save money; patients were placed in nursing homes, transferring an increasing proportion of the costs to individuals. Two NHS funding streams still exist: the first for everyone who needs nursing care, and the second for an extremely limited number of people.

1. NHS-funded nursing care

In a nursing home, the 'board and lodging' and 'personal care' components are means-tested, but the state contributes to the cost of nursing care for everyone. This is known as NHS-funded nursing care (NHS FNC). The rate in 2024 is £235.88 a week. An assessment for this must be done by an NHS nurse prior to placement.

2. NHS continuing healthcare

Individuals are assessed against criteria to decide whether they are entitled to free care for the rest of their lives. To qualify, an individual must have a 'primary health need', and the nature, complexity, and unpredictability of their conditions are considered. A patient granted NHS continuing healthcare (NHS CHC) is usually bed-bound with multiple problems needing regular skilled nursing, e.g., for pressure sores or tube feeding, unpredictable medical needs, and a very short prognosis.

The assessment is in two stages:

i   Initial checklist. If this is positive,
ii A full assessment is done. This looks at 12 domains (behaviour, cognition, psychological needs, communication, mobility, nutrition, continence, skin integrity, breathing, medication, symptom control, altered consciousness, and special factors).

Geographical variation persists. The right of appeal is often used because of the cost of self-funding (see earlier discussion), particularly if the person needing to fund their care will have to sell their house rather than leaving it to their family. If a patient is granted NHS CHC, the care can be provided at home or in a nursing home. In 2022, around 30,000 people were funded to live in nursing homes.

A patient who is dying in hospital and wants to die at home may be 'fast-tracked' home or to a nursing home with NHS CHC, regardless of means. NHS Digital data shows that on average, 52,000 people were considered eligible for NHS CHC at any one point in 2023/2024, around 18,000 of whom were on fast track.

Financial allowances and benefits (rates in 2024–2025 in England)

Pensions are complicated and always changing. Know the basics, look on the AgeUK website for details, and always suggest that patients get advice from Citizens Advice. Some benefits differ between England, Scotland, Wales, and Northern Ireland. The most important benefit for you to know about is the Attendance Allowance (AA); suggest that people put in a claim it if it may be applicable.

State Pension

The new State Pension was introduced in 2016 to replace the basic State Pension. Those already getting the basic Pension continue to get that. New claimants get the new State Pension, which is paid to women and men at age 66. Since 2011, there is no longer a compulsory retirement age in the UK, so people can choose to defer their pension, although some jobs have an age limit set by law, e.g. the fire service. People need at least 10 qualifying years on their National Insurance (NI) record. The full pension is £221.20 a week. The SPA is currently set to rise to 67 between 2026 and 2028 and then to 68 between 2044 and 2046.

Pension Credit

Pension Credit gives people extra money if they are over SPA and on a low income, topping their income up to £218.15 if they are single and £332.95 for a couple. The rules are complicated – a Carer's Allowance counts as income, but AA does not. It is estimated that a million pensioner households are not claiming the Pension Credit they are entitled to. Even if the amount paid is small, it is a gateway to other support, e.g. reduced council tax and a Winter Fuel Payment.

Over 80 pension

This is paid to people of 80 or over with little or no State Pension, making this up to £101.55 a week.

Council tax reductions and exemptions

Council tax helps pay for local services like policing and refuse collection. Reductions for a single-person household or low-income households depend on the local council's policy. People with severe dementia who are getting AA are exempt; if they live with one other person, a 25% discount can be claimed.

Housing benefit

This is a means-tested benefit to help with paying rent. Help with paying for a mortgage may be available as part of Pension Credit.

Attendance Allowance

This is a non-means-tested benefit paid to a person who needs help with personal care at 65+; there is a qualifying period of 6 months, unless there is a prognosis of <6 months when the payment can be made at once, even if the claimant does not currently need help. The higher rate (day and night) is £108.55 a week, and the lower rate is £72.65 (day or night).

Carer's Allowance

The Carer's Allowance (£81.90 a week) is paid to a carer who earns less than £151 a week (after deductions) and provides more than 35-hr of care a week to a person in receipt of a qualifying benefit, e.g. AA. NI contributions are paid to protect the pension rights of working-age carers. Carers receiving State Pensions should apply for Carer's Allowance but cannot receive the full amount of both as they are classified as 'overlapping benefits'. Any extra money is paid as a Carer Addition to Pension Credit. In 2021, 1.3 million people claimed Carer's Allowance in Great Britain, but only 70% (around 900,000) got a payment because of the 'overlapping benefits rule' or other income. Among pensioners claiming, 90% get no payment!

Prescription charges, sight tests, and dental care

If you are 60+, you are entitled to free prescriptions and sight tests. You get free sight tests at 40 if there is glaucoma in the family. Free dentistry is available if you receive Pension Credit (and can find an NHS dentist).

Blue badge

This helps a person with a range of disabilities, or someone who drives them, to park more conveniently and cheaply. They are greatly sought after and only issued by local councils; beware of scams.

Blind Person's Allowance

A person who is registered blind or severely visually impaired can claim this regardless of age or income. It is added to a person's tax-free Personal

Allowance and is £3070. It can be transferred to a spouse if the person does not pay tax.

Keeping warm

- Winter Fuel Payment is an annual benefit for people above the SPA; £250–600 depending on circumstances. It was non-means tested but from winter 2024 is restricted to those on Pension Credit.
- The Warm Homes Discount Scheme, run by most energy suppliers, is an automatic annual payment of £150 towards the electricity bills of people on Pension Credit.
- Cold weather payments, £25 a week for each 7-day period of very cold weather between 1 November and 31 March, are paid to those on Pension Credit.

The war in Ukraine led to a dramatic rise in energy costs in 2022. The UK government introduced additional payments to mitigate the effects, but long-term plans are needed. Energy use must be reduced because of climate change, but the rise in costs must be managed.

Concessions

Older people get concessions for bus and rail travel and entry to places of entertainment, but there are local variations in age qualifications and generosity. At SPA, people in England can apply for a free national bus pass. In London, free off-peak travel is available for residents with a 60+ Oyster photocard (£20), and there is no charge for the Freedom Pass at 66 years. A free television licence is available to people over 75 on Pension Credit, and reductions are available for blind people, those in care homes, and sheltered housing.

Christmas bonus

An annual £10 is added to the State Pension.

Hardship funds

These are organised locally; what is available, and the name varies, e.g., 'Household Support Fund' or 'Local Assistance Scheme'. Means-tested discretionary loans, grants, or vouchers may be available for clothing, home repairs, redecoration, bedding, furniture, etc. An increasing number of people of all ages rely on food banks; pet food may be available too.

Funeral Expense Payment

This is available to the person arranging the funeral if they are on Pension Credit or other qualifying benefits. It covers fees and costs of up to £1,000 but will not usually cover all the costs.

REFERENCES AND FURTHER READING

ONS *National population projections* (2020). www.ons.gov.uk/peoplepopulationandcommunity/populationandmigration/populationprojections/bulletins/nationalpopulationprojections/2020basedinterim#uk-population

ONS *Census data* (2021). www.ons.gov.uk/census

Our World in Data *Life expectancy increased at all ages.* https://ourworldindata.org/its-not-just-about-child-mortality-life-expectancy-improved-at-all-ages

London Datastore *London's diverse population* (2019). https://data.london.gov.uk/dataset/london-s-diverse-population-

The Migration Observatory. Cangiano A. *The impact of migration on UK population growth* (2023). https://migrationobservatory.ox.ac.uk/resources/briefings/the-impact-of-migration-on-uk-population-growth

ONS *Profile of the older population living in England and Wales in 2021 and changes since 2011* (2023). www.ons.gov.uk/peoplepopulationandcommunity/birthsdeathsandmarriages/ageing/articles/profileoftheolderpopulationlivinginenglandandwalesin2021andchangessince2011/2023-04-03

The King's Fund *What is happening to life expectancy in England?* (2022). www.kingsfund.org.uk/publications/whats-happening-life-expectancy-england

ONS *Health state life expectancies by national deprivation deciles, England: 2018 to 2020* (2022). www.ons.gov.uk/peoplepopulationandcommunity/healthandsocialcare/healthinequalities/bulletins/healthstatelifeexpectanciesbyindexofmultipledeprivationimd/2018to2020

ONS *Health state life expectancy at birth and at age 65 years by local areas, UK* (2019). www.ons.gov.uk/peoplepopulationandcommunity/healthandsocialcare/healthandlifeexpectancies/datasets/healthstatelifeexpectancyatbirthandatage65bylocalareasuk

Department for Work and Pensions (DWP) *Family Resources Survey 2021–22 Disability data tables* (2023). https://www.gov.uk/government/statistics/family-resources-survey-financial-year-2021-to-2022

RNIB *Key statistics about sight loss* (2021). https://media.rnib.org.uk/documents/Key_stats_about_sight_loss_2021.pdf

Ministry of Housing, Communities and Local Government *English Housing Survey Home adaptations report* 2019–20 (2021). https://assets.publishing.service.gov.uk/government/uploads/system/uploads/attachment_data/file/1000070/EHS_19-20_Home_adaptations.pdf

DWP Households below average income statistics (2024). https://www.gov.uk/government/statistics/households-below-average-income-for-financial-years-ending-1995-to-2020

DWP *Pensioners' Incomes Series: financial year 2020 to 2021* (2022). https://www.gov.uk/government/statistics/pensioners-incomes-series-financial-year-2020-to-2021

Stott, AJ (2021) The longevity society. *Lancet Healthy Longevity* 2: e828–e835, doi: https://doi.org/10.1016/S2666-7568(21)00247-6.

The Ferret *Is the UK state pension the worst in the developed world?* (2022). https://theferret.scot/claim-uk-pension-worst-developed-world-half-true

DWP Family Resources Survey 2021-22 Care data tables (2023). https://www.gov.uk/government/statistics/family-resources-survey-financial-year-2021-to-2022

Department for Levelling Up, Housing and Communities *English Housing Survey. Older People's Housing 2020–21* (2022). https://assets.publishing.service.gov.uk/government/uploads/system/uploads/attachment_data/file/1088802/EHS_Older_people_s_housing_2020-21.pdf

Carehome.co.uk *Care home stats: number of settings, population & workforce* (2022). www.carehome.co.uk

LaingBuisson *Care homes for older people UK market report 34th edition* (2024) - limited data from their website. https://www.laingbuisson.com/shop/care-homes-for-older-people-uk-market-report-34ed

Hertfordshire social services. www.hertfordshire.gov.uk/services/adult-social-services/care-and-carers/arranging-and-paying-for-care/paying-for-your-care-costs.aspx

NHS Continuing Healthcare and NHS-funded Nursing Care Report Q3 2023/24 Report, England. https://www.england.nhs.uk/statistics/wp-content/uploads/sites/2/2024/02/CHC-and-FNC-Report-Q3-2023-24_YE14w.pdf

Nuffield Trust *Care home bed availability* (2023). www.nuffieldtrust.org.uk/resource/care-home-bed-availability

ONS *Life expectancy in care homes, England and Wales 2021–2022* (2023). www.ons.gov.uk/peoplepopulationandcommunity/birthsdeathsandmarriages/lifeexpectancies/articles/lifeexpectancyincarehomesenglandandwales/2021to2022#toc

The King's Fund *Integrated care systems explained: making sense of systems, places and neighbourhoods* (2022). www.kingsfund.org.uk/publications/integrated-care-systems-explained

BMA (2023) *Integrated care systems.* www.bma.org.uk/advice-and-support/nhs-delivery-and-workforce/integration/integrated-care-systems-icss

The Health Foundation *Health care funding* (2024). www.health.org.uk/publications/long-reads/health-care-funding

UK Health Security Agency. Ferguson B, and Belloni A. *Ageing and health expenditure* (2019). https://ukhsa.blog.gov.uk/2019/01/29/ageing-and-health-expenditure

Nuffield Trust *Who organizes and funds social care?* (2023). www.nuffieldtrust.org.uk/news-item/who-organises-and-funds-social-care-1

Age UK *Briefing: Health and care of older people in England in 2019* (2019). www.ageuk.org.uk/globalassets/age-uk/documents/reports-and-publications/reports-and-briefings/health--wellbeing/age_uk_briefing_state_of_health_and_care_of_older_people_july2019.pdf

The Health Foundation *How many hospital beds will the NHS need over the coming decade? Projections: General and acute hospital beds in England, 2018–2030* (2022). www.health.org.uk/publications/reports/how-many-beds-will-the-nhs-need-over-the-coming-decade

The Health Foundation *Why are delayed discharges from hospital increasing?* (2023). www.health.org.uk/publications/long-reads/why-are-delayed-discharges-from-hospital-increasing-seeing-the-bigger

Gordon A L, Dhesi J. (2023) *Resolving the health and social care crisis requires a focus on care for older people* BMJ 380 https://doi.org/10.1136/bmj.p97

RCP *The UK is facing a crisis in care for older people* (2022). https://www.rcp.ac.uk/news-and-media/news-and-opinion/rcp-warns-the-uk-is-facing-a-crisis-in-care-for-older-people/

BGS *Clinical research methods for studies of older people* (2019). www.bgs.org.uk/resources/clinical-research-methods-for-studies-of-older-people

NHS Digital *Adult Social Care Activity and Finance Report, England, 2022-23* (2023). https://digital.nhs.uk/data-and-information/publications/statistical/adult-social-care-activity-and-finance-report/2022-23#

ONS Census 2021 *Unpaid care by age, sex and deprivation, England and Wales* (2023). www.ons.gov.uk/peoplepopulationandcommunity/healthandsocialcare/socialcare/articles/unpaidcarebyagesexanddeprivationenglandandwales/census2021

DWP Family Resources Survey 2021-22 Tenure data tables (2023). https://www.gov.uk/government/statistics/family-resources-survey-financial-year-2021-to-2022

House of Commons *Research briefing Informal carers* (2022). https://researchbriefings.files.parliament.uk/documents/CBP-7756/CBP-7756.pdf

NHS Digital *Adult Social Care Activity and Finance Report, England - 2021-22 Chapter 5 Carers* (2022). https://digital.nhs.uk/data-and-information/publications/statistical/adult-social-care-activity-and-finance-report/2021-22/carers

WEBSITES OF USEFUL ORGANISATIONS

Age UK: www.ageuk.org.uk

Citizens Advice Bureau: http://www.citizensadvice.org.uk

Carers UK: http://www.carersuk.org

DHSC: https://www.gov.uk/government/organisations/department-of-health-and-social-care

NHS Social Care and Support Guide: http://www.nhs.uk/conditions/social-care-and-support-guide

Care Information Scotland: http://www.careinfoscotland.scot

Government information on pensions and benefits www.gov.uk and search for individual benefits

The Care Quality Commission England: www.cqc.org.uk

Health Inspectorate Wales: www.hiw.org.uk

The Care Inspectorate of Scotland: www.careinspectorate.com

Northern Ireland Regulatory and Quality Improvement Authority: www.rqia.org.uk

ONS: https://www.ons.gov.uk/

Scottish government statistics: https://statistics.gov.scot/data_home

All websites were accessed in August 2024.

3

The science of ageing

Ageing scenarios

The global population is ageing rapidly. A longer life is a blessing if the added years are spent in health. Tallis described four possible outcomes of increased longevity, shown in Figure 3.1:

- Scenario A, the current situation: people tend to be relatively healthy until their late 60s, when chronic disabilities start to accumulate until death.
- In Scenario B, both morbidity and death are postponed.
- Scenario C is the best outcome in which life expectancy is increased and there is 'compression of morbidity' into the final months of life.
- Scenario D, the worst case, is where life expectancy increases, but there is no delay in the age at which limiting disabilities start to accrue, so more years are spent in poor health.

The medicine and science of ageing should aim to achieve C, with B being the next best option.

What is ageing?

The characteristic features have been recognised since antiquity.

- Look online for a vase from Cerveteri (480 BCE). Herakles, who finally overcame age and death to achieve immortality, is keeping Geras at bay with a club. Look at Geras – what features suggest his age?
- Look at portrayals of old age in Renaissance art, e.g. Portrait of an Old Man (Pietro Cardinal Bembo), Titian, 1546, in the Budapest Museum of Fine Arts. 2000 years later, how does the artist depict old age?

However, we are only just beginning to understand the underlying processes involved in ageing.

There has been an explosion of research on ageing across a wide range of disciplines (Figure 3.2), but unifying hypotheses on the mechanisms still elude us.

There are many definitions of ageing. Read the three definitions and note how they differ:

1 A phenomenon of increasing risk of failure with the passage of time.
2 A progressive generalised impairment of function resulting in a loss of adaptive response to stress and a growing risk of age-related disease.
3 The process that progressively converts physiologically and cognitively fit healthy adults into less fit individuals with increasing vulnerability to injury, illness, and death.

Could these apply to an old car, yeast, a giant redwood, and a middle-aged man?

The first is reliability theory – an all-systems approach that includes the car – and is useful in relating to the non-biological sciences. The second is from a biological perspective and applies to all living organisms (yeast and sequoia as well as man). The third is a medical approach and just relates to man. Note that the latter two definitions do not mention time.

Reliability models

- Are useful for distinguishing between markers of age (passage of time) and markers of ageing (deleterious changes).
- There are two groups of system failures: catastrophic or degradation, depending on redundancy.

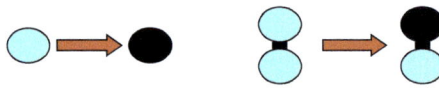

No redundancy   Redundancy

- The reliability of a complex system depends on the arrangement of the components and the amount of redundancy (Figure 3.3).

A shows a series, Ss = $p1p2...pn$. In a series, system failure depends on the weakest link. In the body, each component can be represented by an organ, e.g. the heart, brain, and kidneys. In B, the components are arranged in parallel, e.g. many cells in an organ. C is a series-parallel with equal redundancy, e.g. two kidneys and D is a series-parallel with distributed redundancy, e.g. different organs with different amounts of reserve.

- The reliability of a system in series Ss is a product of the reliability of its components. If a system is built of 458 components by the age when 99% of the components are still functioning, the system has only a 1% chance of remaining functional. Thus, premature failure is critical.
- Failure kinetics in biological systems, like the failure rate of technical products with time, follows a 'bathtub curve'.

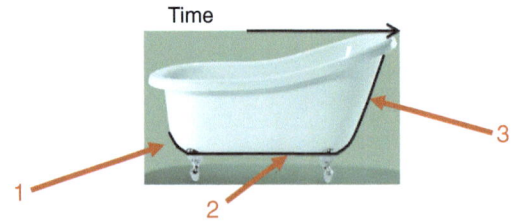

Time

Geriatric Medicine and Elderly Care: Lecture Notes, Ninth Edition. Claire G. Nicholl, K. Jane Wilson, and Shaun D'Souza.
© 2025 John Wiley & Sons Ltd. Published 2025 by John Wiley & Sons Ltd.
Companion website: www.wiley.com/go/lecturenotesgeriatricmedicine9e

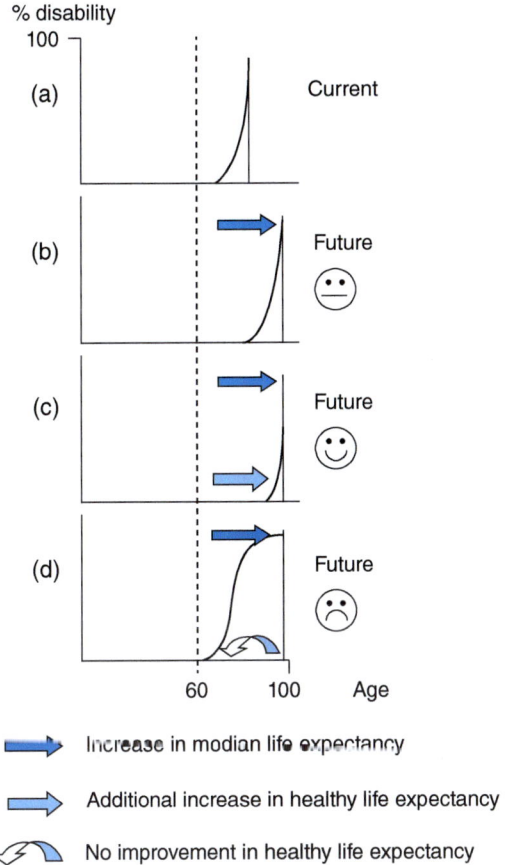

Figure 3.1 Theoretical ageing scenarios after Tallis.

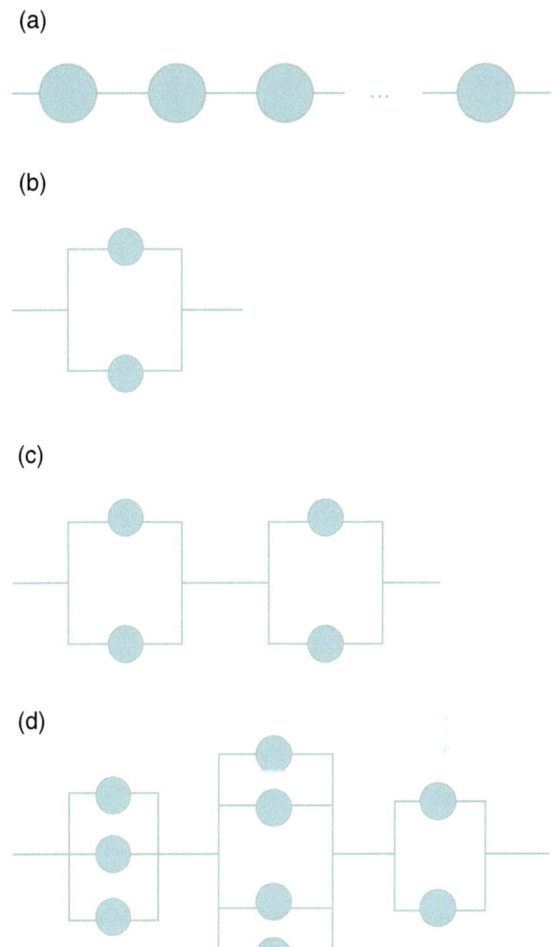

Figure 3.3 Components in a system.

1 Some individual units will fail early due to defects and blunders (the highest rate results in very early pregnancy loss and extends to neonatal mortality).
2 Some will fail during the prolonged period typically called normal life.
3 Others (we hope most) will last until they wear out (old age), and here even some things may be replaceable, e.g. hips (or tyres).

The ageing process

Cells, tissues, and organs all change with age and eventually, their function begins to deteriorate. The processes that determine ageing are very complex. There are two major groups of theories:

1 Programmed self-destruction
2 Stochastic (random events)

An injured cell will swell, burst, and release its contents, causing an inflammatory and immune cascade, but when a cell dies a normal death, it shrivels up and is consumed by nearby cells so fast that it never gets a chance to spill its contents. Wyllie named this apoptosis (pronounced apotosis), from the Greek for 'falling off' as in leaves from a tree. An array of intracellular and extracellular signals can trigger the cell to enter the process of programmed cell death. Apoptosis occurs from the earliest stages of development (e.g. leading to the separation of fingers), is highly active during growth, and continues throughout life. Aberrant regulation of apoptosis contributes to cancer, autoimmune disorders, neurodegenerative diseases, and systemic viral infection.

Individual cells can undergo programmed death, but there has been debate as to whether multicellular organisms carry programmes to

Molecules - genetics, biochemistry
Cells - cell biology
Tissues, organs, and systems - CVS, respiratory, neurological, GI, blood,
 endocrine, urogenital, bones and joints, muscles, immune system — physiology, pathophysiology
Organisms (yeast to man, lifespan, models) comparative and experimental biology, mathematics
Populations - epidemiology
Ecosystems - social gerontology

Figure 3.2 Substrates and disciplines for studies on ageing. CVS, cardiovascular system.

self-destruct ('a ticking clock'). Ageing as a predetermined, genetically controlled process is supported by the characteristic lifespans of different species.

Genetic theories

There are several broad genetic theories:

Mutation accumulation theory (Medawar, 1952)

- Mutant genes that kill or reduce vigour before reproductive age are selected out – those that exert their effect later are not.
- Over successive generations, late-acting deleterious mutations will accumulate, leading to increased mortality in later life.

Disposable soma theory (Kirkwood, 1977)

- Organisms divide their finite energy between reproduction and the maintenance of the non-reproductive aspects (soma).
- They invest in the repair of somatic cells for durability over a typical lifetime.
- There is a trade-off between life span and reproduction, e.g. *Drosophila*, subject to high extrinsic mortality, prioritises reproduction; the elephant, the converse.

Theory of antagonistic pleiotropy (Williams, 1957)

- Pleiotropy, the production by a single gene of two or more apparently unrelated effects, is common, as most proteins have multiple roles in different cell types, e.g. in Werner syndrome, a single gene mutation results in many effects.
- Antagonistic pleiotropy describes the situation where a gene increases the odds of successful reproduction and fitness early in life but decreases fitness in later life. Such genes are not eliminated by natural selection, e.g. ob/ob mouse.
- Genes controlling apoptosis and cellular senescence may be other examples – pathways that are essential for the development, viability, and fitness of young organisms may contribute to ageing phenotypes (Campisi 2003), e.g. the *p53* gene directs damaged cells to stop reproducing, resulting in cell death and helping to avert cancer, but it also suppresses the division of stem cells, limiting their availability for repair and renewal of ageing tissues.

Experimental models of genetics and ageing

Genes that affect lifespan have mainly been studied in:

- Yeast – fungal genomes diverged from animals 1500 million years ago, but many genes and the proteins they produce are conserved.
- *Caenorhabditis elegans*, a free-living 1 mm soil nematode. As background information, larvae hatch 24 hours after fertilisation, go through four larval stages, and mature by 72 hours. If food is limited, after the L2 moult, a larva enters an alternative third larval stage called a dauer (enduring) larva and may spend 2 months in this dormant phase. The adult worm lives for 3 weeks, with maximum egg production in the first 4 days. During ageing, it displays a number of human ageing phenotypes, including sarcopaenia, a decline in sensory and cognitive capacities, and a weakened defence against pathogens. By week 3, it moves less, stops feeding and dies.
- *Drosophila*.
- Mice and rats.

Genetic lifespan extension in experimental models

Manipulation of single genes can have dramatic effects.

- Lifespan in yeast, *C. elegans* and *Drosophila* can be doubled (e.g. *C. elegans* by *daf-2* mutations, which encode an ortholog of the insulin/insulin-like growth factor 1 [IGF1] receptor).
- The average lifespan of mice can be increased by about 20% by mutations that reduce mTOR (mechanistic target of rapamycin) production.

Genetics and lifespan in humans

No genes have been found that have such a dramatic effect on the lifespan of man. There are many genes that cause diseases, but the effect of genes on ageing is harder to unravel; to some extent, healthy ageing is the avoidance of diseases.

Genes that cause ageing in humans

There are single genetic disorders that cause premature ageing (progeria). These are 'segmental ageing' syndromes, as they do not result in all the typical features of ageing, but it is likely that some of the mechanisms involved will be relevant to normal ageing. There are two main groups: those caused by defects in DNA repair pathways or telomere maintenance, and those affecting the nuclear membrane, the laminopathies.

- **Werner's syndrome** is a rare, autosomal recessive progeria of adulthood. Characteristic features include premature greying and hair loss, an aged appearance, cataracts, skeletal changes, dyslipidaemia, insulin-resistant diabetes, premature atherosclerosis, and a propensity to cancer. Death occurs at around 50 years old. It is caused by truncating mutations in a *RecQ helicase/exonuclease* gene on chromosome 8p. The normal helicase unwinds, separates, and repairs damaged DNA and may be important in maintaining telomeres. It also regulates the transcription of a key enzyme controlling the synthesis of NAD+, which has a role in mitochondrial homeostasis. NAD+ levels are depleted in Werner syndrome and the Werner models in *C. elegans* and *Drosophila*. In these models, NAD+ repletion delays accelerated ageing and extends lifespan.
- **Hutchinson–Gilford syndrome** is an exceedingly rare, sporadic, autosomal dominant progeria of childhood. Characteristics include small stature, an abnormal face with a beaked nose and small mouth, baldness, severe atherosclerosis, bone and joint abnormalities, and loss of subcutaneous fat. Death occurs around 14 years from MI or stroke. It is usually due to a silent substitution from glycine GGC to glycine GGT in codon 608 of the lamin A (*LMNA*) gene on 1q, which activates a cryptic splice donor site to produce abnormal lamin A, known as progerin. This is truncated and retains a farnesyl moiety that is removed in normal lamin A. The nuclear fragility of lamin A-deficient cells increases apoptosis and may exhaust stem-cell-driven regeneration. Telomere shortening is also seen. Lonafarnib, a farnesyltransferase inhibitor, increased lifespan by 1.6 years in a clinical trial, but eventually gene therapy to inhibit aberrant splicing is likely to be developed.

Evidence for a genetic effect on normal human ageing

- Twin studies suggest about 25% of the variation in human longevity is genetically determined.
- Many nonagenarians and centenarians live independently and avoid age-related diseases until the very last years of their lives (Scenario C in Figure 3.1).

- The environment and lifestyle appear more important until the ninth decade. Once individuals enter their 80s, genetic effects become more apparent, particularly in males. For centenarians, the genetic effect may account for up to 33% for women and 48% for men.
- There are five longevity hotspots, or 'blue zones' named after the blue circles the researchers drew on the map when looking at regions where people appear to live long, healthy lives (Sardinia, Okinawa, Nicoya, Loma Linda, and Ikaria). Both a healthy lifestyle and genetic factors may be important, but there are issues with the accuracy of records. Some believe Jeanne Calment, who died at 122 years of age in 1997 (the world record for longevity), was in fact her daughter.

Which genes are important for longevity in humans?

Ageing is polygenic, with many genes having a small effect. Candidate genes are identified from experimental models and genome-wide association studies (GWAS) looking for single nucleotide polymorphisms (abbreviated SNPs, pronounced snips) associated with longevity. These studies are limited by the relatively small pool of centenarians. To increase the number of 'older people' included, some groups have reduced the age threshold, and signals tend to be lost.

- Supercentenarians have the same gene variants that increase disease risk in people with average life spans. The supercentenarians, however, appear to have other gene variants that promote longevity.
- Some of the gene variants that are associated with longevity are involved with basic cellular maintenance including DNA repair, telomere maintenance and protection from free radicals. Other genes affect vascular health by sensing nutrient levels, influencing lipid levels, insulin resistance, and inflammation, and reducing the risk of heart disease, the main cause of death in older people.
- Common polymorphisms associated with long lifespans are found in the *APOE* (apolipoprotein E), *FOXO3* (forkhead family of transcription factors), *CETP* (cholesteryl ester transfer protein), *IGF1R* (IGF1 receptor), and *IL-6* (interleukin 6) genes, but they are not found in all individuals with exceptional longevity.
- The list of longevity-associated polymorphisms is growing as new associations are identified. A recent example (if you want to follow the science as it evolves) is a longevity-associated variant of the *BPIFB4* family (Bactericidal/permeability-increasing protein fold or *BPI* fold gene, family B member 4). Carriers of this variant have few cardiovascular complications. New techniques enable the effects of the variant and its mechanism of action to be investigated. Gene therapy in mouse models of disease prevents the onset of atherosclerosis and diabetic complications and 'rejuvenates' the immune system (Cattaneo).
- One of the problems in the literature is that once a polymorphism has been linked, e.g. to ageing, if the association is NOT subsequently confirmed, it is hard to 'unlink'.

The contribution of stochastic events to ageing

Ageing processes appear to be due to a combination of genetic predisposition, genetic changes, and random or stochastic events. In *C. elegans*, although genotype determines the mean lifespan of a population, individual longevity has a large random element, with several-fold differences observed even within an isogenic population in a uniform environment.

- The biochemistry of the cell is noisy. All cellular processes – transcription, translation, protein folding, every enzymatic reaction and all the inbuilt regulatory mechanisms – are subject to random errors.

- The workings of cells get noisier as they get older, and this might contribute to increasing cellular dysfunction with age.
- Stochastic theories claim that ageing is caused by random accumulated injuries from external stressors, e.g. ultraviolet light, radiation, and physical damage, and endogenous stressors, e.g. toxic by-products of metabolism such as free radicals, etc.

Rate of living theory (Pearl, 1928)

- A broad inverse correlation between lifespan and metabolic rate, i.e. live fast, die young, would be explained by the faster accrual of errors.

Free radical theory (Harman, 1956)

- Macromolecular damage due to free radicals is the major cause of ageing, with the mitochondria being both the main source and target.

Effects of the environment and lifestyle

The most robust way of increasing lifespan in animal studies is through calorie restriction. However, many environmental and lifestyle factors have a major effect on both ageing and disease. These include air and water pollution, smoking, under and overnutrition, exposure to pathogens, and exercise. New challenges which may be relevant to ageing include the ubiquity of microplastics in our food chain and the increasing proportion of ultra-processed food in the diet. Social integration and mental health are also increasingly recognised to affect ageing in humans.

Psychosocial theories of ageing

These focus on the mental and emotional as well as social aspects of growing old. Erikson suggests that the primary psychosocial task of late adulthood (65 and beyond) is to maintain **ego integrity** (holding on to one's sense of wholeness) while avoiding despair (as there is too little time to begin a new life course). Those who succeed develop wisdom, which includes accepting the life one has lived and the inevitability of death. Some regret is common when reflecting on whether different choices might have led to a happier life. Older people often reminisce and review their life, perhaps in search of its meaning.

Three major psychosocial theories are disengagement, activity, and continuity.

1 **Disengagement (Cummings and Henry):** ageing is a process of mutual withdrawal in which older adults voluntarily slow down by retiring, as expected by society. However, in economically developed societies, a long retirement in relatively good health means that this is not typical.
2 **Activity (Havighurst):** the opposite, sees a positive correlation between keeping active and ageing well. Proponents of activity theory hold that mutual social withdrawal runs counter to Western ideals of activity, energy, and industry; evidence supports the benefits of ongoing engagement.
3 **Continuity (Atchley):** older adults typically maintain the pattern of activities and behaviours from their earlier lives despite changing circumstances.

Growing old means different things for different people. Physical and mental health, income and companionship have a marked effect. Individuals who led active lives as young and middle adults will probably remain active, while those who were less active may become more disengaged as they age. Disengagement may also be seen in previously active people in the late stages of chronic disease and terminal illness.

Effects of disease

As increasing age is the biggest risk factor for acquiring disease and death, it is difficult to distinguish the changes of ageing from the changes associated with pathology.

- Many degenerative processes develop over decades and are so universal that it is difficult to determine whether this is ageing or pathology.
- Diseases we think of as 'modern' scourges of ageing were present in antiquity. CT scans of mummies from four continents found arterial plaques in every population studied, from pre-agricultural hunter-gatherers in the Aleutian Islands to the ancient Puebloans of the Southwestern United States (Thompson et al. 2013).
- There is also a direct interaction – ageing promotes disease, and vice versa; diseases and/or their treatments may accelerate ageing processes.

Many biochemical pathways are affected by ageing, but the main proximal cause of these changes remains unknown. We are in an era of phenomenology – a myriad of changes have been described, but it is unclear which are causative, which are secondary and how they fit together.

The ageing cell

In 2013, to bring some structure into a very confusing field, a European group proposed nine hallmarks of molecular and cellular ageing. Hallmarks are factors that are consistently linked to the ageing process and can be manipulated experimentally to both increase and decrease the ageing process. The group added three more in 2023.

Hallmarks of ageing

1 Genomic instability.
2 Telomere attrition.
3 Epigenetics.
4 Loss of proteostasis.
5 Deregulated nutrient sensing.
6 Mitochondrial dysfunction.
7 Cell senescence.
8 Stem-cell exhaustion.
9 Altered intercellular communication.
10 Disabled macroautophagy.
11 Dysbiosis (an imbalance in the gut microbiome).
12 Chronic inflammation.

Around the same date, a different model, the seven pillars of ageing, was proposed by the US NIH geroscience group. 'Pillars' is perhaps a misnomer, as the model makes it clear that the processes are highly intertwined. It seems confusing that the pillars appear to differ from the hallmarks, but they incorporate most of the processes, just aggregated differently: (i) Macromolecular damage (includes genomic instability and telomere attrition), (ii) Stem cells and regeneration, (iii) Metabolism (includes nutrient sensing and mitochondrial dysregulation), (iv) Epigenetics, (v) Inflammation (includes cell senescence), (vi) Maladaption to stress, and (vii) Proteostasis (includes macroautophagy).

1. Genomic instability

There is an increased tendency for alterations in the genome during the life cycle, driven by a large variety of endogenous and exogenous insults. Multiple changes are seen.

- Chromosomal aneuploidy (variable chromosome number), somatic mutations, translocations, deletions, and gene disruptions by the insertion of viruses and transposons are all more common with ageing.
- Increased somatic mutations are also seen in mitochondrial DNA.
- DNA repair systems are also less efficient.

DNA damage leads to dysregulation of gene expression, dysfunctional mitochondria and cellular responses that may lead to apoptosis or cell senescence, resulting in stem-cell depletion.

2. Telomere attrition

Telomeres are non-coding repeat sequence caps at the end of chromosomes.

- They protect the coding region from damage and prevent the ends from fusing with neighbouring chromosomes when cells divide.
- Telomeres also act as an ageing clock, controlling the number of divisions a cell can make. When cells divide, DNA polymerase cannot continue to the end of the DNA, so telomeres become shorter every time a cell divides. Eventually, when they reach a critically short length, the cell cannot divide any more, leading to apoptosis or a state of cell cycle arrest known as cellular senescence. This is the explanation for the finite number of divisions that normal cells can undergo in tissue culture, the Hayflick limit, and the telomere theory of ageing.
- Germ cells and stem cells express telomerase, a reverse transcriptase that rebuilds the telomeres, so these cells can keep dividing, but telomerase is inactivated or expressed at a very low level in most somatic cells. Telomerase-deficient mice appear prematurely aged, and telomerase reactivation results in the rejuvenation of some tissues. However, telomerase reactivation would not be a simple solution to ageing, as telomerase is expressed in most human cancers and plays a crucial role in the immortality of cancer cells.

As well as replicative shortening, telomeres can be lengthened and shortened by other processes. A new mechanism by which some T cells elongate their telomeres has been described recently. Antigen-presenting cells were able to transfer telomeres in extracellular vesicles to the T cells. Sampling may also affect the measured length as telomeres are usually measured in mixed white cells from blood samples. If the leukocyte population changes, e.g. because of margination or cell death, the telomere length from subsequent samples may be different.

It is now accepted that telomere length can be modulated by environmental and lifestyle factors throughout the life course, from in-utero development onwards, by factors including infection, stress, nutrition, smoking, alcohol use, and some drugs. Commercial blood tests are available to get your telomere length tested and compared to an age-matched sample to 'assess your biological age'. This is too simplistic, but telomere length may be a composite marker of ageing and cumulative stress.

3. Epigenetics

Epigenetic changes affect gene expression by turning genes on and off. There are several mechanisms:

- DNA methylation turns genes off.
- Histone modification makes the sections of the genome spooled on histones unavailable for transcription.
- Non-coding RNA can attach to mRNA and mark it for degradation.

Many factors throughout life lead to epigenetic changes, including the intrauterine environment (maternal malnutrition has a major effect on adult vascular health), nutrition, exercise, smoking, alcohol, drugs, and infections. In ageing, the pattern of which genes are on and off changes. Monozygotic twins display few epigenetic differences at 20 years, but differences become more pronounced with age, a phenomenon termed 'epigenetic drift'. Overall DNA methylation decreases with age, and a variety of epigenetic clocks have been proposed to predict chronological and biological age.

4. Loss of proteostasis

Proteostasis requires proteins to be made (through translation, folding, post-translational modification, and shuttling to the correct compartment) and then degraded correctly. There are several mechanisms by which cells degrade damaged or unwanted proteins.

- Multiprotein complexes in the endoplasmic reticulum (ER) identify, remove, ubiquitinate, and deliver misfolded proteins to the 26S proteasome for degradation in the cytosol, a process known as ER-associated degradation, or ERAD. Several steps in the ERAD pathway are facilitated by molecular chaperones.
- The UPR, or unfolded protein response, is a transcriptional response that is activated by the accumulation of misfolded proteins in the ER. It slows protein translation, reducing the protein load in the ER while simultaneously up-regulating factors that facilitate the folding or clearance of misfolded molecules.
- Autophagy or self-engulfment, lysosomal targeting, and phagocytosis (engulfment of waste products by other cells) can also be used as proteostatic degradation mechanisms.

Ageing cells accumulate damaged and misfolded proteins, which have deleterious consequences, including compromised structure and enzymatic activity, and direct toxicity.

- Proteins can be damaged by a wide range of biochemical processes. Oxidative, reductive and nitrosative stress produce carbonylation, glycation, glutathionylation, sulfhydration, nitration, and nitrosylation, and other reactions include racemisation, isomerisation, and all kinds of molecular breaks, adducts, substitutions, insertions, and deletions.
- All protein degradation pathways become less efficient with ageing. Misfolded proteins tend to aggregate and are implicated in the pathogenesis of many diseases, including Alzheimer's.
- Lipofuscin is an autofluorescent brown-yellow intralysosomal polymeric substance composed of crosslinked protein residues, lipids, and iron. It cannot be degraded, so it accumulates with age, particularly in long-lived cells, where it spills over into the cytosol. It was thought to be an inert marker of ageing, but may have deleterious effects on the proteasome, autophagy, and lysosomal degradation, and by providing a reservoir of metal ions, it may lead to reactive oxidative species (ROS) generation and apoptosis. It has been implicated in the pathogenesis of age-related macular degeneration.
- Age also affects the number or function of cellular pumps (a family of proteins called multidrug resistance pumps) that enable toxic products to be removed from cells.

5. Deregulated nutrient sensing

This is very complex, but a lot of work has focused on the manipulation of four main interacting pathways that affect lifespan in experimental models and mediate the lifespan extension seen with calorie restriction. When nutrients are abundant, mTOR and insulin-like growth factor 1 signalling (IIS) work together to maintain an anabolic state, whereas in low-energy conditions, AMPK (adenosine monophosphate-activated protein kinase) and sirtuins promote catabolism.

i **mTOR** has a key role in sensing nutrients in the cell. It forms the catalytic subunit of two distinct protein complexes: mTORC1 (mTOR Complex 1), which has a central role in cell growth, and mTORC2, which is involved in cell survival and proliferation. mTORC1 controls the balance between anabolism and catabolism in response to environmental changes. When amino acids are available:
- It promotes the synthesis of lipids and nucleotides.
- It shifts glucose metabolism to glycolysis.
- It suppresses protein catabolism through autophagy.
Reduced expression of the homologues of mTOR in *C. elegans* (daf-15), *Drosophila* and mice extend lifespan and mTOR inhibition with rapamycin (used clinically as sirolimus) extends life span in all these experimental models. The mechanism by which mTORC1 inhibition slows ageing in mammals is still not clear and is multifactorial. It may reduce proteotoxic stress, increase autophagy and the removal of cell debris, and have a role in renewing stem cells.

ii **Insulin/IIS** is another highly conserved pathway with a role in nutrient sensing and effects on lifespan. A rise in blood glucose stimulates insulin release. Insulin binds with its tyrosine kinase receptor, and conformational changes result in autophosphorylation. This activates a docking protein, insulin receptor substrate (IRS), on which phosphatidylinositol-3-kinase (PI-3K) is attached, phosphorylating PIP2 (phosphatidylinositol-biphosphate) to PIP3. PIP3 acts as a docking site for PDK1 (phosphoinositide-dependent protein kinase 1) which activates AKT (also known as protein kinase B). AKT plays a role in four key downstream processes:
- Protein synthesis via mTOR.
- Glycogen synthesis.
- Regulation of gluconeogenic and adipogenic genes through the transcription factor FOXO.
- Translocation of the insulin-sensitive glucose transporter GLUT4 to enable glucose uptake.
In *C. elegans*, a mutation in *daf-2*, the homologue of insulin/IGFR doubles its life expectancy to around 6 weeks. Mutations in *age-1* (also known as *daf-23*), the homologue of PI3K, and *daf-16*, the homologue of FOXO, also affect lifespan. The daf-2 pathway is one of the mechanisms that allows the worm to suspend its development when the environment is harsh. The situation is more complex in man, but the insulin pathway is important in diabetes and cancer, which have links with ageing.

iii **AMPK** is activated when intracellular AMP/ADP (adenosine monophosphate/diphosphate) levels rise, e.g. in response to low glucose or exercise.
- Activated AMPK phosphorylates several substrates to have rapid effects on metabolism and growth.
- It phosphorylates transcriptional regulators that have a longer-term effect on metabolism.
- It controls mitochondrial homeostasis by triggering the removal of existing defective mitochondria and replacing them with new ones.
In *C. elegans*, the loss of *aak-2*, the gene encoding the homologue of the AMPK protein, decreases lifespan, and increased expression of *aak-2* increases lifespan. Overexpression of a constitutively active form of AMPK increases lifespan, as does metformin, an indirect AMPK agonist. In humans, exercise, calorie restriction and metformin all activate AMPK.

iv **Sirtuins**, or silent information regulators (SIRTs), are a family of nicotinamide adenine dinucleotide (NAD+)-dependent lysine deacetylases that can regulate gene expression by directly deacetylating histones. Mammals have seven sirtuins (the analogue of *sir2* in yeast), located in different intracellular compartments, which have a wide range of actions.
- Sirtuins detect low intracellular energy levels by sensing NAD+.
- Low-energy levels also activate AMPK, and the pathways may work together to maintain energy balance.

Sirtuins hit the headlines when SIRT1 was reported to extend the lifespan of yeast, *C. elegans*, *Drosophila* and mice. There was also great interest in resveratrol (a polyphenol in red wine), which was claimed to be a SIRT1-activator. However, a paper in 2011 found that the increased lifespan in worms and flies was attributable to confounding genetic backgrounds and doubt has been cast on whether resveratrol acts via SIRT. Multiple papers on the cardioprotective effects of resveratrol have been retracted (Dipak Das). There is still debate in the literature, but GSK spent billions on SIRT-activating compounds and no clinical drugs resulted. Despite this, resveratrol supplements are still widely available online.

Interest has switched to SIRT6, which extends lifespan in *Drosophila* and mice, but so many pathways that might affect ageing have been proposed that it is hard to unravel what might be important. Meanwhile, SIRT6 activators from seaweed can be bought for £430 a year online.

6. Mitochondrial dysfunction

The traditional view of the role of mitochondria in ageing was the free radical theory, which proposed that ROS produced during aerobic metabolism were responsible for damage to macromolecules such as DNA, proteins, and lipids, which led to the deterioration of cells and tissues and, ultimately, the entire organism. However, in experimental models, there is no clear correlation between the reduction or enhancement of oxidative damage and lifespan. For example, the *SOD-2* (*C. elegans* mitochondrial superoxide dismutase) loss-of-function mutation, which is predicted to increase oxidative damage, extends lifespan. However, several linked mechanisms do implicate mitochondria in cell senescence and ageing.

- Levels of mitochondrial DNA (mtDNA) mutations increase with age, but as mitochondrial genomes are present in multiple copies in cells, extremely high levels of somatic mutations would be needed to have an effect. A mouse model with extensive mtDNA mutations, which has features of premature ageing and a short lifespan, appears to have an abnormality of stem cells that develops in embryogenesis.
- Mitochondrial function is less efficient in ageing tissues. This could be due to:
  - An increase in age-dependent mitochondrial damage.
  - A decline in the removal of damaged mitochondria.
  - A combination of these.
- There are several mechanisms by which cells deal with damage to mitochondria. Low-level stress leads to signals from the remaining healthy mitochondria, perhaps by the mitochondrial UPR to the cell nucleus, to alter the transcriptional response to improve the intracellular environment. If there is some mitochondrial damage, the affected area can be removed into a mitochondrial-derived vesicle, or if the mitochondrion is damaged beyond repair, the whole organelle can be removed by mitophagy.
- Mitochondria might play a role in 'inflammageing' the activation of the innate immune system that is seen with ageing. Molecules that are released from the cell are thought to trigger an immune response. Mitochondria, derived billions of years ago from the endosymbiosis of alpha-proteobacteria into eukaryotic cells, may be a source of these molecules, termed damage-associated molecular patterns (DAMPs).

7. Cell senescence

Cell senescence is the irreversible arrest of growth and proliferation that occurs when cells experience a variety of insults. In cell culture, this occurs when a cell reaches its Hayflick limit. The number of senescent cells in tissues increases with chronological ageing in experimental animals, humans, and progeroid syndromes.

- Numerous factors, such as oxidative damage, telomere shortening, protein aggregation, hyperproliferation, the expression of oncogenes, irradiation, and chemical agents, can trigger a DNA damage response in cells. This may lead to:
  - Senescence.
  - Apoptosis.
  - Necrosis.
  - Autophagy.
    A variety of factors that are not well understood determine which route a cell will take.
- Senescent cells are generally resistant to apoptosis but can be induced to do this; more usually, they are removed by a variety of immune system cells.
- Cellular senescence is an example of antagonistic pleiotropy. It performs an essential role in embryogenesis and wound healing and may act as an anti-tumour mechanism, but in later life, appears to be deleterious.

The senescence-associated secretory phenotype

Chronically senescent cells remain viable but acquire morphological and phenotypic changes, including the secretion of pro-inflammatory cytokines (especially IL-6 and IL-8), chemokines, growth modulators, and proteases, termed the senescence-associated secretory phenotype (SASP), which affects other cells in a paracrine manner.

- SASP gene expression can be regulated by epigenetic changes, mTOR and DAMPs, indicating that all these mechanisms interact. Senolytic drugs, which direct senescent cells into apoptosis, are one of the ways that are being studied to reduce ageing.
- The senescent cell secretome also reduces an anti-ageing protein, alpha Klotho. Klotho, named after the youngest of the Three Fates who spins the thread of human life, is a protein from the glycosidase family with little enzymatic activity that appears to be a cofactor for fibroblast growth factor. It can be membrane-bound or circulating. Serum levels fall with age in humans and are predictive of mortality. Reduced Klotho accelerates ageing in mice, and overexpression increases mouse lifespan. Polymorphisms in humans are associated with longevity. It is not known how it modulates ageing, but it has several effects (cytoprotection, anti-apoptosis, reduction in cell senescence, antifibrosis, and improved autophagy), all of which might contribute to tissue protection and regeneration. In young animals, circulating alpha Klotho, maintains the mitochondria in stem cells so that they are available if muscle fibres are damaged. When Klotho levels fall in old age, there is increasing damage to mitochondrial DNA, ROS accumulate, and stem cells become less efficient or even senescent, so they are not available for tissue repair and exacerbate inflammageing.

8. Stem-cell exhaustion

The initial cells resulting from cell division in the zygote are totipotent and form the embryo and the placenta. After 4 days, the inner cell mass of the blastocyst becomes pluripotent embryonic stem cells and can no longer form the placenta. These differentiate into endoderm, mesoderm, and ectoderm, and the cells become multipotent stem cells with the ability to form cells of just that germ layer apart from mesenchymal stem cells that remain pluripotent.

- Somatic or adult stem cells persist in the tissues throughout life, but as noted, most have a restricted range of differentiation.
- Their numbers, function, and distribution may depend on intrauterine development.
- Neural stem cells give rise to neurons and glia.

- Haemopoietic stem cells form all the cellular components of the blood.
- Skin stem cells form keratinocytes and bone, cartilage, and fat cells.
- Mesenchymal stem cells can produce a wide range of cell types.

It is possible to reverse the differentiation in tissue culture and redirect differentiated cells to become pluripotent. The local environment, or 'stem-cell niche', is important for the maintenance of the stem cells. During ageing, the regenerative potential of stem cells declines, and this is one mechanism by which the response to tissue injury is impaired. The worsening function of stem cells depends on changes in the cells themselves and their niche. The changes in the stem cells are like those in all cells, including DNA damage, mitochondrial dysfunction, epigenetic changes, and impaired proteostasis. The presence of senescent cells in the tissue produces inflammageing in the niche, which impairs stem-cell proliferation and regeneration.

9. Altered intercellular communication

The change in signals between cells with ageing tends to be pro-inflammatory and includes SASP, secretion of ROS and leakage of molecules through gap junctions. This leads to the activation of the nuclear factor kappa light chain enhancer of activated B cells (NF-kB), which, despite its name, is present in most cells. Its activation in the hypothalamus inhibits the production of gonadotrophin-releasing hormone. This reduction may contribute to osteoporosis, sarcopaenia, and skin changes.

The existence of circulating factors that affect ageing, such as Klotho, is demonstrated by blood exchange, in which blood from older animals appears harmful to younger animals and blood from young animals appears to have some rejuvenating effects on older ones.

10. Disabled macroautophagy

Autophagy is a cellular process to eliminate molecules and organelles to maintain cellular homeostasis. There are three main types of autophagy:

i   **Macroautophagy** was thought of as a bulk clearance mechanism, but there are separate pathways for aggregated ubiquitinated proteins, glycogen, lipids, mitochondria, the ER, components of cell nuclei, lysosomes themselves and pathogens. These are all taken up by specific receptors into an autophagosome, which then fuses with the lysosome. It is activated by AMPK and inhibited by mTOR. Macroautophagy declines with age in experimental models.

ii   **Microautophagy** involves direct invagination of the lysosome membrane.

iii   **Chaperone-mediated autophagy** clears proteins with a characteristic pentapeptide moiety and nucleic acids.

All three mechanisms result in the delivery of unwanted material to the lysosome for degradation and recycling.

In most experimental models, increased autophagy is seen in mutations with delayed ageing, and vice versa. However, it should be noted that there are some models in which 'excessive' autophagy shortens lifespan. The importance of lysosomal function is seen in clinical diseases. Major lysosomal defects usually present in infancy, e.g. Pompe disease, where lysosomal glycogen cannot be degraded and accumulates in the lysosomes. Less dramatic age-related declines in autophagy may contribute to common age-related findings such as fat accumulation in hepatocytes and pathology such as metabolic dysfunction-associated steatotic liver disease (MASLD).

The role of autophagy in proteostasis has been studied in more detail because of the importance of removing soluble oligomers – which may be toxic – and aggregated misfolded proteins, which occur in some diseases associated with ageing, such as Alzheimer's disease.

In *C. elegans*, *Drosophila*, and mice, genetic or pharmacological manipulations that increase autophagy generally reduce protein aggregation and associated pathology and improve longevity, whereas interventions that impair autophagy result in more protein aggregation and shorten lifespan.

Autophagy also plays a role in removing other macromolecules. Glycation, the non-enzymatic reaction of free-reducing sugars with amino groups on nucleic acids, proteins, and lipids, leads to the formation of advanced glycation end products (AGEs). These glycated molecules can lose function, be involved in cross-linking, or activate inflammation, ROS generation, and apoptosis by binding with their receptor, RAGE. Autophagy has a role in removing AGEs.

Impaired autophagy may result in impaired mitophagy, contributing to stem-cell decline and failure to clear nucleic acid fragments, which might contribute to autoimmunity.

11. Dysbiosis

The normal human adult gut contains about 10^{14} bacterial cells with more than 1,000 different bacterial species. The four bacterial phyla of Firmicutes, Bacteroides, Proteobacteria and Actinobacteria account for 98% of microorganisms. These include bacteria that are protective as well as some that could be potentially harmful.

When they are in balance, the microflora provide:

- A barrier effect or resistance to colonisation.
- Several metabolic functions, such as producing short-chain fatty acids from undigestible fibres, which have local effects on the colon wall.
- Systemic effects, particularly on the immune system after absorption.

Ageing is associated with a variable degree of gut microbiome dysbiosis (imbalance) due to the loss of beneficial bacteria, overgrowth of pathogenic bacteria, or loss of bacterial diversity. This can lead to barrier dysfunction, leading to a higher systemic level of bacterial endotoxins, which may be a driver of inflammageing, as described below. Italian and Chinese centenarians were found to have a more diverse and less pro-inflammatory microbiota than healthy older people.

12. Chronic inflammation

Acute inflammation is an essential response to injury, enabling tissue repair. However, a common feature of ageing tissues is low-level chronic inflammation, known as inflammageing. This is believed to further drive the ageing process. Chronic inflammation appears to be more common in older people with frailty and sarcopaenia.

Inflammageing is mediated by:

- Soluble mediators, including the range of cytokines and other components of the SASP.
- Cells such as macrophages, microglia, and T cells.

Older people typically have higher serum CRP, IL-6, and TNF-alpha (tumour necrosis factor) but worse adaptive immunity, particularly reduced T helper cell function and poorer T cell responses. Thymic involution and attenuated T-cell-mediated immunity predispose to the reactivation of quiescent infections, such as TB and varicella. There seems to be a decline in delayed-type skin hypersensitivity reactions to injected antigens (anergy) in many frail, aged subjects. Autoantibodies occur more often (e.g. antiphospholipid antibodies, rheumatoid factor) in older people, but their significance is uncertain.

A variety of stimuli may sustain inflammageing including pathogens (non-self) – although the inflammation is usually described as 'sterile' as no pathogens are detectable, endogenous cell debris and aberrant molecules (self), and the gut microbiota (quasi-self). Excess nutrients are also thought to drive chronic inflammation in disordered metabolism, a parallel process known as metaflammation.

Ageing tissues

Ageing tissues are composed of ageing tissue-specific cells and ageing connective tissue. Ageing connective tissues have extensive cross-linkages due to chemical changes, e.g. disulphide bonds in collagen and elastin, which cause increased stiffness and reduced elasticity or compliance, especially in the skin, elastic laminae of the blood vessels, tendons, and the lens of the eye. All the inputs and outputs from the tissue, e.g. arterioles, venules, lymphatics, and nerves, have their own ageing processes.

Declining function

Many physiological parameters decline with age, but the magnitude of the decline is hard to estimate. Data is usually based on cross-sectional rather than longitudinal studies, and the elderly cohort will include more individuals with diseases that may affect function, e.g. impairment of renal function because of hypertension or diabetes, or whose sedentary lifestyle in retirement has caused cardiorespiratory fitness to decline through disuse. To be attributable to ageing per se, a phenomenon must be universal, intrinsic, and progressive. Watching the London Marathon will reveal that many 70- or even 80-year-olds are fitter than most people in their 30s and 40s

Endpiece

The science of ageing has exploded in the last 30 years but is an exceptionally confusing field. The world's bestselling popular book on ageing is *Lifespan: Why We Age and Why We Don't Have To*, coauthored by David Sinclair, Professor of Genetics at Harvard. It is worth reading a cool review of the book by Professor Charles Brenner. Brenner highlights problems that arise when positive results are feted and negative ones are ignored. It is a cautionary tale; the search for the elixir of life is now funded by billions of dollars, and social media ensures that everyone can 'benefit' from the latest advances, for a price. Money might be better spent on a good diet, exercise, maintaining a healthy weight, getting enough sleep, the increasingly occasional glass of red wine, and finding socially stimulating hobbies to enjoy.

📖 REFERENCES AND FURTHER READING

Gavrilov L, Gavrilova NS (2004). *Why we fall apart.* https://engineering. purdue.edu/~ee650/downloads/Why-we-fall-apart.pdf. https://www. researchgate.net/publication/3000762_Why_we_fall_apart_Engineering%27s_reliability_theory_explains_human_aging#fullTextFileContent

Weinert BT, Timiras PS (2003) Review of genetic theories of ageing *J. Appl. Physiol.* https://doi.org/10.1152/japplphysiol.00288.2003.

Oshima J, Martin GM, Hisama FM (2021) *Werner syndrome* - Gene reviews. https://www.ncbi.nlm.nih.gov/books/NBK1514

Gordon LB, Brown WT, Collins FS (2019) *Hutchinson-Gilford Progeria Syndrome* - Gene reviews. https://www.ncbi.nlm.nih.gov/books/NBK1121

Aging Atlas Consortium. Aging Atlas: a multi-omics database for aging biology. *Nucleic Acids Res.*, gkaa894. doi: 10.1093/nar/gkaa894.

Campisi J (2003) Cellular senescence and apoptosis: how cellular responses might influence aging phenotypes. *Experimental Gerontology* 38: 5–11. https://www.sciencedirect.com/science/article/pii/S0531556502001523

Cattaneo M, Beltrami AP, Thomas AC, et al. (2023) The longevity-associated BPIFB4 gene supports cardiac function and vascularization in ageing cardiomyopathy. *Cardiovasc. Res.*: cvad008. doi: 10.1093/cvr/cvad008.

Heinz M, Cone N, Da Rosa G, et al. (2017) Examining supportive evidence for psychosocial theories of aging within the oral history narratives of centenarians. *Societies* 7:8. doi:10.3390/soc7020008.

Thompson RC, Allam AH, Lombardi GP (2013) Atherosclerosis across 4000 years of human history: the Horus study of four ancient populations. *Lancet* 381:1211–1222. doi: 10.1016/S0140-6736(13)60598-X

López-Otín C, Blasco MA, Partridge L, et al. (2013) The hallmarks of aging – leading edge review. *Cell* 153:1194–1217. doi: 10.1016/j.cell.2013.05.039.

López-Otín C, Blasco MA, Partridge L, et al. (2023) Hallmarks of aging: an expanding universe. *Cell* 186:243–278. doi: 10.1016/j.cell.2022.11.001.

Kennedy BK, Berger SL, Brunet A (2014) Geroscience: linking aging to chronic disease (the seven pillars of aging). *Cell* 159:709–713. doi: 10.1016/j.cell.2014.10.039.

Goh J, Wong E, Soh J, et al. (2021) Targeting the molecular and cellular pillars of human aging with exercise. *FEBS J.* doi: 10.1111/febs.16337.

Singh PP, Demmitt BA, Nath RD et al. (2019) The genetics of aging: a vertebrate perspective. *Cell* 177:200–220. https://pubmed.ncbi.nlm.nih.gov/30901541/

Vaiserman A, Krasnienkov D (2021) Telomere length as a marker of biological age: state-of-the-art, open issues, and future perspectives. *Front Genet.* 11. doi: 10.3389/fgene.2020.630186.

Jin M, Huang JD (2023) New mechanism to promote long-term T-cell immunity by telomere transfer from antigen-presenting cells. Cell Mol. Immunol. 20:117–118. doi: 10.1038/s41423-022-00949-z.

Pérez-Torres ME, Soto EV, Castrejón-Tellez E et al. (2020) Oxidative, reductive, and nitrosative stress effects on epigenetics and on posttranslational modification of enzymes in cardiometabolic diseases. *Oxid. Med. Cell. Longevity.* doi: 10.1155/2020/8819719.

Bernabeu E, McCartney DL, Gadd DA, et al. (2023) Refining epigenetic prediction of chronological and biological age. *Genome Med.* 15:12. doi: 10.1186/s13073-023-01161-y.

Hoppe T, Cohen E (2020) Organismal protein homeostasis mechanisms. *Genetics* 215:889–901. doi: 10.1534/genetics.120.301283.

Pan H, Finkel T (2017) Key proteins and pathways that regulate lifespan. *J. Biol. Chem.* 292:6452–6460. doi: 10.1074/jbc.R116.771915

Saxton RA, Sabatini DM (2017) mTOR signaling in growth, metabolism, and disease. Cell 168:960–976. doi: 10.1016/j.cell.2017.02.004.

Kumari R, Jat P (2021) Mechanisms of cellular senescence: cell cycle arrest and senescence associated secretory phenotype. *Front. Cell Dev. Biol.* 9. doi: 10.3389/fcell.2021.645593.

Zhu Y, Langhi Prata LGP, Wissler Gerdes EO (2022) Orally-active, clinically-translatable senolytics restore α-Klotho in mice and humans. *eBioMedicine* 77:103912. doi: 10.1016/j.ebiom.2022.103912.

Mehdipour M, Amiri P, Liu C, et al. (2022) Small-animal blood exchange is an emerging approach for systemic aging research. *Nat. Protoc.* 17:2469–2493. doi: 10.1038/s41596-022-00731-5.

Aman Y, Schmauck-Medina T, Hansen M, et al. (2021) Autophagy in healthy aging and disease. *Nat. Aging* 1:634–650. doi: 10.1038/s43587-021-00098-4.

Ragonnaud E, Biragyn A (2021) Gut microbiota as the key controllers of healthy aging of elderly people. *Immun. Ageing* 18:2. doi: 10.1186/s12979-020-00213-w.

Sinclair DA, LaPlante MD (2019). *Why We Age and Why We Don't Have To.* Simon and Schuster. ISBN 1501191977, 9781501191978.

Brenner C (2023) A science-based review of the world's best-selling book on aging. *Arch. Gerontol. Geriatr.* 104:104825. https://doi.org/10.1016/j.archger.2022.104825.

All websites were accessed in August 2024.

4

Core geriatric medicine

Distinctive features of illness in older patients

Illness in older people is usually a continuum of conditions found in middle age, but the impact of the illness will be modified by the context of ageing physiology, loss of fitness, and the person's social situation (see Figure 4.1).

Ageing physiology

Ageing changes are seen in *all organs* (go through the body in your mind), including the brain, special senses, and peripheral nerves. For each organ, think about the specific cell types, connective tissue, and blood supply. Typically, ageing tissues show cell loss, resulting in atrophy, scarring with fibrosis, depletion of stem cells, loss of elasticity in the connective tissue, and atheroma in the blood supply. The pattern and extent of the changes depend on genetics and the accumulated effects of environment, lifestyle, and chance, so in a group of octogenarians, there will be more variation than in a group of young adults. Cellular changes result in a gradual physiological decline. Impaired homeostasis is revealed by physiological stressors and results in problems when the environment becomes more challenging, or pathology supervenes. For example:

- Fasting glucose is minimally higher in older people, but after a meal, the rise is greater.
- Older people are more susceptible to extreme heat or cold.
- In extreme old age, a minimal challenge, such as maintaining BP on standing up may be overwhelming.
- A minor infection may result in delirium and acute kidney injury.

Think about the variable effects of ageing when you do ward rounds. You will see people in their 60s who have multiple problems, and some very sprightly 85-year-olds.

Fitness and thresholds

Older people show great variation in fitness, from exceptional individuals who run marathons in extreme old age to those who struggle with walking and need help with activities of daily living.

- Most physiological parameters, such as muscle strength, decline from adulthood.
- Because of considerable reserve, this is often not apparent if an individual has an undemanding lifestyle. However, eventually, a threshold is reached, and a task can no longer be performed, e.g. getting out of a chair without arms.

- The concept is important. It explains why even limited exercise in old age can be beneficial, as it may keep performance just above a threshold, and why rehabilitation can restore function (see Figure 4.2).

Social factors

- There have been very marked changes in society, even since the first edition of this book!
- Most women work. The younger generation has less time available for caring for older relatives, although many provide hours of care (see Chapter 2).
- 'Old' covers a wide age range, sometimes arbitrarily divided into 'young old' and 'old old', but the definition of what is considered 'old' varies.
- Old age is still a time of loss of family, friends, income, housing, mobility, independence, status, health, and life itself. There may be practical solutions for some issues. However, often what is most appreciated is support and a little of your time to hear about how things were.
- Changing attitudes towards professions (the church and the law, as well as medicine), numerous scandals, and concerns about funding have made people much less trusting of medical care.
- There is huge variation between people of the same age – silver surfers with high disposable income and opportunities for travel versus people who are impoverished, or chronically sick, and those with unexpected caring responsibilities. There is a strong relationship between health and social deprivation (see Chapter 2). The effect of an illness on an individual is affected by their social capital as well as their material wealth.

Multiple pathologies and aetiologies

Older people often have more than one disease. There are several reasons for this:

- The prevalence of many diseases increases with age (e.g. stroke, Parkinson's disease, Alzheimer's disease), so the fact that an older person has several diseases may simply reflect this.
- Some chronic diseases have complications affecting several systems (e.g. diabetes may lead to heart, eye, kidney and nerve problems) or predispose to other disorders (e.g. infections).
- A single risk factor may predispose an individual to several diseases (e.g. smokers are more likely to have chronic bronchitis, oral and lung cancer, heart disease, strokes, gangrene, macular degeneration, osteoporosis and bladder cancer).
- One problem may have several causes; e.g. falls are usually multifactorial (previous stroke+cognitive impairment+poor vision+osteoarthritis of the knees, etc.).

Geriatric Medicine and Elderly Care: Lecture Notes, Ninth Edition. Claire G. Nicholl, K. Jane Wilson, and Shaun D'Souza.
© 2025 John Wiley & Sons Ltd. Published 2025 by John Wiley & Sons Ltd.
Companion website: www.wiley.com/go/lecturenotesgeriatricmedicine9e

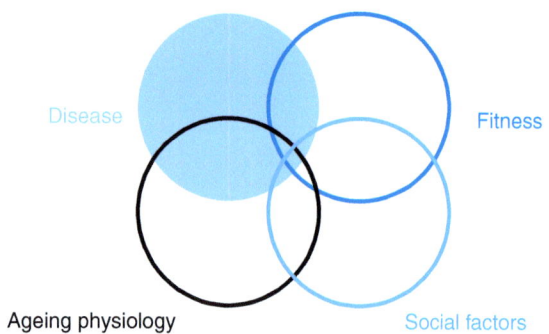

Figure 4.1 Interaction between disease, ageing physiology and the individual's fitness and social situation.

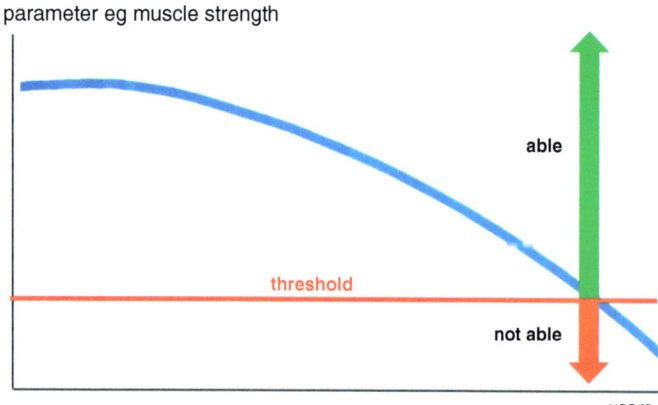

Figure 4.2 The importance of thresholds.

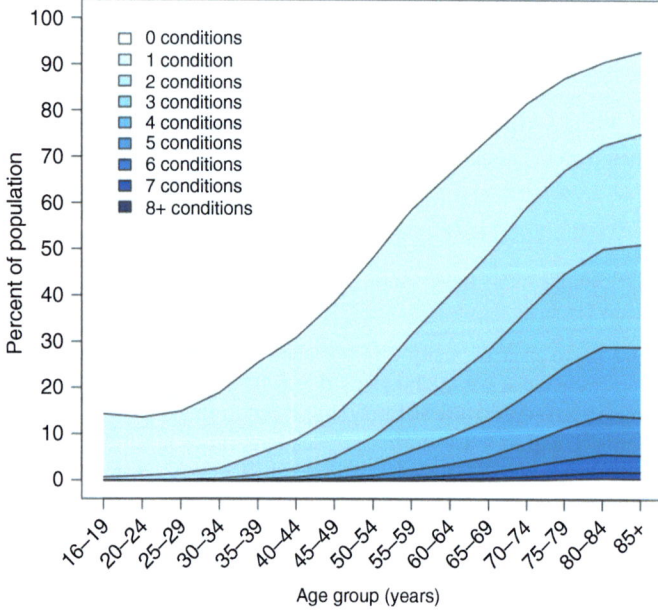

Figure 4.3 Number of chronic conditions by age group – Schiøtz et al. (2017) / Springer Nature / CC BY 4.0.

- The usual situation is that an older person has multiple comorbidities. Data on multimorbidity in Denmark from a cross-sectional prevalence study of 1.4 million people is shown in Figure 4.3. More than half of the population aged 65+ had at least two chronic conditions.

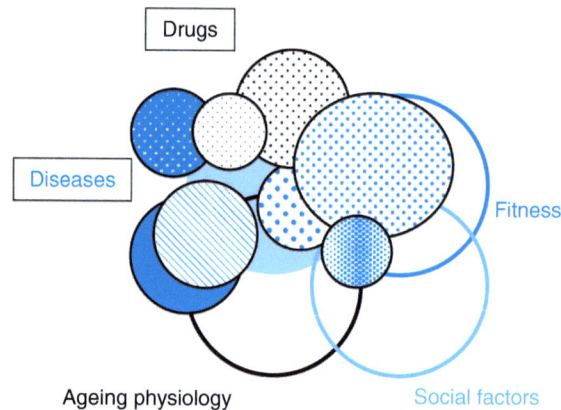

Figure 4.4 The complex interaction between ageing physiology, social factors and fitness with multiple pathologies and the drugs that are prescribed.

Multimorbidity was more prevalent in women and people with low educational attainment.
- As discussed later, multiple diseases lead to the prescription of many drugs (see Figure 4.4).

Risk factors

Risk factors for disease may have different predictive values in middle age and old age. The independent centenarian who still smokes and the 85-year-old with a cholesterol level of 8 mmol/L presumably have 'protective' genes. Hypertension has been established as a risk factor for cardiovascular disease into the ninth decade, but over 30 years since the first drug trials which included older people, there is still debate about who to treat and the target blood pressure.

Susceptibility to disease

Nosocomial *C. difficile* is more common in frail older people than in middle-aged people, so antibiotic formularies typically differ according to age. The most striking recent example has been the dramatic association between increasing age and death from COVID-19.

Cohort effects

- There has been a higher rate of TB in UK-born older people, thought to be due in part to reactivation of the disease in survivors from the pre-drug era, whose immunity declined with age, but numbers have been small and are falling as the cohort dies.
- Post-polio syndrome will also disappear.
- Age-standardised mesothelioma rates are finally beginning to fall in Europe and the US.
- If COVID infection has widespread long-term sequelae (there is some data for changes in the brain), this will pose a new challenge.

Multiple medications

As older people have multiple medical problems, they are often on multiple drugs (see Chapter 5).

Differential diagnosis

Although the range of possible diagnoses may be similar at any age, age is important in deciding what is most likely. For example, the commonest causes of fits, jaundice, and anaemia will be different in neonates, children, young adults, and older people (see Table 4.1).

Table 4.1 Probable causes of fits and jaundice in different age groups.

Age	Probable cause	
	Fits	**Jaundice**
Neonate	Birth trauma and hypoxia	Physiological
Baby/toddler	Fever	Biliary atresia
Child/teenager	Epilepsy	Hepatitis A
Young adult	Drugs, alcohol, or withdrawal	Drugs and alcohol
Middle age	Brain tumour	Gallstones
Old age	Stroke	Carcinoma of the pancreas

Altered response to disease

Many older people present in the same way as middle-aged people, e g crushing central chest pain in an MI. However, this is not always the case, making diagnoses in frail older people a challenge. There may be:

- Missing symptoms, e.g. lack of pleuritic pain, fever and thirst in pneumonia.
- Missing signs, e.g. lack of neck stiffness in meningitis.
- Non-specific presentation (see frailty syndromes below).

Consequences of immobility

The presenting condition is often complicated by the consequences of immobility:

- Incontinence.
- Dehydration.
- Pressure sores.
- Hypothermia.
- DVT.
- Hypostatic pneumonia.
- Muscle wasting.
- Loss of BP regulation.

Frailty

Frailty is a clinically recognisable state of vulnerability that results from an ageing-associated decline in functional reserve.

Frailty is defined as a syndrome of physiological decline in older people, which makes them particularly vulnerable to adverse outcomes and deterioration in physical health after major stressors.

- Frail older patients often present with an increased burden of symptoms, including weakness and fatigue, medical complexity, and reduced tolerance to medical and surgical interventions.
- An individual's degree of frailty is not static; it can improve, but a cycle of worsening frailty is more common.
- Older people with frailty risk dramatic declines in well-being after a minor event.

- There is a wide range of prevalence figures for frailty, depending on the population and definition used. Typical figures are that >10% of people aged 65+ and 35% of those aged 85+ living at home, and around 50% in a nursing home (probably now higher as more people stay at home for longer) live with frailty.
- Risk factors for frailty include being female, having a low educational level, being from a low socioeconomic group, multimorbidity and having a BMI < 20 or >30 (note the 'fat frail' tend to be missed).
- Patients with frailty are likely to present with one of the 'frailty syndromes' ('geriatric giants').
- People do not like being labelled as 'frail'.

Models of frailty

There are two main models:

- **The phenotype model** is based on five characteristics: unintentional weight loss, exhaustion, low energy expenditure, slow walking speed, and weak grip strength (Fried et al.). Using this, people can be classified into broad groups as fit (none of the 5 characteristics), prefrail (1–2), or frail (3–5). Sarcopaenia is discussed in Chapter 10.
- **The cumulative deficit model** includes a variety of symptoms, signs, disabilities and diseases (Rockwood).

Frailty, by either definition, predicts disability, hospitalisation, and death. Frailty, disability and multimorbidity overlap but are not synonymous.

Assessing frailty

Rockwood devised a visual Clinical Frailty Scale (CFS), which is self-explanatory (see Figure 4.5). NHS England has taken it up, and it is widely used in hospitals for individual patients and clinical research. It can be carried out by all members of the multidisciplinary team (MDT) with minimal training. Other assessments (see Appendix) include the PRISMA 7 questionnaire (patient-reported), the Timed Up and Go test, and gait speed (both have good sensitivity but poor specificity, so they are good for ruling out frailty).

The English GP contract has mandated the identification and management of those aged ≥65 with frailty in primary care since 2017. To manage the workload, an Electronic Frailty Index (eFI) is used. The eFI is based on the cumulative deficit model and includes 36 deficit variables (clinical signs, symptoms, diseases, disabilities, and impairments), which are obtained from primary care electronic health records.

- The data is collected routinely and already in a database, so this is a rapid, cheap method of stratifying the population.
- However, this population screening tool has been used to label individuals. A significant number of older people are now coded as 'frail' on their GP records. This was not the intention – when the eFI identifies an individual who 'may be living with severe or moderate frailty' they should have a clinical assessment to confirm this (NHS England).
- In a study of 350 community-dwelling older people, with a median age of 80, there was only a moderate correlation between the eFI and both the CFS (ρ = 0.59, 95% CI 0.49 to 0.65) and phenotype model (ρ = 0.51, 95% CI 0.42 to 0.59).
- Data on over two million patients in the Royal College of General Practitioners' network using eFI gives a prevalence of frailty in 10% of adults aged 50–64 (moderate to severe in 3%) and 70% in adults aged 75–84 (moderate to severe in 30%).
- Studies have **NOT** shown benefits from population screening for frailty, perhaps because too many people are identified as frail, and frailty is so complex.
- The evidence for treating frailty is limited – there is some benefit from exercise but little evidence for nutrition. Amongst the drug

Clinical Frailty Scale

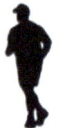 **1 Very Fit** - People who are robust, active, energetic and motivated. These people commonly exercise regularly. They are among the fittest for their age.

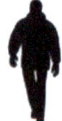 **2 Well** - People who have no active disease symptoms but are less fit than category 1. Often, they exercise or are very active occasionally, e.g. seasonally.

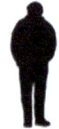 **3 Managing Well** - People whose medical problems are well controlled, but are not regularly active beyond routine walking.

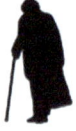 **4 Vulnerable** - While not dependent on others for daily help, often symptoms limit activities. A common complaint is being "slowed up", and/or being tired during the day.

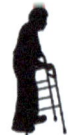 **5 Mildly Frail** - These people often have more evident slowing, and need help in high order IADLs (finances, transportation, heavy housework, medications). Typically, mild frailty progressively impairs shopping and walking outside alone, meal preparation and housework.

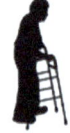 **6 Moderately Frail** - People need help with all outside activities and with keeping house. Inside, they often have problems with stairs and need help with bathing and might need minimal assistance (cuing, standby) with dressing.

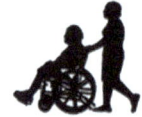 **7 Severely Frail** - Completely dependent for personal care, from whatever cause (physical or cognitive). Even so, they seem stable and not at high risk of dying (within ~ 6 months).

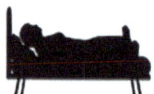 **8 Very Severely Frail** - Completely dependent, approaching the end of life. Typically, they could not recover even from a minor illness.

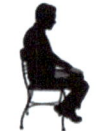 **9 Terminally Ill** - Approaching the end of life. This category applies to people with a life expectancy <6 months, who are not otherwise evidently frail.

Scoring frailty in people with dementia

The degree of frailty corresponds to the degree of dementia. Common **symptoms in mild dementia** include forgetting the details of a recent event, though still remembering the event itself, repeating the same question/story and social withdrawal.

In **moderate dementia**, recent memory is very impaired, even though they seemingly can remember their past life events well. They can do personal care with prompting.

In **severe dementia,** they cannot do personal care without help.

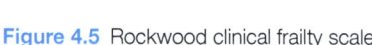

Figure 4.5 Rockwood clinical frailty scale.

candidates, vitamin D should be replaced in those with low levels and is recommended for all adults in the UK in the winter. Testosterone should be reserved for hypogonadal men if the benefits outweigh the risks, and growth hormone should not be used.

However, recognising frailty in an individual should alert the doctor that their patient may decline rapidly and prompt dialogue with the patient. Targeted interventions could include falls assessment, medicine review, and anticipatory care planning. It may improve the recognition that a non-specific illness may have a serious cause and potentially a poor outcome.

Frailty syndromes

Non-specific presentations are common. The 'geriatric giants' – the big 'I's – or 'frailty syndromes' as they have been rebadged – are commonly seen in frail older people in the ED:

- **I**ntellectual failure (acute or chronic confusion).
- **I**ncontinence (if this is new, why?).
- **I**mmobility ('off her feet').
- **I**nstability (falls).
- **I**atrogenic disease.
- **I**nability to look after oneself (functional decline).
- **I**nanition (exhaustion due to malnutrition, similar to 'failure to thrive' in paediatrics).

All these vague and dull-sounding clinical pictures, often labelled 'social problems' in the ED or medical records, are almost never due to social problems and can be due to a wide range of serious and treatable conditions – if you look – such as MI, stroke, PD, etc.

The expectation dichotomy

Older people sometimes have quite different expectations and wishes about their health from members of their own family. There can also be very different attitudes towards serious illness between families.

Late presentation

Some older people present very late in their illness. They may have a limited medical understanding or be frightened of the implications of symptoms, so that treatable conditions or warning signs, e.g. urinary incontinence, rectal bleeding or swollen ankles, are overlooked. The difficulty of accessing primary care without the internet and the reduction in face-to-face consultations may be especially challenging. Older people may have poor expectations of health care, fuelled by friends and family, earlier experience of health care professionals, and increasingly, the poor service. It might now be rare to hear, 'What do you expect at your age?' but that is the reality. The inadequacies of health care in the UK became clear to many in 2023. It seemed to become accepted that an old person who had fallen would be left on the floor for hours waiting for an ambulance, despite data linking both a long lie and delay to surgery for a fractured hip to death.

Something must be done!

Conversely, some older patients – and often their families – have very unrealistic expectations. Not all families are prepared to accept that a visibly frail 96-year-old should be allowed to die peacefully at home, managed by their GP (RIP Queen Elizabeth II), and demand admission for investigation, IV antibiotics, renal dialysis or even intensive care.

The clinical assessment of the older patient

Just as with younger patients, this consists of history, examination, and investigations.

Occam's razor or Lear's beard?

In younger adults, Occam's razor may be applicable – a single disease may be sought to explain all the symptoms and findings. However, in a frail older person, it is more helpful to think of 'Lear's beard' (see Figure 4.6). The science of clinical geriatrics is to find and classify all the nesting birds; the art is deciding which ones to deal with, and how, and which ones to leave alone.

The complexity of the typical frail older patient and the single-problem focus that is used in most other specialities led Rubenstein and others to codify the clinical approach traditionally used in geriatric medicine and develop the concept of comprehensive geriatric assessment.

Comprehensive geriatric assessment

Comprehensive geriatric assessment (CGA) is usually defined as a multidimensional, interdisciplinary diagnostic process which identifies medical, social, and functional needs to develop a coordinated and integrated plan for treatment and long-term follow-up. Its use needs to be modified according to the setting. In primary care, the information can be gathered over several visits, and in the ED, the focus must be on the urgent aspects, but it is always holistic. Evidence for its efficacy is best for patients in hospital.

- Older people who had CGA rather than routine care were more likely to be living at home and less likely to be admitted to a nursing home a year after admission but there was no difference in mortality or need for help for everyday activities (Ellis et al., 29 studies, 13,766 people over 65 in 9 countries).
- Older people who had CGA in the community did not have a significantly lower risk of death or nursing home admission, but there was low-quality evidence for a lower risk of hospital admission (Briggs et al., 21 studies, 7893 frail older people in 10 countries across 4 continents).

CGA involves data gathering across 5 domains and favours the use of standardised scores (see Table 4.2).

History taking

The approach is the same as in other specialities with some nuances:

- Ask the patient themselves, but they have more history to remember and may be confused, so corroborate with the ambulance sheet (often the most accurate) and old records.
- You will often need a collateral history: consider calling the family/warden/GP. Ask permission if possible, but otherwise, this is in their best interests.
- Think about how to address your patient: you will seem impossibly young and informally dressed for a doctor! A clear introduction and formal approach will help. This may need repeating each time you see the patient.
- Enable your patient to communicate: for lip readers, make sure you are not in front of a window and that your face is lit, use a communicator if needed or write down key questions, and use short direct questions if there is confusion. If language is an issue, a staff member may be able to translate, but using a translating service is best practice.

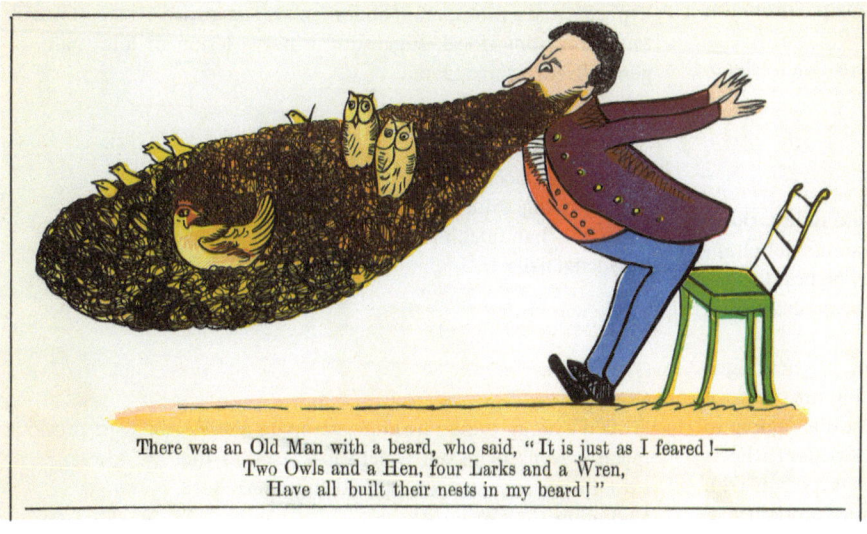

There was an Old Man with a beard, who said, "It is just as I feared!—
Two Owls and a Hen, four Larks and a Wren,
Have all built their nests in my beard!"

Figure 4.6 'Lear's beard'. *Source*: Chronicle/Alamy Stock Photo.

Table 4.2 Domains of CGA.

Domain	Components	Suitable tools
Physical health	Main diagnosis	History, exam and investigations
	Co-morbid conditions	Clinical frailty score
	Medications	STOPP/START
	Nutrition	Weight
		MUST score or
		Mini nutritional assessment (MNA)
Psychological and cognitive health	Cognition	AT4/MoCA
	Mood	Geriatric Depression Score
	Quality of life	SF36
Functional capacity	Activities of daily living	Barthel
	Continence and skin	Waterlow
	Gait and balance	Tinetti
	Activity status	Timed up and go
Social networks	Support networks	Social support scale
	Care resources	
Environment	Home Facilities	Liaison with family
	Telehealth	

STOPP/START, screening tool of older persons' prescriptions and screening tool to alert to right treatment; MUST, malnutrition universal screening tool; AT4 - rapid screen for delirium; MoCA, Montreal cognitive assessment; SF36, short form 36 - a health staus survey.

- Family history is less relevant if you have lived into your 80s.
- A detailed social history is more important.
  - What could they do before they became ill? (essential for rehabilitation)
  - Tobacco and alcohol history (older people may be regular drinkers)
  - Home environment and support (e.g. stairs – is there a toilet up and downstairs? – details of aids, grabrails, care packages, and informal care). (You may feel that this is 'not your job' but this knowledge may help you get an older person out of an over-crowded ED and avoid admission.)
  - Driving and foreign travel (the most unlikely-looking patients may do both; malaria has been misdiagnosed as 'flu' in older sunseekers returning from the Gambia).
- A full medication history (prescribed and bought 'over the counter' – OTC)
- Systems review, including cognition, mood, continence, falls, sleep, and pain.

Examination

Approach your patient gently and explain what you are doing. Don't start by pulling the sheet off a confused old lady to examine her chest, as she will grab it back to preserve her modesty. It may be best to start with her feet – you will learn a lot; she will get used to you examining her – and you can work upwards.

Learn what is typical of a frail older patient. Some physical signs have different significance, e.g. small pupils in a young unconscious adult are likely to be due to an opiate overdose, whilst this finding in a nonagenarian may reflect the usual pupil size in a patient who is unconscious for another reason. Impaired upgaze in a person with parkinsonism in their 50s is a strong indicator of progressive supranuclear

palsy (PSP) but is non-specific in old age. Likewise, wasting of the small muscles of the hand is more often due to disuse than neck pathology.

Gait

- Aided or unaided.
- Foot drop.
- Lack of arm swing.
- Shuffling or striding.
- Stable or unstable.
- Difficulty up/down from the chair.
- Parkinsonian or multi-infarct.

Face

- Parkinsonian (lack of expression).
- Depression.
- Hypothyroidism, anaemia, and vitiligo.
- Angular stomatitis (often due to ill-fitting dentures).
- Orofacial dyskinesia.
- Ptosis: symmetrical ('age-related') or unilateral (eye surgery or Horner's).
- Basal-cell carcinoma.
- Facial palsy.

Sensory loss

Simple tests of acuity and fields, especially in fallers.

Conversation

- Dyspnoea.
- A good account of circumstances, plausible but with obvious lacunae, or very limited.
- Drowsiness or inattention may suggest delirium.
- Mood.
- Hearing: repeat whispered numbers; a hearing aid that doesn't whistle when handled needs a new battery.
- Speech: dysphasia, dysarthria, dysphonia.
- Emotional lability.
- Abnormal content.

Musculoskeletal system

- Stiff neck.
- Tentative handshake of rotator-cuff atrophy, difficulty getting in/out of sleeves.
- Stiff hips/knees.
- Kyphosis and a protuberant abdomen are suggestive of osteoporosis.
- Muscle wasting: focal, suggesting a nerve lesion or joint pain, or generalised in sarcopaenia.

Self-neglect

- Dirty hands/face/body.
- Dirty clothing, evidence of incontinence.
- Unshaven, hair unkempt.
- Neglected nails.

Nutrition

- Oral health.
- Obesity.
- Protein–energy undernutrition: compare the weight with previous records, signs of recent weight loss, clothes that are too large, or extreme cachexia with a scaphoid abdomen.
- Hydration.

Skin

- Ulcers: due to pressure, diabetes, venous, or arterial disease.
- Scratch marks suggesting pruritis (most commonly due to dry skin)
- Abnormal bruising (anticoagulants, low platelets, frail capillaries, steroids, falls, abuse).

Feet

- Oedema (immobility, right heart failure, low albumin, calcium channel blockers).
- Poor perfusion (check pulses).
- Fungal infection (treat this as its a portal of entry for cellulitis, especially in diabetes and peripheral vascular disease).
- Corns, ingrowing toenails, and onychogryphosis all make walking painful.

Formal examination

- Extrasystoles: common and seldom significant, but AF is important to find and manage.
- Neglected breast cancer.
- Displaced apex beat: often due to chest deformity, which also affects the typical radiation of murmurs.
- Lying and standing BP.
- Abdomen: ribs tend to sit over the pelvis, so it is hard to ballot kidneys, distended bladder, and faecal impaction.
- Reduced up-gaze: common, doubtful significance.

Investigations

Be systematic – think *why* do we do tests?

1 General screening (often done in older patients because of multimorbidity).
2 Confirm diagnosis.
3 Look for complications.
4 Baseline for therapy
 - TIP for exams – work your way through the labs.
   ○ Full blood count FBC
   ○ Urea electrolytes and creatine (U&Es), glucose (G), liver function (LFTs), bone function (BFTs), thyroid stimulating hormone (TSH), and C reactive protein (CRP).
   ○ Urine dip, blood cultures, if pyrexial
   ○ CXR, other imaging, as indicated.
   ○ ECG or ECHO if there is heart failure.
 - FBC, U&Es, G, LFTs, BFTs, TSH, CRP, urine dip, CXR, and ECG would be a reasonable screen for most older people admitted to the hospital. Add specific tests for diagnosis. Add iron studies, B12, and folate for anaemia; a myeloma screen; ESR and PSA (for men) for back pain; B12, folate and CT/MRI head for cognitive impairment; and a lipid screen and HbA1c for vascular disease.

Problem list

At the end of your history and examination, write a problem list. This should include your main diagnosis, comorbidities, and functional problems. It must include what matters to the patient. If you are unsure of the cause of a finding, say so, e.g. 'large bruise on the left forearm, cause unclear'. This is a 'work in progress', so it will not be perfect, but you must document your thoughts. The list will be amended by your seniors, as results come back, and by the team.

Advantages and disadvantages of 'labels'

Be circumspect before labelling people. It is part of the doctor's job; the label usually helps the patient to understand what is causing their symptoms and helps clinicians to manage the condition. For example, the Alzheimer's Society campaigns for people with dementia to be given a diagnosis, as without this they cannot access support. However, labels can be unhelpful: a 93-year-old care home resident with impaired glucose tolerance labelled 'diabetic' may be refused Christmas cake. It is difficult to shake off an incorrect label, so, if in doubt, remain descriptive, e.g. 'breathless with a shadow on CXR', pending further investigation.

Management plan

The end of your clerking must include your management plan; this is easier and more likely to be comprehensive if you have a good problem list.

The multidisciplinary process

CGA involves input from other members of the MDT. They will assess the patient, and discussion and planning will take place in regular ward MDT meetings. There will usually be daily brief meetings between the doctors, nurses, and therapists, and longer meetings a couple of times a week. The size of the team and disciplines will vary, but typically include a junior and senior doctor, a nurse, a physiotherapist (physio), an occupational therapist (OT), a care manager, and perhaps a pharmacist. As the junior doctor, you will be expected to give a thumbnail sketch of each patient's medical problems, progress, and outstanding investigations, contribute to the discussion (e.g. you may know the views of the patient and carers), and document the discussion and plan in the medical record.

CGA should enable the team to work with the patient to:

- Look for functional impairment amenable to intervention.
- Improve independence.
- Choose interventions to preserve the quality of life.
- Optimise the environment.
- Predict and communicate outcomes with the patient and family.
- Enable the patient to stay at home for as long as possible.
- Plan for the future.

Rehabilitation

A technically successful intervention is of limited value if the patient does not recover the ability to enjoy a worthwhile quality of life. However, rehabilitation is not always appropriate, and palliation may be the best way to manage severe disability.

Rehabilitation is defined as the restoration of the individual to their fullest physical, mental and social capability. It takes several forms:

- Restoration to full activity after a severe illness (e.g. abdominal surgery or MI).
- Restoration of maximum achievable function following a specific impairment (e.g. stroke or hip fracture or amputation).
- Facilitating the achievement of as much independence as possible despite progressive impairment (e.g. PD, and worsening hip disease).

Rehabilitation is an active process, and the MDT, including the patient and carer, must share common goals and objectives.

Principles of rehabilitation

It is essential to know what the patient could do before the current illness:

- Full assessment of the patient's problems before the process starts.
- Goals must be realistic, with defined endpoints.

- Logical step-by-step approach to achieve the set goals.
- A continuous process – 'every activity is a therapeutic opportunity', i.e. rehabilitation does not just occur face-to-face with a therapist, but with all interactions with the extended team of health care workers.
- Maintenance is needed to maintain improvement (not available on the NHS – recommend ongoing home exercises or a community group, e.g. Otago falls prevention exercises).
- If progress is not as good as anticipated, look for factors that may be interfering.

Rehabilitation settings

Rehabilitation can take place in a wide range of settings:

- Acute hospital wards (includes orthopaedic wards).
- Rehabilitation ward in an acute hospital.
- Intermediate care ward in a community hospital.
- Stroke units, wherever situated.
- Outpatient therapy departments.
- Geriatric day rehabilitation and falls unit.
- Psychiatric counterparts of the above.
- Primary-care premises.
- Care homes.
- Sheltered flats.
- Community groups, e.g. stroke clubs, keep-fit classes.
- Patient's own home (e.g. a home-based exercise programme).

Rehabilitation from an acute illness

Hospital admission is often needed for an acute illness, e.g. pneumonia, not just for investigations or IV drugs, but because the associated weakness makes patients unable to attend to their bodily needs (nutrition, fluid intake, bowel, bladder, hygiene, etc.) unassisted. They may feel too unwell to get out of bed. Unless there is adequate support at home, early admission is essential to prevent dehydration, incontinence, constipation, pressure ulcers, contractures, and loss of confidence, which would necessitate protracted rehabilitation.

However, in hospital, older people become deconditioned and may become institutionalised. 'Reablement' is low-level rehabilitation and is often sufficient to get people back to their previous level of function after an acute illness, but an older person usually needs longer to recover than a younger person. This may be obvious to the reader, but is not always obvious to the patient, family, and medical attendant.

The rehabilitation team

- Patient.
- Family and friends.
- Nurses.
- Therapists (physios, OTs, speech and language therapists – SLTs).
- Doctors.
- Care manager or discharge planner
- Pharmacists (who advises on all aspects of drugs and are especially helpful for planning drugs to take out – TTOs).
- Dietitians (assess, diagnose, and treat dietary and nutritional problems)

In specialist areas:

- Podiatrists (inpatient service often limited to those with severe diabetes and peripheral vascular disease).
- Orthotists correct problems or deformities in nerves, muscles, and bones with a range of aids, such as splints.
- Clinical psychologists (psychology degree and PhD, focus on health-related psychological difficulties).
- Prosthetists create and fit artificial limbs.

The roles of therapists

Therapists are core team members in hospital and community settings. They are experts in their areas. They use a holistic approach to assess the patient, plan and implement tailored treatment programmes, and evaluate outcomes. They often supervise therapy assistants and the nursing team to deliver treatment. They may provide advice and practical training to carers, especially if the patient has dementia.

Physiotherapy

- Physios focus on mobility and functional problems.
- If a patient can walk, this is usually regarded as the best chest physiotherapy.
- Remobilisation is achieved by suitable exercises (passive, assisted, or resisted) combined with functional exercises such as sitting, sit-to-stand, transfers and walking (see Figure 4.7).
- Provide and adjust mobility aids (see Chapter 11). Most walking aids are measured with the patient's arm hanging by their side from the wrist crease (radial styloid). Walking sticks relieve pain by taking some weight and aid balance by widening the base. A tripod is more cumbersome than a simple cane, but it stays standing if not needed temporarily. Zimmer frames need lifting, whilst rollator frames have wheels at the front and are pushed. Two frames may be needed – for upstairs and downstairs. Some frames fold. They may have baskets, trays, seats, or forearm rests (gutter frames) to take weight if hand or wrist function is limited or painful.
- Specialist areas include assessments to prevent admission from ED, falls prevention (strength and balance training), stroke, orthogeriatrics, PD, community cardiac and pulmonary rehabilitation, chronic musculoskeletal pain and prehabilitation for older people before major elective surgery.

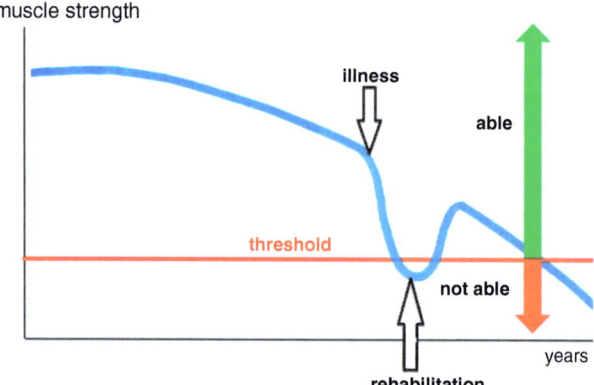

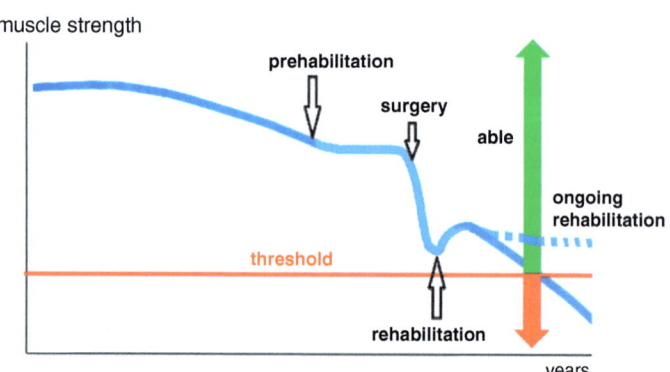

Figure 4.7 Restoring functional independence with rehabilitation and prehabilitation.

Occupational therapy

- OTs focus on promoting independence in activities of daily living (ADLs).
- The aim is to help the person recover the ability to manage day-to-day tasks. In inpatients, this tends to be basic functions such as washing, dressing, eating and toileting.
- Provide or recommend equipment or changes to the environment to enable independence (see Figures 4.8 and 4.9).
- Identify hazards at home and work with the patient and their family to overcome them.
- Specialist areas are like those above. Working in the community with people affected by stroke, acquired brain injury, and early dementia gives more opportunities for working on instrumental activities of daily living (IADLs), such as helping people manage transportation, shopping, and meal preparation.

The right equipment and environment can be game-changing. In our example, if physiotherapy cannot improve quadriceps strength enough for the person to get up from a chair with no arms, changing the chair can enable this. The family may need to buy a new chair, and the OT may provide chair raisers or advise on a chair with a rising seat. A perching stool in the kitchen may enable the person to continue preparing meals. So even when there is irremediable impairment, simple measures can reduce disability and handicap.

There are long waits for community OT. Self-help options include the Disabled Living Foundation AskSARA website, which has a free online, guided self-assessment tool with links to product suggestions and advice. Products that are well-designed and attractive are most likely to be accepted. Advice about aids is also available from Living Made Easy, Independent Living Centres, the Age UK Factsheet on disability equipment and home adaptations, and Which? Reviews.

Wheelchairs (see Chapter 11 for more detail) may be provided free on long-term loan from the NHS. In the hospital, OTs may be able to arrange for a wheelchair. In the community, the local wheelchair service will provide advice. Manual chairs are self-propelling (with big wheels) or attendant-propelled. The Red Cross may loan them. Adequate padding is crucial. There is a huge range of electric wheelchairs and mobility scooters, but older people usually buy these.

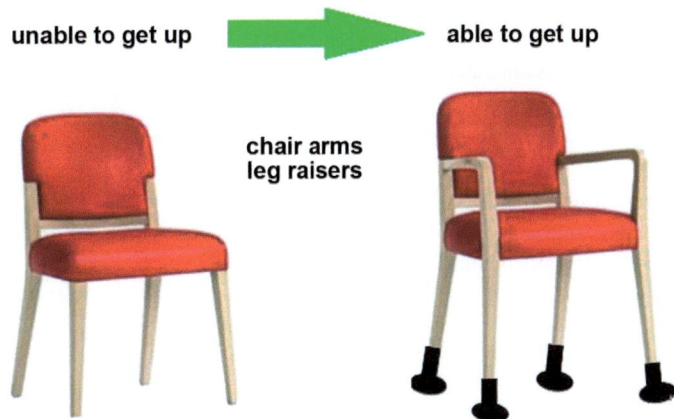

unable to get up ➡ able to get up

chair arms
leg raisers

Figure 4.9 The role of simple changes in promoting independence. *Source*: a) Foton/Adobe Stock.

Nurses, physios, and OTs work closely. If a patient is struggling to transfer, the physio will advise on whether a hoist is needed or if it is safe to transfer them with two nurses. The therapy will aim to get the person as mobile as possible, perhaps walking with a frame, but much of the practice is done by the nursing team. If a hoist is needed on discharge, the OT will check what will fit at home and arrange this.

Speech and language therapy

- SLTs focus on people with difficulty communicating, eating, drinking, and swallowing.
- Communication difficulties include dysphonia (often in PD), dysarthria and dysphasia (typically after a stroke).
- Inpatient therapy prioritises dysphagia (most often due to dementia and stroke). Bedside assessment involves looking at the patient's swallow and trialling different textures of food and drink to see which is least likely to be aspirated. However, recent evidence suggests that thickener is of limited or no benefit. Specialist tests include an x-ray of swallowing (videofluoroscopy) or a fibreoptic endoscopic evaluation of swallowing (FEES).

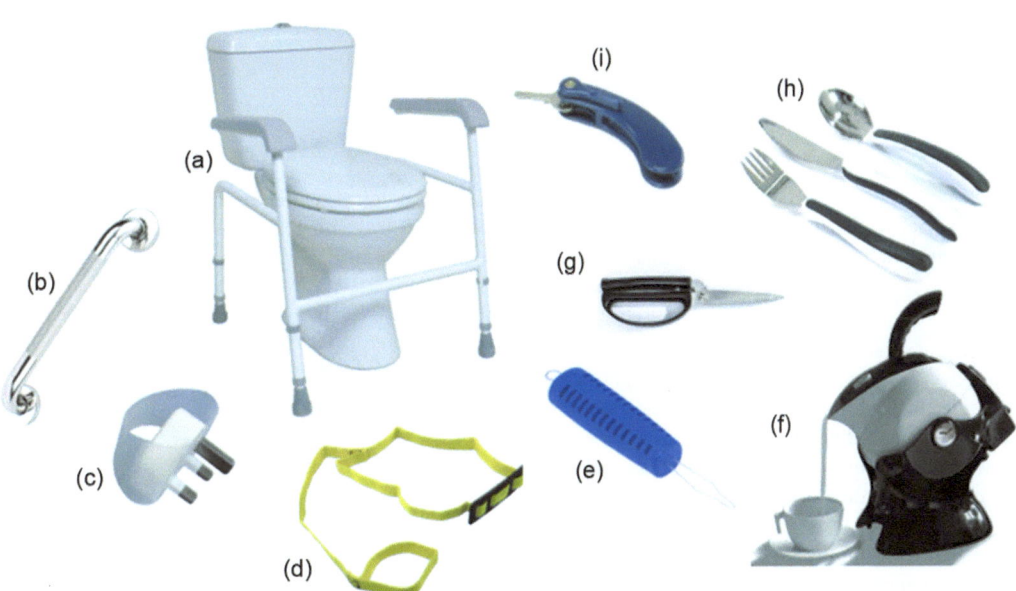

Figure 4.8 Aids to help with ADLs. (a) toilet frame, (b) grab rail, (c) plug pull, (d) leg lifter (to get legs into the car or bed), (e) buttonhook, (f) tipping kettle, (g) self-opening scissors, (h) wide handled cutlery, and (i) key turner.

Barriers to rehabilitation

If the patient is not making progress as expected, look for a reason:

- Poor motivation (patient or carer).
- Unrealistic expectations.
- Depression.
- Delirium/dementia.
- Communication difficulties.
- Sensory deprivation.
- Loss of body image, sensory ataxia, and disordered visuospatial perception.
- Co-morbidities (arthritis, heart failure, post-COVID exhaustion).
- Suboptimally treated pain.
- Poor nutritional state.
- Pressure ulcers and contractures.
- Hidden agendas – 'If I improve, I will be a burden'.

The discharge process

Discharge planning starts prior to elective admissions and on admission for emergencies. The NHS plan says that all patients in acute beds should have twice-daily multidisciplinary reviews. These must be brief, or all day is spent meeting!

- After the first meeting, the patient is given an 'expected date of discharge' (EDD) when they are likely to be ready to leave.
- The EDD is changed as needed.
- As the patient improves, the MDT should describe the function and likely needs of the person on discharge rather than prescribing exact post-discharge care.
- If it is likely that care will be needed, the patient is sent home with reablement, so that decisions about long-term support or care are made when the patient has recovered and is in a familiar place. This is known as 'Home first/Discharge to assess'. Financial discussions should take place after discharge.
- A few patients are discharged to a rehabilitation bed (in a community hospital or care home with therapy).
- Direct discharge to a nursing home for long-term care (e.g. after a major stroke) or end-of-life care may be needed.

The discharge planner liaises with the patient, any unpaid carers, and the care hub to plan initial care on discharge. The senior nurses on the ward keep the required documentation, ensure that the family is kept informed, and oversee the entire process. The aim is to discharge the patient safely as soon as they are 'medically optimised'.

Discharge planner

Traditionally, this was a social worker but is now usually a specialist nurse outside the ward team, with links to social services in a 'transfer of care hub'.

Case conferences

Most discharges are handled in the MDT, but if the situation is extremely complex and discharge is proving difficult, a formal case conference may be held. This must be planned at a time to suit the family and community contributors and will include a wider range of people, e.g. the patient if possible or their advocate, all key family members, others from the community such as their community psychiatric nurse (CPN), the warden from their sheltered accommodation, and a social worker, in addition to senior members of the usual ward MDT. Success may depend on the skills of the individual chairperson. Try to attend as a learning experience.

WHO International Classification of Functioning, Disability and Health

Disability is considered a universal experience – everyone is likely to experience some degree of disability in their life through a change in their health or environment. The ICF can be used to describe an individual or to make comparisons between different countries.

- **Impairment**: loss of structure or function, e.g. a weak limb after a stroke.
- **Activity limitations (disability)**: the resulting loss of ability to perform an activity, e.g. walking.
- **Participant restrictions (handicap)**: the ensuing limit on the person's role, e.g. being unable to cook or take part in leisure activities.

Because people function in society, environmental factors make up the physical, societal, and attitudinal environment in which people live. Several of the components can be graded. Figure 4.10 shows the schema, and Figure 4.11 shows how it can be used to describe back pain in an older lady in a standardised way.

The ICF also provides a framework to consider the levels at which intervention can improve quality of life and highlights the role of environmental factors and social legislation in enabling participation (see Table 4.3).

Ethical issues and ageism

The whole area of denial of access to high-class care versus overaggressive and futile intervention is complex and one of the fascinations of geriatric medicine. Ageism still exists, but there is less systematic ageism as most guidelines no longer have fixed upper age limits. The importance of frailty rather than chronological age is increasingly recognised (see Chapter 21). Whilst it is true that frail older people do not always do well in an acute hospital environment, some of the other proposed options may amount to covert rationing. Always ask yourself, 'Would I be happy with this for my grandma?' There is concern that 'frailism' may become a covert form of ageism.

Sources of information

Use your medical school or hospital library, mainstream journals (BMJ, Lancet, NEJM) and librarian support for searches, e.g. PubMed and Cochrane Library.

National guidelines

- NICE guidelines – www.nice.org.uk: a place to start, but often convoluted or niche. Clinical knowledge summaries (CKS) are more user-friendly.
- SIGN guidelines (Scottish) – www.sign.ac.uk: also becoming very long.

Specialist society guidelines

- The British Geriatrics Society website – www.bgs.org.uk: useful resources e.g. in the Silver Book II, see the scope of geriatrics if you are considering a career. The journal is Age & Ageing.
- The American Geriatrics Society: free resources listed. The journal is JAGS. https://www.americangeriatrics.org/publications-tools

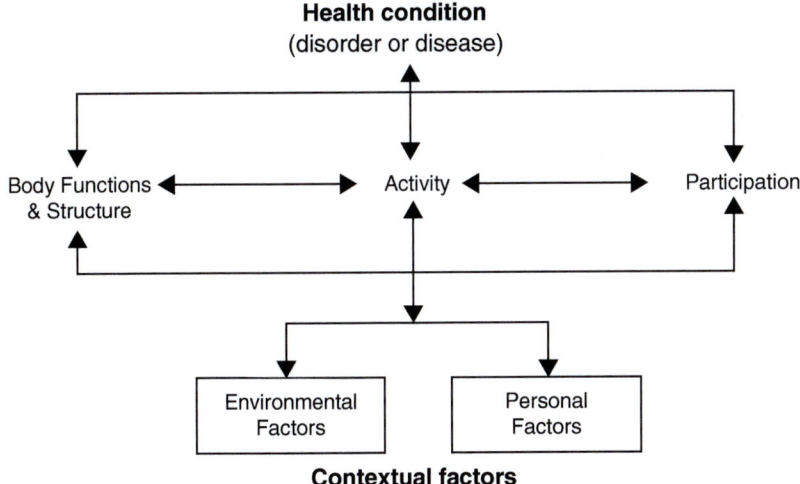

Figure 4.10 The ICF schema.

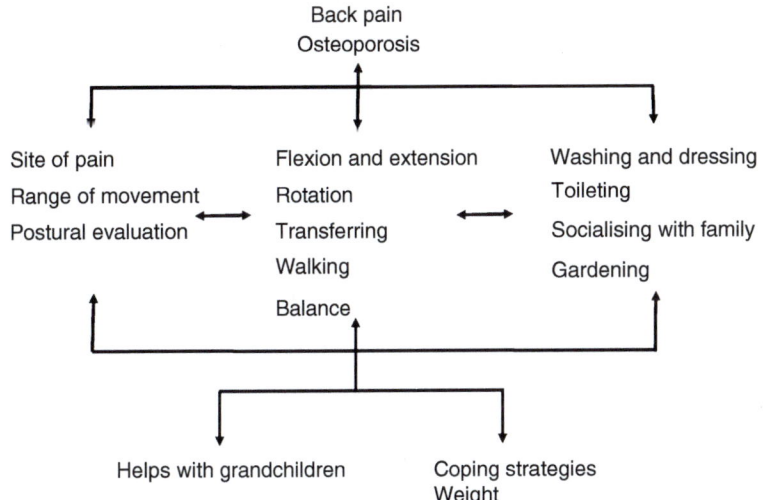

Figure 4.11 The ICF describing the effect of back pain from vertebral fractures on Mrs JB, a 78-year-old grandmother.

- UK, European or US societies for organ-based problems, e.g. British Thoracic Society guidelines for the use of oxygen and European Society of Cardiology management of valvular heart disease.

Medically focused

Excellent but not free – check if your Trust has a subscription.

- UpToDate: US-based, but very popular.
- BMJ Best Practice.

Recommended by juniors

Geeky Medics: https://geekymedics.com
Life in the fast lane: https://litfl.com/library

Research trials

www.clinicaltrials.gov is a website and online database of clinical research studies and information about their results. The purpose of http://ClinicalTrials.gov is to provide information about clinical research studies to the public, researchers, and healthcare professionals.

Table 4.3 ICF Framework for Intervention and Prevention.

	Intervention	Prevention
Health condition	Medical management Drugs	Health promotion Nutrition Immunisation
Impairment	Medical management Drugs Surgery	Prevent the development of further activity limitations
Activity limitation	Rehabilitation Assistive devices Personal assistance	Prehabilitation Prevention of the development of participation restrictions
Participation restriction	Suitable housing Public education Anti-discrimination law Universal design	Environmental change Employment strategies Accessible services Universal design Lobbying for change

NHS

An A-Z of conditions to inform patients – explains the patient pathway. https://www.nhs.uk/conditions
NHS Inform Scotland: https://www.nhsinform.scot/illnesses-and-conditions

Patient

A UK-based information website with more journalistic input and adverts unless you subscribe, but easy to read and good articles for patients and medics. https://patient.info

Patient-support societies

Almost all conditions have one! 'Google' and see. Information for patients, often more holistic than a medical textbook and clearly explained, is a good starting point for students. Information for professionals is usually wide-ranging and up-to-date. Print information for patients to supplement consultations.

- Alzheimer's Society (for all types of dementia): www.alzheimers.org.uk Section 'for GPs' is especially helpful.
- Parkinson's UK: www.parkinsons.org.uk

Old age charities

Reliable, clear information, particularly about support and benefits

- Age UK: www.ageuk.org.uk
- Carers UK: www.carersuk.org
- HelpAge International: www.helpage.org

📖 REFERENCES AND FURTHER READING

Sinclair AJ, Morley JE, Vellas B et al. (Editors) (2022). Pathy's principles and practice of geriatric medicine hardcover ISBN-13 978-1119484202. Wiley-Blackwell.

Tadros G (Editor) (2024). Handbook of old age liaison psychiatry paperback. ISBN-13 978-1108408516. Cambridge University Press.

Schiøtz ML, Stockmarr A, Høst D et al. (2017). Social disparities in the prevalence of multimorbidity – a register-based population study *BMC Public Health* 17: 422, doi: 10.1186/s12889-017-4314-8.

Douaud G, Lee S, Alfaro-Almagr F et al. (2022). SARS-CoV-2 is associated with changes in brain structure in UK biobank. *Nature* 604: 697–707, doi: 10.1038/s41586-022-04569-5.

British Geriatrics Society. *Frailty Hub*. www.bgs.org.uk/resources/frailty-hub-patient-information.

Fried LP, Tangen CM, Walston J et al. (2001). Frailty in older adults: evidence for a phenotype. *Journals of Gerontology. Series A, Biological Sciences and Medical Sciences* 56: M146–M157. https://pubmed.ncbi.nlm.nih.gov/11253156

Rockwood K, Mitnitski A (2007). Frailty in relation to the accumulation of deficits. Journals of Gerontology. Series A, Biological Sciences and Medical Sciences 62: 722–727, doi: 10.1093/gerona/62.7.722.

Kojima G, Iliffe S, Taniguchi Y et al. (2017). Prevalence of frailty in Japan: a systematic review and meta-analysis. *Journal of Epidemiology* 27: 347–353, doi: 10.1016/j.je.2016.09.008

Romero-Ortuno R, Wallis S, Biram R (2016). Clinical frailty adds to acute illness severity in predicting mortality in hospitalized older adults: an observational study. *European Journal of Internal Medicine* 35: 24–34, doi: https://doi.org/10.1016/j.ejim.2016.08.033.

Rockwood Clinical Frailty Scale www.bgs.org.uk/sites/default/files/content/attachment/2018-07-05/rockwood_cfs.pdf

NHS England Electronic Frailty Index https://www.england.nhs.uk/ourwork/clinical-policy/older-people/frailty/efi

Fogg C, Fraser SDS, Roderick P et al. (2022). The dynamics of frailty development and progression in older adults in primary care in England (2006–2017): a retrospective cohort profile. *BMC Geriatrics* 22: 30, doi: 10.1186/s12877-021-02684-y.

Walsh B, Fogg C, Harris S et al. (2023). Frailty transitions and prevalence in an ageing population: longitudinal analysis of primary care data from an open cohort of adults aged 50 and over in England, 2006–2017. *Age and Ageing* 52: afad058, doi: 10.1093/ageing/afad058.

Brundle C, Heaven A, Brown L et al. (2019). Convergent validity of the electronic frailty index. *Age and Ageing* 48: 152–156. ISSN 0002-0729, doi: 10.1093/ageing/afy162.

Brack C, Kynn M, Murchie P et al. (2023). Validated frailty measures using electronic primary care records: a review of diagnostic test accuracy. *Age and Ageing* 52: afad173, doi: 10.1093/ageing/afad173.

Orkaby AR, Callahan KE, Driver JA et al. (2024). New horizons in frailty identification via electronic frailty indices: early implementation lessons from experiences in England and the United States. *Age and Ageing* 53: afae025, doi: 10.1093/ageing/afae025

Lears beard. www.royalacademy.org.uk/copyright-policy

Ellis G, Gardner M, Tsiachristas A et al. (2017). Comprehensive geriatric assessment for older adults admitted to hospital. *Cochrane Database of Systematic Reviews* (9): CD006211, doi: 10.1002/14651858.CD006211.pub3.

Briggs R, McDonough A, Ellis G et al. (2022). Comprehensive geriatric assessment for community-dwelling, high-risk, frail, older people. *Cochrane Database of Systematic Reviews* (5): CD012705, doi: 10.1002/14651858.CD012705.pub2.

Crocker TF, Ensor J, Lam N et al (2024). Community based complex interventions to sustain independence in older people: systematic review and network meta-analysis. *BMJ* 384: e077764, doi: 10.1136/bmj-2023-077764

WHO ICF elearning tool. https://www.icf-elearning.com/wp-content/uploads/articulate_uploads/ICF%20e-Learning%20Tool_English_20220501%20-%20Storyline%20output/story_html5.html

INFORMATION FOR PATIENTS AND FAMILIES

- Some charities and general resources are listed above.
- The Disabled Living Foundation https://asksara.livingmadeeasy.org.uk/about-ask-sara
- Living Made Easy https://livingmadeeasy.org.ukchecking

All websites were accessed in August 2024.

5

Drugs and prescribing

In paediatrics, drug doses are adjusted for age or weight. In adult medicine, most drugs are prescribed for a '70 kg man'. If your patient is a frail woman aged 85 with sarcopaenia, she may weigh 45 kg. There are many reasons to reduce drug dosage, as described below, but remember weight. Check your trust guidelines for paracetamol. For adults weighing 41–49 kg, the usual dosing is 500 mg to 1 g tds.

Key physiological changes of ageing that affect drugs

- Reduced gastric acid secretion, delayed gastric emptying, and slower gut motility.
- Liver mass and perfusion decline by around a third, and microsomal oxidation (CYP3A4) is reduced, although liver function tests usually stay within the normal range.
- Decreased muscle mass, resulting in an increased proportion of body fat and a reduced proportion of body water.
- Renal perfusion and function decline progressively with age – check the estimated glomerular filtration rate (eGFR) online.
- Increased blood-brain barrier permeability.

Pharmacokinetics and pharmacodynamics

Pharmacokinetics (what the body does to the drug – absorption, distribution, metabolism, and excretion) and pharmacodynamics (what the drug does to the body) are both affected by these changes.

Pharmacokinetic factors

- **Delayed gastric emptying and drug absorption**: reduced active absorption of iron and calcium, increased absorption of levodopa due to reduced dopa-decarboxylase in the gut wall.
- **First-pass metabolism**: *increased* bioavailability of drugs that would typically have an extensive hepatic first pass in younger people, e.g. atorvastatin, morphine, and verapamil, and reduced activation of pro-drugs that are activated in the liver, e.g. perindopril, so *lower* bioavailability.
- **Drug distribution**: increased serum concentration of water-soluble (polar) drugs, e.g. digoxin, gentamicin, morphine, lithium, and alcohol, as volume of distribution (Vd) is lower, increasing the risk of toxicity; a higher Vd and a longer half-life of lipid-soluble drugs, e.g. diazepam, increasing the risk of accumulation.

- **Protein binding**: reduced plasma albumin rarely causes an issue except in acute illness or severe chronic disease, but circulating levels of highly protein-bound drugs such as ibuprofen and phenytoin will be higher.
- **Brain concentrations**: some drugs may get into the brain more easily or not be as efficiently pumped out (e.g. domperidone, loperamide), but it is unclear whether this has clinical significance.
- **Drug clearance**: important for renally excreted drugs, especially with a narrow therapeutic index, e.g. digoxin and lithium, and for drugs with high hepatic extraction, e.g. pethidine and lidocaine.

Pharmacodynamic factors

- The same concentration of drug at its site of action has a different effect because of changes in receptor numbers or balance, post-receptor changes or other physiological factors.
- Complex; poor correlation between receptor number and effect.
- Usually, there is greater sensitivity, e.g. more sedation and increased postural sway with benzodiazepines, more confusion with anticholinergic drugs, and increased anticoagulation with warfarin, but the peak diuretic response to furosemide is reduced.

Other ageing changes

The many other changes and impaired homeostasis of ageing interact with medication; e.g. bruising is more common with a DOAC because of capillary fragility; any drug that causes dizziness is more likely to result in a fall because of impaired vascular tone and a reduced righting response.

There may be practical issues with taking a drug correctly due to impaired vision, swallowing, motor function, hand–eye coordination, health literacy, and cognition. These include reading and understanding the instructions, handling the packaging, preparing the medication, using devices such as inhalers or injectors, or forgetting to take the drug.

As a result of all these factors for *each drug*, there is:

- Greater susceptibility to side effects.
- More likelihood of adverse effects.
- When these occur, they are more likely to have serious sequelae.

Many older people are on *multiple drugs*, so there is:

- More chance of side effects and adverse drug reactions.
- More risk of drug interactions.
- More likelihood of problems with adherence, especially if confused.
- They may be on a drug to treat the side effects of another!

Geriatric Medicine and Elderly Care: Lecture Notes, Ninth Edition. Claire G. Nicholl, K. Jane Wilson, and Shaun D'Souza.
© 2025 John Wiley & Sons Ltd. Published 2025 by John Wiley & Sons Ltd.
Companion website: www.wiley.com/go/lecturenotesgeriatricmedicine9e

When problems arise, there are often many causes (see box).

Joan Smith does not get out much because of her arthritic knees. She spends most of her day in her chair and is taking furosemide because of ankle swelling. She is prescribed a non-steroidal anti-inflammatory drug (NSAID):

- She decides indigestion is normal at her age (based on multiple symptoms and her expectations).
- She has haematemesis (more prone to side effects).
- She collapses (impaired homeostasis, worsened by her furosemide).
- She fractures her hip (co-existing osteoporosis).
- She is not found until the next day (social factors – she lives alone).
- She is admitted but has complications (need for swift management to avoid complications of immobility).
- Antibiotics are prescribed (iatrogenic – third-generation cephalosporins should be avoided unless essential).
- She develops *C. difficile* diarrhoea, that increases the length of her admission and from which she may die.

Was the NSAID indicated initially?

Trends in drug prescribing

The number of prescribed drugs has increased; more drugs are available over the counter (OTC) in supermarkets as well as pharmacies, and more people take herbal remedies and supplements.

In primary care in England, the total number of prescription items dispensed each year grew until 2019 but has remained stable since (1.04 billion in 2021/22) with atorvastatin being the most often prescribed and apixaban accounting for the biggest cost. In 2019–2020, the NHS spent £20.9 billion on drugs (NHS Digital). The number of drugs a person takes increases markedly with age (Figure 5.1).

- About half of the over-75s take five or more medicines.
- By 80, more than a third of all people are on eight or more medicines.

In 2022, there were over 876,000 people on 10 or more medicines, and over 349,000 of these people were 75+.

The drugs that are prescribed to a greater proportion of older people include those liable to result in dependence or withdrawal and likely to cause confusion (see Figure 5.2). This does not necessarily equate to bad prescribing. In 2020, the modal (most common) age at death was 87 years for males and 89 years for females, so some of the opiate use will be for end-of-life care, but each prescription needs consideration.

Polypharmacy

Polypharmacy refers to the use of multiple medications by a patient. There is no standard definition, and the number ranges from ≥ four drugs (WHO) to > nine (NHS Scotland). Evidence-based clinical guidelines often recommend several drugs for a single disease (see box on cardiac guidelines), so polypharmacy is almost inevitable in older people with several diseases.

Cardiac guidelines in many countries, including the NICE Guidelines for treatment after MI, recommend multiple drugs:

- Beta-blocker (if reduced ejection fraction)
- Aspirin.
- Clopidogrel or ticagrelor.
- ACE inhibitor (ARB if intolerant).
- Statin.
- With heart failure: loop diuretics, spironolactone, and dapagliflozin for HFpEF/HFmrEF.
- With diabetes: insulin in the acute phase, usual treatment later.
- With AF: DOAC.
- With angina: calcium channel blocker or nicorandil.
- With COPD….
- To prevent peptic ulceration….

It may be more helpful to consider:

- **Appropriate polypharmacy**: evidence-based prescribing for an individual with multiple conditions where medicines use has been optimised to maintain good quality of life, improve longevity, and minimise harm from drugs.

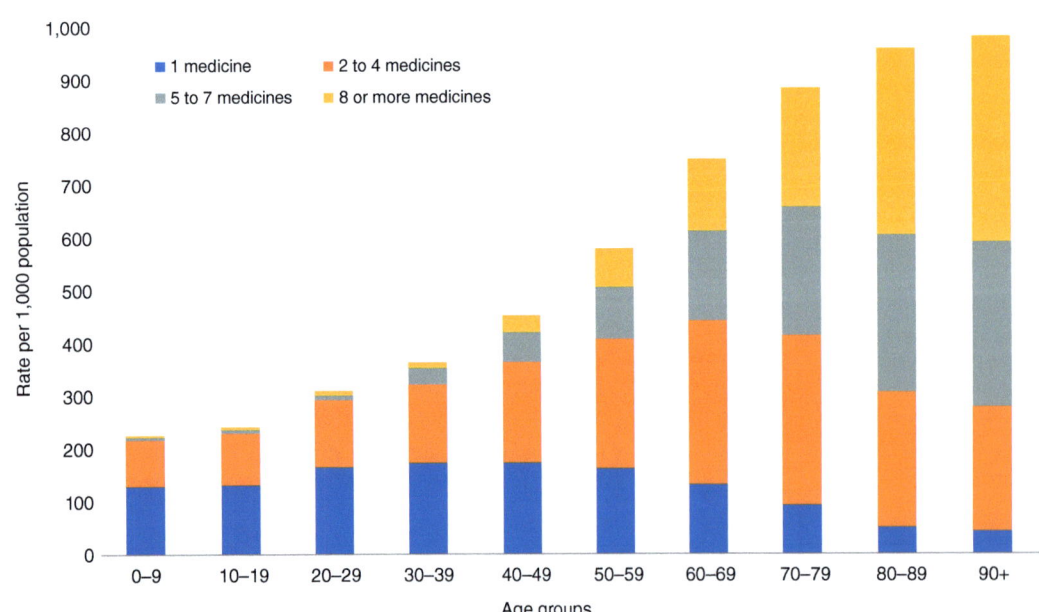

Figure 5.1 Distribution of the number of medicines by age. *Source*: Adapted from primary care in England in 2019.

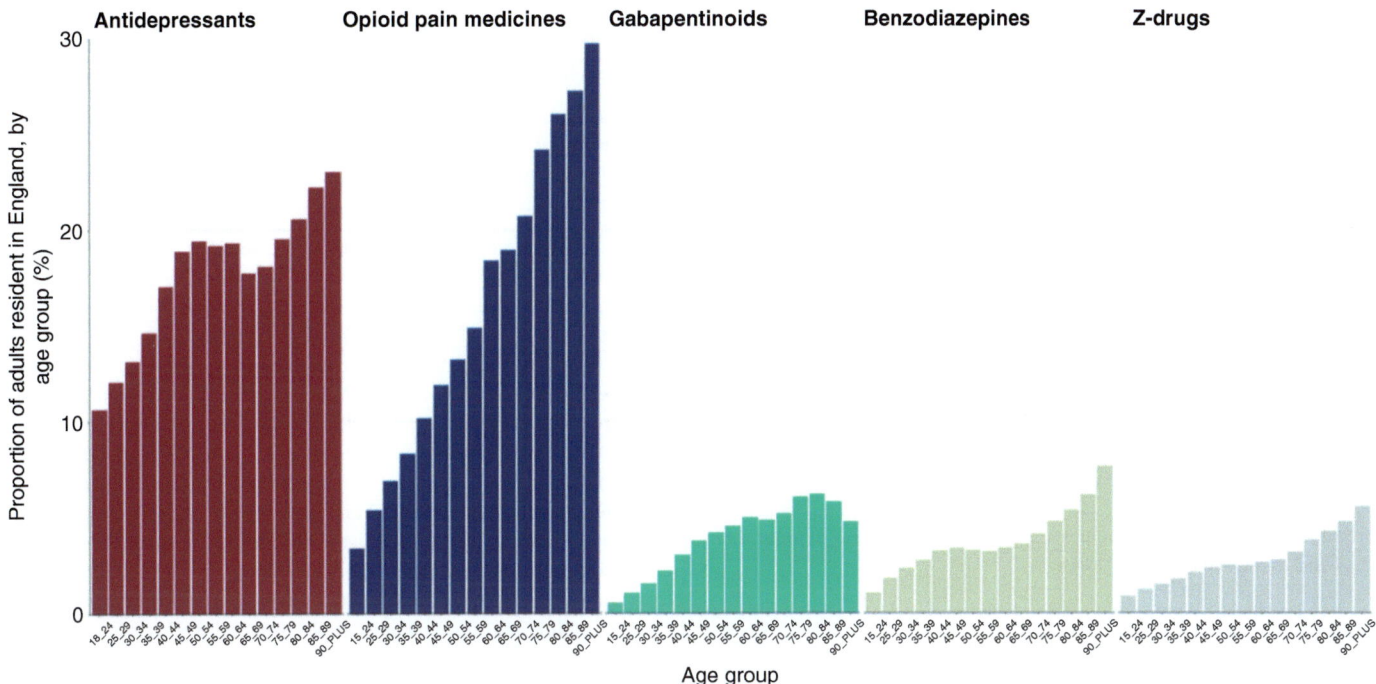

Figure 5.2 Proportion of adults receiving a prescription in 2017–2018, by age group and class of medicine (England). The youngest band is 18 to 24 years old. Then, 5-year bands are shown from 25 to 89 years, with the oldest group being 90 years and above.

- **Problematic polypharmacy:** multiple medications are prescribed inappropriately, or the intended benefit of the medication is not realised. Treatments are not evidence-based, or the risk of harm is likely to outweigh the benefit, or one or more of the following apply:
  - The drug combination is hazardous because of interactions.
  - The 'pill burden' is unacceptable to the patient or makes concordance difficult.
  - Medicines are being prescribed to treat the side effects of others, although alternatives are available.
  - A prescribing cascade may ensue when an adverse drug event is misinterpreted as a new medical condition and a subsequent drug is prescribed to treat it.

Terminology

PIMs (potentially inappropriate medicines) and PPOs (potential prescribing omissions) are commonly found in older people.

An adverse drug reaction (ADR) is an unintended, harmful response to a drug.

Type A 'augmented' reactions are predictable, e.g. bleeding on warfarin, dry mouth with tricyclics.

Type B 'bizarre' reactions are idiosyncratic, e.g. anaphylaxis with penicillin.

Type C 'continuing' osteonecrosis of the jaw with ongoing use of bisphosphonates.

Type D 'delayed' abnormal liver function weeks after a course of co-amoxiclav.

Type E 'end of use' withdrawal symptoms from benzodiazepines.

Alternative classifications are based on the relationship to dose, time, susceptibility (DoTS), and severity.

Adverse events (AEs) are any untoward medical events that occur during drug studies but are not necessarily caused by the drug.

Predictable ADRs are often referred to as side effects, but the Medicines and Healthcare Products Regulatory Agency (MHRA) uses adverse drug reactions and side effects synonymously. The British National Formulary (BNF) lists all types of ADR as side effects, by frequency of occurrence.

Hospital admissions due to adverse drug reactions

There is a range of figures in the literature; many quote Pirmohamed (2004), who found that 5.2% of admissions were caused by ADRs. His team has repeated a similar study (2021) and found a higher rate. In a prospective review of all medical admissions over a month in Liverpool ($n = 1187$), ADRs were the primary or contributing cause of 16.5% of total admissions. Those with an ADR were taking more drugs (10.5 versus 7.8, $p < 0.01$), had more comorbidities and had a mean age of 73. The top 5 drugs implicated were diuretics, steroid inhalers, anticoagulants, proton pump inhibitors, and antiplatelet drugs. 40% of ADRs were classified as avoidable or possibly avoidable. The higher figure may reflect better ascertainment of ADRs and increased multimorbidity and polypharmacy.

Adverse drug reactions often present as one of the frailty syndromes through multiple mechanisms.

- **Intellectual failure:** anti-cholinergic burden, hyponatraemia, sedation.
- **Instability:** low BP, sedation, arrhythmias, neuropathies, cerebellar toxicity.
- **Immobility:** extrapyramidal effects, sedation.
- **Incontinence:** bladder irritation, urine retention and overflow, diuresis, relaxation of prostatic smooth muscle, sedation.
- **Inanition:** anorexia, oral candidiasis, nausea, vomiting, sedation, constipation, diarrhoea, abdominal pain, Candida.

Medicine wastage

The cost of wasted medicines is huge. The oft-quoted figure of £300 million dates from 2010! Another problem is that nearly half of the people admit to throwing prescriptions away, so if the drugs were needed, their health would suffer. One-third to half of all medicines for long-term conditions are not taken. This is a loss to the individual, the health care system, and the country. This is one of the reasons that a full discussion is needed when prescribing. If the person does not intend to take the drugs, do not prescribe them.

Prescribing tools

Several tools are available to help with the systematic review of patients' drugs and to reduce PIMs and PPOs.

STOPP/START

Earlier prescribing support tools were not widely used in Europe as they reflected American practice. The STOPP/ START (Screening Tool of Older Persons' potentially inappropriate Prescriptions/ Screening Tool to Alert Doctors to the Right Treatment) are evidence-based criteria that have shown benefits for individuals in hospitals and the community. Early studies showed that START found prescribing omissions in 60% of hospital admissions and that STOPP would save a significant proportion of the drug budget in Ireland. A meta-analysis (2015) found that most studies were ineligible for inclusion and only evaluated four RCTs. The drug regimens of 1,925 patients from four countries in acute ($n = 2$) and long-term care ($n = 2$) met STOPP criteria, which reduced PIM rates in all four studies. There was evidence of a reduction in falls, delirium, hospital length-of-stay, care visits and medication costs, but no evidence of improvements in quality of life or mortality.

The tool was updated in 2015. There has been criticism that the criteria lack clarity. The use of a computerised version did not show benefit. In a multi-national, parallel arm, prospective, randomised, open-label, blinded endpoint-controlled trial at six European medical centres, 1,537 older medical and surgical patients with multi-morbidity and polypharmacy were randomised to SENATOR software-guided medication optimisation plus standard care or standard care alone. The uptake of software-generated medication advice was poor and did not reduce ADRs during the admission. For tools to work, they must be used; too much information causes overload for the prescriber and possibly a failure to think!

STOPPFall

The Screening Tool of Older Persons' Prescriptions in those with a high Falls risk is a deprescribing tool developed by European experts that focuses on fall-risk-increasing drugs, or FRIDS. Two facilitators created an initial list of medications from recent systematic reviews, and this was then amended in a Delphi process. Agreement was reached for 14 classes of medication, the top three being benzodiazepines, antipsychotics, and benzodiazepine-related drugs. For more detail, see Chapter 11.

STOPPFrail

This is a similar tool designed for use for older people approaching the end of life (Version 2 2021).

Anticholinergic burden

Many drugs have anticholinergic (antimuscarinic) properties.

- Some are prescribed for their anticholinergic effect, e.g. oxybutynin for an overactive bladder.
- Others have their intended effect on another receptor but also have antimuscarinic effects.

M_1, M_4, and M_5 receptors are found in the CNS; M_2 receptors are in the heart, especially the AV and SA nodes; and M_3 receptors are widely distributed in smooth muscle, but drugs are rarely selective for one receptor subtype.

In older people, anticholinergic drugs are associated with confusion (particularly if there is preexisting cognitive impairment or dementia), dizziness, and falls. If several drugs with anticholinergic activity are prescribed, the effect is additive. There is evidence that the long-term total anticholinergic burden (ACB) is a risk factor for developing cognitive impairment, dementia, and death. Many scales are available, but note that there is variation in the way some drugs are classified. Drugs are prescribed for a specific indication and have other side effects and contraindications, so one approach is, where there are alternatives, to prescribe the one with the lowest cholinergic burden. For example, if an antipsychotic is essential, risperidone carries a lower cholinergic burden than olanzapine or quetiapine. Paroxetine is the most anticholinergic of the SSRIs. There is a link to a recommended ACB calculator on the RCGP website.

Levodopa equivalence calculators

Stopping regular oral medication in patients with Parkinson's disease (e.g. perioperatively or in acute illness when the patient cannot swallow) produces rapid deterioration and can be dangerous; several common PD drugs have no non-oral equivalent. A specialist opinion should be sought, but in the interim, use a levodopa equivalence calculator.

- They convert the patient's medication to a levodopa equivalent dose (LED) to give as dispersible Madopar via a nasogastric tube or as a rotigotine patch.
- Apomorphine infusions or Duodopa via a PEG-J (percutaneous gastrostomy with jejunal extension tube) should be continued.
- Entacapone, selegiline, rasagiline, and amantadine can be omitted safely.
- Check your local guidance; otherwise, use OPTIMAL, which is endorsed by the BGS and updated annually. The other common calculator is the 'PD nil-by-mouth medication dose calculator'.

Practical prescribing

Be aware that the riskiest time for unintended changes in medication is when a patient moves between care settings (see box).

The transition between care settings

- On admission, confirm medication with the GP record.
- Never write up a drug if you don't know what it is! Check.
- Do you think the person has been taking their drugs? If they are 'on' 4 antihypertensives, consider writing up 1 or 2 and observe. You can add the others the next day IF needed.
- Improve your discharge summary by ensuring every drug has a listed problem. If a drug was stopped, state why.
- After discharge, a primary care review is needed. A patient started on ramipril, may continue taking their home stock of enalapril.
- The ward and community pharmacy teams provide great support. Some doctors find pharmacists' extreme precision with drug charts a frustration. Avoid this! Pharmacists save many doctors' registrations.

Reviewing the drugs

When you encounter a patient, they are usually on many drugs already. Before you add new drugs, rreview these, especially on every transition of care. For each drug, consider:

- Does the likely benefit outweigh the risk? This is not straightforward. For example, an 84-year-old man who has been on long-term warfarin for stroke risk reduction secondary to AF has dementia, is prone to falls, and is found to have an unexpected INR of 7.2: A patient with AF needs to fall **nearly 300 times** in 1 year for the risk of a subdural to be greater than the benefit of preventing a stroke with anticoagulation therapy. However, falls may result in other injuries, such as hip fractures and severe lacerations where blood loss on anticoagulation may be significant. Regardless of the falls, he may have a major gastrointestinal bleed or a spontaneous intracranial haemorrhage. If he is approaching the end of his life, it may be right to stop anticoagulation. Otherwise, changing to a DOAC given by a carer may be safer and avoid the need for monitoring. Document what you have done and why and if possible, explain this to the patient and his family.
- Still indicated? (Oxybutynin, sulphonylureas, etc. are often continued with little evidence of efficacy and may be causing undetected harm.)
- 'Nicest' drug for the job? (e.g. clarithromycin has fewer gastric side effects than erythromycin.)
- Is a drug causing the symptoms? (e.g. nausea or confusion due to codeine; furosemide and fludrocortisone are an illogical combination.)
- Could a single agent replace two? (e.g. an ACE inhibitor for hypertension with CCF.)
- Is the formulation/route of administration the best? (Syrups and patches may help.)
- Are the timings appropriate? (Once- or twice-a-day options aid adherence for the patient and carer.)
- Aids to administration? (e.g. spacers for inhalers, no childproof tops, Medicines Administration Record – MAR chart.)
- Aids to adherence? (e.g. Dosette box.)
- Regular or 'as required'? (Analgesics are usually best taken on a regular basis, but efficacy is poor for chronic pain.)
- Does the patient understand the medications and any precautions? (Supply written information and record advice given, e.g. for a sore throat on carbimazole.) It is not just older people that do not understand their medication – in a poll of 3,000 adults, only a third said they understood the package insert.
- Cheapest, if there are equivalents? (e.g. proton pump inhibitors.)
- Check against STOPP criteria and check the anticholinergic burden.

Deprescribing

Stopping a drug (intentionally) is called deprescribing.

- This should be discussed with the patient and carer, if possible. This is important, so they appreciate that it is for their benefit, not to save money!
- A slow withdrawal may be needed.
- If a drug is stopped, record why.

Social prescribing

Social prescribing enables GPs, nurses, and other primary care professionals to refer people to a range of local, non-clinical services to support their health and well-being. Although there is limited evidence for efficacy in older people (see the excellent review by Percival), anecdotally, a huge range of activities, e.g. exercise groups, rambling clubs, guided museum visits and choirs for people with dementia, have much to offer. This is particularly true for chronic conditions like pain and anxiety, where long-term medication is often not effective.

Should a new drug be started?

Review your patient's problem list and prioritise the treatable.

- Drugs are prescribed for cure, disease modification, symptom control, and primary or secondary prevention.
  - Symptom control is essential at all ages.
  - Cure and disease modification are desirable if the benefits outweigh the risks. There is a difference between an antibiotic for pneumonia and chemotherapy for cancer or DMARDs for rheumatoid arthritis.
  - When the aim is prevention, the 'patient' is not ill, and the balance of benefits and risks will be different in older people. If a condition hasn't developed, is it likely to? Life expectancy is shorter, but if events are more common, the benefit may be greater.
- Frailty is more important than age per se; there is a substantial difference between prescribing for a frail nursing home resident and an active community dweller.
- What does the patient want? Concordance is essential if the patient is to try to adhere to the regimen.
- Use familiar drugs; the latest cardiac medication should initially be used by cardiologists!
- Start low; go slow, but increase the dose until it is in the therapeutic range or side effects develop.
- Use generic names unless bioavailability is crucial or when using a slow-release preparation.
- Give a drug for a long enough time before deciding it is ineffective, e.g. antidepressants.
- Look for side effects and interactions.
- In prevention, consider the overall burden of pathology and drugs, but avoid therapeutic nihilism.
- Check against START criteria.

Sick day rules

If a patient develops severe diarrhoea, vomiting, or fever, they may become dehydrated and some drugs that are normally tolerated may cause harm. AKI develops rapidly in older people. The most common offenders are tablets for diabetes, diuretics, drugs affecting angiotensin and NSAIDs. Consider recommending that patients withhold these until they have been better for 24–48 hours.

The evidence base for prescribing in older people

The treatment of hypertension and statin use are discussed. Remember, the evidence base for prescribing is often lacking, as older people are rarely enrolled in trials and typical older people are NOT included.

Antihypertensive drugs

The management of HT shows the challenge of evidence-based practice for people over 80 years old. The best evidence for using drugs comes from randomised, double-blind, placebo-controlled trials.

- A key issue is whether the trial subjects reflect the people doctors treat every day.
- The 'older group' in a study may have a mean age in the 70s or even 60s.
- People with multiple comorbidities, frailty, cognitive impairment, and those who live in institutions are almost never included in trials.

In HYVET, the HYpertension in the Very Elderly Trial (Bulpitt), the patients were in their 80s, with a mean age at baseline of 83.6 years. The target BP was 150/80 mmHg. The trial showed mortality benefits for the fit community-dwelling participants. Following this, most guidelines recommended treating high blood pressure to this target in people in their 80s if they were reasonably fit.

SPRINT, the Systolic blood PRessure INTervention trial, was another trial that changed practice (2015 and subsequent publications). After this, many guidelines were changed to aim for tighter control. The trial compared a standard target of <140 mmHg with a tight control of <120 mmHg in people with increased cardiovascular risk. In those aged 75+, age itself was a sufficient cardiovascular risk for inclusion.

- The intensive treatment produced a mortality benefit even in people aged 75+ and those with 'frailty'.
- However, rates of SAEs – hypotension, syncope, electrolyte abnormalities, and acute kidney injury or failure – but not of injurious falls, were higher in the intensive-treatment group.

It is important to consider what is meant by 'old' and 'frail', and the risks of treatment as well as the benefits. Data is not always easy to find; there are 121 papers on the SPRINT website.

- The prespecified older group, n = 2636, mean age 79.9 years, is older than in many studies but younger than many people considered for treatment.
- Inclusion criteria (living in the community, expected survival of at least 3 years) and exclusion criteria (including stroke, diabetes, a cardiovascular event within 3 months, 1-min standing SBP <110 mmHg) excluded many people with comorbidities.
- Frailty was a post-hoc analysis based on a frailty index.
  ○ Frailty was associated with self-reported falls and all causes of hospitalisation (supporting the validity of the definition).
  ○ In the whole study population of 2,560 participants (27.5%), with a mean age of 68.3 years were classified as frail.
  ○ This was similar to the proportion considered frail in the older group (30.9%).
  ○ Usually, frailty increases with age. The younger group may have been selected for 'frailty' as they needed an additional cardiovascular risk factor for inclusion, but this supports the idea that the older group were relatively robust.

Older age and frailty (at all ages) were associated with an increased risk of an SAE for syncope, hypotension, and falls. There was no evidence of 'differential risk' associated with intensive treatment between older and younger adults. The authors suggest that these results should reassure clinicians that treating patients ≥75 years old to an SBP goal of <120 mmHg does not result in 'excess risk' of SAEs for syncope, hypotension, or falls versus patients aged 50–74. However, as the *absolute risk* of adverse effects is greater with age, the same increase in *relative risk* with tighter control will result in more events in the older group.

Large observational studies of older people have shown that SBP <130 mmHg is associated with excess mortality without significant reductions in cardiovascular risk. For example, in a study of 416,000 primary care patients over 75 years using electronic records, BP <130/80 was associated with excess mortality. HT was not associated with increased mortality at ages above 85 or at ages 75–84 with moderate/severe frailty, perhaps due to the complexities of co-existing morbidities.

As a result of limited data and different interpretations of the same evidence, international guidelines for managing hypertension in people

Table 5.1 Risk of cardiovascular events in a cohort study of statins for primary prevention according to age and presence of diabetes.

Age and presence of diabetes	Risk of cardiovascular events in those taking statins
75–84 with diabetes	↓
>85 with diabetes	← →
75–84 without diabetes	← →
>85 with diabetes	← →

over 80 are inconsistent. The most common target SBP is <150 mmHg, but several countries, including Australia and Canada, have adopted a target of <120 mmHg. Guidelines focus on age, but varying age bands are used. Frailty is mentioned in some, but there is no consensus.

A 2019 review suggests treating the fit, deprescribing in the very frail, and using CGA and clinical judgement in those in between.

Statins

In comparison with treating HT in old age, there is less evidence for both the benefits and harms of statins. The UK is an outlier in Europe and North America, as NICE effectively recommends statins for anyone aged 75–84, as QRISK3 assigns everyone aged 75–84 a 10-year cardiovascular risk score of >10%.

- The only clinical trial specifically in older people, the Prospective Study of Pravastatin in the Elderly at Risk (PROSPER), included patients aged 70–82 years (mean 75 years) and showed benefit from statins but only in the secondary prevention group.
- The results of a large (n = 46,864, median follow-up, 5.6 years) retrospective cohort study of statins in patients aged 75+ without clinical cardiovascular disease (2018) are shown in Table 5.1.
- A 2019 meta-analysis of RCTs of statins included an analysis of outcomes in patients aged > 75 years (n = 14,483; median follow-up: 4.9 years). Each 1 mmol/L reduction in LDL-C (low-density lipoprotein cholesterol) was associated with a significantly decreased risk for major vascular events and major coronary events. However, this was only the case in patients with pre-existing vascular disease.

A more evidence-based approach would be:

- Not to start statins for primary prevention in the over-75s, unless there is coexisting diabetes, when there is evidence of benefit to the age of 85. Consider deprescribing those already on statins after discussion.
- Start or continue a statin in patients ages >75 who have known vascular occlusive disease. There is no good evidence on when to stop; consider the biological age, patient preference, etc.

Empowering your patient

Proposed management should always be discussed with the patient, if possible or their families (with their agreement or in their best interests). When people are ill in the hospital, recognise that the patient–doctor power imbalance is at its most extreme and repeat explanations as needed. In community settings, encourage patients and their families to use resources such as information from patient support groups and the Choosing Wisely website. This has several helpful links and encourages people to use the BRAN questions about any proposed treatment.

1 What are the **Benefits?**
2 What are the **Risks?**
3 What are the **Alternatives?**
4 What if I do **Nothing?**

Particularly when treating older people, there are many uncertainties. This needs to be acknowledged.

Summary: the overall picture

- Would non-drug therapies be better, e.g. respiratory rehabilitation, social prescribing?
- If there are multiple drugs, are they all essential?
- Consider deprescribing.
- Avoid drugs to treat the side effects of another drug.
- Look for potential interactions.
- If the patient has renal/hepatic failure, do not rely on memory; check every drug they are taking in the British National Formulary (BNF).
- The patient will change. Always review their medication. Consider the individual's comorbidities, degree of frailty, and life expectancy, and discuss their wishes. Is secondary prevention still appropriate?

REFERENCES AND FURTHER READING

Drenth-van Maanen AC, Wilting I, Jansen PAF (2020) Prescribing medicines to older people—how to consider the impact of ageing on human organ and body functions. *British Journal of Clinical Pharmacology* 86: 1921–1930, doi: 10.1111/bcp.14094.

DHSC *Good for you, good for us, good for everybody. A plan to reduce overprescribing to make patient care better and safer, support the NHS, and reduce carbon emissions* (2021) https://assets.publishing.service. gov.uk/government/uploads/system/uploads/attachment_data/ file/1019475/good-for-you-good-for-us-good-for-everybody.pdf

Taylor S, Annand F, Burkinshaw P et al. (2020) Dependence and withdrawal associated with some prescribed medicines: an evidence review. Public Health England, London https://assets.publishing. service.gov.uk/government/uploads/system/uploads/attachment_ data/file/940255/PHE_PMR_report_Dec2020.pdf

Pirmohamed M, James S, Meakin S, et al. (2004) Adverse drug reactions as cause of admission to hospital: prospective analysis of 18 820 patients. *BMJ* 329: 15, doi: 10.1136/bmj.329.7456.15

Osanlou R, Walker L, Hughes DA et al. (2022) Adverse drug reactions, multimorbidity and polypharmacy: a prospective analysis of 1 month of medical admissions. *BMJ Open* 12: e055551. doi: 10.1136/ bmjopen-2021-055551

O'Mahony D, O'Sullivan D, Byrne S et al. (2015) STOPP/START criteria for potentially inappropriate prescribing in older people: version 2. *Age Ageing* 44: 213–8. doi: 10.1093/ageing/afu145.

Hill-Taylor B, Walsh KA, Stewart S et al. (2016) Effectiveness of the STOPP/START (screening tool of older Persons' potentially inappropriate prescriptions/screening tool to alert doctors to the right treatment) criteria: systematic review and meta-analysis of randomized controlled studies. *Journal of Clinical Pharmacy and Therapeutics* 41: 158–169, doi: 10.1111/jcpt.12372.

O'Mahony D, Gudmundsson A, Soiza RL et al. (2020) Prevention of adverse drug reactions in hospitalized older patients with multimorbidity and polypharmacy: the SENATOR randomized controlled clinical trial. *Age and Ageing* 49: 605–614, doi: 10.1093/ageing/ afaa072.

Seppala LJ, Petrovic M, Ryg J et al. (2021) STOPPFall (screening tool of older persons prescriptions in older adults with high fall risk): a Delphi study by the EuGMS task and finish group on fall-risk-increasing drugs. *Age and Ageing* 50: 1189–1199. doi: 10.1093/ageing/ afaa249

Anticholinergic burden calculator: www.acbcalc.com

Levodopa equivalence calculators:

- PD 'Nil by Mouth' Medication Dose Calculator (www.pdmedcalc. co.uk)
- OPTIMAL Parkinson's calculator and guideline (www.parkinsonscal culator.com)

Percival A, Newton C, Mulligan K et al. (2022) Systematic review of social prescribing and older adults: where to from here? *Family Medicine and Community Health* 10: e001829, doi: 10.1136/fmch-2022-001829.

Beckett NS, Peters R, Fletcher AE et al. (2008) Treatment of hypertension in patients 80 years of age or older. *New England Journal of Medicine* 358: 1887–1898, doi: 10.1056/NEJMoa0801369

Wright JT for the SPRINT research group. (2015) A randomised trial of intensive versus standard blood pressure control. *New England Journal of Medicine* 373: 2103–2116, doi: 10.1056/NEJMoa1511939.

Pajewski NM, Williamson JD, Applegate WB et al. (2016) SPRINT Study Research Group. Characterizing frailty status in the systolic blood pressure intervention trial. *Journals of Gerontology A* 71: 649–655. doi: 10.1093/gerona/glv228

Sink KM, Evans GW, Shorr RI et al. (2018) Syncope, hypotension, and falls in the treatment of hypertension: results from the randomized clinical systolic blood pressure Intervention trial. *Journal of the American Geriatrics Society* 66: 679–686 doi: 10.1111/jgs.15236

Benetos A, Petrovic M, Strandberg T (2019) Hypertension Management in Older and Frail Older Patients. *Circulation Research* 124: 1045–1060 https://doi.org/10.1161/CIRCRESAHA.118.313236.

Masoli JAH, Delgado J, Pilling L et al. (2020) Blood pressure in frail older adults: associations with cardiovascular outcomes and all-cause mortality. *Age Ageing* 49 (5): 807–813, doi: 10.1093/ageing/afaa028

Wright JT, Whelton PK, Johnson KC for the SPRINT Research Group (2021) SPRINT revisited. *Hypertension* 78: 1701–1710. doi: 10.1161/ HYPERTENSIONAHA.121.17682.

Masoli JAH, Sheppard JP, Rajkumar C et al. (2022) Hypertension management in older patients - are the guideline blood pressure targets appropriate? *Age and Ageing* 51: afab226, doi: 10.1093/ ageing/afab226.

Ramos R, Comas-Cufi M, Marti-Lluch R et al. (2018) Statins for primary prevention of cardiovascular events and mortality in old and very old adults with and without type 2 diabetes: retrospective cohort study. *BMJ* 362: k3359. https://www.bmj.com/content/362/bmj.k3359.

Cholesterol Treatment Trialists' Collaboration (2019). Efficacy and safety of statin therapy in older people: a meta-analysis of individual participant data from 28 randomized controlled trials. *The Lancet* 393: 407–415. https://www.ncbi.nlm.nih.gov/pmc/articles/PMC6429627

INFORMATION FOR PATIENTS AND FAMILIES

Choosing Wisely UK https://www.aomrc.org.uk/wp-content/uploads/ 2023/08/CWUK_patient_leaflet_100120.pdf

Patient. Information on medicines. https://patient.info/medicine

All websites were accessed in August 2024.

6

Surgery

Introduction

An increasing number of frailer, older patients are undergoing surgical procedures, in line with advances in surgical technique and anaesthetic management and coupled with changes in patient expectations. In England, 2.5 million people over the age of 75 underwent surgery between the years 2014 and 2015, as opposed to just under 1.5 million between 2006 and 2007. An increasing number of older people are undergoing emergency laparotomies; in 2019–2020, 55% were aged 65+ and 18% were 80+. Older patients have longer hospital stays and higher 30-day and 90-day mortality rates than younger people.

The outcome of surgery depends on the following:

- Patient (age, diagnosis, co-morbidities, frailty, and social support).
- Procedure.
- Degree of urgency.
- Perioperative support.

Emergency or elective surgery

Some operations are essential if the patient is to have a chance of survival and reasonable function, e.g. repair of a fractured hip or resection of a colonic cancer. The fracture is repaired as an emergency. The cancer will be removed as an emergency if there is perforation of the bowel or obstruction, but semi-electively otherwise. If the risk of surgery is too high, non-operative management is used. The balance depends on the situation and custom and practice. For example, it is considered so painful to die with a broken hip that surgery is usual, often regardless of high operative risk, as part of a palliative (pain control) approach.

These indications for surgery contrast with operations that may be desirable to improve quality of life, e.g. a knee replacement, which is always elective and for which the patient will need to be fit for the demands of the procedure.

For individuals over 75 years old, the 30-day mortality for emergency surgery is 10–30%, depending on the procedure, around three times the risk of elective surgery.

The type of surgery is a major factor in terms of outcomes. Very frail patients can have cataract surgery under local anaesthetic. Less invasive options have been devised as alternatives to very major procedures, e.g. endovascular aneurysm repair (EVAR) for aortic aneurysm, endoscopic stapling of pharyngeal pouches, laparoscopic parathyroidectomy, and percutaneous endoscopic colopexy (PEC) for recurrent sigmoid volvulus.

Assessment of the risks of surgery

Anaesthetists and surgeons use a variety of validated preoperative risk scores. They can be useful for communicating with patients and colleagues:

- Help with shared decision-making.
- Aid in the identification of patients with a risk of significant morbidity and mortality who need tailored perioperative management plans.

The ASA and conventional risk factors

Anaesthetists have long used the ASA (American Society of Anaesthesiologists) scoring system, which correlates well with postoperative complications and mortality. It is limited by variability in the individual anaesthetist's assessments of problems and focuses on conventional risk factors. Risk factors include:

- Cardiac: MI in the preceding 3 months, reduced ejection fraction, valve disease;
- Respiratory: COPD, current smoking;
- Neurological: stroke during the preceding 3 months, dementia;
- Metabolic: diabetes, steroids, renal failure, obesity, alcohol use;

and the severity of illness such as shock or sepsis.

It has been known for years that the cumulative effect of multimorbidity and the loss of physiological reserve with ageing predispose to poor outcomes.

Impact of multimorbidity

In older patients with hip fractures, the presence of three or more comorbidities predicts mortality (Figure 6.1), with pneumonia and heart failure being the most common postoperative complications.

Impact of frailty

Frailty and multimorbidity are interrelated (some frailty scores involve summing chronic diseases) but cardinal features of frailty, including functional decline and the reduced ability to maintain homeostasis under physiological stress, make it particularly relevant for surgery.

Increasing frailty is associated with worse outcomes, regardless of the type of surgical procedure (Figure 6.2), although the magnitude of the impact of frailty varies, with the starkest effect for colorectal procedures. A large retrospective cohort study found that highly frail patients had

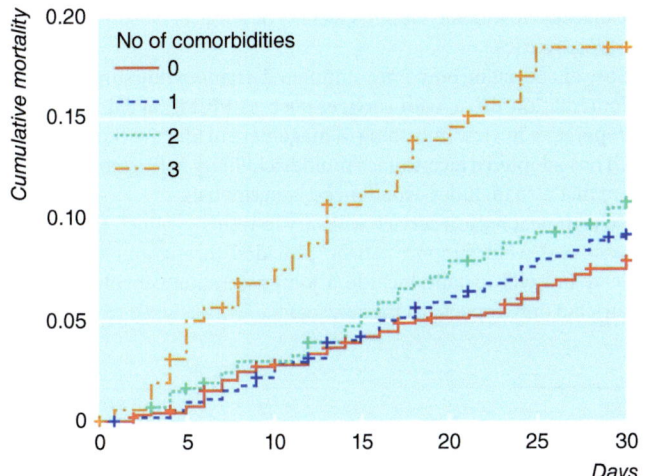

Figure 6.1 The effect of the number of comorbidities on death after surgery for a hip fracture. *Source*: Roche et al. (2005) / BMJ Publishing Group Ltd.

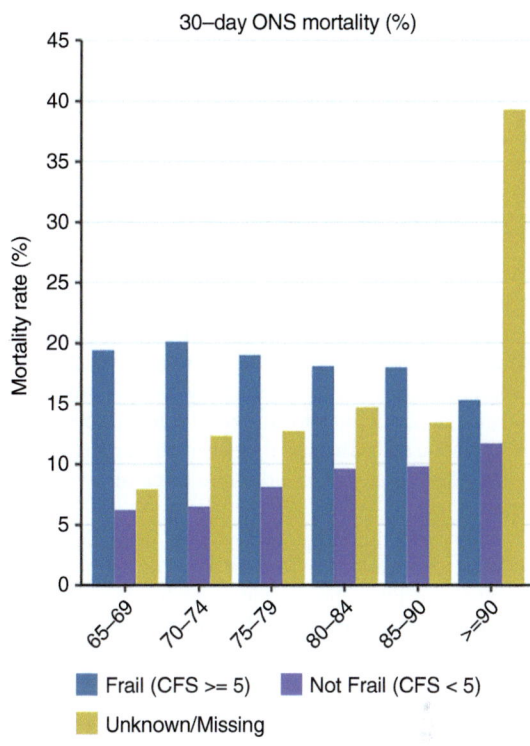

Figure 6.3 30-day ONS mortality after emergency laparotomy by age and Rockwood clinical frailty score (CFS). *Source*: Adapted from NELA 2021.

four times the mortality rate of less frail patients. Other studies have suggested an overall complication rate of between 13 and 19% in frail older patients, compared to the overall complication rate (for both frail and robust) of 2% (retrospective database review using ACS NSQIP [American College of Surgeons National Surgical Quality Improvement Program] data – see the later discussion). In addition, frail older patients have a higher median length of hospital stay, significantly contributing to the economic healthcare burden.

Laparotomy is one of the riskiest types of emergency surgery. The National Emergency Laparotomy Audit (NELA) included 21,846 patients from 177 hospitals in England and Wales in 2021. Fifty-five per cent were 65 or older, of whom a third were living with frailty (clinical frailty score,

CFS ≥ 5). Eighteen per cent were 80 or older, nearly half of whom had frailty. The risks of surgery increase with age, but frailty has a greater impact, particularly in the 'younger old' where it may not be recognised (Figure 6.3). If a patient is frail, they are at elevated risk, regardless of their conventional risk score.

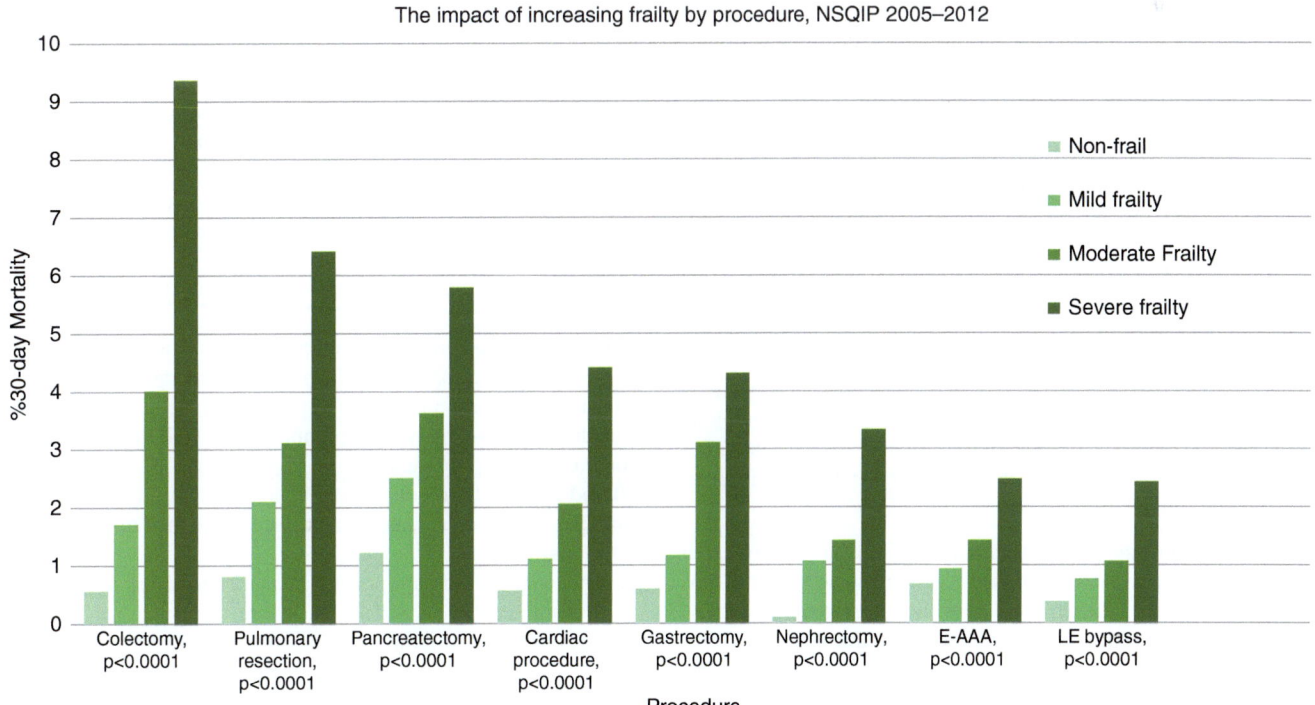

Figure 6.2 Impact of frailty on surgical outcomes. EAAA - endovascular abdominal aortic aneurysm repair, LE bypass - lower extremity (arterial) bypass. *Source*: Mosquera et al. (2016) / with permission of ELSEVIER.

Surgical risk scores

In 2023, there were more than 20 risk scores available in addition to the ASA. The validity of risk calculators is highest in scores that incorporate the type of procedure and a measure of frailty, in addition to conventional risk factors.

ACS NSQIP risk calculator

One of the best is the universal ACS NSQIP surgical risk calculator, although its predictive accuracy varies according to procedure. The ACS NSQIP score (pronounced Nesquip) is user-friendly (you can try it out for yourself on the website). It includes 'geriatric characteristics' such as cognition and the use of mobility aids. It provides colour-coded percentage predictions for the risk of death, severe complications, postoperative delirium, and the risk of discharge to institutional care. It is a useful visual tool to aid in the discussion of surgical risk with a patient.

Not all patients awaiting surgery will want to be made aware of their 'risk of serious complications', especially those unfortunate individuals who feel they have little choice (most notably for cancer surgery). However, a compelling number find such information useful when deciding whether to go ahead with elective surgery.

Improving outcomes for frail older patients

This work was initiated by enthusiasts and has since been driven by service evaluation and national audits.

- Irvine and other geriatricians pioneered holistic care for hip fracture patients from the 1960s onwards; trials in the 1980s suggested benefit, and this was taken up by some units, but not in a systematic manner.
- In 2003, a team at Guy's and St Thomas' Hospital in London conceived, implemented, and evaluated the effect of input from a geriatrician-led multidisciplinary team throughout the surgical pathway, starting with elective orthopaedics. They named the service POPS (now standing for Perioperative medicine for Older People having Surgery).
- The National Hip Fracture Database was set up in 2007 as a joint venture between the BGS and the British Orthopaedic Association. Financial incentives were used to drive collaboration, and the subspecialty of orthogeriatrics became established in most parts of the UK. Initially, outcomes improved but worsened over the COVID-19 pandemic, and as the NHS has struggled since.
- A turning point was the National Confidential Enquiry into Patient Outcome and Death after Surgery in the over-80s (2010). This highlighted serious deficiencies and found that only 37% patients (295/786) had received 'good' care. Its report, 'An Age Old Problem', recommended increased input from geriatricians and a greater focus on syndromes such as frailty and delirium. One initiative that resulted is the annual NELA.

The POPS group and others have continued to produce research showing benefit from a comprehensive geriatric assessment (CGA) approach in different surgical specialties including general surgery, urology, and vascular surgery, and in a variety of settings. Improved outcomes include reductions in postoperative morbidity, mortality and length of stay (typically 3–4 days) for elective and emergency surgery. The role of the geriatrician in surgical liaison is now advocated by the UK's Royal Colleges of Surgeons, Anaesthetists, and Physicians, as well as the BGS. It is gaining traction internationally, and geriatric medicine

has expanded to include the subspecialty of 'surgical liaison' in addition to 'orthogeriatrics'.

These encouraging outcomes stimulated a nationwide surgical liaison implementation drive, with services such as PRIME at Addenbrooke's (Perioperative Review Informing Management of Elective Surgery 2014), which has adopted a face-to-face multidisciplinary approach harnessing a team that also includes experienced anaesthetists.

Each surgical liaison service will vary in terms of which patients can be seen and what support can be provided throughout the surgical pathway but will usually include a joint assessment involving both a geriatrician and a specialist therapy team.

Pre-surgical optimisation

Emergency surgery

The amount that can be achieved preoperatively depends on the urgency of the surgery. Prior to emergency surgery, it is essential to manage heart failure, salt and water depletion, respiratory infection, and severe anaemia as rapidly as possible. The volume depletion associated with a fractured hip is easy to underestimate, and more aggressive fluid replacement prior to surgery improves the outcome.

Elective surgery and prehabilitation

In major elective surgery prehabilitation, the practice of enhancing functional capacity before surgery, has been shown to improve outcomes, including reducing length of stay, postoperative pain, and postoperative complications. Interventions include:

- **Stop smoking:** a Cochrane review of eight clinical trials of smoking cessation programmes on pulmonary and overall complications concluded that intervention 4–8 weeks prior to surgery with nicotine replacement therapy was likely to reduce the risk of any complication (RR 0.70; 95% CI 0.56–0.88).
- **Incentive spirometry:** using this breathing training aid to strengthen inspiratory muscles and minimise atelectasis reduces postoperative chest infections.
- **Own equipment:** check whether patients use support such as continuous positive airway pressure (CPAP) at home and compel them to bring in their machine on admission.
- **Improve fitness:** may be achievable before a colonic resection but is often not practical if the surgery is for chronic pain, e.g. knee replacement.
- **Improve nutrition:** through supplementation/nasogastric tube, if necessary.
- **Optimise management:** note co-morbidities, but balance gain from investigations, e.g. an echocardiogram, against a delay whilst awaiting this test. If there is a history of COPD, would a course of steroids be needed prior to surgery? Low preoperative SaO_2 is more predictive of outcome than spirometry.
- **Blood review:** (particularly haemoglobin, albumin, renal function, and HbA1c if diabetic) and correct electrolytes, anaemia, etc.
- **Optimise drugs:**
  - Anticoagulant and antiplatelet agents: depends on the indication, the individual's risk, and the procedure, but usually stop warfarin a week before and swap to therapeutic LMWH, e.g. enoxaparin to bridge, stop direct oral anticoagulants 2 days before, and stop clopidogrel a week before (limited data).
  - Stop non-essential drugs, particularly if they will add to delirium.
  - Diabetics may need a reduction in usual insulin dosing on the day of surgery or insulin on a sliding scale.

- ○ Plan which drugs should be taken on the morning of surgery with a little water (long-term beta-blockers, drugs for PD).
- **Assess cognition:** to assess the risk of postoperative delirium; forewarn the patient and family and provide written information; this reduces distress and possibly complaints, and enables the family to help with reorientation after surgery.
- **Swab for MRSA:** eliminate if present.
- **Pre-op therapy input:** plan walking aids and appliances.
- **Pre-op social work input:** if a package of care will be needed.
- **Special considerations:** e.g. stoma nurse.
- **The mode of anaesthesia:** will be discussed with the patient, such as explaining why a spinal anaesthetic approach may be preferable to a general anaesthetic (e.g. in those with poor respiratory function and chronic lung disease) or when local anaesthesia with sedation is more desirable.
- **A bespoke care plan:** is then created, which will often include a risk stratification score such as the ACS NSQIP, which produces mortality and morbidity data that can help inform discussion.
- **Plan the position on the list:** to minimise the length of fasting and avoid overnight stays, if possible.
- **Plan the location of early postoperative care:** e.g. an ICU or a high-dependency bed.
- **Explain and check understanding:** ensure the patient has a grasp of their diagnosis and treatment plan (feedback suggests that patients really value this component).

Anaesthetic care

The skill of the anaesthetist is as important as the surgeon in ensuring a good outcome; frail older people are usually assessed pre-operatively by a senior anaesthetist, who will decide whether general or regional anaesthesia is appropriate.

- Ageing affects the pharmacokinetics and pharmacodynamics of many anaesthetic drugs.
- Pre-medication is often avoided, and reduced doses are needed for many drugs.
- During surgery, the aim is to avoid episodes of excessive hypotension after induction, hypoxia, large blood loss, or the combination of hypertension and tachycardia after noxious stimulation.
- Patients need diligent care of their pressure areas and maintenance of their body temperature.

Delirium is more likely after prolonged surgery. Reducing the 'depth' of anaesthesia has been studied in terms of delirium risk, but results have been inconclusive. However, the bispectral index (BIS) may be monitored by placing four electrodes on the forehead to monitor the EEG and frontalis activity. Similarly, there is surprisingly little evidence that regional rather than general anaesthesia reduces delirium, although it reduces respiratory complications. Using non-opiate analgesics and avoiding benzodiazepines may be beneficial. Meta-analysis suggests that the use of dexmedetomidine (an alpha$_2$ adrenoceptor agonist often used as a sedative intraoperatively) is useful in reducing postoperative delirium.

Postoperative care

Postoperative analgesia requires care to maximise pain relief with minimal sedation or respiratory depression. Other measures include support and encouragement, early mobilisation, careful fluid and electrolyte balance, removing the urinary catheter as soon as possible, maximising nutrition with dietetic support, avoiding constipation, minimising sleep deprivation and using non-drug measures as the first line for confusion.

Postoperative complications

Surgery has inevitable consequences, including a tissue inflammatory response, exposure to a variety of drugs, a period of immobility, pain, and atelectasis if a general anaesthetic is required; in a proportion of people, these lead to complications.

Postoperative complications are often predictors of *long-term* mortality and survival. This is in addition to the short-term challenges of managing these complications. Common medical complications of surgery (rather than 'surgical' complications, e.g. wound infection) are listed in the box, and those that are particularly common in older people are discussed in more detail.

'Medical' postoperative complications

1. **Respiratory infection:** resulting from atelectasis due to poor inspiration because of pain (abdominal surgery) or sedation.
2. **Venous thromboembolism:** DVT and PE are common after surgery, estimated at 10–40%, but adequate prophylaxis reduces clinical thrombosis to 1–2%.
3. **Acute kidney injury:** usually occurs within 2 days of surgery and strongly predicts poor outcomes.
4. **Delirium:** commonest on days 3 or 4 and following orthopaedic rather than general surgery, possibly related to cerebral fat embolism. See Chapter 8 for other causes; drug toxicity, and abrupt withdrawal from drugs, or unrecognised preoperative high alcohol intake are common. Other precipitating factors include intra-operative blood transfusion, hyponatraemia due to bladder irrigation during prostatectomy, sensory deprivation, pain, bladder distension, and constipation.
5. **Vomiting:** many causes, including ileus, but check the drug chart for codeine.
6. **Cardiac failure:** occurs in 5–10% of surgical patients over 65, multifactorial, exacerbated by overenthusiastic fluid replacement and increased ADH secretion due to surgery and pain.
7. **MI:** occurs in 1–4% of cases, half are painless, may present as 'failure to thrive' postoperatively. Compare new and preoperative ECGs.
8. **Stroke:** in 3% of patients over 80 undergoing surgery.
9. **Pressure ulcers:** assiduous prevention is best (see Chapter 19).
10. **Deconditioning:** minimise by prehabilitation and early mobilisation

---

Pulmonary complications

- **Procedure-related factors:** are most predictive of postoperative pulmonary complications – PPCs. Procedures close to the diaphragm with upper abdominal incisions (such as cholecystectomy), emergency surgery, use of general anaesthesia, need for blood transfusion, and long operations are all associated with a higher risk of PPCs.
- **Patient-related factors:** age, chronic lung disease, cancer, comorbidities, obesity, frailty.

Common pulmonary complications

- **Pneumonia:** about 1 in 5 people having major abdominal surgery get a chest infection. Pneumonia is associated with a mortality rate of

30%. The incidence is 14 times higher in ventilated patients. Aspiration is a common cause of pneumonia in patients with postoperative ileus, but there is no benefit from inserting a nasogastric tube before vomiting occurs.

- **Atelectasis:** small studies had suggested that CPAP might reduce postoperative morbidity, but PRISM, an open-label randomised trial in 4,800 patients after major abdominal surgery, found that CPAP did not reduce pneumonia, reintubation, or death. CPAP has a role in managing respiratory failure after surgery but is not recommended prophylactically.
- **Bronchospasm:** more common in asthmatics but can be triggered by some anaesthetic agents.
- **Venous thromboembolism** (VTE): rates of deep vein thrombosis (DVT) and its serious sequel of pulmonary embolism (PE) (see Figure 6.4) vary widely in the literature (from 1 to 30%). The incidence depends on the age of the patient, the type of surgery, the adequacy and duration of prophylaxis, and particularly whether the clot presents as a clinical problem or is discovered on imaging as part of a trial. Many patients with lower limb fractures start to develop a DVT because of the trauma *prior* to surgery. As the length of stay decreases, VTE is more likely to occur after discharge. A 2023 meta-analysis (22 studies, 1.86 million patients, mixed surgery) found that of blood clots occurring within 4 weeks after surgery, 47% occurred by the first, 74% by the second, and 90% by the third week after surgery. The overall rate of clinical VTE was 1.1%.

The choice of regime for VTE prevention has expanded since the 1990s (when LMWH was introduced), with fondaparinux (a synthetic pentasaccharide that inhibits factor 10), DOACs, and a return to aspirin amongst the options.

In the UK, because of the substantial risk after hip surgery, prophylaxis is usually continued at least 28 days after the operation. NICE guidance is complex, e.g. after elective hip replacement:

- LMWH for 10 days, followed by aspirin (75 mg or 150 mg) for a further 28 days or
- LMWH for 28 days combined with anti-embolism stockings (until discharge) or
- Rivaroxaban for 5 weeks.
- Apixaban for 5 weeks if none of the above can be used.

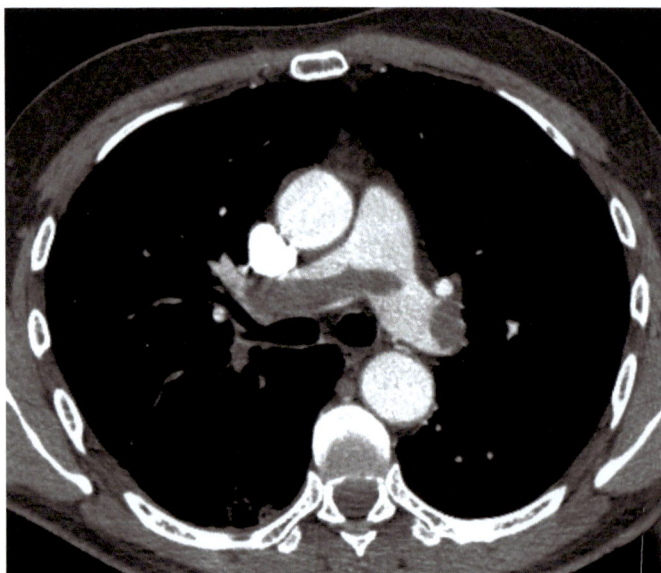

Figure 6.4 CT scan of the chest with contrast showing major bilateral pulmonary emboli.

Factors such as whether the patient can self-inject may affect the choice. Consult your local guidelines.

After fragility fracture of the pelvis, hip and proximal femur offer VTE prophylaxis for a month (if the risk of VTE outweighs the risk of bleeding) with either:

- LMWH, starting 6 to 12 hours after surgery or
- Fondaparinux sodium, starting 6 hours after surgery, providing there is low risk of bleeding.

Consider pre-operative VTE prophylaxis if surgery is delayed beyond the day after admission. Give the last dose no less than 12 hours before surgery for LMWH or 24 hours before surgery for fondaparinux.

The management of postoperative respiratory complications does not differ greatly from that in a non-surgical context. Close collaboration with surgical colleagues is needed to ensure that families receive an overall picture of a patient's current clinical state rather than simply that 'the operation went well'.

Renal complications

Postoperative acute kidney injury (AKI) is associated with an eightfold increase in 30-day mortality. Even small increases in serum creatinine levels are independently associated with poorer outcomes. AKI is most likely to occur in the first day or two after surgery. 80% of those experiencing postoperative AKI have at least one period of perioperative haemodynamic instability (usually hypotensive episodes).

- **Patient-related factors** are important, especially pre-existing intrinsic renal disease and diabetes. Look for common factors such as post-renal obstructive causes (prostatic hypertrophy or urethral strictures), which may have been well tolerated prior to surgery.
- **Procedure-related factors** may also play a part - laparoscopic techniques cause iatrogenic increases in intra-abdominal pressure, which may constrict renal vasculature, affecting blood flow.

Fluid management and drugs

As one might expect, careful fluid balance management is key in minimising the risk of postoperative renal failure. Over-enthusiastic IV fluid resuscitation can predispose to increased intra-abdominal pressure and poor wound healing, as well as exacerbating heart failure. Goal-directed fluid therapy is the gold standard, but is much easier to implement in an intensive care setting. The choice of intravenous fluids must also be carefully considered – the overuse of normal saline can predispose to hyperchloraemic metabolic acidosis, so balanced crystalloids (e.g. Hartmann's solution) are recommended (though trial evidence is limited). Nephrotoxic drugs are another cause or contributor to AKI – review the drug chart. Drug doses may need reducing, e.g. dalteparin. Non-steroidal painkillers should be avoided, ACE inhibitors and ARBs (angiotensin receptor blockers) should be held, and tight glycaemic control has been found to be beneficial, particularly in cardiac surgery.

Neurobehavioural complications

Postoperative delirium is the presence of cognitive change, variable consciousness, and/or perceptual disturbance in the postoperative period. Symptoms are identical to delirium in any context, with agitation and hallucinations being the most troublesome for patients; one must take care not to miss the 'hypoactive' group. There are several theories proposed to describe the pathophysiological process, including neuro-inflammation associated with the release of inflammatory mediators such as CRP and IL-6.

Postoperative delirium is extremely common and is experienced by up to 50% of vulnerable older patients. It increases all-cause mortality by up to 10% and length of hospital stay by 2–3 days. It is often distressing for patients and their relatives.

Given the consequences, it is important to recognise those most at risk prior to surgery and address any modifiable risk factors (a key task for a preoperative optimisation team).

Predisposing factors for postoperative delirium

- Age.
- Nursing home residency/functional dependence.
- Pre-existing cognitive impairment.
- Psychiatric disorders, including alcohol misuse.
- Cerebrovascular disease.
- End-stage renal failure.
- Low albumin.
- High ASA score.
- Electrolyte abnormalities.

In medical inpatients, studies have shown that a multidisciplinary, comprehensive approach leads to sizeable reductions in both the incidence and duration of delirium. It would be reasonable to extrapolate this to a surgical cohort. When preventative measures fail, postoperative delirium is managed like delirium in other settings, but surgical wounds, drains, and intravenous lines provide extra challenges. In addition to good general nursing, reorient the patient often if this helps them, or reassure and encourage them.

It is good practice to supply written information about the concept and treatment of delirium to patients and relatives if this was not done prior to surgery. Encourage relatives to visit as early as possible to help with orientation. Trials with low-dose antipsychotics suggest they do not reduce the incidence of delirium but may reduce the duration of symptoms.

The future

Unfortunately, the implementation of surgical liaison and pre-surgical optimisation is still extremely limited in the UK. In 2019, a survey suggested that only 1% of UK hospitals had a surgical liaison service for older patients. This will increase, but it will be years before it is available to most patients.

- The surgical community has recognised that operating on increasingly frail patients challenges the limits of their usual practice.
- In a survey in 2013, 85% of surgical trainees believed support from geriatric medicine was necessary but, in most cases, it was inadequate.
- Liaison is harder to organise for an emergency than elective surgery, but NELA recommends that all over 65s with frailty and all those over 80 who need an emergency laparotomy should have an assessment by a consultant geriatrician. This target is currently not met, and will not be soon, given the shortage of geriatricians.

If safe care is to be provided, there will need to be more emphasis on older people in undergraduate and postgraduate training in *all* specialities, an expansion in the number of geriatricians, and financial incentives to drive the changes.

📖 REFERENCES AND FURTHER READING

American College of Surgeons *NSQIP Surgical Risk Calculator* https://riskcalculator.facs.org/RiskCalculator

American Society of Anesthesiologists (2020) *ASA Physical Status Classification* https://www.asahq.org/standards-and-practice-parameters/statement-on-asa-physical-status-classification-system

Roche JJW, Wenn RT, Sahota O, et al. (2005) Effect of comorbidities and postoperative complications on mortality after hip fracture in elderly people: prospective observational cohort study. *BMJ* 331:1374. doi: 10.1136/bmj.38643.663843.55

Mosquera C, Spaniolas K, Fitzgerald TL (2016) Impact of frailty on surgical outcomes: the right patient for the right procedure. *Surgery* 160:272–280. doi: 10.1016/j.surg.2016.04.030.

Royal College of Anaesthetists *National Emergency Laparotomy Audit (NELA)* www.nela.org.uk

Golden DL, Ata A, Kusupati V, et al. (2019) Predicting postoperative complications after acute care surgery: how accurate is the ACS NSQIP surgical risk calculator? *The American Surgeon* 85:335–341. doi: 10.1177/000313481908500421.

Harari D, Hopper A, Dhesi J, et al. (2007) Proactive care of older people undergoing surgery ('POPS'): Designing, embedding, evaluating and funding a comprehensive geriatric assessment service for older elective surgical patients. *Age and Ageing* 36:190–196. doi: 10.1093/ageing/afl163.

RCP *National hip fracture database* www.nhfd.co.uk

NCEPOD Elective & Emergency Surgery in the Elderly: An Age Old Problem (2010) www.ncepod.org.uk/2010eese.html

Shipway D, Koizia L, Winterkorn N, et al. (2018) Embedded geriatric surgical liaison is associated with reduced inpatient length of stay in older patients admitted for gastrointestinal surgery. *RCP Future Health Journal* 5:108–116. doi: 10.7861/futurehosp 5-2-108.

Thomsen T, Villebro N, Møller AM (2014) Interventions for preoperative smoking cessation. *Cochrane Database of Systematic Reviews*. doi: 14651858.CD002294.pub4.

Douketis J. (2023) Perioperative management of patients receiving anticoagulants. *UpToDate*. https://www.uptodate.com/contents/perioperative-management-of-patients-receiving-anticoagulants/print.

Zeng H, Li Z, He J, et al. (2019) Dexmedetomidine for the prevention of postoperative delirium in elderly patients undergoing noncardiac surgery: a meta-analysis of randomized controlled trials. *PLoS One* 14(8): e0218088. doi: 10.1371/journal.pone.0218088.

Miskovic A, Lumb AB (2017) Postoperative pulmonary complications. *British Journal of Anaesthesia* 118:317–334. doi: 10.1093/bja/aex002.

EuroSurg Collaborative (2020) Timing of nasogastric tube insertion and the risk of postoperative pneumonia: an international, prospective cohort study. *Colorectal disease* 22:2288–2297. doi: 10.1111/codi.15311.

Prism Trial Group (2021) Postoperative continuous positive airway pressure to prevent pneumonia, re-intubation, and death after major abdominal surgery (PRISM): a multicentre, open-label, randomised, phase 3 trial. *The Lancet Respiratory Medicine* 9:1221–1230. doi: 10.1016/S2213-2600(21)00089-8.

Singh T, Lavikainen LI, Halme ALE, et al. (2023) Timing of symptomatic venous thromboembolism after surgery: meta-analysis *British Journal of Surgery* 110:553–561. doi: 10.1093/bjs/znad035.

Anderson D, Dunbar M, Murnaghan J, et al. (2018) Aspirin or rivaroxaban for VTE prophylaxis after hip or knee arthroplasty. *New England Journal of Medicine* 378:699–707. doi: 10.1056/NEJMoa1712746 (arthroplasty=joint replacement).

NICE guidance on *Reducing the risk of hospital acquired VTE* NG 89 (2018), last updated 2019. www.nice.org.uk/guidance/ng89/chapter/recommendations#interventions-for-people-having-orthopaedic-surgery

Bramley P, McArthur K, Blayney A, et al. (2021) Risk factors for postoperative delirium: an umbrella review of systematic reviews *International Journal of Surgery* 93:106063. doi: 10.1016/j.ijsu.2021.106063.

Jin Z, Hu J, Ma D (2020) Postoperative delirium: perioperative assessment, risk reduction, and management. *British Journal of Anaesthesia* 125:492–504. doi: 10.1016/j.bja.2020.06.063.

Shipway DJH, Partridge JSL, Foxton CR, et al. (2015) Do surgical trainees believe they are adequately trained to manage the ageing population? A UK survey of knowledge and beliefs in surgical trainees. *Journal of Surgical Education* 72:641–647. doi: 10.1016/j.jsurg.2015.01.019.

The updated CPOC/ BGS Guideline for Perioperative Care for People Living with Frailty Undergoing Elective and Emergency Surgery (2021) www.bgs.org.uk/sites/default/files/content/attachment/2021-09-28/Guideline for Perioperative Care for People Living with Frailty Undergoing Elective and Emergency Surgery.pdf

Perioperative care for older people undergoing surgery POPS network https://www.popsolderpeople.org

All websites were accessed in June 2024.

7

Neurology

Age changes and clinical examination

1 A full neurological examination can be an ordeal for both a frail older patient and their doctor. Patience and understanding are required by both, and compromise will often be needed.
2 Much can be gained by simple observation. The patient's memory and speech during history-taking and their ability to walk to and get onto the examination couch may give you clues to the underlying pathology.
3 Ageing changes and co-morbidities, e.g. arthritis, may confuse the clinical picture. Gait becomes slower and less regular in pattern with feet closer together, less firm heel strike, and more time with both feet on the ground. One-third of 'normal' over-80-year-olds have a shuffling gait, and almost half have a flexed posture, even in the absence of Parkinson's disease.
4 Muscle wasting is commonly due to disuse, making it difficult for some individuals to rise from a chair without help. Wasting of the small muscles of the hand does not automatically have the sinister connotations of the same finding in young subjects.
5 Reflexes may be difficult to elicit because of other pathologies, e.g. osteoarthritis. Ankle jerks are difficult to elicit in almost 1/3 of older people. Abdominal reflexes are almost universally absent.
6 Pupils are often small and react sluggishly, and cataracts are common, so examination of the fundi is often difficult (even after mydriasis).
7 Slight changes in sensation may be difficult to find – moving from abnormal to normal is easier for patients to detect. Vibration sense is often lost or not understood, so position sense is usually a better test to employ (but fixed joints may make even this difficult).
8 Do be gentle with your patients if you want their cooperation. If necessary, break the examination down into stages and do not expect perfection from yourself or your patient.

Symptomatic classification of neurological disease in older people

1 **Headache:**
  - Raised intracranial pressure, but fewer than 10% of patients with brain tumours present with headache alone.
  - Pain radiating from cervical spondylosis.
  - Giant-cell arteritis – tender temporal arteries, tenderness over proximal muscles, high ESR/CRP.
  - Psychological – but the prevalence of 'tension' headaches decline with age; consider depression.
  - Paget's disease of the skull is occasionally painful when active – often obvious.
  - Migraine, but new onset is unusual over 50 years.
2 **Pain in the face:**
  - Trigeminal neuralgia – the mean age of onset is around 50 years; it rarely starts in old age.
  - Dental problems – increasing as NHS dentistry is so hard to access.
  - Sinusitis.
  - Giant-cell arteritis (pain on chewing).
  - Post-herpetic neuralgia (look for post-inflammatory pigmentary change in a trigeminal dermatome).
3 **Hemiparesis:**
  - Stroke
  - Space-occupying lesion.
4 **Paraparesis:**
  - Cord compression – either a vascular or space-occupying lesion.
  - CSF/CNS infection.
  - Guillain–Barré syndrome (GBS).
  - Pressure from disc prolapse, bone, or collection of pus.
5 **Unsteadiness:**
  - Neuropathy.
  - Proximal myopathy.
  - Cerebellar disease.
  - Drug-induced.
  - Cerebrovascular disease.
  - Middle-ear disease.
  - Myxoedema.
6 **Rigidity/immobility:**
  - Parkinson's disease.
  - Drugs – especially phenothiazines/antipsychotics.
  - Disuse (e.g. after a stroke).
  - Joint/bone problems.
  - Spasticity of stroke, multi-infarct/vascular dementia.
7 **Asymmetrical weakness:**
  - Nerve entrapment.
  - Motor neurone disease.
  - Diabetes – mononeuritis.
8 **Clouding of consciousness:**
  - Meningitis, encephalitis, or sepsis at any site.
  - Raised intracranial pressure.
  - Drugs (sedatives, hypnotics).
  - Biochemical disturbances.

Geriatric Medicine and Elderly Care: Lecture Notes, Ninth Edition. Claire G. Nicholl, K. Jane Wilson, and Shaun D'Souza.
© 2025 John Wiley & Sons Ltd. Published 2025 by John Wiley & Sons Ltd.
Companion website: www.wiley.com/go/lecturenotesgeriatricmedicine9e

- Delirium.
- Lewy body dementia.

9 Coma:
- Stroke (large lesions in the cerebral hemispheres, even small lesions in the brain stem).
- Space-occupying lesion.
- Seizures.
- Drugs (sedatives, hypnotics, alcohol).
- Poisoning (accidental – remember carbon monoxide, self-harm and iatrogenic).
- Biochemical disturbance (do not miss hypoglycaemia).

10 Involuntary movement:
- Parkinson's disease.
- Drugs (anti-parkinsonian treatment, neuroleptics).
- Essential tremor.
- Vascular disease (in old age, choreiform movements and hemiballismus are usually due to stroke).
- Epilepsy.
- Cerebellar disease.

Conditions seen in older patients

These are loosely grouped by aetiology, but some presentations have many causes.

Vascular disease

See Chapter 8 for vascular dementia and Chapter 9 for stroke.

Trauma

Low-trauma skull fractures

If a patient falls on the ward and sustains a head injury or facial bruising routine x-ray is not helpful, but check for diplopia (fractured orbit), request neurological observations, and get an urgent CT head scan if they become drowsy (risk of extradural, subdural, or cerebral contusion), or if they are taking anticoagulant medications.

Subdural haematoma

This is more common in old age because of the increased frequency of falls, and it is said that cerebral atrophy allows the continued oozing of blood into the subdural space after a traumatic head injury. Bleeding occurs from the tearing of the bridging veins that cross from the cortex to the dural venous sinuses.

- A subdural haematoma (SDH) may be asymptomatic, cause mild unilateral weakness, intellectual impairment, seizures, or loss of consciousness.
- Clinical features of acute SDH occur within hours; those of a chronic subdural may manifest over weeks.
- A fluctuating course or disproportionate drowsiness in a patient with an appropriate fall history would suggest the diagnosis.
- Increased use of anticoagulants in old age (e.g. for atrial fibrillation) exposes more patients to the risk of subdural bleeding, especially if prone to falls, drinking to excess, or poor INR control on warfarin. Prompt reversal of coagulopathy should be undertaken.

The diagnosis is confirmed by a head CT and is characterised by a crescent-shaped collection of blood over one hemisphere, with or

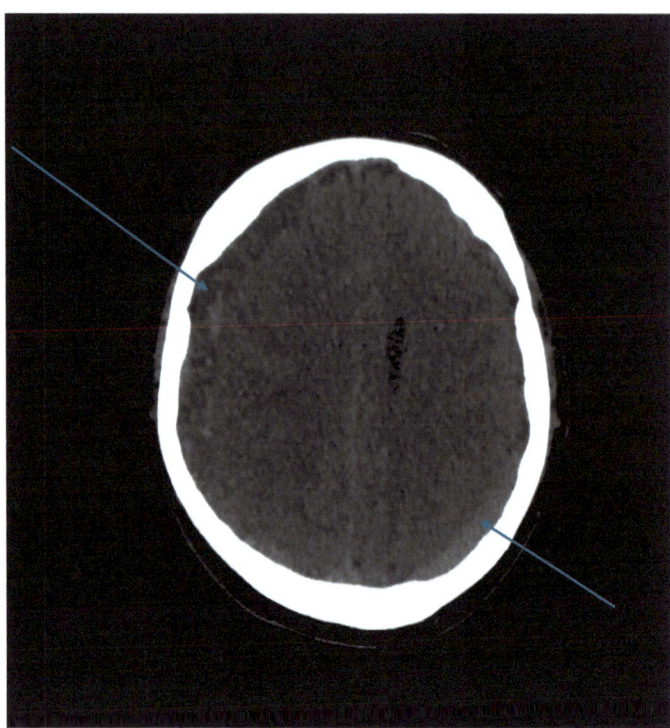

Figure 7.1 Bilateral subdural collections with acute on chronic appearances. Note that the patient was confused and unable to lie straight in the scanner.

without associated midline shift. No randomised trials have compared surgery with conservative management for patients with SDH, but limited observational data suggests that patients with acute SDH who are clinically stable and have small haematomas can be managed non-operatively.

Neurosurgical intervention is considered in those subacute or chronic SDHs that are expanding and causing neurological deficits. The hardest decisions are whether and when to operate. The appearance of the blood alters with time (acute SDH – hyperdense lesions [see Figure 7.1], chronic – diffusely hypodense), but it can be hard to be precise about when the SDH occurred. A hemicraniotomy to relieve cerebral swelling may be needed for acute SDH after rapid medical optimisation, which may include intubation, head-of-bed elevation, and hyperosmolar treatment to reduce intracranial pressure. Chronic SDH may be managed by either burr hole evacuation or twist-drill craniotomy with drain placement. The benefits of surgery are less certain in patients who have preexisting cognitive impairment, dementia, or multiple medical comorbidities. Find out as much as possible about the patient's prior functional performance from carers or relatives – this will inform discussions with the neurosurgeons.

Complications include re-accumulation of the haematoma after evacuation, seizures (consider prophylactic anticonvulsant drugs such as levetiracetam), persistent neurological deficit, coma, and death. Such cases often result in a coroner's inquest requiring the attendance of senior clinical staff.

Degenerative diseases

Spine

Spinal cord compression

Cord compression may be secondary to a prolapsed disc, trauma, pressure from a tumour, osteophytes (especially cervical spondylosis) or collapsed vertebrae (usually metastatic disease, especially prostate cancer or osteoporosis), discitis (vertebral osteomyelitis) or an epidural abscess. Iatrogenic causes include the formation of an epidural haematoma after a lumbar puncture. A fall may be the precipitating event in a patient who had asymptomatic pathology. Plain x-rays can be difficult to interpret, especially in the cervical spine, where degenerative changes are very common.

The motor effect of a cord lesion depends on the level.

- A very high neck lesion gives upper motor neuron (UMN) signs in the arms and legs (spastic quadriparesis) and can also cause diaphragmatic paralysis.
- Lower in the neck, compression leads to nerve root or lower motor neuron (LMN) signs in the arms, but UMN changes in the legs.
- A thoracic lesion will lead to spastic paraparesis with UMN signs in the legs. A sensory level, if present, will help locate the region for further investigation; it is usually several segments below the level of cord compression. Patients with cervical and thoracic lesions often have an irritable bladder due to the loss of supraspinal inhibition.
- Lumbo-sacral lesions present with LMN signs and sensory loss as the cord ends at L1/2 and the spinal roots (cauda equina) then continue down the spinal canal to their exit foramina. Urinary retention is common as the bladder does not empty. Check for anal tone and saddle anaesthesia (use a neurotip in the perianal area).

Sudden onset of compression of the cord or cauda equina is an emergency, and rapid investigation is essential if intervention (surgery or radiotherapy) is to avoid permanent damage. MRI is better than CT for diagnostic purposes. Check that there is no contraindication to MRI, e.g. a non-compatible cardiac pacemaker.

Treatment of spinal cord compression depends on the cause. Malignant cord compression is often due to bone metastases from a prostatic, breast or lung primary. In about 10% of patients, a spinal metastasis is the first manifestation of an unknown primary. A course of steroids (typically dexamethasone, with gut protection) is usually prescribed as soon as this diagnosis is suspected (sometimes even before confirmation by imaging). Radiotherapy is then considered. A Cochrane review of interventions for metastatic spinal cord compression found that decompressive surgery may benefit those with a single area of compression, but only if under the age of 65 years.

Complications of spinal cord compression can be devastating and include aspiration pneumonia, particularly in those needing assisted ventilation due to higher cervical lesions. Prevention of pressure ulcers requires careful nursing attention, regular turning, and suitable pressure-relieving mattresses. Bladder disturbances and sexual dysfunction are also common. If an inpatient, ensure that the patient has adequate protection against venous thromboembolism.

Cervical myelopathy

This is spinal cord dysfunction from compression in the neck, commonly due to degenerative changes termed spondylosis (secondary to osteophytes, disc protrusion, and ligament hypertrophy), often at C5/6, C6/7, or multiple levels. Patients present with progressive pain and stiffness in the limbs, imbalance, loss of dexterity, falls, and incontinence. Patients with sensory changes in both hands are often misdiagnosed as having carpal tunnel syndrome. The diagnosis is confirmed by MRI of the cervical spine, and surgery may be considered.

Lumbar canal stenosis

This is usually due to a congenitally narrow spinal canal but presents in middle or older age when osteophytes or a disc encroach on the cauda equina. It may present with weak legs or intermittent pain in the buttocks and legs when walking. It can be distinguished from peripheral vascular disease as patients find climbing stairs easier than walking on a flat surface (because the spine is flexed), the discomfort takes longer – around 10 min – to improve with rest, and there may be sensorimotor signs. Pain control and exercise are essential. There is no unambiguous evidence that surgery is beneficial, and 10–20% of people undergoing surgery report side effects of the procedure. If surgery is chosen, a meta-analysis suggests that microdecompression may provide better pain relief than traditional decompressive laminectomy.

Brain

Primary dementias

See Chapter 8.

Parkinson's disease and related disorders

Parkinson's disease is a progressive neurodegenerative condition first described by James Parkinson in 1817. Key features include slow movements, stiffness, tremor and postural instability. The term 'parkinsonism' is used to describe this group of movement symptoms or conditions that include these features. The term 'parkinsonian' is used descriptively, e.g. a parkinsonian tremor or a parkinsonian disorder.

The commonest cause of primary parkinsonism is Parkinson's disease (PD), which is a syndrome with the commoner sporadic form, and rarer familial forms. Most cases of secondary parkinsonism are due to drugs or vascular disease. Other neurodegenerative disorders, sometimes known as 'Parkinson's plus syndromes', can be mistaken for PD early in their course, but have a more extensive pathology that determines their clinical features (see Figure 7.2).

PD and related disorders are covered in detail. UK geriatricians often run a multidisciplinary movement disorder service for older people, sometimes in conjunction with neurology colleagues. This is a well-established subspecialty of geriatric medicine.

Parkinson's disease

PD is an idiopathic degenerative condition with progressive death of the dopaminergic neurons of the substantia nigra (SN) in the basal ganglia.

- The neurons appear to die by apoptosis, which may be triggered by mitochondrial impairment and oxidative stress.
- Symptoms appear when around 80% of the dopamine has been lost and are due to a lack of dopamine and a relative excess of acetylcholine.
- PD is thought to occur in genetically susceptible individuals exposed to an environmental trigger, but the nature of both components is still unknown (chronic low-dose pesticide exposure remains a favoured environmental risk factor in the literature). Over 20 genes have been identified in the rarer familial forms of PD, which tend to be younger-onset and have a variety of inheritance patterns.
- The postmortem finding of Lewy bodies (intracytoplasmic inclusion bodies containing abnormally aggregated alpha-synuclein) restricted to the substantia nigra is pathognomonic (Figure 7.3).
- Alpha-synuclein is thought to have a role in DNA repair. When alpha-synuclein aggregates in the Lewy bodies, normal cellular transport may be disrupted, and its lack in the nucleus may be a factor in causing the death of the neuron.
- The prevalence of PD increases with age (from around 250 per 100,000 aged 60–64 to 1,700 per 100,000 aged over 80). Patients should be asked whether they would donate their brain tissue to the PD brain bank posthumously.

Clinical features

PD is one of the most common neurological disorders, affecting around 1% of those over 60. It is 1.5 times more common in men than in women. High caffeine intake and smoking are associated with a lower risk of PD.

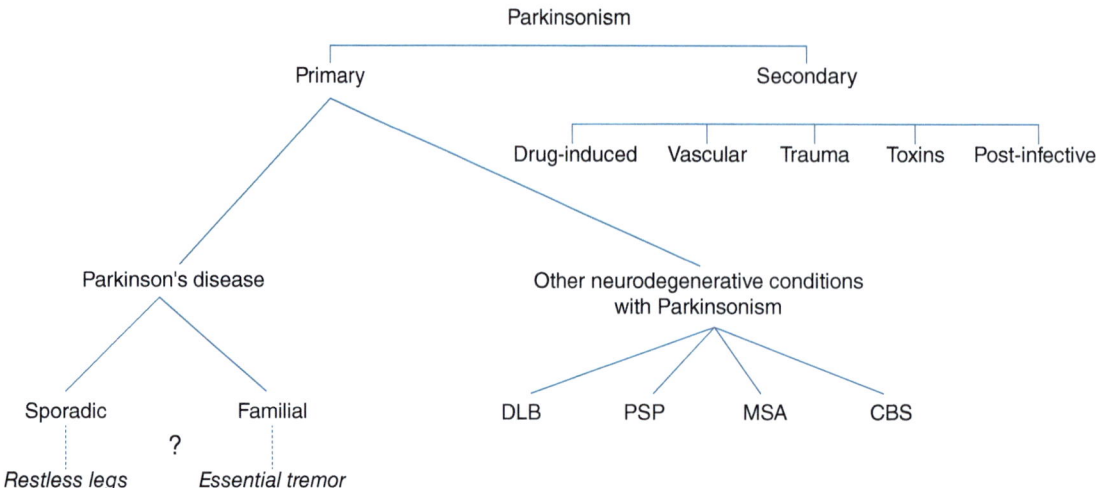

Figure 7.2 The classification of parkinsonian syndromes. DLB - dementia with Lewy bodies, PSP - progressive supranuclear palsy; MSA - multiple system atrophy; CBS - corticobasal syndrome (assume that these can be formatted under the Figure).

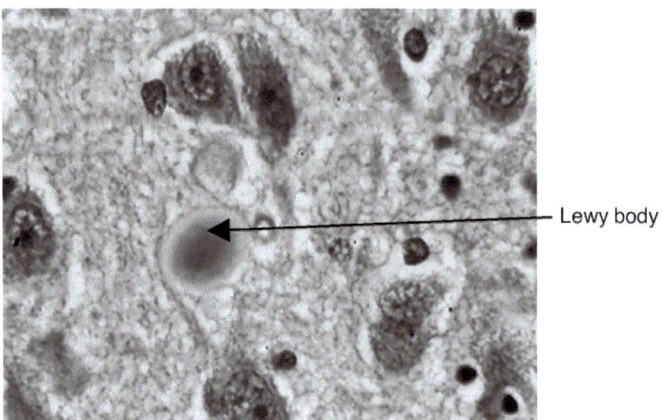

Figure 7.3 Immunohistochemistry for alpha-synuclein showing positive staining of an intraneuronal Lewy body in the substantia nigra in Parkinson's disease.

It can be difficult to make a diagnosis of PD in the early stages, especially in the very old, who may 'normally' have some features of extrapyramidal rigidity. Many cases diagnosed in life, even by experts (perhaps 10%), are not confirmed as PD on post-mortem examination.

Motor features

The triad of classical symptoms and signs are:

1 Poverty of movement (akinesia, bradykinesia),
2 Regular tremor at rest (5/sec, 'pill-rolling') and
3 Muscle rigidity of extrapyramidal type ('lead pipe' or 'cogwheel', which describes rigidity in the presence of tremor).

- The tremor may be obvious, is usually a rest tremor, and may be unilateral (especially in the early stages).
- Bradykinesia may be apparent as paucity of facial expression (parkinsonian facies) and fine movements such as doing up shirt buttons are difficult. Handwriting may get smaller during the completion of a sentence (micrographia). Speech is soft (dysphonic), monotonous and becomes dysarthric.
- The stiffness may be misinterpreted as arthritis, and although PD does not affect the sensory system, joint stiffness, particularly in bed at night, may be painful.
- The gait is characteristic with a flexed posture, tendency to shuffle, loss of arm swing, and impaired postural reflexes, which make the patient likely to fall. Stopping, starting, and turning pose the most difficulty, and if a walking frame is needed, the wheeled type is usually recommended.

Whilst the motor symptoms form the basis of the diagnosis, it is now accepted that non-motor symptoms contribute to morbidity and may be present early in the disease.

Non-motor features

Problems relating to the bladder, bowels, digestion, sleep, and mood often complicate PD. These features were thought to be secondary to chronic disability, but several studies have shown that the paravertebral sympathetic ganglia, the enteric system, and the epicardium are affected by synuclein pathology, i.e. these are non-motor features of the disease.

- Olfactory dysfunction. Seen in up to 90% of patients, it can predate diagnosis by years and hence is a useful preclinical biomarker.
- Neuropsychiatric – More than 50% of older patients with PD develop PD dementia (PDD) as the disease progresses. This resembles dementia with Lewy bodies (DLB). Lewy body disease (LBD) encompasses PDD and DLB. (Tip to remember – LBD is the umbreLla term.) Depression is also common, and psychosis (most commonly visual hallucinations) may result from an associated dementia, depression, or the PD drugs. Rivastigmine may be helpful. Confusion may limit continuation of levodopa treatment. Drug adherence issues can be tackled by using dosette boxes and PD medication clocks/alarms.
- Autonomic disturbance is common, with dysphagia, drooling, bowel dysfunction (especially constipation), weight loss, bladder dysfunction, sexual dysfunction, postural hypotension, and excessive sweating. Midodrine is the first line for correcting postural hypotension if modifying the PD regimen is unsuccessful.
- Sleep disturbance (hypersomnolence) is not just a consequence of difficulty turning over in bed due to nocturnal akinesia. Other factors include rapid eye movement (REM) sleep behaviour disorder, restless legs syndrome, an inverted sleep–wake cycle, and nightmares.

Other symptoms may include pain because of immobility, dystonia and falls. Osteomalacia and osteoporosis add to the disability (prescribe vitamin D).

Diagnostic tests

There is no routine diagnostic test, but this may be about to change (see alpha-synuclein assay).

- A positive response to levodopa strongly supports the diagnosis. This is made more reliable by choosing a standard measurement to repeat after treatment is started, e.g. measuring the time to walk a set distance (10 m), a tap test – the number of pronations and supinations the patient can achieve in a minute tapping on a desk – or documentation of handwriting (micrographia), which should be seen to improve.

- A DAT (dopamine transporter) scan will help confirm clinical suspicion. The scan uses injectable radiopharmaceutical ioflupane, which binds to pre-synaptic dopamine transporters. The signal is detected by single-photon emission computed tomography (SPECT), which uses gamma cameras to create a pictographic representation of the distribution of dopamine transporters in the brain. This will distinguish PD (where the cells die so the amount of receptor falls) from essential tremor (ET) (appearance resembles healthy controls). It is suggested that DAT imaging can identify those with PD earlier in the disease trajectory as it can detect the loss of only 30% of dopamine-producing brain cells, as opposed to the 80% loss that triggers clinical sequelae. It cannot distinguish between PD, PSP or MSA (see later). It can distinguish between Alzheimer's disease and LBD.
- A test for misfolded alpha-synuclein may become available soon. The study was conducted at 33 sites around the world and included testing the CSF of 1,123 participants. Results showed that the tool – called the alpha-synuclein seeding amplification assay (αSyn-SAA) – can confirm the presence of abnormal alpha-synuclein with a high degree of accuracy. 93% of people with Parkinson's who took part in the assay were proven to have abnormal alpha-synuclein.

Multidisciplinary management

All patients with PD benefit from a multidisciplinary treatment package, of which drug treatment is only one part. As the disease progresses, the relative emphasis of the components will change.

Learn the following list – suitably modified; it will provide an outline of how to manage most chronic conditions at any age, from MS to COPD! Management options include:

1 **Education and support:** encourage all patients and carers to join the Parkinson's Disease Society (other support groups are available).
2 **Continuity of care:** chronic progressive diseases are best managed in settings promoting continuity of care to enable the patient and clinician to develop a working relationship and to assess the benefits and side effects of treatment. In many areas, there is a PD clinic run by a geriatrician, neurologist, or both, often with a nurse specialist. The nurse may visit the patient at home and give telephone advice between appointments. Specialist PD nurses are often the first point of contact for both inpatients and those in the community.
3 **Therapy:** assessment and treatment:
   - **Physiotherapy:** work on posture, gait, and falls prevention.
   - **Occupational therapy:** maintaining skills, home modification, etc.
   - **Speech and language therapy:** speech, facial expression, swallowing.
4 **Dietetic input:** advice on supporting nutrition and protein spacing (see Table 7.1).
5 **Assess whether the patient meets the criteria for benefits**
6 **Legal advice:** lasting power of attorney, driving regulations (inform the insurer and DVLA on diagnosis), advance directive, etc.
7 **Maintenance of general health and fitness:** people with a chronic disorder often attribute all their symptoms to it and neglect other possible causes and their general health.
8 **Treat other problems:** e.g. cataracts and in-growing toenails that impair gait; refer appropriately.
9 **Maintenance of morale and mood** (consider complementary medicine, antidepressants, and support from a clinical psychologist if available).

Drugs

Research is aimed at finding 'neuroprotective' drugs to prevent cell death, but no current drugs or supplements achieve this.

Drug treatment aims to restore transmitter balance in the basal ganglia and hence control motor symptoms (see Figure 7.4), most often by enhancing dopaminergic transmission. Antimuscarinic drugs can be useful in younger patients with tremors but are rarely used in older patients because they are likely to cause confusion and memory impairment. Details of drugs used in the management of PD are given in Table 7.1.

Levodopa is the mainstay of treatment across all age groups. In frail older people, if PD is already affecting motor function, levodopa is typically started on diagnosis.

Table 7.1 Drug management for Parkinson's disease.

Mechanism	Name	Prescription tips
Replenish striatal dopamine	Levodopa with peripheral dopa-decarboxylase inhibitor • Sinemet® (co-careldopa) • Madopar® (co-beneldopa)	Start low, increase slowly balancing response with side effects, with meals initially to reduce nausea, later before meals as drug competes for absorption with amino acids from a protein meal. Can use slow-release preparation from the start or to cover the night; dispersible preparation if swallowing a problem. About 85% of patients respond to levodopa.
	Duodopa®	Direct duodenal infusion of levodopa
Catechol-O-methyl transferase inhibitor (COMTI)	• entacapone • tolcapone • opicapone	Entacapone, used with levodopa to reduce end-of-dose deterioration (more 'off time' reduction), may colour the urine red. Tolcapone only used if entacapone unsuitable, as tolcapone occasionally causes severe hepatotoxicity.
Monoamine oxidase-B inhibitor (MAO-BI)	• selegiline • rasagiline • safinamide	Used as early monotherapy or with levodopa to reduce end-of-dose deterioration. Give in the morning as a mild stimulant.
Dopamine agonists	Non-ergoline: • ropinirole • pramipexole • rotigotine (transdermal) • apomorphine (sub cut)	Increase dose slowly, as hypotension can occur in the first few days. The therapeutic effect is mediated via the D_2 receptor; other effects depend partly on their activity at other dopaminergic receptors. Higher risk of hallucinations when compared to other drug classes. Ropinirole and pramipexole are licensed for monotherapy or with levodopa. Eye checks recommended with pramipexole, so ropinirole gaining market share (it is also cheaper). Rotigotine patch for monotherapy in early PD. Apomorphine used subcutaneously via a pen or pump under specialist supervision (usually as an inpatient initially) for intractable fluctuations.
Anti-glutamatergic	• amantadine	Consider when dyskinesias are not managed by modifying existing therapy.

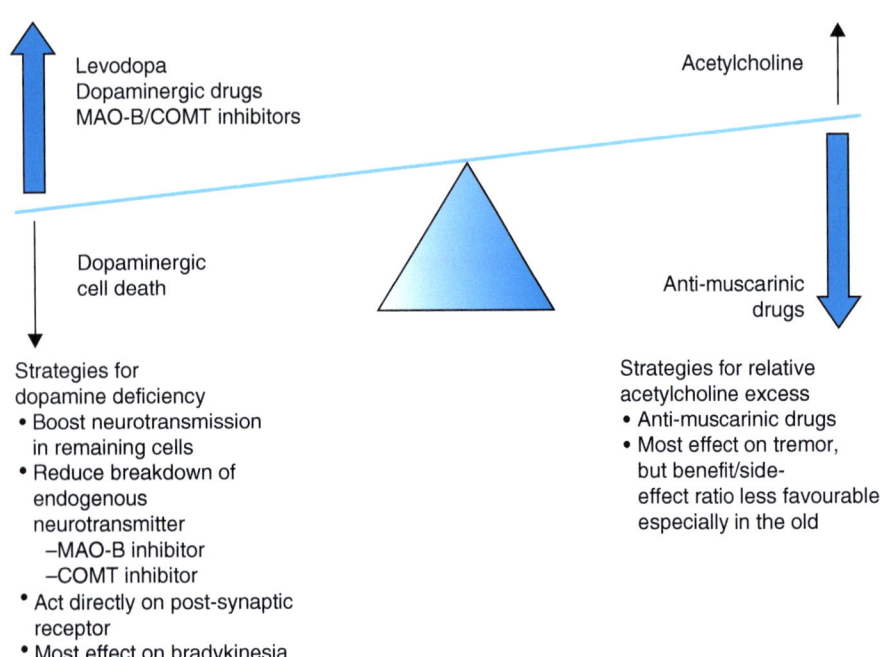

Figure 7.4 Strategies for treating the transmitter imbalance in PD. MAO-B, monoamine oxidase-B; COMT, catechol-0-methyl transferase.

Levodopa preparations usually provide excellent benefits that last for hours after a dose, within days to a few weeks of starting treatment. However, after a few years, the effects of levodopa become more short-lived. Problems may be predictable at first. For example, soon after a dose, there may be involuntary movements (peak-dose dyskinesia), and as the next dose becomes due, the effect of the previous dose may wear off so that the patient becomes rigid, immobile, and frozen or 'off'. These effects can be improved by juggling doses and timing, but eventually, despite complex bespoke drug regimens, the 'on-off' motor fluctuations can become severe and random. The patient may alternate between being 'on' for short periods and having 'offs' and disabling dyskinesias.

Long-acting dopamine agonists are another choice for initial treatment and are used more in younger patients. There are two groups of agonists; ergot and non-ergot-derived, but serious side effects have almost stopped new prescriptions of drugs in the ergot family.

Practical tips

PD medication regimes are now almost always informed by PD specialists, both in the community and inpatient settings. Always have a low threshold to discuss before changing drug regimens, which have been carefully honed over time.

- Combination preparations may help adherence, e.g. levodopa and carbidopa plus entacapone (Stalevo).
- When any other dopaminergic agent is added to levodopa, consider reducing the dose of levodopa.
- If a PD patient is nil by mouth for any reason other than 'gut failure', use a nasogastric tube to avoid missing any drug doses. The development of a transdermal drug delivery system is an attractive option for those patients who cannot tolerate oral medications (such as during an acute illness or perioperatively). Rotigotine transdermal patches are used for this purpose and are a useful alternative to nasogastric administration (see Chapters 5 and 7).
- If a neuroleptic is needed, consider clozapine (but remember it needs special precautions) or quetiapine, but involve your PD team before doing so.
- All dopaminergic drugs should be withdrawn gradually to avoid neuroleptic malignant syndrome (life-threatening fever, unstable BP, and rigidity).

Drug side effects

In older patients, the dose of levodopa or dopamine agonists is often limited by neuropsychiatric problems (confusion, hallucinations). Younger patients tolerate higher doses without confusion, but dyskinesias tend to be dose-limiting.

Dopamine-induced nausea is common. Domperidone was previously used extensively to treat this symptom and is still used, but this drug now carries a caution in older patients due to the risk of cardiac complications, so check an ECG and use a low dose.

All dopaminergic drugs and advanced PD itself can cause sudden sleepiness, so warn drivers and consider the use of modafinil to help promote wakefulness.

A minority of PD patients develop impulse control disorders on dopamine replacement therapy, including pathological gambling, binge eating, hyperlibidinous behaviour and punding (aimless repetitive behaviour), and may need to have the dose reduced at the expense of motor function. Cognitive behavioural therapy can be offered to those for whom dopamine reduction is not successful.

New drugs

Trials continue apace to evaluate non-drug management, to compare current drugs/formulations, and to look at new therapies. Promising drugs include:

- Istradefylline, an adenosine A_{2A} receptor agonist (as an adjunct to reduce 'off' time), is approved in the US and Japan and is awaiting evaluation by NICE.
- Pimavanserin, a 5-HT_{2A} inverse agonist for L-dopa-induced psychosis, is approved in the US.
- Ambroxol (currently used as a cough medicine) increases glucocerebrosidase and improves alpha-synuclein clearance. It is in a Phase 3 trial at University College, London as a PD modifier.
- Long-acting glucagon-like peptide-1 (GLP-1) receptor agonists – Phase 2 studies of exenatide and lixisenatide showed a slowing of deterioration. A Phase 3 study of exenatide is in progress.

Invasive treatments

More invasive procedures are offered in specialist centres but are not usually recommended for/available to frail older patients.

- **Intra-duodenal infusion:** when motor fluctuations become disabling, levodopa/carbidopa gel (Duodopa) can be delivered directly into the duodenum over 24 hours via a PEG (percutaneous endoscopic gastrostomy) with a long tube into the jejunum and a portable pump. This is relatively easy to insert, but it is prone to problems with the delivery system and is very expensive.
- **Continuous subcutaneous apomorphine infusion:** effective but limited by skin reactions and cost.
- **Neurosurgery:** pallidotomy saw a resurgence in the 1990s but has been replaced by deep brain stimulation.
- **Deep brain stimulation:** DBS, particularly of the subthalamic nuclei, is useful for biologically fit patients with disabling motor fluctuations or intractable tremors refractory to optimal medical treatment. (NB: Patients with electrodes in situ must have bipolar, not unipolar, diathermy during surgery to avoid heat trauma to the brain.) The use of DBS may allow the clinician to reduce dopaminergic drugs.
- **MRI-guided focussed ultrasound:** MRgFUS allows accurate ablation of deep brain structures while the patient is conscious to monitor the results. It is still being evaluated, but it appears most useful for tremor.
- **Transplantation** with foetal adrenal tissue did not fulfil expectations but may eventually become a reality with cultured cells once fundamental issues such as how to 'turn off' dopamine production from transplanted cells have been solved; initial trials where the grafts 'took' produced ghastly results due to dopamine excess.
- **Gene therapy:** this is another area where initial encouraging results have not yet translated into clinical treatments. Adeno-associated virus (AAV) and lentivirus vectors with the genes of interest are delivered by bilateral intraputaminal injection. Two approaches have been tried:
  1 Enhance dopamine production or modulate other transmitters, e.g. with ProSavin, a lentiviral vector designed to deliver three key enzymes in the dopamine synthetic pathway: GTP-cyclohydrolase 1, tyrosine hydroxylase and aromatic amino acid decarboxylase; and AAV2-glutamic acid decarboxylase, which makes GABA.
  2 Restore neurotrophic signalling with the glial neurotrophic factor analogue AAV2-neurturin.

Small trials have shown acceptable safety, persistence of the introduced genes, and some efficacy, but this has been limited by inadequate delivery. Techniques are being developed to conjugate drugs and larger molecules to microbubbles, which can be given systemically and enabled to cross the blood–brain barrier in the desired brain region by temporarily opening it with MRgFUS.

Life expectancy

Idiopathic PD is not considered a fatal disease, and patients with normal cognitive function are thought to have a near-normal life expectancy. However, associated complications (i.e. aspiration risk, cognitive impairment) can reduce life expectancy by 1–2 years. The advanced stages may be distressing, with the patient being robbed of mobility, cognitive function, swallowing and sphincter control. Enormous amounts of support for both carers and patients are needed at this stage. Pneumonia is the leading cause of death in patients with PD.

Secondary parkinsonism

Secondary parkinsonism is a syndrome with many causes. The most common are:

1 **Drugs:** the most frequent being neuroleptics, but also antihistamines and commonly used dopamine antagonists such as metoclopramide. It is usually symmetrical, and the tremor is less marked. Some patients with drug-induced parkinsonism have subclinical nigral pathology, which becomes clinically evident when dopamine blockers are prescribed. In this group, stopping the drug does not lead to the resolution of the parkinsonian symptoms. Imaging dopamine transporter receptors with SPECT can help identify these patients; if the SPECT scan is abnormal, the patient will respond to levodopa therapy.

2 **Vascular disease:** the latter stages of vascular (multi-infarct) dementia, i.e. rigidity with dementia. The gait is shuffling (marche à petits pas) but without the forward shift of the centre of gravity seen in PD, sometimes referred to as 'lower body parkinsonism'.

3 **Trauma:** repetitive head trauma, e.g. in ex-boxers and other contact sports.

4 **Virus:** post-encephalitic.

5 **Toxins:** contaminated illegal drugs – MPTP (1-methyl-4-phenyl-1,2,3, 4-tetrahydropyridine) – and case reports associated with Ecstasy.

Patient with parkinsonism often gain little benefit from levodopa therapy and adverse effects, e.g. increased confusion and falls secondary to postural hypotension, are common.

Other brain degenerations with parkinsonism

This is a group of neurodegenerative conditions, sometimes referred to as Parkinson's plus syndromes, that feature rigidity, akinesia and postural instability but have other features as there is wider brain pathology.

In addition to parkinsonism:

- In dementia with Lewy bodies (DLB), dementia and psychiatric phenomena predominate.
- Progressive supranuclear palsy (PSP) is associated with abnormal eye movements and early falls.
- In multiple system atrophy (MSA), cerebellar and autonomic deficits develop.
- Corticobasal syndrome (CBS) is the least common, features include dystonia, and patients may be troubled by an alien limb.

These conditions have no diagnostic tests in life, and clinicopathological correlations are variable, so they may also be syndromes.

Dementia with Lewy bodies

Dementia with Lewy bodies (DLB) is the most common, and features of parkinsonism overlap with dementia and psychiatric phenomena (see Chapter 8). Brain pathology shows Lewy bodies identical to those in PD but scattered throughout the cortex.

The other conditions described here are all rare, usually sporadic, and have a rapid onset and inexorable progression leading to profound disability and death, often from aspiration pneumonia, within 6–10 years. Management is supportive and symptomatic – levodopa is usually tried and may have limited benefit for a brief period or be of no benefit.

Progressive supranuclear palsy

Progressive supranuclear palsy (PSP) (Steele–Richardson–Olszewski syndrome) is characterised by paralysis of eye movements (initially upward gaze but not specific until other eye movements are involved). Other differences from PD are a symmetrical onset, axial rigidity, and lack of tremor.

- The patient typically has an extended neck, raised eyebrows, and walks as if 'sniffing the air'.
- There is marked instability and frequent falls (often the first complaint), dysphagia, speech difficulties and dementia.
- There is variation in the degree to which cognition, behaviour, and language are affected early in the condition.

Rowe gives an excellent account of how to distinguish PD from PSP, use a patient-centred multidisciplinary approach to support the patient and their carers, and a practical guide to using drugs for symptom relief.

Multiple system atrophy

Multiple system atrophy (MSA) (formerly known as Shy Drager syndrome) is characterised by parkinsonian features, cerebellar, and autonomic problems including urogenital dysfunction and corticospinal signs (hyperreflexia and upgoing plantar responses) of varying severity. There are two main forms:

- MSA-P with predominant parkinsonism.
- MSA-C with predominant cerebellar features (previously olivopontocerebellar atrophy).

The protein alpha-synuclein accumulates in the glia rather than in the neurons, as it does in PD and the 'MSA-P' subtype, which can be misdiagnosed as PD. However, at onset, rigidity and autonomic features are more prominent, whilst tremor is rare. Cardiovascular autonomic dysfunction distinguishes the condition from PSP. There are often cerebellar signs. Symptomatic management to minimise postural hypotension is important: avoid diuretics and hypotensives, keep hydrated, try compression stockings (TEDS), head-up tilt in bed, caffeine, fludrocortisone, and midodrine. (See Chapter 11 for more discussion about postural hypotension.)

Corticobasal syndrome

Corticobasal syndrome (CBS) is a clinical entity with many different underlying pathologies, including corticobasal degeneration, which is a tauopathy characterised by progressive nerve cell loss and atrophy of multiple areas of the brain, including the cerebral cortex and the basal ganglia. It typically presents in the 6th decade.

- Symptoms may be unilateral at first and include poor coordination, akinesia, rigidity, and dystonia.
- CBS can cause alien limb syndrome: a limb (usually the arm) feels foreign to the patient and may have observable involuntary movements.
- Cognitive and visuospatial impairments, apraxia, hesitant speech, myoclonus, and dysphagia develop. Clonazepam may help with myoclonus.

Other conditions allied to PD

There are several conditions that can be misdiagnosed as PD, have overlapping pathophysiology or clinical features. Conditions that were thought of as discrete disease entities are now recognised as syndromes. This may explain why, for example, there is occasionally overlap between patients with 'PD' and 'ET', although the typical clinical findings are different and do not merge with the passage of time.

Essential tremor (ET)

ET is one of the most common neurological problems (seen in about 5% of people over 65).

- It often starts in middle age and gradually worsens.
- Characterised by postural tremor, exacerbated by movement and stress.
- The tremor is bilateral but is often noticed more in the dominant hand.
- This can include a head tremor and a 'quivering' voice if the larynx is affected.
- Can be mistaken for the pill-rolling tremor of PD, but other parkinsonian features are absent.

ET used to be tagged 'benign' but can be disabling and embarrassing. It can cause functional problems such as drinking from a cup, writing, or using a computer. It may respond to small amounts of alcohol, beta-blockers (nonselective, e.g. propranolol are best), low-dose primidone or topiramate. Up to 50% of cases are familial, but the clinical presentation and course are variable. ET is now recognised as a syndrome. This probably explains why it has been difficult to consistently identify a linked gene. One of the best candidates is *LINGO1*, which codes for a transmembrane protein that is upregulated in the cerebellum of some PD and ET patients. Some families with dystonic tremor have extra copies of the gene. This is an active research area that may lead to a better classification of tremor syndromes.

Restless Legs Syndrome (RLS, also called Ekbom's syndrome)

This is characterised by a profound desire to move the legs and motor restlessness, which is worse at night and often associated with periodic limb movements, resulting in poor sleep. There is a familial trend, and RLS affects up to 10% of the population. RLS is more common in PD patients – it is hypothesised that some aspect of brain dopamine function is altered in RLS. However, deficits are not seen on DAT scan imaging. Dopamine agonists such as ropinirole, pramipexole or rotigotine taken before bed are licensed for severe cases; an alternative is an alpha-2-delta calcium channel ligand, like gabapentin (off-label). Low-dose opiates can be used as a last resort. RLS is associated with iron deficiency – consider this eminently treatable cause – check ferritin in everyone with relevant symptoms.

Motor neuron disease

Motor neuron disease (MND) is the umbrella term for a group of disorders of unknown aetiology characterised by progressive degeneration of motor neurons in the cortex and the anterior horns of the brainstem and spinal cord. It generally presents as a rapidly progressive fatal neurological disease producing paralysis of the muscles involved in limb movement, swallowing, and breathing. The average time to diagnosis is around 18 months, and from diagnosis to death, is 14 months. It usually presents in the 6th and 7th decades and may be misdiagnosed initially in older people who more commonly have MND mimics, such as:

- Benign fasciculation (cramp).
- Vascular disease causing UMN lesions.
- Cervical radiculomyelopathy which gives UMN and LMN signs (but sensory signs too).
- Cervical myelopathy and unrelated peripheral neuropathy (but sensory signs too).

Most cases are sporadic, but around 10–15% are familial. The most common familial form of MND (amyotrophic lateral sclerosis) has been linked to variants in several genes, most commonly *C9ORF72*. In MND, cognition usually remains normal, sensory changes are absent, and sphincter control is retained. However, a small subgroup develops frontotemporal dementia (FTD).

MND tends to be focal in onset, affecting:

- **Limb muscles (70%):**
  - Amyotrophic lateral sclerosis (ALS) is the commonest form, with mixed UMN and LMN signs.
  - Pure UMN presentation, primary lateral sclerosis (carries a better prognosis).
  - Pure LMN presentation, progressive muscular atrophy.
- **Bulbar muscles (25%):** speech deteriorates before swallowing; bulbar and pseudobulbar (emotional lability) features.
- **Respiratory muscles (5%).**

There is no specific diagnostic test; however, an electromyogram (EMG) can detect LMN disorders and can be a useful aid to diagnosis, together with nerve conduction studies. Muscle creatine kinase (CK) may be elevated (muscle damage from denervation), but this is too non-specific to be diagnostic.

Patients usually present with an asymmetrical weakness of the hands or foot drop, and examination reveals brisk reflexes in a wasted limb with muscle fasciculations. Those with predominantly distal signs affecting legs and mobility tend to have a slower progression of their disease.

The management is supportive and multidisciplinary. Advance planning is important. Certain interventions have proven beneficial. Patients with a good quality of life and bulbar function should be referred for:

- Non-invasive ventilation which has been shown to improve quality of life and give a median survival benefit of 7 months.
- Riluzole (a glutamate release inhibitor), which is postulated to provide protection against motor neurone damage. This prolongs the time to ventilation but is of limited benefit (improves median survival by 2–3 months). Common side effects include abdominal pain, diarrhoea and vomiting, dizziness and drowsiness. It should be stopped if the patient develops neutropaenia.
- Edaravone, an antioxidant approved in the US for use in ALS, appears to slow disease progression. It was initially given intravenously, but an oral formulation is now available. It is not licensed in Europe, and the ADORE trial of oral edaravone in Europe has been halted as it did not meet its primary endpoints.
- Muscle relaxants such as baclofen can help with spasms, and botulinum injections can be considered for contractures.
- Those with a bulbar presentation fare much less well, especially with the onset of speech and swallowing problems, of which the patient is only too aware. Such patients should be considered for early PEG tube placement to support nutrition and hydration. The patient will normally be able to be fully involved in deciding on such a course of action.
- Many areas have specialist nurses who can greatly improve symptom control and provide education and support. The MND website has excellent information sheets for professionals, e.g. tackling 'excess' saliva ('sialorrhoea', really the difficulty in swallowing saliva), and for the patient, covering difficult areas such as 'How will I die?'

Normal pressure hydrocephalus

Normal pressure hydrocephalus (NPH) is a condition with enlarged cerebral ventricles and normal opening pressure on lumbar puncture. It can follow haemorrhage, infection (meningitis), or malignancy, all of which can impair CSF drainage via the arachnoid granulations or cervical lymphatics, but the cause is often unknown; degeneration of the reabsorption mechanisms may contribute. Idiopathic NPH usually occurs in the over-60s; it is postulated that as it develops, abnormal CSF flow must sporadically increase the CSF pressure. The aetiology is unknown.

NPH can be asymptomatic, but some patients present with the insidious onset of a triad of

1 Intellectual failure,
2 Unsteadiness (with broad-based gait or gait apraxia), and
3 Early urinary incontinence.

Diagnosis is suggested by CT, with ventriculomegaly without widened sulci. However, variations in the relative degree of ventricular enlargement to cerebral atrophy in normal ageing and dementia and the high prevalence of the cardinal symptoms in the older population make NPH a difficult diagnosis. As with most neurological conditions, an MRI carries a higher diagnostic yield. MRI features of disproportionately enlarged subarachnoid space hydrocephalus (DESH) have been proposed as a marker for a good response to shunting, but this is controversial.

By the time of diagnosis, the CSF pressure is normal. In specialist centres, external lumbar CSF drainage and flow studies are used to try to improve the prediction of outcome from a ventriculoperitoneal shunt; temporary improvement of symptoms following a 'therapeutic' tap is thought to predict a good outcome.

It is estimated that NPH accounts for 1–5% of dementia cases, but it is one of the few potentially reversible causes of cognitive and gait impairment. However, shunting has risks and may not lead to improvement.

Of 560 cases of dementia seen at the Mayo Clinic from 1990 to 1994, 1% had suspected NPH, but none of those treated with ventriculoperitoneal shunting improved. In a small series with functional MRI before and after CSF drainage, motor function improved but cognition did not. Subjects with short-duration gait problems are most likely to benefit. A meta-analysis found that the mean rate of shunt complications (including death, infection, seizures, shunt malfunction, and subdural haemorrhage) was 38%.

The Cochrane review (from 2002) found no evidence from randomised controlled trials to support shunt procedures in older patients. However, there has been increasing evidence that shunt placement can be beneficial. The updated Cochrane review (2024) included 140 participants with an average age of 75 years. The authors concluded there was evidence for improvement in gait speed and reduction in disability at less than six months after the procedure, but the effect on cognitive function was uncertain. No patients died but adverse events were common. Longer term follow up is needed, but this offers some support for shunting in carefully selected patients.

Epilepsy

Epilepsy has a bimodal age curve, with a high incidence in infants and then a sustained rise from middle age, so that nearly half of new-onset seizures occur in individuals over the age of 65 years. The incidence rises to 150 in 100,000 people aged over 70 years. Both incidence and prevalence are likely to continue to rise as the population ages.

Causes of seizures in older people include:

- **Stroke disease:** commonest cause (up to 50%), usually 3–12 months after the event; higher risk after haemorrhagic stroke and with larger infarcts.
- **Tumours (5%), primary brain tumours, metastases:** in >40% of cases, the first presentation of the cancer.
- **Trauma:** following a head injury, contusion, or SDH.
- **Primary dementias:** e.g. advanced Alzheimer's disease.
- **Drugs or alcohol:** (excess or withdrawal).
- **Other causes:** biochemical disturbance (severe hyponatraemia, hypocalcaemia).

Seizures occurring in old age are usually 'focal' (previously termed partial) seizures as they arise from a localised area of brain damage, e.g. scar tissue following a stroke. In most cases, consciousness is impaired, a 'focal impaired awareness seizure' (previously known as a complex partial seizure). Seizure activity may spread to both sides of the brain and result in a 'focal to bilateral tonic-clonic seizure', or 'convulsion'. A focus in the temporal lobe is relatively uncommon in old age, so features such as olfactory auras and automatisms are not often seen.

Investigation

Investigate for an underlying cause.

- An EEG can support a diagnosis of epilepsy but cannot rule it out, as the yield of specific epileptiform activity is less than half that in a younger population.
- MRI scanning is preferred to CT.

Management

There is a lower threshold to start treatment after a single unprovoked fit in an older person, as underlying brain structural damage is likely. Care is needed with antiepileptic drugs (AEDs), also known as anti-seizure medications (ASMs); monotherapy is preferred, as older patients are more susceptible to adverse effects (including cognitive impairment and ataxia).

- Carbamazepine or sodium valproate were the traditional first-line drugs, but levetiracetam (Keppra) and lamotrigine both have better continuation rates at 1 year, and the patient is more likely to be seizure-free.
- Check the rest of the patient's medication; some drugs increase the chances of a seizure, and the older AEDs have many interactions. Avoid ciprofloxacin for a post-fit chest infection because it is epileptogenic, as is tramadol, and care is needed with antidepressants.
- Rectal diazepam or buccal midazolam are recommended for urgent treatment of prolonged or recurrent seizures in the community.
- The newer AEDs with low drug–drug interaction potential (lacosamide, brivaracetam, and eslicarbazepine acetate) may have advantages for older people, but there is little data at present.

Seizures may result in injuries such as fractures because of underlying osteoporosis (which can be related to AED use). Recovery may be prolonged by postictal symptoms, especially confusion and focal weakness (Todd's paresis), which may last for 24 hours or even, and occasionally, days. The psychological and social consequences are at least as great as in younger patients. Patients and their families need a full explanation and education; this is best managed by an epilepsy specialist nurse as part of a team. Signpost to a patient support group, e.g. the Epilepsy society. Think about safety – especially when planning a discharge home. Consider portable/wristband seizure detection alarms and home modifications. Check whether advice on driving is relevant – do not assume that your patient is a non-driver.

Status epilepticus

Status epilepticus (SE) is a life-threatening neurological condition defined as *five* or more minutes of continuous seizure activity or repetitive seizures without regaining consciousness between episodes. The mortality rate is 50% in the over-80s.

- SE has a twofold increased incidence in the older people, and co-morbidity may complicate therapy and worsen the prognosis.
- An acute or previous stroke is the most common aetiology.

Non-convulsive SE (NCSE) has a wide range of clinical presentations, ranging from confusion to obtundation. It is most common in elderly patients who are critically ill and in the setting of a coma.

- Exclude hypoglycaemia.
- EEG is the only reliable method of diagnosing NCSE.
- The goal is to stop the seizure activity as soon as possible.

The first-line treatment is intravenous lorazepam or buccal midazolam. If this is unsuccessful, intravenous levetiracetam or sodium valproate are next in line. Phenytoin is used less commonly – it requires cardiac monitoring and wide-bore IV access. If treatment fails, refer the patient to the ICU for consideration of a general anaesthetic agent and definitive airway protection.

Infectious diseases of the CNS

Meningitis

In bacterial meningitis, less than 10% of cases but over 20% of deaths occur in patients aged 80 or older, with a case fatality rate of 50%.

- Delays in diagnosis may occur if the symptoms are vague, and signs, especially neck stiffness, can be difficult to interpret because of the frequency of cervical spondylosis.
- Examination of the CSF is essential; however, only perform an LP after a CT scan (papilloedema is often absent in elderly patients with raised intracranial pressure, and fundoscopy is often difficult because of eye pathology).
- If the patient is on clopidogrel or a DOAC, consider the risks and benefits and discuss with haematology, e.g. whether a platelet transfusion should be given prior to LP to reduce the risk of epidural haematoma.

As in younger adults, *S. pneumoniae* is the most common pathogen, but in old age, this is followed by *Listeria*, and other atypical organisms must always be considered. In the White population in the UK, tuberculous meningitis is more common in older people than in middle-aged people. Ceftriaxone plus amoxicillin (to cover *Listeria*) with dexamethasone is a suitable empirical treatment for bacterial meningitis until culture or PCR results are available. Steroids and broad-spectrum antibiotics should be stopped if the LP suggests viral meningitis when aciclovir should be started.

Encephalitis

Headache, fever, confusion, and malaise are followed by focal signs, seizures, and coma.

- Herpes simplex (HSV1) and Herpes zoster (particularly when a cranial dermatome is involved in shingles) are the most common causes, followed by enteroviruses and in France, *Listeria* is also common.
- Consider the possibility of encephalitis early, as the mortality rate can be as high as 70%.
- Autoimmune encephalitis is a differential diagnosis.
- EEG is helpful if it shows focal abnormalities (high-voltage periodic lateralising epileptiform discharges), particularly in the temporal lobes. MRI is the most sensitive imaging, but it can be normal. A lumbar puncture often reveals a high protein level and lymphocyte count. CSF PCR has improved the identification of the causative organism, with a 95% sensitivity rate. Aciclovir is effective and reduces mortality to under 30% in Herpes encephalitis.

Poliomyelitis

There has not been a case of polio caught in the UK since the mid-1990s because of the polio vaccination programme. As of 2024, only two countries still have endemic polio (Afghanistan and Pakistan) and cases have recently been reported in Gaza.

- You will still see older people with the sequelae of polio in the UK – usually a flaccid, wasted, weak leg with absent reflexes (pathology is damage to the anterior horn cells).
- If the damage occurred in childhood, the limb may be small.
- An ankle-foot orthosis (AFO) is often worn for foot drop.

About half the survivors (now mainly from the epidemics in the 1940s and 1950s) will develop post-polio syndrome (PPS), which begins 30–40 years after the acute illness and is slowly progressive. Common problems include fatigue, cold intolerance, joint deterioration with pain, new weakness, muscle pain and atrophy, dysphagia and dysphonia, sleep apnoea and respiratory failure. The aetiology is unclear, and treatment is primarily supportive, although non-fatiguing strengthening exercises may reduce weakness over the short term. Drugs have not been beneficial in controlled trials.

Herpes zoster

Herpes zoster (shingles) is a reactivation of the varicella virus, which has lain dormant in the dorsal root ganglia since an earlier attack of chicken pox. Prior to the shingles vaccination programme (introduced in the UK in 2013 for people over 70), 1 in 5 people who had had chicken pox developed shingles. Patients do not 'catch' shingles from other people with chicken pox or shingles, but a susceptible person can catch chicken pox from someone with active shingles. Patients with shingles are isolated in hospital to protect care staff. Two shingles vaccines are used in the UK – Zostavax, a live vaccine given as a single dose, and Shingrix, a recombinant vaccine given as two doses 6 months apart. Shingrix was reserved for people with immunocompromise, but the national programme is moving to use Shingrix for everyone and by 2033, all people over the age of 60 will be offered this vaccination at 60 years. A recent study has suggested that Shingrix may reduce the risk of dementia, but confirmation is needed.

Clinical features

- Pain in the distribution of the dorsal root with paraesthesia and hyperaesthesia usually precedes the rash by a couple of days, although the illness may be painless.
- The characteristic rash, like that of varicella, follows the sequence papules–vesicles–pustules–crusts, and then ceases to be infectious. The dermatome affected is thoracic in over 50% of cases but is trigeminal in 10–15% and, less commonly, affects the geniculate ganglion (Ramsay–Hunt syndrome), where Bell's palsy may be the first manifestation.
- Anteriorly, the rash does not cross the midline, but posteriorly, it follows the posterior primary ramus a few centimetres across the spinous processes. Sometimes more than one adjacent dermatome is involved, but it is very seldom bilateral.
- Less common complications include muscle wasting in the relevant segment, an internal rash in the same segment (e.g. the bladder), a mixed varicella–zoster eruption, meningoencephalitis, and eye involvement.

Management

Management involves attention to hydration, pain relief and general health, plus aciclovir 800 mg five times daily by mouth. Aciclovir has been shown to shorten the length and severity of the disease. It is now available directly from a pharmacy in England. Famciclovir has the advantage that it can be given once daily. The pain may be severe, and appropriate analgesia should be given, including considering neuropathic agents. A Cochrane review in 2013 concluded that corticosteroids were ineffective in preventing post-herpetic neuralgia, but NICE (2024) suggests consideration of oral corticosteroids in the first 2 weeks following rash onset in immunocompetent adults if pain is severe, but only in combination with antiviral treatment.

Ophthalmic zoster

This occurs when the virus is reactivated in the ophthalmic division of the trigeminal nerve. It requires urgent ophthalmological referral to check for corneal ulceration, with a view to local atropine, and/or aciclovir ointment in addition to systemic antivirals.

Post-herpetic neuralgia

Continued burning neuropathic pain for months or years afflicts more than half of elderly patients following an attack of shingles. It is often severe, debilitating, and intractable. It responds better to tricyclic antidepressants, gabapentin, pregabalin, topical capsaicin or lidocaine patches than to conventional analgesics.

Intracranial neoplasms

Metastases are more common than cerebral primaries. In 50% of cases, cerebral metastases are solitary. Glioblastoma is the most common primary brain tumour in adults. Primary lesions may be amenable to surgery, radiotherapy, or chemotherapy, depending on site and nature – advice will be needed from the neuro-oncology multidisciplinary team (see Chapter 18), but outcomes are poor.

Cerebral metastases are most commonly from the lung or breast. Palliative treatment with dexamethasone will often be beneficial in both untreatable primaries and secondaries. The window of symptom relief will be of value to both the patient and their families and may help them come to terms with the prognosis.

Deficiency/toxicity states

The B group of vitamins maintains neurological integrity. Deficiencies can have central effects, e.g. cognitive impairment, and peripheral effects, e.g. neuropathy. Neurological complications may arise before other systems are affected, e.g. subacute combined degeneration of the cord may precede a macrocytic anaemia. In B_{12} deficiency, the findings depend on whether spinal cord damage ('combined' degeneration of the pyramidal tracts and dorsal columns) or neuropathy dominates (see Chapter 17).

Always consider deficiency states (including myxoedema), as they can be easily confirmed and treated. The 'tea and toast' diet may produce a normal weight but is short of vitamins and minerals. Toxicity and deficiencies may occur together, as in the case of alcohol abuse. Alcohol is a neurotoxin (central and peripheral), and many alcoholics have a poor diet and malabsorption with multiple nutritional deficiencies, including vitamins B_1 (thiamine), B_2 (riboflavin), B_3 (niacin), B_6 (pyridoxine) and C, magnesium, zinc, and folate.

Drugs should also be considered as a cause for many neurological conditions, e.g.:

- **Parkinsonism:** secondary to neuroleptics.
- **Ataxia:** secondary to anticonvulsant toxicity.
- **Tardive dyskinesia:** secondary to neuroleptics.
- **Peripheral neuropathy:** especially antineoplastic drugs, occasionally statins, nitrofurantoin, colchicine, and amiodarone.
- **Seizures:** drugs that lower the fit threshold include ciprofloxacin, tramadol, and antidepressants.

Previous surgery may also be relevant, e.g. thyroidectomy, and gastrectomy or ileal resection, the latter two leading to B_{12} malabsorption.

Neuropathies

Damage to nerves usually takes the form of symmetrical damage to all the nerves (a typical peripheral polyneuropathy), damage to a single nerve usually because of compression or entrapment, or damage to a peripheral nerve trunk, then another, until several are affected (mononeuritis multiplex). Neuropathies can be axonal or demyelinating and affect motor or sensory function, or both (see Figure 7.5). Axonal degeneration is a dying-back process affecting the longest large-diameter fibres first (hence glove and stocking), while demyelination can occur anywhere along the nerve and is patchier. Small-fibre neuropathies affect pain, temperature, and autonomic function.

Peripheral neuropathies

The list of possible causes of neuropathy is very long, but more common causes include:

- **Diabetes:**
  - Diabetic sensorimotor polyneuropathy is very common, chronic, symmetrical, length-dependent and caused by microvascular damage reflecting total hyperglycaemic exposure. It occurs with retinopathy and nephropathy.

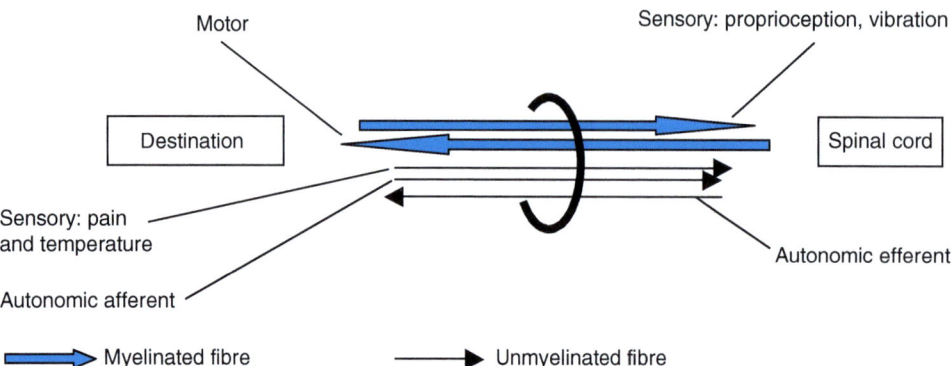

Myelinated fibre   Unmyelinated fibre

Figure 7.5 Peripheral nerve.

○ Diabetic autonomic neuropathy can occur with impaired glucose tolerance and may affect the cardiovascular, gastrointestinal, and urogenital systems. Impaired sweating with dry feet is a factor in foot ulceration.

○ Diabetic amyotrophy is rare – weakness in the thighs, hips, buttocks, and legs, with pain and muscle wasting usually in the front of the thigh caused by ischaemic nerve injury secondary to microvasculitis.

○ Diabetic mononeuritis multiplex – is very rare and may be immune-mediated.

- **Alcohol.**
- **Paraneoplastic sensory neuropathy:** due to immunological damage distant from the primary malignancy.
- **Vitamin deficiencies**.
- **Drugs**.
- **Paraprotein-associated**.
- **Hypothyroidism**.
- **Vasculitis**.
- **Post-inflammatory:**
  ○ **Acute:** Guillain-Barré syndrome (commonest acute-onset), described below.
  ○ **Chronic:** chronic inflammatory demyelinating polyradiculoneuropathy, CIDP
- **Hereditary motor and sensory neuropathy (HSMN)** (Charcot–Marie–Tooth disease) is a group of inherited peripheral neuropathies with considerable clinical and genetic heterogeneity. There are two common forms in adults:
  ○ **Type 1:** demyelinating, affecting the glia-derived myelin.
  ○ **Type 2:** axonal. Type 2 D is caused by mutations in glycyl–tRNA synthetase (GARS), the first *tRNA synthetase* gene to be linked to a disease.

Most patients have symptoms by the age of 20, but these may be mild, progression is slow and there are late-onset cases, so HSMN may occasionally be recognised for the first time in old age. These subtypes can be distinguished by electrophysiological or neuropathological studies. Inheritance can be autosomal dominant, recessive, or X-linked. HSMN is characterised by distal symmetrical polyneuropathy, with slowly progressive weakness and atrophy (particularly peroneal muscular atrophy) resulting in foot drop, secondary steppage gait, and pes cavus. Sensory impairment tends to be less severe, but the presentation and course are variable.

Entrapment neuropathies

These are common mononeuropathies.

Carpal tunnel syndrome

This is due to compression of the median nerve in the wrist. Look for reduced sensation over the thumb, index finger, middle finger and lateral aspect of the ring finger plus the lateral palm, plus wasting of the thenar eminence, and weakness of the abductor pollicis brevis and thumb opposition. Mild symptoms can be managed by wearing a splint at night. Steroid injections may give temporary relief, but if there are signs of nerve damage, refer for nerve conduction studies and then surgery.

Meralgia paraesthetica

This is not serious, but if you recognise it, the patient will be grateful for the reassurance! It is the entrapment of the lateral cutaneous nerve of the thigh under the inguinal ligament, commonly in obese people, resulting in numbness and tingling in the anterolateral thigh.

Guillain–Barré syndrome

This often occurs 1–3 weeks after a viral infection (respiratory or gut, especially *Campylobacter jejuni*) and usually takes the form of a rapidly ascending polyneuropathy. Although it is relatively rare, it was the first condition where carbohydrate mimicry between the human ganglioside GM1 and the *C. jejuni* lipo-oligosaccharide was shown to induce the production of pathogenic autoantibodies and the development of GBS.

The commonest pattern in Europe and North America is acute, ascending, inflammatory demyelinating polyradiculoneuropathy (AIDP). In other areas, axonal neuropathy is most common. Motor features (flaccid paralysis with reduced reflexes) dominate, but there may be some sensory involvement, including severe pain, which may be puzzling until the weakness develops. By the third week of the illness, 90% of patients are at their weakest. Investigations include LP (CSF is usually cellular with high protein) and nerve conduction studies. Treatment consists of support, intravenous immunoglobulin, or plasma exchange and ventilation if respiratory muscles are involved. The Miller–Fisher variant is characterised by paralysis of the eye muscles, areflexia and ataxia; a characteristic antibody, anti-GQ1b IgG, is present. If the initial progressive phase lasts longer than 6 weeks, the polyneuropathy is termed 'chronic', i.e. CIDP. Steroids may be useful.

Autoimmune conditions

Myasthenia gravis

Myasthenia gravis (MG) is a chronic autoimmune disease that affects skeletal muscle and causes painless weakness, which worsens with use. It is rare, with an annual incidence of around 3 per 100,000, and affects 1 in 5,000 people.

- The overall incidence is similar for men and women. It has a bimodal age distribution that differs according to sex; women usually present under the age of 40 and men in their 60s.

- In 80–90% of cases, MG is caused by IgG antibody blockade of nicotinic acetylcholine receptors (AChR) at the post-synaptic neuromuscular junction (NMJ) of skeletal muscle. The antibodies activate complement, and the membrane attack complex damages the NMJ and reduces the number of AChR. Three to seven per cent of patients have antibodies to muscle-specific tyrosine kinase (MuSK); other antibodies are less common.
- MG usually presents in one of three different patterns:
  1 Ocular, causing ptosis or diplopia,
  2 Oropharyngeal with dysphagia and dysarthria, or
  3 Generalised weakness (often proximal and asymmetric).
- The hallmark of MG is muscle weakness that worsens after periods of activity and improves after rest. The degree of weakness varies. Clinical signs include ptosis, diplopia, facial muscle weakness (mask-like face), dysarthria, dysphagia, limb weakness, and respiratory failure. The 'ice pack' test is based on the principle that neuromuscular transmission is more efficient at lower temperatures – it is 80% sensitive in those with ptosis.
- Patients often feel at their best in the mornings, with increasing muscle fatigue throughout the day.
- Overall, 15–20% of patients will experience a 'myasthenic crisis', an exacerbation with respiratory muscle weakness necessitating mechanical ventilation (unless extremely frail) whilst plasma exchange, IV immunoglobulin, and high-dose steroids are given. Occasionally, this is the first presentation.
- Intercurrent infection may precipitate a crisis. In people with MG, COVID-19 increases the risk of myasthenic crisis, respiratory failure, and lung damage. Cases of new-onset MG have been reported after COVID, but it is difficult to prove causality.
- Myasthenia may be drug-induced (penicillamine, aminoglycosides, checkpoint inhibitors).
- The diagnosis is usually clinical, supported by serological and electrophysiological testing (including repetitive nerve stimulation). The Tensilon test is rarely used. A CT chest is used to rule out thymic enlargement, and an MRI brain is needed in ocular MG to rule out other conditions.
- Thymus hyperplasia occurs in 75%, and 10% develop a thymoma. Some centres are offering early thymectomy, but the risk–benefit ratio is generally unfavourable for those over 65 years old.
- Most patients live normal lives, so 'gravis' is historic. Ongoing treatment is usually with pyridostigmine, an oral acetylcholinesterase inhibitor. A 'cholinergic crisis' due to excessive medication is very rare.
- If pyridostigmine monotherapy is not effective, prednisolone is added, titrated up, and then tapered; the combination with steroids is successful in 70% of cases.
- Immunomodulation with azathioprine is third line.
- Other immunosuppressants may be used in refractory cases and new options include C5 complement inhibitor MAbs, e.g. eculizumab.
- Patients with myasthenia should avoid drugs that can worsen symptoms, including antibiotics such as aminoglycosides, fluroquinolones, macrolides, beta-blockers, and neuromuscular blocking drugs (therefore, a senior anaesthetic assessment is essential if a patient needs surgery). Various websites and fact sheets are available that highlight these medications. http://www.myaware.org/drugs-to-avoid is a good starting point.

Myasthenic syndrome (Eaton Lambert)

This can present in a similar way and often causes proximal leg weakness, so the patient finds it difficult to get out of a chair. There is often an underlying cancer, most often small-cell lung carcinoma. Autoantibodies are directed against voltage-gated calcium channels of the P/Q type in the muscle.

Other autoimmune conditions

The neuropathies (AIDP and CIDP) are discussed above.

Autoimmune encephalitis is a rare differential diagnosis in older patients with acute encephalitis or subacute psychiatric presentations.

Autoimmune paraneoplastic conditions are discussed in Chapter 18.

Multiple sclerosis very rarely presents in old age and is not considered here. However, if patients do develop MS in old age, they are usually misdiagnosed initially. If things do not fit, have a low threshold for referring to a neurology colleague. Patients with long-term disability – often spastic paraparesis, are seen. Remember, they will be expert patients and listen to them.

📖 REFERENCES AND FURTHER READING

Uno M, Toi H, Hirai S (2017) Chronic subdural hematoma in elderly patients: is this disease benign? *Neurol. Med. Chir. (Tokyo)* 57:402–409. doi: 10.2176/nmc.ra.2016-0337.

Zainab F, Tomkins-Lane C, Carragee E et al. (2016) Surgical versus non-surgical treatment for lumbar spinal stenosis. *Cochrane Database Syst. Rev.* 2016, Issue 1. Art. No: CD010264. doi: 10.1002/14651858. CD010264.pub2.

Funayama M, Nishioka K, Li Y et al. (2023) Molecular genetics of Parkinson's disease: contributions and global trends. *J. Hum. Genet.* 68:125–130. doi: 10.1038/s10038-022-01058-5.

Schaser AJ, Osterberg VR, Dent SE, et al. (2019) Alpha-synuclein is a DNA binding protein that modulates DNA repair with implications for Lewy body disorders. *Sci. Rep.* 9:10919. doi: 10.1038/s41598-019-47227-z.

Siderowf A, Concha-Marambio L, Lafontant D-E, et al. (2023) Assessment of heterogeneity among participants in the Parkinson's progression markers initiative cohort using α-synuclein seed amplification: a cross sectional study. *Lancet Neurol.* 22:407–417. doi: 10.1016/S1474-4422(23)00109-6.

NICE (2017) *Guidelines for Parkinson's disease in adults.* www.nice.org.uk/guidance/ng71/chapter/Recommendations#pharmacological-management-of-motor-symptoms.

NICE CKS (2022) *Parkinson's disease.* https://cks.nice.org.uk/topics/parkinsons-disease

Van Laar AD, Van Laar VS, San Sebastian W, et al. (2021) An update on gene therapy approaches for Parkinson's disease: restoration of dopaminergic function. *J. Parkinsons Dis.* 11(s2):S173–S182. doi: 10.3233/JPD-212724.

Shanker V (2019) Essential tremor: diagnosis and management. *BMJ* 366:l4485. doi: 10.1136/bmj.l4485.

Siokas V, Aloizou A-M, Tsouris Z, et al. (2020) Genetic risk factors for essential tremor: a review. *Tremor* 10:4. doi: 10.5334/tohm.67.

Rowe JB, Holland N, Rittman T (2021) Progressive supranuclear palsy: diagnosis and management. *Pract. Neurol.* 21:376–383. doi: 10.1136/practneurol-2020-002794.

Goh YY, Saunders E, Pavey S, et al. (2023) Multiple system atrophy. *Pract. Neurol.* 23:208–221. https://pn.bmj.com/content/practneurol/early/2023/03/16/pn-2020-002797.full.pdf.

Wilson D, Le Heron C, Anderson T (2021) Corticobasal syndrome: a practical guide. *Pract. Neurol.* 21:276–285. doi: 10.1136/practneurol-2020-00283.

Dharmadasa T, Scaber J, Edmond E, et al. (2022) Genetic testing in motor neurone disease. *Pract. Neurol.* 22:107–116. https://pn.bmj.com/content/22/2/107.

Pearce RK, Gontsarova A, Richardson D, et al. (2024) Shunting for idiopathic normal pressure hydrocephalus. *Cochrane Database of Systematic Reviews* 2024(8): Art. no. CD014923. doi: 10.1002/14651858.CD014923.pub2.

Graff-Radford NR (2020) *Normal Pressure Hydrocephalus*. https://www.uptodate.com/contents/normal-pressure-hydrocephalus

Lee SK (2019) Epilepsy in the elderly: treatment and consideration of comorbid diseases. *J. Epilepsy Res.* 9:27–35. doi: 10.14581/jer.19003.

NICE guideline 217 (2022) *Epilepsies in children, young people, and adults*. www.nice.org.uk/guidance/ng217/chapter/5-Treating-epileptic-seizures-in-children-young-people-and-adults#focal-seizures-with-or-without-evolution-to-bilateral-tonic-clonic-seizures

van Soest TM, Chekrouni N, van Sorge NM, et al. (2022) Community-acquired bacterial meningitis in patients of 80 years and older. *JAGS* 70:2060–2069. doi: 10.1111/jgs.17766.

Taquet M, Dercon Q, Todd JA, et al. (2024) The recombinant shingles vaccine is associated with lower risk of dementia. *Nat Med.* doi: 10.1038/s41591-024-03201-5

NICE CKS Management of shingles (2024): cks.nice.org.uk/topics/shingles/management/management/

Petitgas P, Tattevin P, Mailles A, et al. (2022) Infectious encephalitis in elderly patients: a prospective multicentre observational study in France 2016–2019. *Infection*. doi: 10.1007/s15010-022-01927-3.

Behrman S, Lennox B (2019) Autoimmune encephalitis in the elderly: who to test and what to test for. *Evid. Based Ment. Health* 22:172–176. doi: 10.1136/ebmental-2019-300110.

INFORMATION FOR PATIENTS AND FAMILIES

Parkinson's UK: www.parkinsons.org.uk

PSP Association: www.pspassociation.org.uk

Epilepsy Society: www.epilepsysociety.org.uk

Motor neurone disease association: http://www.mndassociation.org/index.html and http://www.mndassociation.org/professionals

GAIN supports people with GBS and inflammatory neuropathies. https://gaincharity.org.uk

National Institute of Neurological Disorders and Stroke website: a fantastic website with patient-friendly (hence student-friendly) material on a whole variety of neurological diseases you didn't know existed as well as the standard topics. www.ninds.nih.gov

All websites were accessed in July 2024.

8

Old-age psychiatry

Age-related changes

1 Brain weight decreases by 20% from its young adult weight by the age of 90.
2 Selective neuronal loss of 5–50%, and cells tend to shrink.
3 Reduction in synapses in the frontal lobes of 15–20%.
4 Lipofuscin accumulates in some cells (significance uncertain).
5 Plaques and tangles are found in aged brains, but seldom in middle-aged ones.
6 Granulovacuolar degeneration can often be found in the hippocampus and occasional vascular amyloid deposits are seen in cortical blood vessels.
7 All these changes are more pronounced in Alzheimer's disease (AD), but this disease is not just 'exaggerated ageing'.
8 Performance in intelligence testing, learning ability, short-term memory and reaction time tend to decline with age, but often not significantly until around the age of 75.
9 The physical and social concomitants of ageing, particularly loss of abilities and relationships, (e.g. forgetfulness and sadness after bereavement) are so common that they are often accepted as normal.

The organisation of mental health services for older people

Until recently, general adult psychiatry and psychiatry for older people were separate services. If patients had a mental health issue before the age of 65, when they reached 65 (or 75 in some areas), their care was transferred to their old age psychiatry team. This approach was considered ageist. The NHS Long Term Plan of 2019/2020 and 'move to care', organised by local integrated care systems, are removing this age divide for older people with functional needs (depression, anxiety, and severe mental illnesses). Dementia services will continue to centre on an initial assessment and diagnosis in a memory clinic. The most recent dementia audit was conducted when care was disrupted by the COVID-19 pandemic, but only half of clinics offered post-diagnostic interventions. Traditional ways of providing ongoing support, such as day care, are disappearing.

This change in the organisation may improve services for older people (who are less likely to access talking therapies and specialist services, e.g. for eating disorders), but it could separate the management of depression and dementia, whereas the two often coexist and may cause diagnostic uncertainty early in their trajectories. The main risk is that when staffing and resources are limited, older people will get even less. Any move towards universal services should not constitute a move towards services that lack specialist skills and expertise for older people.

Training in Old Age Psychiatry remains separate. After Core Psychiatry Training (CT1-CT3) and passing MRCPsych, candidates apply for a specialist training post (usually 3 or 4 years for dual accreditation with General Psychiatry).

The purpose of the curriculum in Old Age Psychiatry is to develop consultants who specialise in the assessment, diagnosis, treatment, management, and prevention of mental disorders in:

- People of any age with primary dementia.
- People with mental disorders and physical illness or frailty affecting the management of their mental disorders. This may include people under 65 years of age.
- People with psychological or social difficulties related to the ageing process or end-of-life issues, or who feel their needs may be best met by a service for older people. This would normally include people over 70 years old seen in inpatient, community, hospital liaison, crisis and home treatment, and memory assessment and treatment services.

The three most important psychiatric disorders in older people are the 3Ds: depression, delirium, and dementia. Anxiety is also very common.

The effects of the COVID-19 pandemic

The pandemic, with its long periods of enforced isolation, had an overall negative effect on mental health, with increased anxiety and insomnia. It has increased anxiety and self-harm in younger people but among older people; the greatest effect was on those living with dementia. Death rates were high, particularly among care home residents who have a high prevalence of dementia. Older people with acute COVID may present with delirium. The negative effects of COVID on dementia appear to be twofold – the lack of stimulation, family visits, etc. worsened the rate of cognitive decline, and COVID appears to have a direct neurotoxic effect on damaged brains. The long-term effects are not known.

Geriatric Medicine and Elderly Care: Lecture Notes, Ninth Edition. Claire G. Nicholl, K. Jane Wilson, and Shaun D'Souza.
© 2025 John Wiley & Sons Ltd. Published 2025 by John Wiley & Sons Ltd.
Companion website: www.wiley.com/go/lecturenotesgeriatricmedicine9e

Loneliness

According to Age UK, more than two million people in England over the age of 75 live alone, and more than a million older people say they go over a month without speaking to a friend, neighbour, or family member. This should be a source of national shame.

- Loneliness is a subjective feeling that a person experiences when there is a gap between their actual level of social contact and what they would wish it to be.
- It is not just a lack of contacts, which is 'social isolation', but a perception of a lack of quality in the relationships that they do have. So, a person can be surrounded by people, e.g. in a care home, but still feel lonely.
- Loneliness is associated with poorer physical and mental health and wellbeing.
- It is a risk factor for anxiety, depression, and dementia.
- Social isolation can be addressed by providing a visitor, but loneliness will only be helped if the visitor can make an ongoing and meaningful relationship with the person they are meeting.
- People can be lonely and isolated at any age, regardless of gender or background, but it can be a particular issue for:
  - Older men, who may have previously had most of their social interaction at work.
  - Older LGBTQ+ people who may feel isolated from their same-age peers.
  - People from minority ethnic groups who may feel more isolated because of cultural issues, limited English, and poverty.

If older people are relatively fit, options that get them out of the house, e.g. to join local groups or volunteer, are the most successful, but these are not possible for many frail older people, especially in rural areas where transport is limited. Likewise, suggestions to 'learn to love computers' on the NHS web page about loneliness in older people are frequently unrealistic. Local initiatives may be the most likely to succeed.

Depression

Prevalence

Depression is the most common and most treatable mental illness in people aged 65 and older. It affects one in five people in the community. This figure doubles with a physical illness and trebles in care homes. It is severe in 5%. Unipolar depression is most common, but bipolar disorders make up 5–10% of more severe cases, and the hypomanic phase is often missed. The key is to consider the possibility of a mood disorder. Ask the patient – most will tell you. There is a surprisingly good correlation between a 'Yes/No' answer to the question 'Are you depressed?' and the result of a full psychiatric assessment. NICE recommends two questions, specifically:

- During the last month, have you often been bothered by feeling down, depressed, or hopeless?
- During the last month, have you often been bothered by having little interest or pleasure in doing things?

Screening tools such as the Geriatric Depression Score (see Appendix) may be helpful. Many ill older people in hospitals are anxious, lose their appetite and cannot sleep or concentrate. In the list of features that follows, physical aspects are the least helpful in discriminating between physical and psychiatric disease and anhedonia the most.

Features

- Association with physical illness, especially chronic disease. There is growing evidence for a subtype of depression in later life associated with cerebrovascular disease.
- Somatisation of symptoms, hypochondriasis.
- Pervasive anhedonia ('when did you last enjoy anything?').
- Guilt, worthlessness, and low self-esteem.
- Hopelessness and helplessness.
- Apathy or agitation, anxiety, or delusions (usually mood-congruent).
- Sleep disturbance.
- Withdrawal, poor concentration, and poor memory ('pseudodementia').
- Self-neglect, malnutrition, and dehydration.
- Suicide risk.

Suicide risk

In almost all industrialised countries, men aged 75 years and older used to have the highest suicide rates. Since 2010, this has been superseded by the middle-aged, who may be more affected by factors such as economic downturns or alcoholism. However, suicide attempts by older people have a high fatality rate: they are often long-planned and involve high-lethality methods, older people have less homeostatic reserve and are more likely to live alone. In later life, in both sexes, severe depression is the most common diagnosis in those who attempt or complete suicide. A previous serious attempt, recent bereavement and isolation all indicate ongoing high risk.

In the UK, the greatest reductions in male suicide rates have been seen in men over 75 years of age, from 25 per 100,000 population in 1991 to 13 per 100,000 population in 2022 (see Figure 8.1). The trend in older women is similar, but with rates of about one-third. This is compelling evidence that recognition and treatment of depression by traditional old-age psychiatry services were effective. The trend will need to be monitored in the new all-age services.

Management

Depression is now categorised simply as 'less severe' or 'more severe'. Less severe depression is managed in primary care. More severe depression is often best managed with the help of the local psychiatry service (often termed the 'CRHT' or crisis resolution and home treatment team), involving community psychiatric nurses (CPNs), social workers and a consultant. An urgent referral will be needed if there are psychotic symptoms or a risk of self-harm or suicide. The team usually assesses the patient in their own home and will support them to continue with medication or cognitive behavioural therapy (CBT). Such patients must have a crisis plan.

Supportive management

This is important for everyone with depression.

- Provide information, e.g. Depression UK, Depression in older adults (RCPsych), and MIND.
- Signpost to relevant peer support groups, e.g. Cruse following bereavement.
- General health advice about diet, sleep, and a reminder that alcohol will make a low mood worse.
- Provide advice on activities that improve the sense of well-being (depending on frailty); outdoor activities, e.g. rambling, gardening, and singing, are evidence-based.
- Relieving loneliness: local coffee morning, AgeUK visitor.
- Practical measures, e.g. a benefits check.

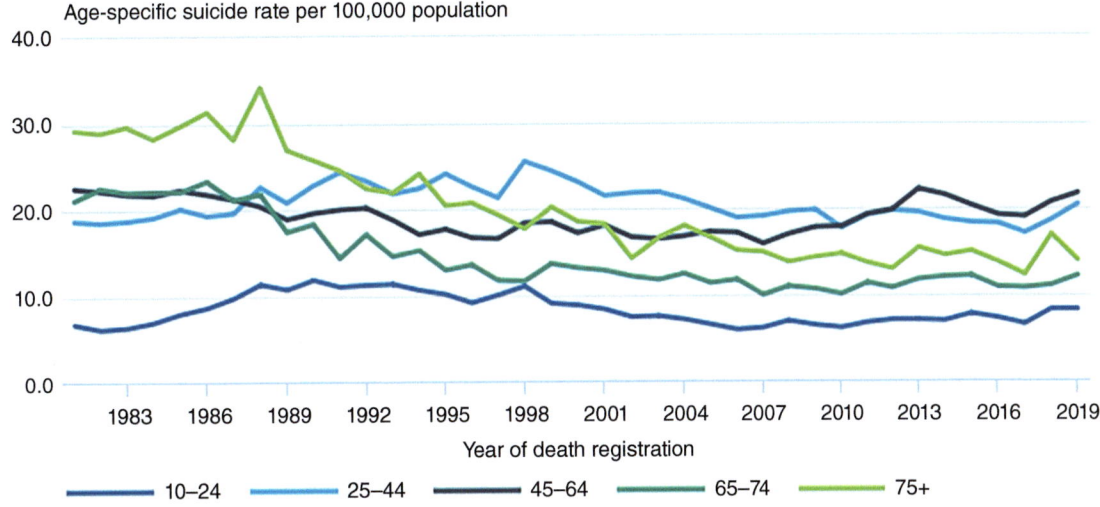

Figure 8.1 Age-specific suicide rates for men in the UK since the 1980s. *Source*: ONS 2019/CC BY 3.0.

- Support families and carers, e.g. respite care or a sitting service such as Crossroads for the patient, before deterioration in the carer's mental health precipitates a crisis.

First-line treatment options for less severe depression include CBT, group exercise, group mindfulness, meditation and counselling, and patient preference is emphasised. Services that are available in different localities vary and usually fall short of what is described on the NICE website. Older people may not be able to use online options or get to groups, so many will be started on antidepressants even if they would have preferred 'short-term psychodynamic psychotherapy'!

Drugs

Antidepressants may effectively treat depression in older adults, but adverse events may be more common because of multiple coexistent medical comorbidities and drug interactions.

Selective serotonin reuptake inhibitors

Selective serotonin reuptake inhibitors (SSRIs) are the drugs of choice; they cause fewer sedating and anticholinergic effects than tricyclic antidepressants. SSRIs are also relatively safe in overdose (compared to tricyclic antidepressants). Bear in mind the following:

- Nausea, diarrhoea, and restlessness can occur.
- To minimise nausea, start at a very low dose and increase gradually over a period of a few weeks. Explain to the patient that any nausea should wear off.
- Monitor for hyponatraemia by checking blood within a month of commencing therapy.
- Consider a PPI for gastric protection but avoid this if the patient is prone to hyponatraemia.
- Give a simple explanation of the chemical basis of depression and explain that depression cannot just be shaken off by 'counting your blessings' or having a bit more moral fibre!
- Explain that SSRIs are different from benzodiazepines, do not usually cause 'dopiness', but will be stopped gradually when no longer needed.
- Strongly reinforce the need to stick with the tablets for at least 6 weeks before expecting the cloud to lift. Information sheets can be useful. Treatment should be continued for a year, or even for life in severe cases. A positive drug response is defined as a 50% reduction in symptoms on a validated depression scale. Current practice is:
  - Start with sertraline at a low dose (25 mg); citalopram is next in line, but higher doses of citalopram can prolong the QT interval, so check a baseline ECG.
  - If weight loss is an issue, use mirtazapine (see the later discussion).
- Unless it is essential to stop treatment at once, e.g. severe hyponatraemia, wean rather than stopping suddenly, and if a change to another drug is needed, look up cross-titration in the BNF.
- Fluoxetine, fluvoxamine, and paroxetine are more likely to be involved in significant drug–drug interactions than sertraline or citalopram.

Other antidepressants

- Mirtazapine is a NaSSA, a noradrenergic and specific serotonergic antidepressant with a tetracyclic structure. It is a presynaptic α2-antagonist, which increases noradrenergic and serotonergic transmission. It stimulates appetite and aids sleep, which can be useful or cause the side effects of weight gain and drowsiness.
- Venlafaxine and duloxetine are SNRIs; serotonin noradrenaline reuptake inhibitors and are other options if the above fail to provide the required response.
- Lithium is helpful as a mood stabiliser in bipolar disorder and as an adjunct treatment for depression, but it has a narrow therapeutic index, and levels must be checked if toxicity is suspected (tremor, ataxia, and impaired renal function). The use of lithium should be supervised by a psychiatrist.

Polypharmacy in older patients can be minimised by using the Screening Tool of Older Persons Prescriptions and Screening Tool to alert doctors to the Right Treatment (STOPP/START).

Electroconvulsive therapy

There are potentially several distinct types of direct brain stimulation that can be used to treat depression, including transcranial direct current stimulation (tDCS), repetitive transcranial magnetic stimulation (rTMS) and electroconvulsive therapy (ECT).

ECT is comparatively safe and effective in severe depression with life-threatening features, with some studies suggesting that over two thirds of patients benefit. The consenting patient is placed under general anaesthesia and given a muscle relaxant, following which an electrical current is passed across the brain, inducing a controlled seizure. ECT is usually given twice a week for up to 12 sessions in total. The Mental Health Act 2007 states that ECT may not be given to a patient with capacity who refuses it and may only be given to an incapacitated patient where it does not conflict with any advance directive, the decision of a donee (the person who has been given a power of attorney), deputy, or the Court of Protection.

Anxiety

Anxiety is very common in older people. It may accompany depression, dementia, and physical illness or may cause physical symptoms (palpitations, breathlessness, giddiness, abdominal discomfort, and bowel fixation). Always consider anxiety or depression in recurrent attendees and in rehabilitation patients who fail to make progress. When severe (Generalised Anxiety Disorder), it decreases social functioning and has a marked impact on health-related quality of life. Treatments include reassurance or cognitive therapy, but if associated with panic attacks or significant impairment to quality of life, try mirtazapine, an SSRI, or pregabalin (an antiepileptic gamma amino butyric acid [GABA] agonist). Beta-blockers and benzodiazepines are less well tolerated in older patients.

Late-onset delusional disorders

The commonest reason for new psychotic symptoms in old age is delirium (see later) but a small proportion of schizophrenia-like psychoses develop for the first time in people over the age of 60 years, termed 'very late-onset'.

- Single women who live alone, especially those who are deaf are most often affected. Isolation is thought to be a significant factor in development of the condition.
- Personality, affect and self-care skills are well preserved and there is no formal thought disorder (e.g. disconnected or knight's move thinking).
- There is often a highly structured system of delusions and hallucinations that may centre on a conspiracy involving the neighbours or have a sexual content.
- The response to antipsychotic drugs is good if concordance can be achieved. Low-dose risperidone can be effective.

Hallucinations

These are the abnormal perceptions of something that is not present. They are likely to be under-reported even in the presence of insight, due to the associated stigma. Sensory and cognitive impairment are significant risk factors in older people, as are sleep deprivation and co-existing medical illnesses.

Causes of hallucinations

- Bereavement.
- Depression.
- Delirium (including drugs, e.g. dopaminergic treatment for Parkinson's disease).
- Dementia.
- Late-onset schizophrenia.
- Poor vision (Charles Bonnet syndrome – no other features of psychiatric illness – patients need explanation and reassurance that this is not a harbinger of mental illness).

The treatment of hallucinations begins with establishing the cause. Ensure that sensory faculties are optimised (glasses, hearing aids). Provide reassurance and consider stopping or reducing medications that may be contributing. Consider the use of antipsychotics in those in whom hallucinations are not due to an underlying reversible cause and those experiencing distress/agitation. Newer antipsychotics (risperidone, olanzapine) are effective, but start with a low dose and ensure that there are no contraindications (perform an electrocardiogram before treatment). Cholinesterase inhibitors such as rivastigmine can be considered when antipsychotics are contraindicated, such as in individuals with PD.

Cognitive changes with ageing

Many old people are subjectively slightly forgetful, and it can be difficult to distinguish normal ageing changes from the earliest stages of pathology.

Age-associated memory impairment is a subjective complaint of forgetfulness in those over 50 years, with a performance on memory testing one standard deviation below the normal for a young adult. Almost 20% of people over 50 years old meet these criteria, and the significance is uncertain. Older people often compensate well for memory changes using pattern recognition from experience.

Mild cognitive impairment (MCI) has been coined for people who have evidence of memory loss in comparison with those of the same age, confirmed by testing and noticeable to other people. It is not considered a part of the normal ageing process. There is no single accepted definition, but most specialists now agree that there may be subtle impairments in language, attention, reasoning, judgement, reading and writing, as well as memory problems. The American College of Physicians suggests that 20% of the population over 70 may have MCI. Some people with MCI are in the early stages of Alzheimer's or other dementia; others have stress, anxiety, depression or a physical illness; and others may have always had a poor memory. In memory clinic series, depending on the population, definitions and protocols adopted, around 10% of people with MCI progress to dementia per year (compared to around 1% in the normal population).

All definitions of MCI agree that the problems are not severe enough to affect activities of daily living. However, even this is not objective, as different lifestyles place different demands on the individual (see Figure 8.2). Whether or not a person notices cognitive impairment depends on the environment in which they find themselves. In an undemanding situation, a compromised brain may be perfectly adequate for the demands placed on it. In a complex, unfamiliar situation, difficulties become apparent.

It is difficult to pinpoint the onset of dementia because of differences in baseline cognitive abilities, variations in the ageing process, and the gradual onset of the disease process.

Figure 8.3 shows cognitive change with ageing in three normal individuals with different cognitive baselines: an individual with two episodes of acute illness and two individuals who are developing dementia. At the single point in time shown by the arrow, it would be difficult to be certain about what a given level of cognition means for each individual, apart from Person A, who clearly falls below the normal range.

Confusion

Many older people are described as confused. Anyone can become delirious when they are ill, but this is more common in frail older people. Simplistically, delirium is the term used for acute confusion, and dementia describes chronic confusion. The interrelationship between the two is complex.

- Dementia is the biggest risk factor for delirium; a person with dementia typically gets much more muddled when ill and improves to some extent (but not always back to baseline) if they recover.

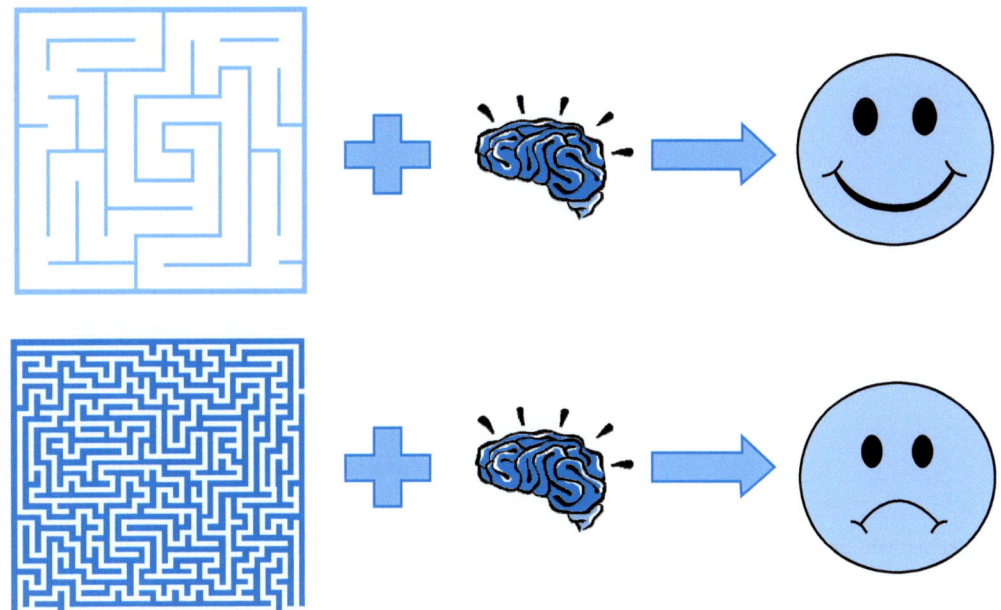

Figure 8.2 The interplay between the brain and the environment. *Source:* © Claire G. Nicholl.

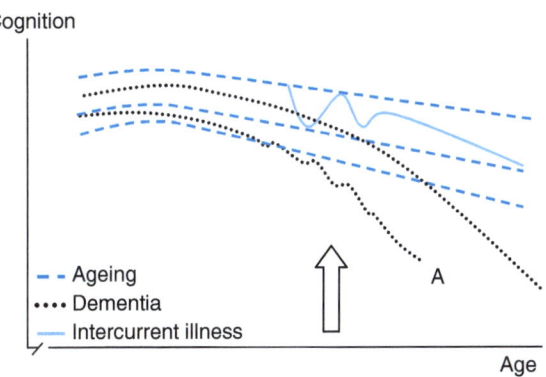

Figure 8.3 Cognitive change with ageing. *Source:* © Claire G. Nicholl.

- Delirium may persist for months (or years, according to some) – when does this become 'dementia'?
- Some of the causes of dementia are reversible.
- Long-term cognitive decline is common after an episode of delirium.
- Dementia with Lewy bodies (DLB) (see later) has features more typical of delirium.

Delirium

Delirium is an acute, fluctuating syndrome of encephalopathy causing disturbed consciousness, attention, cognition, and perception. It usually develops over hours to days and behavioural disturbance, personality changes, and psychotic features may occur.

Delirium is common and occurs in up to half of frail older patients admitted to hospital. Up to 70% of mechanically ventilated intensive care admissions will be complicated by delirium. It is historically under-reported, and research has been hampered by a lack of consistent nomenclature – it is often labelled as 'acute confusional state', 'acute encephalopathy', or 'acute brain failure'. It can be a key component in the cascade of events leading to a downward spiral of functional decline, institutionalisation and eventually death. All-cause mortality is increased by 10–20% for those with delirium.

All patients who are potentially susceptible to delirium should be routinely screened upon admission to hospital. The most commonly used screening methods are the AMTS (Abbreviated Mental Test Score) and CAM (Confusion Assessment Method; see the later discussion). The AMTS is particularly useful due to its simplicity, with no formal training required.

Delirium is typically seen in people with predisposing factors when new precipitating factors are added.

Predisposing factors

- Age.
- Brain vulnerability: previous delirium, depression, cognitive impairment, dementia.
- Multiple comorbidities.
- Multiple drugs.
- Functional impairment.
- Falls (a marker of frailty).
- Sensory impairment/deprivation.
- Alcohol misuse.

Precipitating factors

Intracranial

- Infarction: any stroke.
- Infection: meningitis, encephalitis.
- Injury: head injury with contusion or intracranial blood; fat embolism.
- Post-ictal.

Extracranial

- Infection: commonly chest, urine, and cellulitis.
- Metabolic and nutritional: fluid and electrolyte imbalance, hypoglycaemia, hypo-/hyperthermia, refeeding syndrome, Wernicke's encephalopathy.
- Anoxia: cardiac or respiratory failure, 'silent' myocardial infarction, anaemia.

- Toxic: drugs that cross the blood–brain barrier and alcohol or their withdrawal.
- Stress response.
- Anaesthesia and surgery.

Consequences of illness and hospitalisation

- The severity of the illness.
- Pain.
- Emotional distress.
- Sleep deprivation.
- Unfamiliar environment, exacerbated by the loss of glasses and hearing aids.
- Catheters, drips, etc.
- Urinary retention.
- Constipation.

Pathophysiology

Many neurobiological mechanisms are likely to contribute to delirium, and evidence supporting a common pathophysiological pathway is currently lacking (see Figure 8.4). High-risk individuals demonstrate a failure to cope with an acute stressor. This may be due to the reduction in cholinergic and noradrenergic neuronal pathways and an exaggerated pro-inflammatory response to stress. Vascular factors may also be at play – the older brain is more susceptible to cerebral hypoperfusion.

The precipitating events cause further acute breakdown of network connectivity by increasing inhibitory tone within the brain (GABAergic neurotransmission). All transmitters may be affected, but a frequent pattern is cholinergic hypofunction, dopaminergic excess/stress response, and neuro-inflammation. Pro-inflammatory cytokines released during a systemic inflammatory response may affect the brain and trigger neuronal apoptosis and neurotoxicity. The form of delirium that results – hypoactive, hyperactive, or mixed – depends on which networks are affected. A small study with single-photon emission computerised tomography (SPECT) has shown hypoperfusion in the frontal, parietal, and pontine regions in delirium.

Delirium subtypes

Three subtypes are based on the symptoms.

1 Hyperactive delirium - may present with inappropriate behaviour, hallucinations, or agitation. Restlessness and wandering are common.

2 Hypoactive delirium - may present with lethargy and reduced concentration and appetite. The person may appear quiet or withdrawn. This is more easily overlooked and is very common at the end of life.

3 Mixed delirium - signs and symptoms of both subtypes are present.

Clinical features of delirium

- Onset is typically rapid over hours or days.
- Marked fluctuation: lucid intervals.
- Reversal of the sleep–wake cycle is common.
- Altered consciousness, often described as 'clouding'.
- Inability to sustain, focus or shift attention.
- Disturbed cognition: e.g. disorganised thinking, disorientation.
- Illusions: misinterpretation, e.g. thinking an IV line is a snake.
- Hallucinations: perceptions in the absence of a stimulus.
- Delusions and false beliefs: the patient may deny they are ill and attempt to abscond.
- Fear, bewilderment, restlessness, or hypoactivity.

Management of delirium

- Prevention is the most important aspect. Essentially, optimise the environment by paying attention to orientation, oral intake, and sleep to reduce the likelihood of delirium. Make sure that there is an accurate clock nearby. Inpatients may benefit from families providing bedside photographs of familiar faces. Make sure that the patient has their glasses and hearing aids. Avoid suddenly stopping sedatives and antidepressants unless essential. Use caution with new drugs that cross the blood–brain barrier. Avoid overstimulation.
- Minimise moves around the hospital and ward.
- Identification of high-risk patients and explaining to the family that delirium may occur reduces distress if it does develop.
- Recognition of delirium is key. An algorithm such as the CAM (see box) may help. Agitated delirium is obvious, but hypoactive delirium is easy to overlook.
- Treat the underlying cause(s) and correct additional factors: fluid and electrolyte imbalances and nutritional deficiencies.
- Look for and treat exacerbating factors, e.g. faecal impaction, urinary retention, and pain etc.
- Reassurance and explanation: avoid confrontation; ask the family to sit with the patient. The family may appreciate written information such as the RCPsych leaflet on delirium.

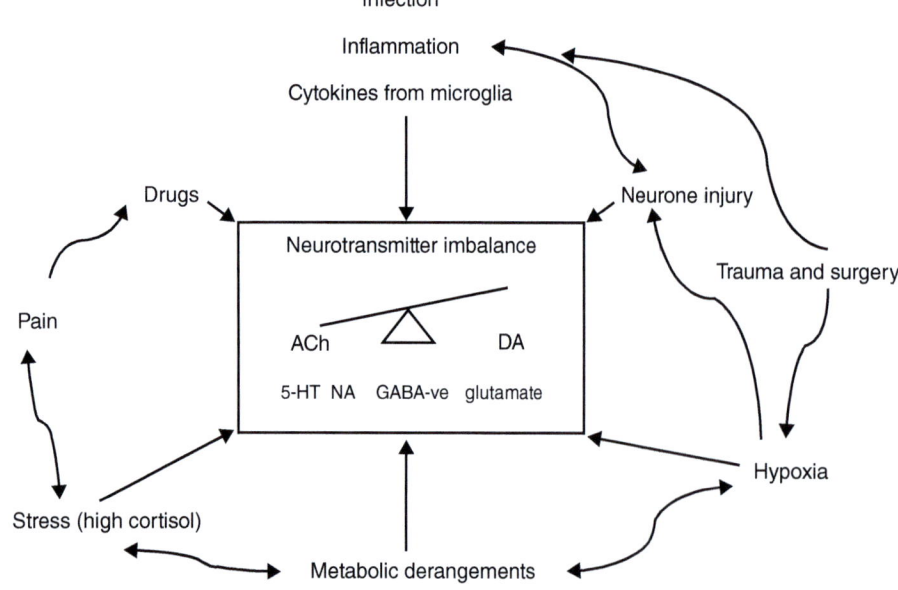

Figure 8.4 How neurotransmitter imbalance may contribute to the pathogenesis of delirium. ACh, acetylcholine; DA, dopamine; 5-HT, 5 hydroxytryptamine; NA, noradrenaline; GABA, gamma-aminobutyric acid. *Source*: © Claire G. Nicholl.

- Avoid complications: nurse sitting with the patient, 1 to 1 'specialling', mattress on the floor to reduce risk of hip fracture, pressure mattress, falls mats.
- The use of regional (rather than general) anaesthesia has been shown to reduce the incidence of postoperative delirium in some types of orthopaedic surgery. Although this conclusion appears intuitively correct, it has not been replicated in other types of surgery.
- Serious restlessness or agitation that results in danger to the patient or others and does not respond to the above nonpharmacological measures: trial haloperidol or risperidone, starting at the lowest dose (increasing, if necessary, in increments after 2 hr). If neuroleptics must be avoided (e.g. in LBD or PD), try low-dose lorazepam. Give drugs orally if possible, (but this will take 30–60 min to start to have an effect) or intramuscularly if it is essential to sedate rapidly for the person's safety.
- Low-dose antipsychotics will not reduce the incidence of delirium but may reduce duration, which nevertheless is likely to positively affect outcomes.

The Confusion Assessment Method (CAM) diagnostic algorithm

Four features are assessed:

1. Acute onset and fluctuating course – need information from a family member or carer.
   Is there an acute change in mental status from the patient's baseline? Does the (abnormal) behaviour fluctuate?
2. Inattention
   Does the patient have trouble keeping track of what is said? Are they easily distracted or do they have difficulty focusing attention?
3. Disorganised thinking
   Is the patient's thinking disorganised, rambling, irrelevant or illogical?
4. Altered level of consciousness
   Is the patient's level of consciousness alert (the only normal answer), vigilant (hyperalert), lethargic (drowsy but easily roused), stuporous (difficult to arouse), or comatose (unrousable)?

The diagnosis of delirium by CAM requires the presence of features 1 and 2 and either 3 or 4. (With training, sensitivity is around 94% and specificity is 89%.)

Complications of delirium

- Distress for the patient and their family.
- Falls.
- Poor nutrition and reluctance to drink.
- Slower recovery and rehabilitation.
- Increased length of stay.
- Nosocomial infections.
- Increased risk of pressure sores.
- Risk of admission to long-term care.
- Accelerated cognitive decline and increased incidence of dementia.
- Increased mortality.

Dementia

Dementia is a clinical and public health problem of enormous magnitude.

Definition

Dementia is a syndrome of *acquired*, *chronic* (lasts months to years), *global* (not just memory or just language problems) impairment of higher brain function in an *alert patient*, which *interferes with the ability to cope* with daily living. There must be evidence of decline over time. This definition satisfies the current International Classification of Diseases (ICD-11) threshold. Dementia is *not* an inevitable part of ageing. In the US, the Diagnostic and Statistical Manual of Mental Disorders is preferred to the ICD and in the current version (DSM-5), the term 'dementia' has been replaced with 'major neurocognitive disorder'.

Causes

Dementias may be classified as primary, where the disease process causes degeneration of brain neurons, or secondary, where the effect on the neurones is due to another pathology. Treatments to slow progression in primary dementias are in their infancy, but secondary dementias may be reversible. Classification of primary dementias is complex and evolving. The clinical features depend on which part of the brain is affected first, regardless of the pathology. Age of onset and early symptoms are helpful, but there is often a period of uncertainty before a diagnosis can be made. Advanced dementia, of any cause, tends to have similar features.

Common causes include:

- Alzheimer's disease (AD), the commonest cause.
- Vascular dementia (VaD).
- Mixed dementia, most often AD with VaD
- Lewy body dementia (LBD) is an umbrella term which includes dementia with Lewy bodies (DLB) and Parkinson's disease dementia (PDD). In practice, LBD and DLB are often used synonymously.
- Frontotemporal dementia (FTD) is more common in people in their 60s.

Rarer causes include:

- Normal pressure hydrocephalus (NPH), which presents with a triad of incontinence, gait dyspraxia, and dementia, probably due to abnormal CSF flow, although by the time CSF pressure is measured, it is in the 'normal' range. It may respond to shunting (see Chapter 7).
- Prion diseases such as familial, sporadic, and variant Creutzfeldt–Jakob disease.
- Huntington's disease, an autosomal dominant trinucleotide repeat disorder in which an excessive number of CAG repeats results in a polyglutamine sequence in the huntingtin protein, which leads to neuronal death. It causes dementia with abnormal movements, usually presenting in middle age, although it can begin in later life.

Other conditions that may present as a dementia include:

- Any major metabolic problem, especially hypo- or hyperthyroidism, hypercalcaemia, hyponatraemia, recurrent nocturnal hypoglycaemia, major organ failure (usually obvious),
- Vitamin deficiencies, especially thiamine, folate and B_{12}, and niacin (B_3) worldwide.
- Toxicity from centrally acting drugs and alcohol.
- Brain tumour, particularly in a frontal lobe.
- Head trauma (either repetitive, e.g. 'punch drunk' syndrome - now known as chronic traumatic encephalopathy - in boxers, and the sequel to a long sporting career heading the ball), or the sub-acute confusion of a subdural haemorrhage following a fall and head injury.
- Neurosyphilis was the most frequent cause of dementia in Western Europe in the 19th century but although syphilis is increasing again, neurosyphilis remains very rare, and HIV is usually diagnosed before dementia develops.

Prevalence

About 950,000 people in the UK are estimated to have some form of dementia (62% of whom have a diagnosis).

- The prevalence is likely to increase to 1.15 million by 2030 (Alzheimer's Society, 2023).
- Dementia is rare under 55 years old, but the prevalence increases dramatically with age to about 2% in those over 65 and rises to about 20% in those over 85 (see Figure 8.5).
- Black and South Asian people are more likely to be diagnosed at a younger age and die earlier from dementia than White people.
- Previous strokes, diabetes, hypertension, and depression increase the risk.
- About 65% of people living with dementia in the UK are women.
- The lifetime risk for AD at age 45 is 1 in 5 for women and 1 in 10 for men.
- In older people, AD accounts for half to two-thirds of cases of dementia.
- An estimated 80% of people living in care homes have dementia.

The increase in prevalence over the last few years has been lower than predicted, perhaps because the cohort of people reaching their 80s were fitter than previous generations. There is concern that rates will rise again more rapidly due to poorer lifestyles in those who are currently middle-aged.

Overview of the clinical course

The onset is insidious, with gradual changes in:

- Memory and concentration.
- Thinking processes such as planning and judgement.
- Language use.
- Orientation.
- Personality.
- Behaviour.

Short-term memory is impaired early; long-term recall is often much better. Thinking becomes rigid and concrete. The condition progresses to obvious memory loss, difficulty managing basic activities of daily living, increasing disorientation and sometimes difficult or distressing behaviour such as night-time wandering, aggression, or apathy. These behavioural and psychological symptoms of dementia (BPSD) cause great distress for carers. A tendency to lose things easily turns into paranoia and even delusions. Constant repetition of the same questions can be very trying. Eventually, the patient can become completely disorientated, no longer recognise close family members, and cease communicating. Functional abilities decline further, and the patient becomes doubly incontinent, bed-bound, and totally dependent. It is hard to maintain nutrition and hydration, and pressure ulcers may develop despite good nursing. The typical disease duration is 8–10 years.

Impact

- Dementia is a devastating condition for the patient while insight is preserved and for their family, who witness the progressive deterioration. For the spouse, this has been likened to 'being bereaved without being widowed'.
- As people live longer, there are more of the 'oldest old', one in five of whom may have dementia, a major cause of dependency and need for institutional care.
- Politicians and society grapple with the economic consequences of health and social care. In the UK, the national cost of dementia is about £25 billion per year (2021), and in 30 years, the cost will increase to over £50 billion per year. Direct costs to social care account for half of this; informal care consumes 41%; and healthcare costs just £1.7 billion (7%). The costs of dementia are greater than the costs of stroke, heart disease and cancer.
- The impact of dementia on other health outcomes is dramatic. A person with a fractured hip and dementia is over 2.5 times as likely to die and 18 times more likely to be discharged to a care home than a person with normal cognition.

In addition to causing considerable morbidity, dementia is a major cause of death in high-income countries. Dementia and Alzheimer's disease are the overall leading causes of death in England and Wales (see Figure 8.6). In 2022, this accounted for nearly 66,000 deaths (11.4% of all deaths), although in men, ischaemic heart disease still tops the list. Note that in the *month* of July 2023, ischaemic heart disease again became the leading cause of death, replacing dementia after 24 months. This may be a 'blip' or evidence of the concern that cardiovascular risk management declined over the pandemic.

Diagnosing dementia

The patient's family will often raise concerns with the GP first, but a survey performed by the Alzheimer's Society (AS) in 2006 suggested that it was difficult to get a diagnosis. In 2012, the then UK Prime Minister David Cameron launched an initiative to improve dementia management. NHS Digital (2023) reported that 62% of people >65 years old with dementia had a formal diagnosis, which represents progress. There is still room for improvement, and many barriers remain to obtaining a diagnosis, some of which are highlighted in the box.

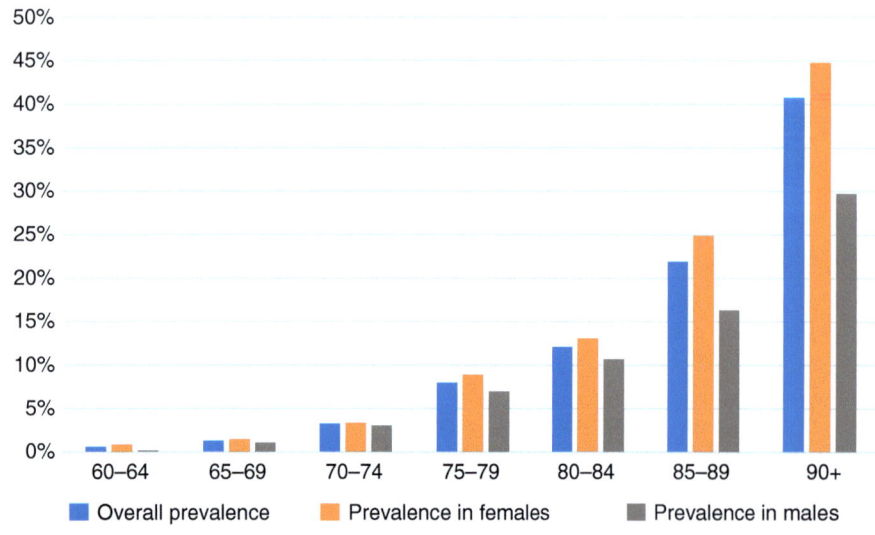

Figure 8.5 Prevalence of dementia in Europe 2018 by age band and sex. *Source*: Adapted from EURODEM data.

Legend: ■ Overall prevalence　■ Prevalence in females　■ Prevalence in males

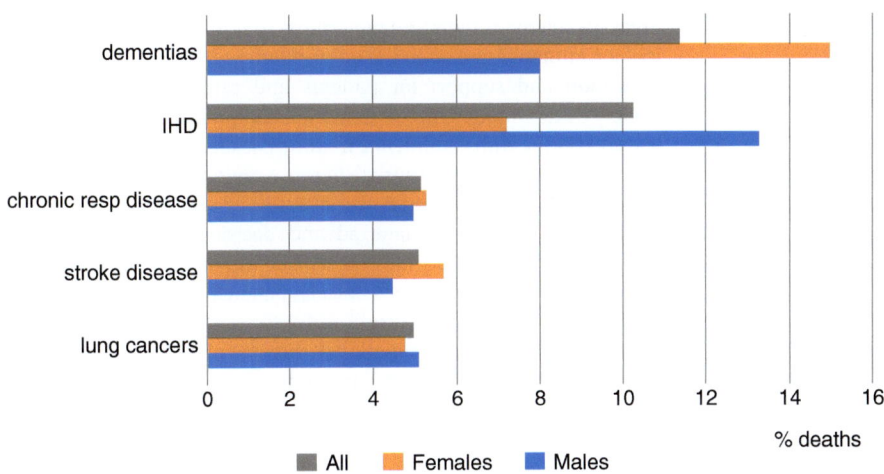

Figure 8.6 Top five causes of death in England and Wales overall and by sex 2022. IHD, ischaemic heart disease. *Source*: Adapted from ONS.

Difficulties in getting a diagnosis of dementia

Doctor factors
- Lack of confidence/training in this area: this is an increasing problem as healthcare professionals narrow their focus of expertise; see also the management of diabetes and PD for other examples of this trend.
- Reluctance to diagnose an 'untreatable illness' (but much can be done; see management discussed later).
- Reluctance (rightly so) to diagnose a progressive degenerative condition in the context of acute illness ± superimposed delirium whilst the patient is in hospital (see Figure 8.3).

Patient/carer factors
- It is necessary to know the previous level of function to identify decline.
- Patients with dementia do not give the best medical histories – they can get disorientated in place or time and may focus on previous problems (e.g. 'It's the doctor... what did I want to say?... Ah, doctor, it's my back').
- Patients are often older and live alone; family may be distant, so corroborative information may be limited. However, if family members are concerned, there is usually a problem, whereas if only the patient is complaining, the potential differential diagnoses widen to include depression or health anxiety.

Environmental factors
- The point at which the person has difficulty coping depends on their environment (see Figure 8.3) and support network, as well as their cognitive abilities.
- Dementia often presents acutely because of a social crisis (e.g. the death of a caring spouse).

The aims of a clinical assessment

Is it dementia?

There is no simple test for dementia. A GP may start assessments with GPCOG scoring (see Appendix) or by using the clock face test, which excludes all but early dementia if completed correctly. In the UK, suitable patients are then referred to memory clinics. A full history, together with a more detailed cognitive function testing method that includes assessments of language, visuospatial skills, and reasoning, such as Addenbrooke's Cognitive Examination (ACE III), usually answers the diagnostic question. The MMSE (Mini-Mental State Exam) is no longer widely used due to copyright law.

However, even in expert hands, there is often uncertainty, which is only resolved with the passage of time. Cognitive scores are affected by education, language fluency, impaired hearing and vision, acute illness, dysphasia, and low mood. These conditions must be optimised or allowed for, as must psychiatric problems like depression, schizophrenia, and mania.

What type of dementia is it?

The next step is to identify the cause. Subtyping is important – the cause may be reversible (e.g. hypothyroidism), treatment may slow disease progression (e.g. treating hypertension in VaD), specific treatment may be available (e.g. AD), genetic counselling may be required (e.g. familial AD) or it may be important to avoid certain medications (e.g. neuroleptics in LBD).

There is no diagnostic test for most of the primary dementias until a post-mortem examination, so the *likely* cause is determined by the *clinical features* and the results of *investigations*. Common conditions such as AD and VaD may co-exist ('mixed dementia') and are probably additive.

History

Progressive deterioration in memory and executive functions (such as reasoning) is usual in AD, experienced over a period of years. VaD classically presents as a 'stepwise' deterioration. Mixed dementia can be difficult to differentiate from its components based on clinical history alone. Hallucinations and delusions are more prominent features of LBD. Parkinsonian features tend to follow the initial cognitive impairment in DLB. Most patients with dementia show some fluctuation, known as 'sun-downing' because the confusion worsens in the evening, but this can be marked in LBD. Younger patients are more likely to have frontotemporal dementia.

Weighted scores, such as the Hachinski ischaemia score (HIS), may improve diagnostic accuracy, and patterns of change found on neuropsychological and language testing add to the diagnosis.

Examination

- Clues from general appearance (self-care or neglect).
- Cardiovascular system; BP, cardiac rhythm; burden of atheroma.
- Neurological system (walk and turn undress, get onto the couch swiftly, follow commands):
  - Stroke disease or other focal problems.
  - Other neurological conditions, e.g. PD.
- Psychiatric state, mood, hallucinations.

Investigations

- Blood tests to exclude reversible causes of cognitive impairment or other major pathologies (blood count, biochemical profile including renal and liver function and calcium, ESR/CRP, thyroid function, B_{12} and folate). NICE recommends syphilis serology and HIV testing if clinically indicated.
- CXR and ECG. An ECG is particularly useful due to cardiac contraindications to acetylcholinesterase inhibitors (arrhythmias).
- A head CT early on is likely to be normal but is useful to exclude space-occupying lesions or a subdural haematoma. Disproportionately large ventricles with little sulcal atrophy raise the possibility of NPH (see Chapter 7). The presence of small vessel disease or previous strokes suggests a vascular component, or at least a 'mixed' picture. In the late stages, a CT scan usually shows cerebral atrophy.
- MRI is more sensitive than CT in documenting volume loss (particularly in the medial temporal lobe and hippocampus in AD) and the amount of vascular damage. Serial scans will show the progression of atrophy.

Investigations in tertiary centres

- CT-SPECT imaging labels presynaptic dopamine transporters and helps distinguish dementia associated with either Parkinson's or DLB.
- Fluorodeoxyglucose positron emission tomography (FDG)-PET can distinguish patients with AD who show a specific pattern of decreased glucose uptake.
- Amyloid PET scanning (to detect amyloid beta deposition) is mainly used for research but also in occasional difficult cases.
- Genetic tests, e.g. for apolipoprotein E (*APOE*) alleles that predispose to AD, are not routine.
- Lumbar puncture, to exclude prion disease or cerebral angiitis, or for biomarkers of Aβ deposition, including CSF Aβ42 (lower than normal) and neuronal injury CSF tau/phosphorylated-tau (increased).

Management

GPs most often refer patients with suspected LBD or frontotemporal dementia, as well as those who are still relatively young. Assessments are then undertaken in specialist memory clinics, often staffed by neurologists or psychiatrists. First assessments are often undertaken within the patient's usual environment. Memory clinics also have access to resources from voluntary agencies such as the Alzheimer's Society.

Management depends on the severity of the dementia and whether the patient lives alone and follows a multidisciplinary, multi-agency assessment. Much of the management is similar, regardless of the aetiology.

Supportive management

The management plan for all types of dementia needs to be tailored to the patient, well-coordinated and evolve as the needs of the patient and carer change. The many options *should* include:

- Coping strategies (diaries, reminder alarms), psychological techniques (CBT), reminiscence work (a life-story book), and validation therapy (an approach where care staff accept the reality of the world as perceived by the person living with dementia but there is no evidence for benefit).
- Optimisation of hearing and vision, and improving general health.
- Treat other conditions that may impair cognition (e.g. anaemia, heart failure).
- Treat risk factors (e.g. hypertension in VaD).
- Take every opportunity to stop inappropriate medications especially those crossing the blood brain barrier and increasing the anticholinergic burden.

- Treat specific symptoms and behaviours (tranquillizers and anxiolytics, unfortunately, are often the only options).
- Education and support for patients and carers: the Alzheimer's Society deals with all types of dementia and produces excellent leaflets and Caring with Confidence training packages; Carers UK.
- Genetic counselling (appropriate in rare early-onset dementias).
- Legal advice (e.g. a Lasting Power of Attorney may obviate the need for the Court of Protection later, advance decisions, etc.).
- Advice on driving (see the Consensus Guidelines, an excellent factsheet from the Alzheimer's Society; patients can pay for a driving assessment at a mobility centre).
- Therapy assessments: occupational therapy, speech and language therapy (for swallowing and communication), and physiotherapy; usually aimed at arranging appropriate care and advising carers rather than treating the patient.
- Assistive 'smart' technology includes pressure mats to turn on lights, fridges, and door monitors to detect movement, automatic fall detectors if the person cannot press the buzzer, and automatic tap cut-off.
- Assessment of benefits and care by social services (see Chapter 2).
- Regular district nurse/CPN support.
- Continence services.
- Sitting services (Crossroads), day hospitals, respite care.
- Optimal provision of long-term care.
- Encourage training for staff in care homes.
- Palliative care in the terminal stages.
- Drugs may be used:
  - For secondary prevention, e.g. aspirin, statins, and antihypertensives may slow the development and progression of VaD.
  - To treat specific symptoms (see debate on antipsychotics in BPSD).
  - To enhance cholinergic transmission, block *N*-methyl D-aspartate (NMDA) receptors or reduce brain amyloid in AD (see later).

Alzheimer's disease

AD is the most common dementia. It is named after Dr Alois Alzheimer, a clinical psychiatrist and anatomist. Alzheimer followed the clinical trajectory of Auguste D, a 51-year-old inmate of an asylum with memory impairment and behavioural problems. Alzheimer studied her brain posthumously, and in 1906, presented his histological findings of brain atrophy with the presence of lesions now described as plaques and neurofibrillary tangles using specific staining techniques.

Pathologically, AD is characterised by:

- Amyloid-containing extracellular plaques.
- Intraneuronal neurofibrillary tangles containing tau protein.
- Neuronal loss.

Pathogenesis

In AD, beta-amyloid (Aβ) is clipped from a normal transmembrane protein, amyloid precursor protein (APP), by two enzymes – beta-secretase and gamma-secretase. Aβ oligomers are produced in the diseased brain at a normal rate but are not cleared efficiently and stick together to form amyloid plaques. According to the amyloid hypothesis (still not universally accepted), the accumulation of Aβ drives the rest of the disease process, including the formation of neurofibrillary tangles (consisting of abnormally phosphorylated tau protein) and cell death. Figure 8.7 shows a simplified scheme for APP metabolism.

Risk factors for Alzheimer's disease

- Age (the most significant risk factor).
- Down's syndrome (the *APP* gene is located on chromosome 21). Affects 75% by age 60.

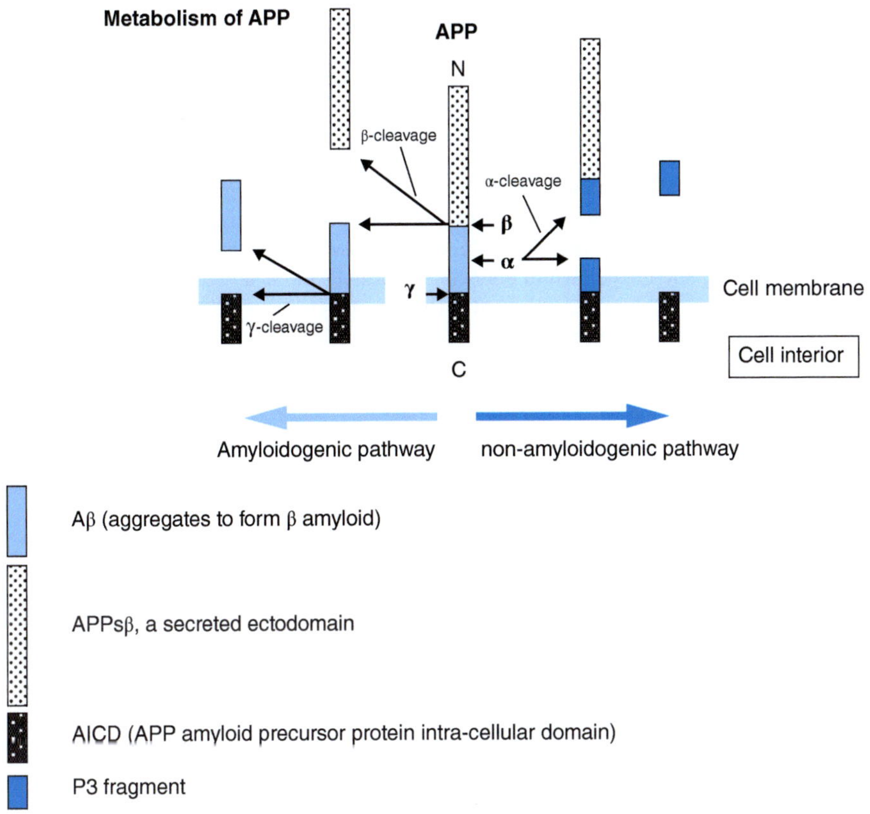

Metabolism of APP

APP

N

β-cleavage

α-cleavage

β

α

γ

Cell membrane

γ-cleavage

C

Cell interior

Amyloidogenic pathway   non-amyloidogenic pathway

Aβ (aggregates to form β amyloid)

APPsβ, a secreted ectodomain

AICD (APP amyloid precursor protein intra-cellular domain)

P3 fragment

Figure 8.7 The metabolism of APP. N and C are the N and C terminus of the polypeptide. Source: Adapted from Cole and Vassar, 2007/Springer Nature/CC BY 4.0.

- Female sex.
- Genetic susceptibility: *APOE e4* (main risk factor for late-onset AD).
- Family history: the estimated lifetime risk of AD in first-degree relatives without a defined underlying genetic risk factor is 25–50%.
- Cerebrovascular disease.
- Hypertension, dyslipidaemia, smoking, midlife obesity, and diabetes.
- Head injury.
- Hearing loss.
- Elevated homocysteine levels (can be decreased by folate, so may be counterbalanced by fruit and vegetables).
- Depression.
- Artificially sweetened soft drinks.

Protective factors for Alzheimer's disease

- Education (partly a threshold effect but confounding with other associations with social class, e.g. a diet high in antioxidants).
- Continued brain activity/cognitive reserve (keep reading, Sudoku, social activity, physical activity).
- A diet rich in foods containing unsaturated fats and antioxidants.
- Vitamin D (variable results; a large observational study in 2023 was positive, but baseline data on the two groups showed differences in ethnicity, rates of depression and MCI).
- NSAIDs and aspirin (no benefit and may be harmful in cognitively healthy older people).
- Hormone replacement therapy (variable results; a 2023 Danish nested case-control study suggested increased dementia).
- Statins (2021 metanalysis suggests benefit; reassure those on statins, but cognition is not a reason for a prescription because of the caveats about observational studies).

Genetics and Alzheimer's disease

There are rare autosomal dominant forms of AD with mutations in three genes, all of which increase brain levels of amyloid: the *APP* gene on

chromosome 21, *presenilin 1* on 14q, and *presenilin 2* on 1q. People with trisomy 21 (Down's syndrome) frequently develop AD from their 40s onwards because of the gene dose effect of APP. Most cases of AD appear sporadic, but there is evidence of a polygenic genetic predisposition in these cases too. The best-established association is with the *ApoE4* gene on chromosome 12. There are three common alleles: *APOE e2*, *APOE e3* and *APOE e4*.

- *APOE e2* is less common and may provide some protection against AD.
- *APOE e3*, the most common allele, appears neutral.
- *APOE e4* increases the risk of getting dementia and getting symptoms at a younger age, but the mechanism is unknown. *APOE e4* is a risk-factor gene; it increases the risk of AD, but some with the e4/e4 genotype never get the disease. However, new data suggests that e4 homozygotes have a very high probability of disease.

Phases of Alzheimer's disease

The National Institute on Ageing and the Alzheimer's Association (NIA–AA) workgroup (2011) has produced guidelines for the diagnosis in three phases:

Phase I – Preclinical Alzheimer's disease (of research interest)

The pathophysiological process of AD (and brain shrinkage) is thought to begin many years before it becomes clinically apparent. Individuals have no symptoms initially, but a subjective cognitive decline may develop. If interventions that delay or arrest the progression of the pathology become available, identifying pre-symptomatic people will be very important.

Phase II – Mild cognitive impairment due to Alzheimer's disease

People in this stage may be slower, less efficient and make errors when completing complex functional tasks such as paying bills, preparing a meal, or shopping. Their loved ones may become concerned; however, they still function independently. Prominent impairment in episodic memory is a strong predictor of progression to AD, but other patterns of cognitive impairment, e.g. visuospatial impairment, can also progress. In this stage, encourage patients to remain as engaged as possible in the following domains: physical activity, cognitive activities, and social engagement. Barriers to participation contributed to cognitive decline during the COVID pandemic.

At this stage, several biomarkers may confirm that the underlying pathology is AD. These are used in research but are being incorporated into the clinical diagnostic process in tertiary neurology centres in the UK.

- CSF amyloid β1 – 42
- CSF phosphorylated-tau181 (ptau)

A reduction in CSF Aβ42 and raised levels of ptau are indicative of Aβ and tau pathologies in AD. Work is in progress to develop highly sensitive blood assays for these markers so that they could be used in routine memory clinic assessments, after appropriate studies on sensitivity and specificity.

Data from amyloid PET scans in older people shows why this is important. In a large population-based study, the proportion of people aged 80 and over with no cognitive problems but a positive amyloid PET is above 40%. In people with MCI and a positive amyloid PET scan, only one-third progressed to AD after nearly 4 years of follow-up. 15% of those with MCI and a negative amyloid PET scan also progressed to AD.

Phase III – Dementia due to Alzheimer's disease

At this point, cognitive deficits start to impact functional independence. How long the patient remains in their own home depends on the robustness of the available family support and the pattern of their dementia. Behavioural problems, falls, urinary, and particularly faecal incontinence, predict institutionalisation.

Clinically, the course of AD is described as going through seven stages, which also form the basis of the Global Deterioration Scale (see Table 8.1).

Variants of Alzheimer's disease

Problems with memory are the most common symptoms of AD. About 1 in 20 people with AD have different early symptoms, or atypical AD. The two most common types are frontal variant AD (FvAD), where typical Alzheimer's pathology starts in the frontal lobes plus posterior cortical atrophy, which starts in the occipital cortex and causes difficulty with object recognition and spatial awareness. People with FvAD are often misdiagnosed as having behavioural variant frontotemporal dementia (see later).

The metabolism of acetylcholine

The rationale for the current drugs used for AD is based on earlier work showing that most neuronal death occurs in cholinergic projections. Cholinergic transmission could be enhanced by increasing the availability of the precursor via direct stimulation of the receptors or by preventing the breakdown of endogenous acetylcholine, and acetylcholinesterase inhibition has provided the best strategy (see Figure 8.8). Anticholinergic drugs should be stopped where possible (see Chapter 5 on the anticholinergic burden of medication).

Drug treatment for AD

Drugs affecting neurotransmitters

Acetylcholinesterase inhibitors
Three acetylcholinesterase inhibitors (AChEIs) are used in AD:

- Donepezil: reversible inhibitor of AChE.
- Galantamine: reversible inhibitor of AChE with nicotinic receptor agonist properties.
- Rivastigmine: reversible, non-competitive inhibitor of AChE and butyryl cholinesterase.

The drugs have limited efficacy and do not benefit all patients, but many (about 60%) get a useful response in terms of memory or behaviour, with around 6 months of better function. There appears to be little clinical difference between the drugs, and most clinicians start with donepezil because of familiarity. Rivastigmine is also available as a patch, which may reduce side effects and help if people dislike tablets.

- Treatment must be recommended by a healthcare professional with expertise in dementia (including consultant psychiatrists, neurologists, geriatricians, GPs, and nurse practitioners), but the first prescription can be made in primary care.
- Indicated for mild and moderate AD.
- The carer's views should be considered, as they will need to support adherence.
- All AChEIs have cholinergic side effects, especially nausea, vomiting and diarrhoea. To minimise these, the drugs are started at a low dose and gradually increased. Care must be taken in cases of sick sinus syndrome, peptic ulcer disease, COPD and urinary retention, and there may be interactions with muscle relaxants used in anaesthesia.

Table 8.1 The phases and stages of Alzheimer's disease.

		Symptoms
Phase I	Stage 1	Persons appear cognitively normal, but pathological changes are happening in the brain.
	Stage 2	Prodromal stage: mild memory loss, but generally this is indistinguishable from normal forgetfulness.
Phase II	Stage 3	Progression into mild cognitive impairment (MCI). Individuals may get lost or have difficulty in finding the correct wording.
Phase III	Stage 4	Mild dementia with moderate cognitive decline and poor short-term memory. Individuals start to struggle with the instrumental activities of daily life and may forget some of their personal history.
	Stage 5	Cognition continues to decline, and at this point, individuals need help in their daily lives. They suffer from confusion and forget many personal details.
	Stage 6	Severe dementia. Requiring constant supervision and care. Patients fail to recognise many of their family and friends and have personality changes.
	Stage 7	Individuals are nearing death. They show motor symptoms, have difficulty communicating, and are incontinent.

Source: Based on the stages first published by the Fisher centre.

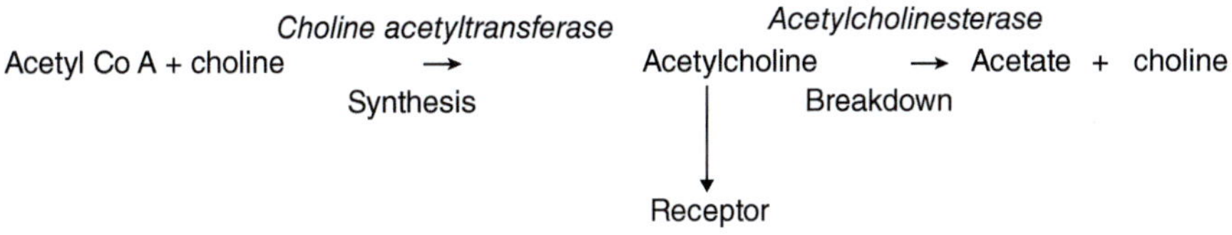

Acetyl Co A + choline → Acetylcholine → Acetate + choline

Choline acetyltransferase   *Acetylcholinesterase*

Synthesis   Breakdown

↓

Receptor

Figure 8.8 The metabolism of acetylcholine.
Source: © Claire G. Nicholl.

- If one drug is not tolerated, try another.
- The drug should be continued if there is a cognitive or behavioural benefit (stable cognition indicates benefit, as decline would be expected).
- Review as needed, at least annually.
- Stop the drug if problems arise, but not because a cognitive threshold is reached.

Memantine

- Memantine is an NMDA receptor antagonist that reduces glutamate-induced neurotoxicity.
- NICE recommends memantine as the first line in severe AD and in moderate AD if there is intolerance or a contraindication to AChEIs; it is the preferred drug in the presence of cardiac arrhythmias.
- Memantine can be added to AChEI in moderate and severe AD. It may be useful for BPSD symptoms.
- Side effects include constipation, and are mild.

Disease-modifying drugs

The goal of treatment is to slow or stop disease progression. One challenge is ensuring that enough drugs get across the blood–brain barrier. Research is ongoing about ways to achieve this by modifying the drugs or physically disrupting the barrier, e.g. by using focused ultrasound.

Anti-amyloid drugs

Beta-amyloid was isolated in 1984, and the amyloid hypothesis of AD was first proposed in 1992 by Hardy and Allsop. Targeting amyloid has been the main recent focus of drug development.

Strategies for treatment based on the Aβ hypothesis include:

- Beta- and Gamma-secretase inhibitors to reduce Aβ production; several beta-site APP cleaving enzymes (BACE inhibitors) have reached Phase III trials, but none have progressed.
- Drugs to inhibit Aβ aggregation.
- Immunotherapy.

Monoclonal antibodies (MAbs) successfully clear amyloid in sequential amyloid PET scans of AD patients, so some of the infused antibodies must be getting across the blood–brain barrier. Different MAbs target Aβ monomers, oligomers (believed to be the most neurotoxic), fibrils, and plaques. Plaques may be broken up, Fc-mediated phagocytosis into microglia may be promoted, and there may be a gradient 'sink' effect with MAbs in the cerebral circulation, removing amyloid fibrils.

It has been harder to show that amyloid removal translates into meaningful improvements in cognition, but increasing evidence suggests that disease progression is slowed, particularly in early disease. The magnitude of improvement is difficult to assess because of the varied responses in the placebo arms, and the improvements are not dramatic.

However, infusion reactions and serious adverse events occur, principally cerebral oedema and amyloid-related imaging abnormalities (ARIA). In the trial of donanemab, clinical improvement was only seen in people with a low or medium tau burden. In the treatment arm, 112 people had to stop the drug due to adverse events compared with 38 on placebo, and three deaths on the drug were related to brain bleeding or swelling. The Alzheimer's Society understandably wants to encourage its supporters, but their account of the trial and timeline for possible drug availability in the UK seem too optimistic.

Two anti-amyloid MAbs are available in the US:

1 Aducanumab, the first to be FDA-approved in 2021, was rarely used due to problems with insurance cover and administration and withdrawn in January 2024.
2 Lecanemab was FDA-approved in 2023. The European Medicines Agency refused approval in July 2024, but granted limited approval in October 2024. In the UK, the Medicines and Healthcare Products Regulatory Agency (MHRA) approved lecanemab (August 2024) for some people with early-stage AD but in draft guidance NICE has not approved its use. This means that UK patients can only access the treatment as a private patient. The decision reflected the limited benefit, risk of serious side effects, limited access to the advanced diagnostics needed and the logistic difficulty of delivering the fortnightly infusions as well as the cost, but the media have just focused on the cost of the drug.
3 Donanemab also got FDA approval in 2024 and the MHRA (October 2024), (TRAILBLAZER-ALZ2) but was not approved by NICE.

> **Other drugs in the trial pipeline for AD (2024) include:**
>
> - Further anti-amyloid MAbs (including remternetug (TRAILRUNNER-ALZ1), which is given as a subcutaneous injection rather than an infusion).
> - ALZ-801, a prodrug of homotaurine, inhibits Aβ42 aggregation into toxic oligomers.
> - Tau therapies, including MAbs.
> - Gene therapy to drive expression of *APOE2*.
> - Anti-inflammatory agents include tyrosine kinase inhibitors, semaglutide, and sargramostim (a synthetic granulocyte-macrophage colony-stimulating factor).
> - Neurotransmitter therapies include dextromethorphan, a sigma 1 receptor agonist, and bupropion to increase its plasma concentration for agitation.

Supplements for AD

A healthy diet may reduce the risk for cognitive decline and dementia, but no food ingredient, vitamin, or supplement has been proven to prevent, treat or cure AD or to benefit cognitive function or brain health. The evidence for lack of efficacy is summarised on the Alzheimer Association website.

Dementia with Lewy bodies

Dementia with Lewy bodies (DLB) accounts for around 6% of all cases of dementia. Think of DLB if your patient seems to have a combination of symptoms of dementia, parkinsonism, neuropsychiatric phenomena (particularly complex visual hallucinations), and postural instability, with wide fluctuations that can even involve conscious level. Always consider this condition in those that are labelled as 'delirium, cause unknown…' Attention, executive, and visuoperceptual functions are affected more than naming and memory abilities. Rapid eye movement (REM) sleep behaviour disorder is another core feature. Vivid dreams are accompanied by the loss of the atonia that is usual during REM sleep, so patients make violent and unpredictable movements as they dream. DLB closely resembles the dementia typically associated with PD. Pragmatically, if cognitive symptoms precede physical symptoms by 1 year, the patient is considered to have DLB; if physical symptoms precede dementia, it is called Parkinson's disease dementia (PDD).

Pathology

Lewy bodies, intracytoplasmic deposits of misfolded α-synuclein, are found throughout the cerebral cortex, whereas in PD they are restricted to the substantia nigra. Coexisting AD pathology is common.

Management

Management is multidisciplinary, and the supportive approaches are like those in AD. The Alzheimer's Society produces relevant information, and there is a Lewy Body Society.

Donepezil or rivastigmine can be prescribed to people with mild, moderate, or severe LBD. Galantamine should be offered if donepezil and rivastigmine are not tolerated. Memantine should be tried if AChEIs are not tolerated or are contraindicated, and it may be useful in agitation and hallucinations. Small trials have suggested low-dose levodopa preparations may improve motor symptoms in a third of patients, especially if relatively young, whilst increasing the risk of known side effects such as hallucinations. Melatonin or low-dose clonazepam may be used in sleep disorders.

Extreme care must be taken with all antipsychotic drugs, as the patient may become drowsy and hypertonic.

The course of DLB tends to be more rapid than Alzheimer's disease, with a life expectancy of between 5 and 8 years after diagnosis.

Frontotemporal dementias

Six patients with frontal dementia were first described by Pick in 1892.

- It is now recognised that frontal dementia is not a single entity but a family of brain disorders in which there is degeneration of the frontal and temporal lobes (see Figure 8.9). The clinical syndromes are known as frontotemporal dementias (FTDs) and the associated pathologies as frontotemporal lobar degenerations (FTLDs) but the terms are often used synonymously.
- FTDs are the most common forms of dementia in people under the age of 60. They cause around 15% of dementias with onset below 65 years old (mean age of onset: 58 years) but can present later, accounting for about 2.5% of all dementias.
- Clinically and pathologically, there is an overlap with conditions that present mainly to neurologists – corticobasal syndrome, progressive supranuclear palsy, and amyotrophic lateral sclerosis.
- FTDs are likely to be underdiagnosed, as neuropathological studies in some populations suggest that 5% of the older population with or

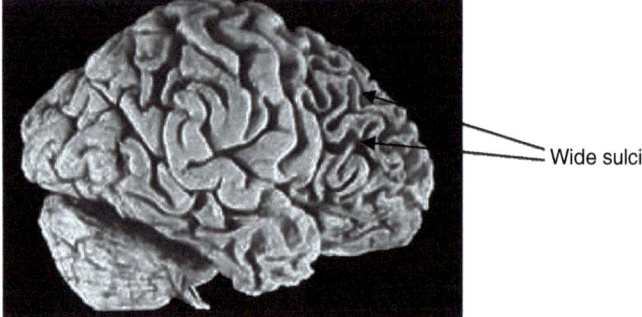

Figure 8.9 Brain showing frontal degeneration. *Source:* Wikimedia Commons: http://commons.wikimedia.org/wiki/File:Frontotemporal_degeneration.jpg

without known cognitive impairment at death has FTLD pathology. Although FTD patients tend to have better scores than AD patients on initial cognitive testing, the course tends to be more rapid, with a mean life expectancy of 8 years.

FTD subtypes

- Behavioural Variant FTD: the most common (Pick's disease); personality changes, apathy, and a progressive decline in socially appropriate behaviour, judgement, self-control, and empathy, with relative sparing of memory.
- FTD, primary progressive aphasia: starts with gradual impairment of language with differing early features. With time, features of the behavioural variant emerge. The videos on the Rare Dementia Support website demonstrate the issues.
  - Nonfluent-agrammatic variant: speech apraxia with impaired grammar.
  - Semantic variant: loss of meaning of words, e.g. 'rose' becomes 'flower' and then 'thing'.
  - Logopenic variant: impaired single-word retrieval.

  Although these conditions are grouped with FTD, there is overlap with AD. The logopenic variant is most likely to have Aβ pathology, and patients may benefit from AChEIs.
- FTD, motor variants: can present as an overlap syndromes with features of amyotrophic lateral sclerosis, or the parkinsonian syndromes corticobasal syndrome or progressive supranuclear palsy.

Pathology

FTLDs are characterised by the loss of neurons, frontotemporal atrophy, gliosis and intraneuronal inclusion bodies consisting of abnormal amounts or forms of protein. The first protein to be identified was tau. Until around 2006, all FTLDs were thought to be 'tauopathies', but it is now known that tau abnormalities account for around 45% of cases (FTLD-tau). Another protein, transactive response DNA-binding protein TDP-43, has been identified in 50% of cases as the TDP-43 'proteinopathies' (FTLD-TDP). In the remaining 5%, the protein that aggregates is an RNA-binding protein fused sarcoma protein (FTLD-FUS). Ubiquitin may also be found in the inclusion bodies, but this is non-specific as ubiquitin is attached to damaged or misshapen proteins as the cell's way of marking them for disposal. Whatever the nature of the inclusion bodies, serotonergic systems are more affected than dopaminergic systems, with cholinergic and noradrenergic pathways being relatively normal.

Around 30% of cases are familial. The most common genetic mutations are found in the microtubule-associated protein tau (*MAPT*), progranulin (*PGRN*) and *C9orf72* genes, and transmission is autosomal dominant. The remainder appear sporadic, but there may be a genetic predisposition.

Clinical features

FTDs are characterised by behavioural and language changes due to the selective atrophy of the frontal and temporal lobes. Symptoms typically include:

- Impaired executive functioning: problems with planning and sequencing, prioritising, multitasking, self-monitoring, and correcting behaviour.
- Perseveration: repeating the same word or activity when it no longer makes sense.
- Social disinhibition: 'private behaviour in public' with no regard for social norms or legal limits; acting impulsively with no regard for the impact on others, e.g. laughing or swearing at a funeral.
- Compulsive eating: gorging on food; taking food from other people's plates.

- Utilisation behaviour: difficulty resisting impulses to use or touch objects; e.g. will pick up a phone receiver when the phone is not ringing and the person does not intend to make a call.
- Aphasia.
- Dysarthria.
- Apathy and abulia: loss of interest and motivation to perform a task.
- Loss of empathy: loss of ability to appreciate how others will feel.
- Dystonia: abnormal postures of the hands or feet.
- Gait disorder: shuffling, frequent falls.
- Tremor: usually of the hands.
- Clumsiness: dropping or difficulty manipulating small objects.

In comparison with AD, memory and orientation tend to be well preserved. There is considerable overlap between the clinical pictures, and as the disease progresses, more symptoms emerge.

Management

This is supportive, as for other dementias. Non-pharmacological options should be attempted first, such as relaxation techniques and exercise, distraction techniques, speech therapy, and encouraging families to try to plan structured daily routines. As these syndromes are rare, patient support groups are invaluable.

SSRIs may be helpful for disinhibition, repetition, overeating and compulsive behaviours. Trazadone can be used for disruptive behaviours and depressive symptoms. The use of antipsychotics and anxiolytics is more frequent in FTD when compared to AD – this reflects the higher rate of behavioural disturbance, particularly in the behavioural variant of FTD.

AChEIs are not proven to be beneficial, and their use is not recommended unless there is diagnostic uncertainty or a syndrome that may be caused by AD, like logopenic PPA, in which a drug trial is reasonable.

Vascular dementia

VaD is caused by brain damage secondary to impairment of the blood supply to parts of the brain. This can happen in several ways.

Pathogenesis

- Multiple strokes (usually thrombotic or embolic but can be haemorrhagic) – 'multi-infarct dementia'– individual strokes may be clinically silent.
- A single stroke in a critical part of the brain, e.g. the angular gyrus or thalamus, especially the left brain.
- Subcortical ischaemic vascular disease (SIVD):
  - Lacunar disease: small, spherical strokes in the deep parts of the brain.
  - Binswanger's disease: damage to small blood vessels in the white matter (myelinated fibre tracts).
  - CADASIL (cerebral autosomal dominant arteriopathy with subcortical infarcts and leukoencephalopathy) is a rare inherited vascular disease linked to abnormalities of a specific gene, *notch3*, on chromosome 19p. It causes multi-infarct dementia, stroke, migraine, and mood disorders. Individuals usually develop symptoms in their 30s and often die by age 65, but older individuals may not be identified. CARASIL is a recessive version with

variants in the serine protease *HTRA1* gene. It may be associated with early alopecia and spondylolisthesis. Carriers are also at risk of an early stroke.
  - Cerebral amyloid angiopathy (CAA): amyloid is deposited in the media and adventitia of small and mid-sized arteries. The deposits weaken the vessel walls and make them prone to bleeding (see Chapter 7). Some cases are familial and some are sporadic. Familial forms tend to present at a younger age. Mutations in different proteins, including beta-amyloid, cystatin C, prion protein, transthyretin, and gelsolin, lead to their aggregation and deposition. In sporadic CAA, beta-amyloid is the commonest and may be associated with AD disease but also occurs in older brains without typical Alzheimer's pathology. Gradient echo MRI (T2*) sequences may demonstrate multiple small, chronic haemorrhagic lesions in patients with CAA who often present with lobar intracranial haemorrhage.

Clinical course

The textbook description of VaD dementia is of stepwise deterioration temporally related to a series of small infarcts, but many cases show slowly progressive cognitive and motor decline. The number of pure VaD cases is small, and many cases are thought to have mixed pathologies (see Figure 8.10). Studies using ^{11}C-PiB to image amyloid and MRI to quantify vascular damage suggest that the effects of the two pathologies are additive. White matter changes can be seen in many people who appear to have no cognitive complaints, but as the total volume of changes increases, cognitive difficulties are more likely.

Risk factors for VaD dementia are like those for stroke and include hypertension, smoking, obesity, high cholesterol, diabetes, atrial fibrillation and a South Asian or African-Caribbean ethnic background.

Symptoms of VaD can be very similar to those of AD. There are often physical signs of vascular damage. Frequent features include:

- Cognition: executive function is often affected more than memory; encoding is more of a problem than retrieval, inattention, and poor concentration.
- Psychological symptoms: apathy and depression, emotional lability, hallucinations, and delusions. Insight may be better preserved.
- Motor: focal neurological signs and findings such as parkinsonian features, pseudobulbar palsy, marche à petits pas, incontinence, and epilepsy.

Treating vascular risk factors is recommended, and the evidence base for the efficacy of antihypertensive medication in reducing dementia risk is increasing as more trials have cognition as an end point. .

FINGER is a Finnish multicentre RCT looking at whether a 2-year multi-domain intervention (diet, exercise, cognitive training, and management of vascular risk factors) could improve cognitive outcomes in a population-based sample, $n = 1,260$, aged 60–77, mean age 68.9, who were at risk of vascular disease and dementia. The trial showed a significant but small benefit on a composite score of cognition. Longer-term follow-up to 7 years reports that 'participants who received the intervention showed cognitive benefits, a 20% lower risk of cardiovascular events, a 30% lower risk for functional decline, a 60% reduced risk of chronic diseases, and a better health-related quality of life, as well as reduced health-care service costs when compared with controls' (see the summary in the European Geriatric Medicine Society – EuGMS – Congress report).

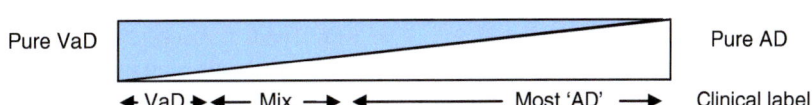

Figure 8.10 Overlap between Alzheimer's disease pathology (AD) and pathology of vascular dementia (VaD). *Source:* © Claire G. Nicholl.

Other large studies have not shown benefit, but either the population was unselected (as in a Dutch study) or the interventions were lifestyle-only (as in a French study). Similar studies are ongoing.

Behavioural and psychological symptoms of dementia

Dementia may manifest as apathy, but up to 90% of patients with dementia will develop BPSD. Wandering behaviour, agitation, disinhibition, aggression, and emotional lability can all occur. Hallucinations can promote paranoia and jealousy. Sexual jealousy is a recognised occurrence, particularly with LBD and can be very upsetting for spouses and carers. The best approach is to try to understand the basis of the behaviour from the individual's perspective, identify an unmet need, and rectify the cause.

- Physical: see delirium; thirst, constipation, pain.
- Psychological: anxiety, depression, boredom.
- Environment: poor facilities (no space to wander, lack of views, no aids to orientation), over- and under-stimulation, disturbed behaviour of others, inadequate numbers, or training of staff.

Dementia support workers and community psychiatry nurses can help support patients prone to such behaviours, which can cause significant difficulties at home, in care facilities and in hospitals.

Drug treatment

Unfortunately, these behaviours often persist in attempts to understand and address the underlying cause.

- No drugs are licensed for long-term management of BPSD, but antipsychotics are widely used.
- Doses are lower than those in schizophrenia, but parkinsonian side effects were common with first-generation drugs like haloperidol.
- Newer atypicals, e.g. risperidone, olanzapine, and quetiapine, are thought to have fewer side effects. However, a meta-analysis of 17 trials (modal duration of 10 weeks) demonstrated that the risk of death (from a variety of causes, including cardiovascular) associated with the drugs was 1.7 times that of placebo.
- Use the lowest dose possible for the shortest time possible; once the patient has settled, aim to reduce, and then stop the drug.
- When prescribing these drugs, explain the rationale and risks to the family and document the discussion. Only use these drugs if symptoms are detrimental to quality of life (not all hallucinations are distressing).

Recognition that dementia is a terminal illness

In early dementia, patients should be supported to live a full life. However, clinicians must recognise when the patient is entering the terminal phase and ensure that the family understands.

- In a study of 323 nursing home residents with advanced dementia, 6-month mortality was high (nearly 25%). Complications such as pneumonia, febrile episodes and eating problems were common and distressing symptoms were frequent.
- In the last 3 months of life, 40% of residents had a burdensome intervention such as hospital admission or tube feeding.
- One-third of patients in nursing homes with end-stage dementia and aspiration are tube-fed in the US. There is no evidence of benefit in terms of nutritional state, pressure ulcers or mortality.
- Family dissatisfaction with care is more likely where the family and carers did not appreciate the clinical course. It is essential to educate relatives about the poor prognosis of people with advanced dementia. Aim

to change to a palliative approach at the right time in a patient's journey to prevent unnecessary suffering for both the patient and family.

- Avoid keeping people 'nil by mouth'; offer food and fluids as the patient can manage. If appropriate and agreed upon, consider the notion of 'comfort feeding' for those with unsafe swallows who are not appropriate for non-oral feeding. This is the best way of preserving quality of life, enjoyment, and social interaction. A speech and language therapist will advise on making eating and drinking as safe as possible, in the knowledge that risk of aspiration cannot be fully eliminated.
- Asking for a second opinion is often advisable and legally desirable in incidences of divided opinion between family and clinical teams.

Transient global amnesia

This is a poorly understood episodic disorder in which there is temporary anterograde amnesia with an acute onset that usually lasts several hours. Most reported cases occur between the ages of 50 and 80. During the episode, the patient can function, e.g. drive, but will then have no recollection of how they got to a place and will be perplexed, repeat questions, and feel disorientated. They remain alert and do not lose self-identity. The episode may follow vigorous activity and be more common in migraine sufferers. Symptoms usually resolve within 24 hr and rarely recur. Transient global amnesia (TGA) is a diagnosis of exclusion, but it is helpful to recognise what it might be. Differentials include intoxication, encephalopathy, stroke, and seizure disorders.

Sleep disorders

Figure 8.11 is a reminder of basic sleep architecture.

Ageing changes

Changes in *sleep architecture* occur with ageing, and sleep quality worsens with more arousals.

1 Increased *sleep latency* – takes longer to fall asleep.
2 Difficulty in staying asleep (*sleep maintenance*) results in *sleep fragmentation.*
3 Decrease in slow-wave sleep (deep sleep) – periods are shorter and less frequent, so REM sleep may not be achieved.
4 Early-morning awakenings are common.
5 Circadian rhythm tends to shift earlier '*advanced sleep phase*' so that people go to bed and wake earlier.
6 Increased daytime somnolence.

In normal sleep, sleep onset occurs with drifting into light sleep (stages 1 and 2) and then deep sleep (3 and 4). Periods of REM sleep when dreaming occur at intervals of around 90–110 min. There is often brief arousal at the end of REM periods, and problems such as pain or the need to pass urine will result in full waking.

Circadian rhythm

There is a 24-hr rhythm of sleep/wakefulness regulated by an intrinsic body clock located in the suprachiasmatic nucleus (SCN).

- Individual periods average 24.2 hr.
- Normally synchronised to the environmental day by light and other cues (zeitgebers).
- The main transmitter is melatonin – pineal release stops by day and starts in the evening to peak at midnight.

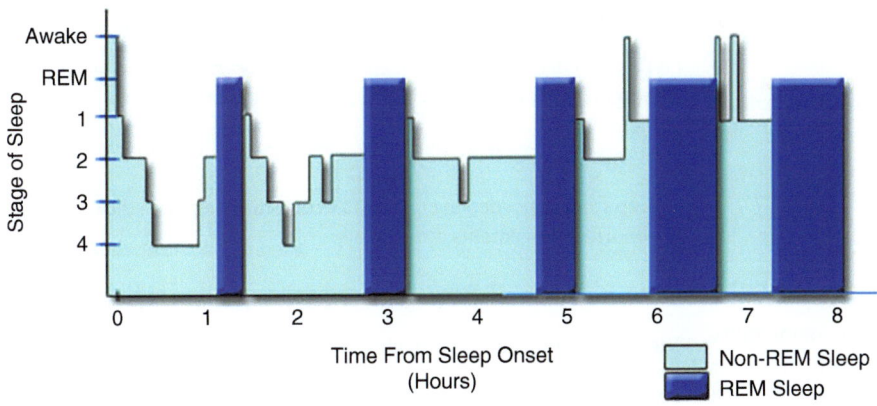

Figure 8.11 Sleep stages through the night. REM, rapid eye movement. *Source*: Pinterest.

- Melatonin is both chronobiotic and soporific (it attenuates wake-promoting signals). Levels fall with ageing.
- Hypocretin 1 and 2 (orexins) are produced by neurons in the posterior hypothalamus and promote waking. Genetic defects in orexin or its receptor cause some cases of narcolepsy. In animal studies, there is a reduction in orexin and the response to it with ageing.
- There are thousands of oscillating genes in all organs, and other physiological functions, e.g. cortisol release, follow this circadian pattern.
- Circadian rhythms are less tight with ageing and ageing may be associated with clock disruption. E.g. from childhood we pass less urine at night (decreased brain arousal, decreased urine production and increased bladder capacity), but these mechanisms are less efficient with age before the additive effect of pathology. Interestingly, nocturnal animals like rats pass less urine during the day!

Poor sleep is multifactorial, with problems due to a variety of conditions superimposed on the physiological changes of ageing and social factors that may impair sleep, such as the lack of daytime physical activity and the loss of a long-term partner. Sixty per cent of older people complain about insomnia. The worst sleep patterns are found in people with dementia.

Primary sleep disorders

Insomnia

The lack of precise definitions hampers comparisons between populations and drugs.

- Insomnia may be due to difficulty falling asleep (increased sleep latency) and staying asleep (sleep fragmentation or sleep maintenance insomnia) or waking too early with daytime tiredness that causes distress or interferes with life.
- Difficulties occur at least three nights a week and last for over a month.
- Studies suggest that in chronic insomnia, there is a hyperactivated state with a chronic stress response.

Sleep-disordered breathing

This becomes commoner with increasing age, but figures for prevalence are very variable depending on the population studied and the definitions used.

Obstructive sleep apnoea

This is the best-recognised type of sleep-disordered breathing.

- Characterised by recurrent complete (apnoea) or partial (hypopnoea) cessation of breathing due to upper airway obstruction. Presents with extreme snoring followed by gasping.

- When obstructive sleep apnoea (OSA) results in intermittent hypoxaemia and arousals from sleep sufficient to result in daytime sleepiness, it is called OSA syndrome – around 4% of those aged 30–60.
- Higher in men, with increasing age and high BMI; gender difference less marked after menopause.
- Adverse consequences include reduced quality of life, increased road traffic accidents, impaired cognition, cerebrovascular, cardiovascular, and metabolic morbidity, and increased mortality.
- Nocturnal continuous positive airway pressure (CPAP) is an established, cost-effective treatment in middle age.
- Pathophysiological factors that increase with ageing include shortening of the mandible, particularly if edentulous; reduced airway dimensions due to loss of muscle and connective tissue elasticity and increased fat; altered central control of breathing; and upper airway muscle dilator dysfunction, so upper airways are more collapsible.
- At an older age, being male and having a high BMI have less effect, daytime sleepiness may be perceived as less of a problem, and other causes of arousal from sleep make the role of OSA less clear.
- There is now RCT evidence for the benefit of treating OSA in older people (but not people in their 80s living with frailty). In the PREDICT trial (2014), 278 patients were randomised, with a mean age of 71, 80% male, a BMI of 33.8, a 12-month duration. The intervention group had reduced objective sleepiness, and improved quality of life. This was confirmed by Martinez-Garcia et al. (2015), in an open RCT of 224 patients, mean age 75, 68% male, BMI 33, and they found some evidence for improvement in behaviour and cognition.

Central sleep apnoea

Rare 1°, and 2° central apnoea are associated with heart failure and stroke, often with periodic respiration (Cheyne Stokes), which can also occur when awake.

Restless legs syndrome

See Chapter 7.

Periodic limb movement disorder

- 80% of people with RLS report periodic limb movements in sleep (PLMS).
- Most people with PLMS do not experience RLS.
- Legs twitch or jerk, brief and repetitive every 10–69 sec.
- Can wake sufferers and partners.
- Probably related to RLS, and the treatment is similar.

REM behaviour disorder

- Normally, in rapid eye movement (REM) sleep, the pons send signals to the spinal cord to paralyse limb muscles.

- If this fails, people can act out their dreams, which is potentially dangerous.
- More common in old age.
- More than 80% go on to develop neurodegenerative disorders, including PD, DLB or multiple system atrophy.
- It may respond to low-dose clonazepam or melatonin.

Assessment of sleep problems

History

A full history is needed to explore the duration and nature of the difficulty with sleep. In older people, factors that impair sleep and drug causes are particularly common. Ask about self-medication – alcohol and over the counter (OTC) antihistamines (anticholinergic). Obtaining a history of sleep-disordered breathing or abnormal movements depends on the partner.

Consider a sleep diary and sleepiness score (Epworth Sleepiness Scale self-rated chance of dozing from 0 (no chance) to 3 (high chance) across a range of activities).

Factors that disturb sleep patterns

- Anxiety.
- Fear.
- Depression.
- Bereavement.
- Delirium.
- Pain from any cause, particularly on turning over in bed.
- Nausea or diarrhoea.
- Discomfort due to constipation.
- Urgency, frequency, nocturia.
- Night sweats.
- Pruritus.
- Restless legs.
- Cramps.
- Nocturnal cough or breathlessness from cardiac or respiratory disease.
- Drugs and alcohol (alcohol initially sedates but then alerts later).
- Drug and alcohol withdrawal (especially benzodiazepines, Z drugs, antidepressants, and opiates).
- Neurological conditions, especially dementia and parkinsonian syndromes.

Medications that can disturb sleep

The neurotransmitters that promote wakefulness are a diverse group, with neuronal projections throughout the brain. These include glutamate, histamine, norepinephrine, dopamine, serotonin, acetylcholine, serotonin, and orexin. The main sleep-promoting neurotransmitters are GABA and adenosine.

- Anticholinergics: suppress REM sleep.
- Acetylcholinesterase inhibitors: may cause vivid dreams.
- Antidepressants: SSRIs suppress REM sleep.
- Levodopa and dopamine agonists: high doses reduce slow-wave and REM sleep and induce wakefulness and insomnia.
- Alpha-blockers: decrease REM sleep, e.g. tamsulosin
- Beta-blockers: reduce melatonin, e.g. carvedilol.
- Sympathomimetics: increase arousal, e.g. salbutamol.
- Theophylline and caffeine (including OTC products): increase sleep latency and arousal.
- Corticosteroids: disrupt circadian rhythms.
- Diuretics: produce the need to micturate.

Examination

Look particularly for factors and conditions that impair sleep and whether chronic conditions like heart failure are optimally controlled.

Special investigations

A sleep study is needed to confirm OSA and may help with the diagnosis of abnormal movements during sleep.

Management of insomnia

The initial approach is to provide information on sleep hygiene.

Sleep hygiene

- Have realistic expectations.
- Maintain activity during the day, avoid or limit daytime napping.
- Exercise >2 hr before bedtime.
- Rise at a regular and early hour.
- Use zeitgebers: morning sun if possible or bright indoor light.
- A regular routine, with an alarm if needed, at weekends too.
- Avoid caffeine and alcohol in the afternoon and evening.
- Do not smoke, especially in the evening.
- Do not go to bed hungry, have a snack or hot milky drink.
- Adjust the environment in the room (lights, temperature, noise, etc.).
- Wind down before bed.
- Do not go to bed too early.
- Do not watch TV, read, eat, or worry in bed. The bed is for sleep and intimacy.
- If you do not fall asleep after 20 min or wake up and can't get back to sleep, try writing down thoughts or go to another room and do a relaxing activity.

After basic advice, some form of CBT is recommended.

Cognitive behavioural therapy for insomnia

This is a structured programme to help an individual identify and replace thoughts and behaviours that cause or worsen sleep problems with habits that promote sound sleep.

- Cognitive part: recognition of causes and acceptance that the person can control negative thoughts that keep them awake.
- Behavioural part: development of good sleep habits and avoidance of behaviours that are likely to impair sleep.
- Approaches include:
  - Stimulus control therapy: to remove factors that condition the mind to resist sleep. Coached to employ basic sleep hygiene.
  - Sleep restriction: to avoid the habit of lying in bed awake. Reduce the time in bed, causing partial sleep deprivation to increase tiredness. Once sleep has improved, time in bed is gradually increased.
  - Relaxation training, e.g. using meditation, imagery, or muscle relaxation.

Sleepio (Big Health) is a self-help sleep improvement programme based on cognitive behavioural therapy for insomnia (CBTI). It can be accessed through a website or an app for iOS and Android devices. The programme is structured around a sleep test, six weekly interactive CBT sessions, and regular sleep diary entries. It uses an artificial intelligence algorithm to provide users with tailored responses. It is NICE-approved and is available without cost in some areas.

Drug treatment for poor sleep

Night sedation should be a last resort for all ages. Short-term prescriptions may be used after acute precipitating events, but insomnia is usually chronic and common drugs cause hangover effects, dependence, and withdrawal when stopped. There are particular risks for older people, particularly frail older women and those with cognitive impairment.

- Risk of falls if they get up at night (multi-factorial: confusion, poor vision, orthostatic hypotension, slip in the toilet if wet). Falls result in fractures.
- Increased confusion due to hangover in the day.
- Balance with carer exhaustion; if a person gets up and wanders at night, it may be the last straw and lead to care home admission.

Treatment of causative factors

Address these first.

- Optimise symptom control of cardiac, respiratory, and neurological conditions.
- Analgesia if pain is an issue.
- Use sedative antidepressants if depression coexists.
  - Trazodone at a low-dose has a sedative effect through blocking $5\text{-}HT_{2A}$, histamine H_1, and α receptors. At higher doses, it blocks serotonin reuptake (antidepressant effect) and is termed a serotonin antagonist-reuptake inhibitor (SARI).
  - Mirtazapine causes sedation by blocking $5\text{-}HT_{2A}$ and H_1 histamine receptors.

Night sedation

Prescribe a trial of sedation with safety measures if needed, such as automatic lights, grab rails in the toilet, etc.

Benzodiazepines

- Benzodiazepines (BZDs) act as positive allosteric modulators on the GABA-A receptor, a ligand-gated chloride ion channel.

Z-drugs

- These are short-acting GABA-A agonists that were marketed as reducing sleep latency without disturbing sleep architecture. Eszopiclone (not approved in the UK) is the active isomer of zopiclone but binds preferentially to the α-3 receptor subtype and appeared to have the best profile in a Lancet review. BMJ Best Practice currently suggests zolpidem 5 mg or 6.25 mg extended-release.
- Despite the early marketing, side effects are similar to those of BZDs, there are similar addiction and withdrawal problems. The side effects suggest that sleep architecture is disturbed, so similar cautions apply.

Drugs that affect circadian rhythm

Melatonin receptor agonists

- Activation of the MT_1 and MT_2 melatonin receptors promotes sleep.
- Melatonin, using modified-release tablets, is licensed for adults over 55 years for up to 13 weeks, but a recent systemic review in all age groups did not show benefit. Arthralgia is the main side effect. Avoid in autoimmune problems or seizures.
- In the US, there are three licensed MT_1 and MT_2 agonists. These reduce adenyl cyclase, and their effect on SCN is thought to lead to sleep. However, ramelteon had low efficacy and high discontinuation rates.

Orexin receptor antagonists

- Suvorexant, seltorexant, lemborexant, and daridorexant are DORAs (dual orexin receptor antagonists), which are thought to modulate the circadian clock. Daridorexant is NICE-approved (2023), and lemborexant is licensed in Europe.
- Early data looks promising, but new drugs for insomnia have often failed to meet expectations or caused harm.

Sleep changes in AD

These are similar to normal ageing but more marked.

- Clinical problems include reduced nocturnal sleep time, sleep fragmentation, nocturnal wandering, and daytime sleepiness.
- Decrease in REM sleep.
- Abnormal circadian rhythm.
- Day/night reversal.
- Sundowning.
- Sleep-related breathing disorders (SDBs) are more common.
- Postulated bidirectional relationship between sleep and AD.

Alcohol excess

Older people are less tolerant of alcohol due to:

- A lower ratio of body fat to water.
- A lower hepatic blood flow and reduced metabolism.
- Increased brain sensitivity.

A given blood alcohol level is likely to be more deleterious in older people than younger people, particularly if there is a cognitive impairment. At any age, repeated excessive ingestion leads to dependency, physical disease, or harm. Consumption peaks at age 55 and declines thereafter, but this may change as the middle-aged, who are used to drinking more than earlier generations, grow older. More people are now dying from alcohol in all age groups (see Figure 8.12), and between 2001 and 2021, the age band with the highest death rate increased by 5 years to 50–55 years. The most striking difference in death rates is the increase seen at older ages. Older people may benefit from a small amount of alcohol, e.g. cardiovascular benefits (increasingly disputed) and improved quality of life. However, the Royal College of Psychiatrists (2015) estimates that 1 in 5 older men and 1 in 10 older women are drinking enough to harm themselves.

Patterns of drinking

Three patterns of harmful drinking are described in older people.

1 Early-onset drinkers or survivors:
   - Males = females i.e. no gender preponderance.
   - Two-thirds of older drinkers have a continuing alcohol problem that began when they were younger.
   - Likely to be resistant to help.
2 Late-onset drinkers or reactors:
   - F > M.
   - Use alcohol to try to assuage loneliness and sadness.
   - Depression is common.
3 Intermittent or binge drinkers:
   - A less common pattern.

Problems linked to alcohol

- Increased risk of falls and osteoporosis resulting in bruising, injury and fractures.
- Self-neglect.
- Acute confusion, anxiety, depression, neuropathy, hallucinations, Wernicke's encephalopathy, dementia, fits.
- Gastrointestinal and liver disease.
- Heart problems, including cardiomyopathy and atrial fibrillation.
- Haemorrhagic stroke.
- Bone marrow suppression.
- Many cancers (especially breast and bowel).
- Hypothermia.
- Interaction with medications.

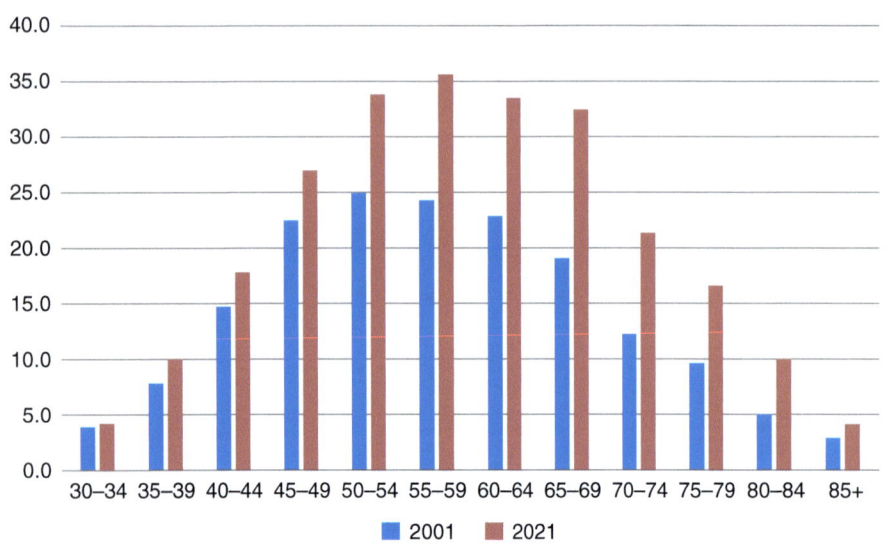

Figure 8.12 Age-specific death rates in UK per 100,000 from alcohol in 2001 and 2021 by age bands. *Source*: ONS/CC BY 3.0.

The usual problem is daily dosing rather than bingeing, so the alcohol problem may not be apparent. People in the age band of 65 and older are most likely to drink daily (10%). The number of higher-risk drinkers increased during the COVID pandemic and has remained higher.

Consider a simple screening tool like CAGE (see Appendix), but this may be less valid for older drinkers.

Carefully consider the routine use of intravenous vitamin supplementation to prevent Wernicke's encephalopathy in susceptible inpatients. Pabrinex was used in UK hospitals but is currently in short supply due to EU problems with manufacturing. The Medicines and Healthcare products Regulatory Agency (MHRA) is developing guidance on the use of other parenteral forms of thiamine. Delirium tremens is managed with chlordiazepoxide (use lower doses in older patients), often using a risk assessment tool such as CIWA (Clinical Institute Withdrawal Assessment for Alcohol).

In cases of problem drinking, it may be possible to reduce intake by checking who is buying the alcohol. The Institute of Alcohol Studies produces a useful fact sheet, and organisations such as Alcoholics Anonymous (AA) offer support.

Substance abuse

The proportion of older people with substance misuse continues to outpace the increase in the proportion of older people in the UK. The 'baby boomer' population born between 1946 and 1964 is at high risk of abusing alcohol and both recreational and prescription drugs, particularly opiates and benzodiazepines. However, only 2% of those in treatment for drug and alcohol addiction (2020–2021) are 65 and over. Be aware and seek advice.

Self-neglect and hoarding

Older people are occasionally encountered living in conditions of extreme degradation, surrounded by piles of things with total disregard for hygiene and self-care: the 'senile squalor syndrome'. Self-neglect is considered in broad terms referring to a person's neglect of their health, hygiene, or surroundings (which includes hoarding).

- The literature is divided as to whether hoarding and squalor are synonymous, distinct, or overlapping syndromes; hoarding can certainly lead to squalor as it becomes difficult to keep things clean. There may be an accumulation of dirt, grime, or even human or animal faeces in a person's home.
- There is also debate as to whether hoarding becomes more common with age or whether older people have simply had longer to accumulate things and may have more difficulty disposing of them.
- A subgroup hoards animals rather than 'stuff' and the Royal Society for Prevention of Cruelty to Animals (RSPCA) may need to be involved.
- Some will be found to have mental illness (dementia, alcoholism, schizophrenia, obsessive-compulsive disorder).
- Others appear normal despite hoarding vast quantities of rubbish. This has been termed the Diogenes syndrome after Diogenes of Sinope, the ancient Greek philosopher who showed his contempt for material things by living in a barrel and refusing offers of help to do otherwise. In this context, the perpetrator is seen to have made a bizarre lifestyle choice rather than having an illness.
- However, many authorities believe that hoarding behaviour is a mental health disorder, and it is included in both the DSM-5 and the ICD-11. The condition may lead to hypothermia, malnutrition, infections, and the risk of pest infections and fire, as well as vigorous protests from neighbours and distress for family members!

Hoarding has become a cause of fascination with TV series in the US and UK. These emphasise the need to fix the problem rather than looking at how and why it has arisen, which may add to the distress and stigma felt by some people who hoard.

- Patients who hoard and do not look after themselves are encountered regularly in geriatric medicine wards.
- The estimated overall UK prevalence is 2.5%, but because hoarding can have severe consequences for older people, including increased risk of falls and making it difficult to manage activities of daily living or even to move around their own home, people who hoard may be overrepresented in older inpatients.
- It is important to establish whether the patient has the mental capacity to decide to live this way and exclude an underlying psychiatric illness (with the help of specialist colleagues).
- Hoarding is one of the behaviours that can constitute self-neglect in the guidance accompanying the English Care Act 2014, so a safeguarding enquiry may be appropriate. If concerns do not warrant safeguarding, support from social services or environmental health may be needed.
- Discharge planning will require good communication with family members and an expert social worker.

Risk factors for self-neglect

- Dementia.
- Depression.
- Bereavement and isolation.
- Disability.
- Alcohol excess.
- Previous psychiatric disorder.
- Learning difficulties.
- Obsessive-compulsive disorder.
- Lifelong difficult personality/eccentricity.

The Mental Capacity Act

In England, if your patient may lack capacity, you must act according to the Mental Capacity Act (see Chapter 21 for more information).

 REFERENCES AND FURTHER READING

NHS England *Community Mental Health Services* https://www.england.nhs.uk/mental-health/adults/cmhs

RC Psychiatry (2022) *Old Age Psychiatry Higher Specialty Training Curriculum* www.rcpsych.ac.uk/docs/default-source/training/curricula-and-guidance/2022-curricula/old-age-psychiatry-curriculum-final-16-june-22.pdf?sfvrsn=73f6e513_4

NICE CKS (2023) *Depression* https://cks.nice.org.uk/topics/depression

Crocco EA, Jaramillo S, Cruz-Ortiz C, et al. (2017) Pharmacological management of anxiety disorders in the elderly. *Curr. Treat. Options Psychiatry* 4:33–46. doi: 10.1007/s40501-017-0102-4.

Badcock JC, Dehon H, Larøi F (2017) Hallucinations in healthy older adults: an overview of literature and perspectives for future research. *Front. Psychol* 8. https://pubmed.ncbi.nlm.nih.gov/28736541/

NICE CKS (2022) *How should I assess a person with suspected dementia?* https://cks.nice.org.uk/topics/dementia/diagnosis/assessment

NICE CKS (2021) *Delirium* https://cks.nice.org.uk/topics/delirium

Poulsen LM, Estrup S, Mortensen CB, et al. (2021) Delirium in intensive care. *Curr. Anesthesiol. Rep.* 11:516–523. doi: 10.1007/s40140-021-00476-z.

Wilson JE, Mart MF, Cunningham C, et al. (2020) Delirium. *Nat. Rev. Dis. Primers* 6:90. doi: 10.1038/s41572-020-00223-4.

Burry L, Mehta S, Perreault MM, et al. (2018) Antipsychotics for treatment of delirium in hospitalised non-ICU patients. *Cochrane Database Syst. Rev.*(6). Art. No.: CD005594. doi: 10.1002/14651858.CD005594.pub3.

Wittenberg R, Hu B, Barraza-Araiza, et al. (2019) *LSE Care Policy and Evaluation Centre (CPEC) Projections of older people living with dementia and costs of dementia care in the United Kingdom, 2019–2040.* www.lse.ac.uk/cpec/assets/documents/cpec-working-paper-5.pdf

Alzheimer's Association Report (2020) *Alzheimer's disease facts and figures* https://alz-journals.onlinelibrary.wiley.com/doi/full/10.1002/alz.12068

Alzheimer Europe (2019) *Estimating the prevalence of dementia in Europe* https://www.alzheimer-europe.org/dementia/prevalence-dementia-europe

ONS (2023) Suicides in England and Wales: 2022 registrations (see section 4 Suicide patterns by age). https://www.ons.gov.uk/peoplepopulationandcommunity/birthsdeathsandmarriages/deaths/bulletins/suicidesintheunitedkingdom/2022registrations#suicide-patterns-by-age

ONS Monthly mortality analysis England and Wales July (2023) Top five causes of death. https://www.ons.gov.uk/peoplepopulationandcommunity/birthsdeathsandmarriages/deaths/bulletins/monthlymortalityanalysisenglandandwales/july2023#leading-causes-of-death

Department of Health and Social Care; *Dementia 2020 Challenge*: 2018 Review Phase 1 https://www.gov.uk/government/publications/dementia-2020-challenge-progress-review

Driving with dementia or mild cognitive impairment (2018) *Consensus Guidelines for clinicians* https://research.ncl.ac.uk/driving-and-dementia/consensusguidelinesforclinicians/Final%20Guideline.pdf

Olmastroni E, Molari G, De Beni N, et al. (2021) Statin use and risk of dementia or Alzheimer's disease: a systematic review and meta-analysis of observational studies. *Eur. J. Prev. Cardiol.* zwab208. doi: 10.1093/eurjpc/zwab208.

Pourhadi N, Mørch LS, Holm EA, et al. (2023) Menopausal hormone therapy and dementia: nationwide, nested case-control study. *BMJ* 381: e072770. doi: 10.1136/bmj-2022-072770.

Tort S, Ciapponi A on behalf of Cochrane Clinical Answers Editors (2020) For cognitively healthy older adults, do aspirin and non-steroidal anti-inflammatory drugs (NSAIDs) help prevent dementia? *Cochrane Clin. Answers.* doi: 10.1002/cca.3177.

Fortea J, Pegueroles J, Alcolea D, et al. (2024) *APOE4* homozygosity represents a distinct genetic form of Alzheimer's disease. *Nat. Med.* doi: 10.1038/s41591-024-02931-w.

Cole SL, Vassar R (2007) The Alzheimer's disease β-secretase enzyme, BACE1. *Mol. Neurodegener.* 22. doi: 10.1186/1750-1326-2-22.

Sims JR, Zimmer JA, Evans CD, et al. (2023) Donanemab in early symptomatic Alzheimer disease: the TRAILBLAZER-ALZ 2 randomized clinical trial. *JAMA* 330:512–527. doi: 10.1001/jama.2023.13239.

Pardridge WM (2020) Treatment of Alzheimer's disease and blood-brain barrier drug delivery. *Pharmaceuticals (Basel)* 13:394. doi: 10.3390/ph13110394.

Roberts RO, Aakre JA, Kremers WK, et al. (2018) Prevalence and outcomes of amyloid positivity among persons without dementia in a longitudinal, population-based setting. *JAMA Neurol.* 75:970–979. doi: 10.1001/jamaneurol.2018.0629.

Meglio M, Ciccone I (2023) Alzheimer Disease Pipeline Update: Inside Look at Promising Agents. *Report from the Alzheimer Association International Conference* https://www.neurologylive.com/view/alzheimer-pipeline-update-inside-look-at-promising-agents

Rea F, Corrao G, Mancia G (2024) Risk of Dementia During Antihypertensive Drug Therapy in the Elderly. *JACC*; 83:1194–1203. doi: 10.1016/j.jacc.2024.01.030

Alzheimer Association. *Alternative treatments* https://www.alz.org/alzheimers-dementia/treatments/alternative-treatments

Taylor J, McKeith IG, Burn D, et al. (2020) New evidence on the management of Lewy body dementia. *Lancet Neurol.* 19:157–169. doi: 10.1016/S1474-4422(19)30153-X. 3.

Greaves CV, Rohrer JD (2019) An update on genetic frontotemporal dementia. J. Neurol. 266:2075–2086. doi: 10.1007/s00415-019-09363-4.

Lee SE (2022) *Frontotemporal dementia: treatment.* https://www.uptodate.com/contents/frontotemporal-dementia-treatment

Price RS (2023) Exploring what progress is being made in the development of health promotion material for vascular dementia: a systematic review of the evidence. *Aging Med. (Milton)* 6:184–194. doi: 10.1002/agm2.12253.

Ngandu T, Lehtisalo J, Korkki S, et al. (2022) The effect of adherence on cognition in a multidomain lifestyle intervention (FINGER). *Alzheimer's Dement.* 18:1325–1334. doi: 10.1002/alz.12492.

European Geriatric Medicine Society Congress (2023) Healthy ageing in a changing world. *Lancet eClinicalMedicine* 64:102263. doi: 10.1016/j.eclinm.2023.102263.

Fisher Centre for Alzheimer's research foundation. Clinical stages of Alzheimers. https://www.alzinfo.org/understand-alzheimers/clinical-stages-of-alzheimers/

Yorkshire and the Humber Clinical Network and London Clinical Network NHS England (2022) *Appropriate prescribing of antipsychotic medication in dementia.* https://www.england.nhs.uk/london/wp-content/uploads/sites/8/2022/10/Antipsychotic-Prescribing-Toolkit-for-Dementia.pdf

McMillan A, Bratton D, Faria R, et al. (2014) Continuous positive airway pressure in older people with obstructive sleep apnoea syndrome (PREDICT): a 12-month, multicentre, randomised trial. *The Lancet Respiratory Medicine* 2: 804–812. doi: 10.1016/S2213-2600(14)70172-9

Martinez-Garcia MA, Chiner E, Hernandez L, et al. (2015) Obstructive sleep apnoea in the elderly: role of continuous positive airway pressure treatment. *European Respiratory Journal* 46: 142–151. doi: 10.1183/09031936.00064214

British Geriatrics Society (2020) *End of life care in frailty: dementia.* https://www.bgs.org.uk/resources/end-of-life-care-in-frailty-dementia

NICE CKS (2022) *Insomnia* https://cks.nice.org.uk/topics/insomnia/background-information

NICE CKS (2021) *Obstructive sleep apnoea syndrome* https://cks.nice.org.uk/topics/obstructive-sleep-apnoea-syndrome

Davidson JR, Dickson C, Han H (2019) Cognitive behavioural treatment for insomnia in primary care: a systematic review of sleep outcomes. *Br. J. Gen. Pract.* 69 (686):e657–e664. doi: 10.3399/bjgp19X705065.

De Crescenzo F, D'Alò GL, Ostinelli EG (2022) Comparative effects of pharmacological interventions for the acute and long-term management of insomnia disorder in adults: a systematic review and network meta-analysis. *Lancet* 400:170–184. doi: 10.1016/S0140-6736(22)00878-9.

Welcome to Sleepio https://www.oxfordhealth.nhs.uk/healthyminds/wp-content/uploads/sites/17/2019/10/Sleepio-info-for-clients.pdf

Institute of alcohol studies (2020) *Alcohol through the life course: older drinkers* https//www.ias.org.uk/wp-content/uploads/2020/12/Alcohol-through-the-life-course-%E2%80%93-older-drinkers.pdf

Royal College of Psychiatrists report CR211 (2018) *Our Invisible Addicts 2nd edition* www.rcpsych.ac.uk/docs/default-source/improving-care/better-mh-policy/college-reports/college-report-cr211.pdf?sfvrsn=820fe4bc_2

Steils N, Woolham J, Manthorpe J et al. (2022) What do we know about hoarding behaviour and treatment approaches for older people? A thematic review. *NIHR Policy Research Unit in Health and Social Care Workforce*, The Policy Institute, King's College London. https://doi.org/10.18742/pub01-083

INFORMATION FOR PATIENTS AND FAMILIES

The Silver Line (0800 4 70 80 90) – a helpline specifically for older people, providing emotional support and advice. www.thesilverline.org.uk

Independent Age If you're feeling lonely, https://www.independentage.org/sites/default/files/2016-11/Advice-Guide-If-youre-feeling-lonely.pdf

The Alzheimer Society: www.alzheimers.org.uk

The Lewy Body Society: www.lewybody.org/

Mind – information on mental health problems: www.mind.org.uk

The Royal College of Psychiatrists (RCPsych), website: www.rcpsych.ac.uk, provides patient information including *Depression in Older Adults, Sleeping well, Alcohol and Depression, Antidepressants, and Cognitive Behavioural Therapy (CBT).*

All websites were accessed in August 2024.

9

Stroke

Notes on stroke services in the UK

Whereas people with strokes are typically managed by neurologists in continental Europe, stroke medicine in the UK is a subspecialty and the training is accessed via a number of higher speciality training pathways with internal medicine, the most common of which is geriatrics, followed by neurology and then acute medicine. If you are interested in a career in stroke medicine, talk to your local stroke team.

Importance

Globally, one in four adults over the age of 25 will have a stroke during their lifetime. Overall rates are highest in China. In Europe, many Eastern European countries have high rates. Stroke is the second-leading cause of death worldwide.

- The lifetime risk of stroke for adults in the UK is one in five.
- Each year, around 100,000 people in the UK have a stroke.
- 30% of these individuals will go on to have another stroke. Stroke is the fourth-biggest killer in the UK, with more than 38,000 stroke-related deaths each year.
- Stroke is the single largest cause of severe adult disability in developed countries, with two-thirds of stroke sufferers leaving hospital with a disability.
- There are 1.3 million stroke survivors in the UK.

The age of onset for a first stroke is falling. The average age is 68 years (median 70) for males and 73 years (median 76) for females. However, most strokes still affect older people, with the largest number of strokes occurring in males aged 70–79 years and in females aged 80–89 years.

The advent and availability of thrombolysis and thrombectomy have improved outcomes over the last 15 years. However, far more lives have been saved by the development of dedicated stroke units. Cost estimates vary widely depending on what is included, but the figures presented to parliament in 2023 were that stroke costs the NHS £3.4 billion a year and social care £2.3 billion in year 1, with another £2 billion on top of that for every subsequent year. As with dementia, the biggest costs fall on individuals providing care, and the UK annual societal cost in 2022 was estimated at £25.6 billion.

Definitions

The term 'stroke' is now used in preference to cerebrovascular accident (CVA).

- A stroke is defined as 'rapidly developing clinical signs of focal disturbance of cerebral function, with symptoms lasting 24 hours or longer or leading to death, with no apparent cause other than of vascular origin'.
- Subarachnoid haemorrhage (SAH) falls within the definition of stroke, but these patients, who are generally younger, are usually cared for by neurology. The rehabilitation (rehab) pathways are the same but are usually delivered by specialist neurorehabilitation teams (NICE includes SAH in the stroke rehab guideline).
- Other cerebrovascular events, such as subdural haematomas or haemorrhagic brain metastases, are not included in the stroke definition, and patients with these are not routinely cared for by stroke teams.
- By definition, transient ischaemic attacks (TIAs) last less than 24 hours and are therefore classified separately, although the causes of TIA and stroke are similar. TIAs are a risk factor for strokes. With the advent of more routine MRI, some patients with TIA are found to have focal damage, but the definition of TIA remains clinical. In general, DWI (diffusion-weighted imaging)-negative TIAs carry a much better prognosis.

Aetiology and pathology

Stroke is a clinical syndrome divided into two broad types – ischaemic and haemorrhagic.

Ischaemic stroke – 85%

Ischaemic stroke (IS) is caused by occlusion of the arterial supply to the brain, which can occur at several levels:

- Extracranial internal carotid or vertebral arteries,
- Large proximal cerebral arteries – large vessel occlusions, or LVOs – (intracranial internal carotids, proximal posterior, middle, and anterior cerebral arteries, intracranial vertebral arteries, and/or basilar artery),

Geriatric Medicine and Elderly Care: Lecture Notes, Ninth Edition. Claire G. Nicholl, K. Jane Wilson, and Shaun D'Souza.
© 2025 John Wiley & Sons Ltd. Published 2025 by John Wiley & Sons Ltd.
Companion website: www.wiley.com/go/lecturenotesgeriatricmedicine9e

Table 9.1 Oxford classification of ischaemic stroke.

Percentage of cases	Clinical	Anatomy/pathology	Outcome
Total anterior circulation infarct (TACI): 15%	All three of: higher cortical dysfunction (e.g. dysphasia), homonymous hemianopia, and unilateral weakness (and/or sensory deficit) of the face, arm, and leg	A large cortical stroke affecting areas supplied by the MCA and ACA. Embolus or spreading thrombus from the ICA	Very poor chance of good function and very high mortality (40% at 30 days and 60% at 1 year) prior to interventions
Partial anterior circulation infarct (PACI): 35%	Two out of three TACI components or higher cerebral dysfunction alone or restricted motor/sensory deficit (e.g. one limb or face, hand, not whole arm)	Branch of MCA or ACA	Fair outcome but very high chance of early recurrence
Lacunar infarct (LACI): 25%	Any one of: pure motor stroke, pure sensory stroke, sensorimotor stroke, ataxic hemiparesis	Occlusion of a deep perforating artery (anterior or posterior circulation)	Lowest mortality and often good recovery
Posterior circulation infarct (POCI): 25%	Any one of: isolated homonymous hemianopia, cranial nerve palsy and contralateral motor/sensory deficit, cerebellar ataxia	Blockage of the posterior circulation supplying the brain stem, cerebellum, or occipital lobes	High chance of good function but also of recurrence in the first year

ICA, internal carotid artery; MCA, middle cerebral artery; ACA, anterior cerebral artery.
Source: Adapted from Bamford et al. (1991).

- Small arteries (also known as perforating, penetrating, or lacunar arteries).

Ischaemic strokes in the carotid territory are grouped as anterior circulation strokes (ACiS); those in brain structures supplied by the vertebrobasilar system are called posterior circulation strokes (PCiS). The clinical differences (see Bamford classification Table 9.1) are due to the part of the brain affected. However, emerging evidence suggests that the mechanisms may be subtly different, partly due to the differences in the vascular trees. PCiS is commoner in younger patients, males, and diabetics.

The underlying pathology in extracranial vessels is usually progressive atherosclerosis and thrombosis in situ; in most cases of LVO, it is atherosclerosis or emboli from atrial fibrillation, whereas in small arteries, the aetiology is a more complex mix of atheroma and endothelial damage. Atheroma in the aorta, carotid, and vertebral arteries is also a source of emboli to distal vessels.

The lack of blood flow results in an ischaemic area of the brain called an infarct. Atheroma is widespread in ageing vessels, so research is looking at whether 'risky atheroma' can be identified. Dual-tracer PET imaging using ^{18}F-FDG identifies plaque inflammation, and ^{18}F-NaF measures active plaque microcalcification (Evans). Prospective studies will look at whether the degree of stenosis or plaque characteristics are better predictors of thrombotic events.

Bamford classification

Validated tools such as the seminal Bamford Classification (see Table 9.1) link the clinical findings to the vascular territory. The study was community-based and recruited patients with a first-ever stroke. Patients had a CT scan, and the classification was based on 543 patients with an infarct.

Rarer causes of ischaemic stroke include:

- Vasculitis.
- Hypercoagulable states such as antiphospholipid syndrome or myeloma.
- Substance misuse.
- Shearing of blood vessel walls (such as an aortic/carotid dissection).
- 'Watershed infarct' from a severe hypotensive episode.
- Back pressure from venous thrombosis.

Substance misuse and dissection are much more common causes of stroke in younger people (vessel walls are stiffer and less likely to shear as you get older). Secondary bleeding, known as haemorrhagic transformation, may occur in an area of the brain damaged by an infarct and can be symptomatic or asymptomatic.

Haemorrhagic stroke – 15%

- Primary intracerebral haemorrhage (PICH) – 10%.
  This was usually due to hypertensive damage to small cerebral arteries, much less commonly due to vascular malformation. However, as hypertension is better managed and the population ages, cerebral amyloid angiopathy (CAA) has overtaken hypertension as the main cause of lobar bleeds seen in many UK services. Bleeds due to hypertension - predominantly in the basal ganglia – have decreased.
- Subarachnoid haemorrhage (SAH) – 5%, most of which are due to a ruptured saccular aneurysm (80%); the remaining 20% are due to arteriovenous malformations, dissections, and anticoagulants.
  The proportion of the types of stroke varies in different parts of the world. UK figures are given above. Globally in 2017, IS constituted 65%, PICH 26%, and SAH 9% of all incident strokes.

Stroke and cancer

There is growing awareness of the link between stroke and cancer. Both are much more common with increasing age, so some of the association is chance, some due to shared risk factors (e.g. smoking and obesity) or common pathogenesis (e.g. oxidative stress and chronic inflammation). However, many cancers increase the risk of stroke directly. The most common mechanism is hypercoagulability, but other mechanisms include nonbacterial thrombotic endocarditis and direct compression of blood vessels. Treatments for cancer, principally chemotherapy and radiotherapy, also increase the risk of stroke, both during treatment (e.g. bleeding due to severe thrombocytopaenia) and years later (e.g. carotid vasculopathy from radiotherapy for head and neck cancer).

There is a wide variety of figures in the literature – rates and types of strokes and cancer vary between countries.

Compared with an age-matched population:

- Patients with a history of active cancer have more strokes. (In a Dutch study, 12% of 2736 patients presenting with ischaemic stroke or TIA had a history of cancer, higher than expected; Turner meta-analysis.)
- Both ischaemic and haemorrhagic strokes are increased.
- In most studies, cancer diagnosis after stroke is more common than would be expected, particularly in cryptogenic stroke. Most cancers are diagnosed within months, suggesting that they were present but unrecognised when the stroke occurred. (Rioux meta-analysis).

At Addenbrooke's Hospital, Cambridge, an occult cancer is considered if an older patient with a stroke has:

- CRP > 30 on presentation.
- A stroke despite being compliant with a direct oral anticoagulant (DOAC) for an indication such as atrial fibrillation.
- No typical risk factors.

There is a low threshold for doing a CT-CAP. The treatment is the same as for a non-malignancy-associated stroke, but the risk-benefit balance will differ, and liaison with oncology is needed. The prognosis is usually poor.

Risk factors for ischaemic stroke

The biggest risk factor for stroke is increasing age. Afro-Caribbean and Southeast Asian ethnicity, a positive family history of stroke, and apolipoprotein E ε2 or ε4 carriage also increase risk, but it is more useful to consider risk factors that can be modified.

Modifiable risk factors

Risk factors for stroke are similar to those for other vascular disease (see Table 9.2), but there is a difference in relative risk. For example, hypertension is more significant for stroke, whereas smoking carries a greater risk for coronary artery disease. Primary prevention looks at overall risk using a score such as QRISK3, which is based on UK data. Discussion about lifestyle and treatment is offered to people with a > 10% risk of having a heart attack or stroke over the next 10 years. Secondary prevention follows similar lines, with a focus on looking for atrial fibrillation (AF), checking the carotids, and tight BP targets. Treating hypertension is paramount in haemorrhagic stroke.

Ischaemic stroke and TIA: recommendations for the primary care practitioner in the Addenbrooke's hospital discharge summary

Risk factor control, medication compliance, and lifestyle modifications are the most important measures to reduce the risk of further strokes. https://cks.nice.org.uk/topics/stroke-tia/management/secondary-prevention-following-stroke-tia.

1 Lifelong single antiplatelet (aspirin or clopidogrel).
   If the patient is on clopidogrel, if an invasive procedure or surgery is planned, change to aspirin 7 days prior to the procedure.

Table 9.2 Modifiable risk factors.

Risk factors	Treatment goals	Management
Hypertension	Aim for 130/80 mmHg, but systolic BP 140–160 mmHg is suggested in frail, older patients (or if the risk from falls exceeds that of stroke).	Diet modification, Reduce alcohol intake and avoid binges. Antihypertensive medications (drugs tailored to individual need; efficacy is more important than drug class, but there is a little evidence for dual ACEI/diuretics; beta-blockers only if IHD is also present).
Smoking	Stop!	Advise quitting and refer for psychological or pharmacology support (nicotine replacement/varenicline).
Atrial fibrillation	Reduce embolic risk	Consider anticoagulation depending on the CHA_2DS_2-VASc score and after assessing bleeding risk.
Carotid artery disease (carotid stenosis)	Ensure appropriate patients are screened promptly and referred to vascular surgery.	Antiplatelet therapy, document the degree of stenosis using carotid Doppler imaging and offer endarterectomy if CT confirms stroke in the ipsilateral hemisphere, function worth preserving and stenosis >70% or >50% in men with cortical symptoms. Asymptomatic stenosis may be stented.
Hyperlipidaemia	'The lower the better' approach	Advise about diet, weight, exercise and consider a statin. For 2° prevention, start statin as soon as possible, regardless of cholesterol. Refer to a specialist if triglycerides/total cholesterol remains high.
Type 2 diabetes mellitus	HbA1c target of <53 mmol/mol	Ensure tight diabetic control, provided it does not compromise health in other ways.
Obesity	Weight loss, BMI 20–25 kg/m²	Calorie restriction with the support of dieticians or weight loss groups

2 Lifelong lipid-lowering therapy (unless not indicated based on clinical judgement).

Target total cholesterol < 3.8, target LDL < 1.8, and target TG < 1.7. Refer for whole genome sequencing if cholesterol > 8.

Please repeat lipids at 3 months; if targets are not achieved, check compliance, and follow the national guidelines (add ezetimibe to statin and then consider PSK9 inhibitors via the lipid clinic).

https://www.england.nhs.uk/aac/publication/summary-of-national-guidance-for-lipid-management

3 Target BP < 130/80 (SBP 140–150 mmHg in severe bilateral carotid artery stenosis). For older and more frail patients, use clinical judgement, as less strict BP control may be needed to avoid falls/side effects.

Repeat BP readings at regular intervals (3 monthly).

A home BP diary is strongly recommended.

Once these targets are achieved, blood tests should be monitored every 6 to 12 months.

We also recommend an opportunistic pulse check and discussion regarding medication adherence at every encounter.

Reducing stroke risk in AF

1.2 million people in the UK have AF which increases the risk of stroke fivefold. This risk is not limited to established AF; it is also associated with paroxysmal AF (PAF) and atrial flutter (see Chapter 12).

An assessment of individual stroke risk (in the presence of AF) is made using the CHA_2DS_2-VASc score (Tables 9.3 and 9.4).

- Anticoagulation is not recommended in patients with non-valvular AF and a CHA_2DS_2-VASc score of 0 if male or 1 if female.
- Depending on patient preference and other risk factors, *consider* anticoagulation for a CHA_2DS_2-VASc score of 1 in males and 2 in females (note this will apply to all patients aged 65+).
- Anticoagulation should be started in patients with a CHA_2DS_2-VASc score of ≥2 if male or ≥3 if female, always balancing risk with bleeding risk.
- Older people are at greater risk of bleeding and stroke. The ORBIT score (see Appendix) has replaced HASBLED for the assessment of bleeding risk.
- Aspirin monotherapy should not be used (especially in the frail, as even 75 mg carries risk with no benefit).

If a decision is made to anticoagulate for non-valvular AF, direct oral anticoagulants (DOACs) are first line; they offer better protection than warfarin, slightly reduced bleeding risk, and are more convenient as they do not require monitoring or dietary restrictions. The drugs occupy the catalytic site of either Factor Xa (rivaroxaban, apixaban, and edoxaban) or thrombin (dabigatran), preventing thrombus development. They are all NICE-approved for this indication. Older subjects (especially those with renal impairment) were underrepresented in the early trials, and there was concern about the lack of reversibility. However, familiarity has established their place. Most older people in AF should be prescribed a DOAC.

There are no head-to-head studies, but clinical data suggest that apixaban, dabigatran, and rivaroxaban have similar rates of any stroke or systemic embolism and rivaroxaban has higher rates of major bleeding than apixaban and dabigatran but lower rates of MI than dabigatran. Make an informed decision about bleeding risk (falls do not confer substantial risk for intracranial bleeding) and discuss this with the patient. Make recommended dose adjustments for renal disease. NHS England recommends edoxaban first as it is the cheapest for the NHS, but the dose must be reduced in moderate renal impairment (many older people).

Edoxaban for non-valvular AF

- Standard dose: 60 mg/day (can be crushed and given in water).
- Reduce dose to 30 mg/day if creatinine clearance is 15–50 mL/min or weight ≤ 60 kg.
- Avoid if creatinine clearance is less than 15 mL/min.
- Very low-dose edoxaban (15 mg) still showed efficacy in Japanese patients aged 80+ for whom standard treatment would not be recommended; bleeding was higher in the treatment group compared with placebo, but this did not reach statistical significance, and overall deaths were similar in both groups (ELDERCARE-AF).

Warfarin with a target INR of 2.5 should be used in valvular AF with a creatinine clearance of less than 15 mL/min, as well as for other indications including metallic heart valves and antiphospholipid syndrome.

Table 9.4 The one-year risk of an embolic event in AF depends on the CHA_2DS_2-VASc score.

CHA_2DS_2VASc score	1-year risk of stroke/TIA/systemic embolism (%)
0	0.3
1	0.9
2	2.9
3	4.6
4	6.7
5	10.0
6	13.6
7	15.7
8	15.2
9	17.4

Table 9.3 The components of the CHA_2DS_2VASc score.

CHADS attribute	Point allocation
Congestive heart failure history	1
Hypertension history	1
Age in years	
<65	0
65–74	1
>75	2
Diabetes mellitus	1
Stroke/TIA history	2
Sex female	1
Vascular disease history (MI, PVD, aortic plaque)	1
Maximum score	9

Transient ischaemic attacks

Overview

Often described as 'mini-strokes', these are transient episodes of neurological dysfunction. Symptoms are like those of a stroke but are defined as lasting less than 24 hours before total resolution.

- Most TIAs last for a few minutes to a few hours (mostly <30 min).
- The recognition of TIAs is vital to preventing impending strokes.
- The risk of ischaemic stroke after a hemispheric TIA is up to 15% in the first month and highest in the first 72 hours post-TIA.

Clinical features

TIAs cause a focal neurological deficit (usually negative symptoms) in a vascular territory suddenly affected by emboli. Thus, patients present with a variety of symptoms, such as:

- Monocular visual loss (amaurosis fugax).
- Facial droop.
- Language disturbance ('dystextia' may pinpoint the exact time of onset on a mobile device).
- Motor symptoms such as unilateral weakness.

As well as presentations attributed to the anterior cerebral circulation, TIAs also occur within the vertebrobasilar territory. This is less common but more easily misdiagnosed and should be considered when patients present with a sudden onset of vertigo, diplopia, ataxia, or true drop attacks (sudden fall due to loss of tone without disturbance of consciousness and with rapid and complete recovery). A vertebrobasilar TIA carries the same risk of a subsequent stroke as an anterior circulation TIA.

TIAs almost never cause transient loss of consciousness (TLoC), and patients with this should not be referred to overstretched acute TIA clinic services.

Pathology

The pathophysiological mechanisms are the same as for ischaemic stroke. They include emboli from an atheromatous plaque in the aorta, common carotid or carotid bifurcation, vertebral arteries, or cardiac embolism. If an early MRI is performed, multiple DWI-positive lesions are quite often seen in different arterial territories, suggesting a cardiac embolic shower – usually due to PAF. More rarely, a vasculitic process or vascular dissection is causative. Risk factors are the same as for stroke.

Management in primary care

Although TIA symptoms have often resolved by the time of presentation to the GP this should still be considered a medical emergency. Given the considerable risk of an impending stroke, aspirin 300 mg is recommended as soon as one is reasonably sure the diagnosis is a TIA, in case there is a delay in being seen in the TIA clinic. Even if the diagnosis is a haemorrhagic stroke, it is unlikely to do harm. This differs from the advice in a suspected stroke, as the patient will be sent to hospital, so aspirin is given after imaging, which excludes a bleed, unless thrombolysis is planned. Refer to a rapid-access TIA clinic with the intention of a specialist assessment within 24 hours. NICE (2021) now discourages the use of risk prediction systems such as the ABCD2 score, as without imaging, such tools have poor discriminatory value. All TIAs are now considered to be high risk for stroke.

If older patients have multiple repetitive events resembling TIAs, a diagnosis of amyloid angiopathy with 'amyloid spells' should be considered, and MRI imaging should be performed to look for microbleeds. Amyloid spells often present with spreading sensory symptoms or speech disruption. If this is not recognised, it is often managed badly by increasing antiplatelet agents, etc.

TIA clinics

Referrals to rapid access TIA clinics, or more accurately 'Suspected TIA clinics', which are usually held daily, are made by primary care or the ED. The role of the TIA clinic is to:

1 Confirm the diagnosis (or – see later – identify another cause for the symptoms).

2 Arrange investigations, including of the brain, carotids, and heart.
- The diagnosis is made on history and imaging. Depending on the clinic, over half of the cases (65% at Addenbrooke's are stroke mimics, most commonly migraine, seizure, syncope, postural hypotension, peripheral vestibular disturbance, transient global amnesia, functional neurological disorder and, most seriously, brain tumours).
- Brain imaging is now almost always diffusion-weighted MRI.
- Carotid Doppler ultrasonography (or either CT or MR angiography) is mandatory following anterior circulation TIA and is used to identify atherosclerotic lesions, which may be amenable to carotid endarterectomy in suitable patients. Carotid stenosis on the relevant side of between 50 and 99% (according to American criteria) would trigger a referral for assessment by a vascular MDT. The consensus is that carotid endarterectomy carries less risk in older patients than carotid stenting. If endarterectomy is indicated, ideally it should be within 7 days of symptoms.
- Cardiac investigations include a 12-lead ECG, rhythm monitoring starting with a 24-hour tape and echocardiography. If the vascular imaging is normal and the patient is not in established AF, a longer period of monitoring the rhythm is essential. This will include a wearable device (e.g. a Zio patch) or an implantable loop recorder, as the priority is to detect PAF and anticoagulate those with no absolute contraindications.

3 Initiate aggressive (appropriate) secondary prevention.
- Dual antiplatelet therapy with either aspirin and clopidogrel or aspirin and ticagrelor should be considered in patients with TIA or minor stroke within 24 hours.
  - Clopidogrel (initial dose 300 mg followed by 75 mg per day) plus aspirin (initial dose 300 mg followed by 75 mg per day for 21 days) followed by clopidogrel 75 mg daily monotherapy OR
  - Ticagrelor (initial dose 180 mg followed by 90 mg twice daily) plus aspirin (300 mg followed by 75 mg daily for 30 days) followed by antiplatelet monotherapy with ticagrelor 90 mg twice daily or clopidogrel 75 mg once daily.
  - If dual antiplatelet therapy is not considered appropriate, clopidogrel at a loading dose of 300 mg, followed by 75 mg daily, should be given.
  - Consider PPI (pantoprazole or lansoprazole) cover with dual antiplatelet therapy; (es/omeprazole may reduce the efficacy of clopidogrel).
- High-intensity statin (e.g. atorvastatin 20–80 mg daily) started immediately regardless of cholesterol.
- BP-lowering treatment (thiazide/long-acting calcium channel blocker/ACE inhibitor to a target clinic systolic pressure <130 mmHg or lower if tolerated.

4 Perform baseline blood tests (FBC, clotting studies, renal, liver and bone function, lipid screen, and TFTs). ESR, CRP, and autoantibodies may be useful if vasculitis is a possibility; any older person with transient visual symptoms should have an ESR for temporal arteritis.

Rapid assessment and intervention are crucial. The EXPRESS (Early Use of Existing Preventive Strategies for Stroke) study in the UK suggested that early intervention could reduce 90-day stroke risk by 80%, and the recent 10-year follow-up showed long-term benefits. Polytherapy, with attention to diet, exercise, and antiplatelet, statin, and antihypertensive therapies, explains these gains.

Stroke presentation

Typically, the onset is abrupt. Attempts are made to establish the exact time of onset (unfortunately impossible if the patient woke from sleep, around 25% of cases). Ask when the patient went to bed or was last seen well. Act fast, as thrombolysis may still be possible (see subsequent text). Occasionally, hemiparesis develops over a few hours, but consider another diagnosis, such as a tumour, if symptoms progress over days or weeks. Other common stroke mimics include hypoglycaemia, Todd's paresis after a partial seizure, hemiplegic migraine, metabolic disturbances, syncope due to postural hypotension in older people, and functional neurological disorders.

Reduced consciousness at presentation usually indicates non-stroke pathology, but a stroke may present with coma if there has been a brain stem infarct or a large cortical infarct compressing the brainstem. Stroke can cause seizures, so patients can present in a 'post-ictal' drowsy phase.

An eyewitness may relate that the patient dropped their cup, developed facial asymmetry and difficulty with speech, and then became unable to stand or even sit properly. The peak time of onset for stroke is in the early hours of the morning, and the patient may describe waking up and trying to get out of bed, only to find themselves unable to walk.

Examination will usually reveal characteristic deficits: in the early stages, the paralysed limbs on the affected side are more often flaccid than spastic, and, in some cases, they stay that way. Facial asymmetry spares the forehead due to its bilateral innervation. In a brain stem stroke, signs are often bilateral, with a mix of UMN and LMN signs, and the pupils may be small. In a major cortical stroke, the cheek on the paralysed side may flap in and out with respiration, and the limbs on that side are likely to have completely lost all tone. Reflexes may be unhelpful at this stage. An almost pathognomonic sign is the conjugate deviation of gaze towards the side of the lesion due to the unopposed effect of the contralateral frontal eye field (remember, the patient 'looks away' from a tumour but 'towards' a stroke). Loss of consciousness points to a severe stroke, but there are no reliable clinical predictors to distinguish haemorrhage from infarction.

Improving stroke recognition and triage

The Face, Arm, Speech, and Time (FAST) mass media campaign in 2009 increased public awareness of stroke and improved stroke triage.

- It was credited with having a significant impact on information-seeking behaviour and emergency admissions.
- However, admissions for stroke fell during the COVID-19 pandemic, and the campaign has been relaunched (see Figure 9.1).
- The ambulance service uses FAST to identify stroke patients and triage them for urgent transfer to a specialist stroke unit.

- Any one of facial asymmetry, arm or leg weakness, or speech disturbance suggests a stroke with a sensitivity of 82% and a specificity for stroke diagnosis of 37%.
- Monoplegia of the arm is the most discriminatory sign in older people; some facial asymmetry is common, and speech disruption and delirium are difficult for paramedics to disentangle.
- FAST performs less well in posterior circulation strokes, and using BE-FAST (adding balance and eyes) improves this.

With the advent of mechanical thrombectomy (MT), clinical scoring systems for LVO are in development, and telemedicine triage at the scene is proving useful in deciding which patients should be taken directly to an MT centre.

Immediate management

There are about 80,000 stroke admissions in England every year. The target ambulance response time for category 2 emergencies like stroke is 18 min but this is not met (April 2023, 28 min). However, most patients with suspected strokes are assessed rapidly and fast-tracked to an acute stroke service. In terms of recovery, 'time is neurone' and such pathways provide access to almost immediate brain imaging and stroke expertise, often on a hyperacute stroke unit. Telemedicine enables 24/7 expert review of patients taken to more remote district general hospitals with similar effectiveness to bedside assessment.

- The purpose of acute treatment of ischaemic stroke is to salvage the viable penumbral tissue around the irreversibly damaged ischaemic core by restoring blood flow (using thrombolysis and possibly thrombectomy) before this tissue also dies.
- Baseline bloods are taken (as for TIAs).
- Stroke severity may be documented using the National Institute of Health Stroke Scale (NIHSS) – see Appendix. This was originally used to determine eligibility for thrombolysis, but this is no longer essential in current guidelines.

Urgent imaging

Brain imaging, including plain CT head and CT angiography, should be performed as soon as possible (at most within 1 hour of arrival at the hospital). On CT head, haemorrhage is immediately apparent as a white

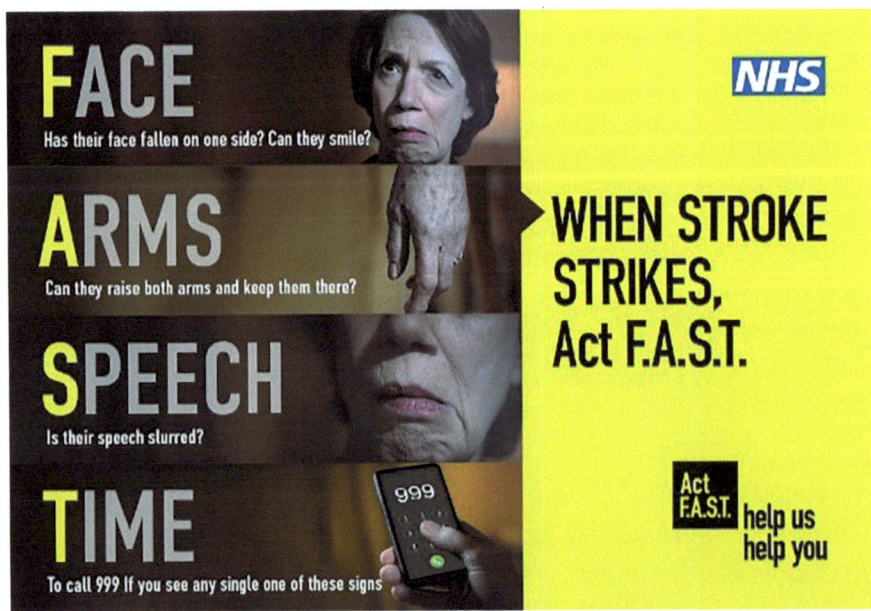

Figure 9.1 Campaign poster to encourage people to act FAST in suspected strokes. *Source*: National Health Service/Public domain.

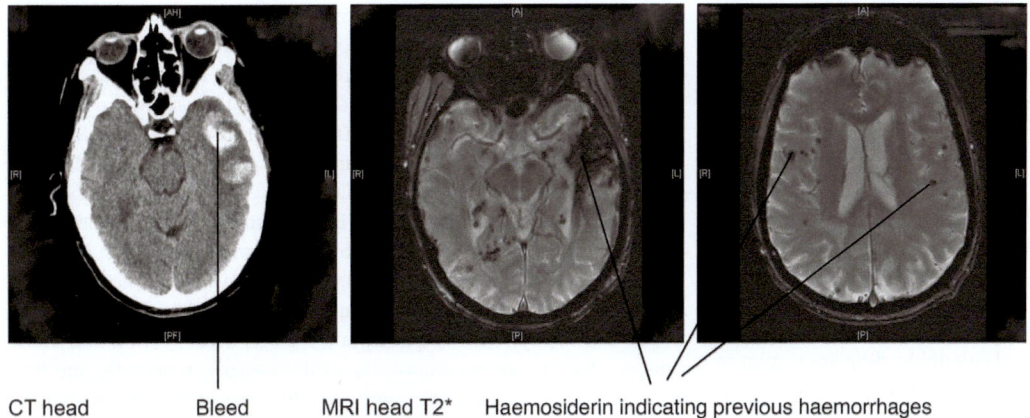

CT head   Bleed   MRI head T2*   Haemosiderin indicating previous haemorrhages

Figure 9.2 CT scan showing a left temporoparietal bleed in a 71-year-old man with prior cognitive decline. An MRI head (T2* imaging) 3 months later shows dense haemosiderin deposition (which appears black) in the area of the previous bleed and multiple small lesions that look like black holes. These represent multiple small bleeds and are characteristic of cerebral amyloid angiopathy.

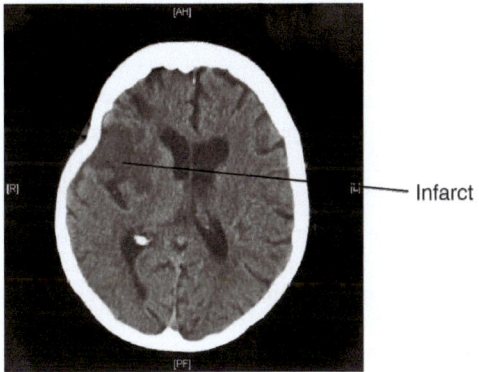

Infarct

Figure 9.3 CT head scan of a 92-year-old woman presenting with left hemiparesis on waking from sleep. Note the irregular area of low attenuation in the right frontal lobe affecting white and grey matter, consistent with a recent right MCA infarct.

area (Figure 9.2). If haemorrhage is excluded, aspirin 300 mg is given, unless the plan is for thrombolysis. The area of low attenuation characteristic of an infarct on a CT scan is often difficult to see in the first 6 hours and may not be apparent for 24 hours (Figures 9.3 and 9.4). Techniques such as CT perfusion are useful for early visualisation and aid decision-making with regard to thrombolysis and MT at later time windows, or when there is an unknown time of onset, to assess whether there is viable brain tissue in the affected area (Figure 7.4). CT angiography is needed if MT is a consideration.

- MRI is more sensitive than CT, especially early after onset, and for imaging the posterior fossa.
- MRI is challenging in an acute stroke, as although image acquisition times are falling, it is more demanding for the patient, and movement artefacts are often significant.
- In some services, acute MRI is used to determine if the patient is suitable for thrombolysis; DWI positive and FLAIR negative images correlate with a patient being within the 4.5-hour window for thrombolysis.
- In a PCS, an MRI is very helpful to determine if vital structures in the brain stem are already damaged, making treatment futile.

Acute treatments for ischaemic stroke

Thrombolysis

Intravenous thrombolysis (IVT) within 4.5 hours of symptom onset is the first-line therapy in patients with acute ischemic stroke, and recombinant tissue plasminogen activator (alteplase) has been the preferred fibrino-

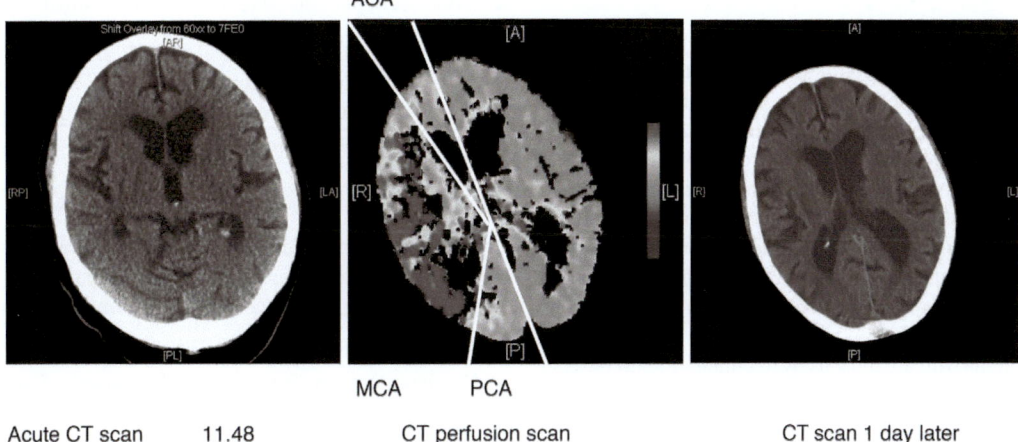

ACA

MCA   PCA

Acute CT scan   11.48   CT perfusion scan   CT scan 1 day later

Figure 9.4 Imaging in an 82-year-old man who developed sudden-onset left hemiparesis at 09.45. The initial CT scan shows that it can be difficult to see early infarction, whereas the CT perfusion scan shows that more than two-thirds of the right MCA territory is affected; the white lines are drawn on to show the area of cortex supplied by the anterior, middle, and cerebral arteries. Although the affected area showed that the contrast time to peak and drain was delayed, only a small area had reduced blood volume, indicating a small infarct within a large penumbra. Thrombolysis produced an excellent clinical response, and minimal long-term damage was sustained, as can be seen from the CT scan the next day.

lytic agent for more than 25 years. Fibrinolytic drugs activate plasminogen to form plasmin, which degrades fibrin and so breaks up thrombi.

- Alteplase is administered intravenously as soon as possible after CT has excluded intracranial haemorrhage (the initial 10% of the dose is given as a bolus and the remainder by intravenous infusion over 60 min). The patient is observed for anaphylaxis. Antiplatelets are delayed for at least 24 hours after thrombolysis, and CT brain imaging is repeated to exclude intracranial haemorrhage.
- Tenecteplase, the thrombolytic of choice for acute MI, was licenced for stroke in April 2024 and NICE approved in July 2024. It is cheaper, has pharmacological (longer half-life) and practical advantages as it is given as a bolus. Overall outcomes and risk of bleeding are similar to alteplase, but it appears more effective at recanalising occluded large vessels. It is fast becoming the thrombolytic of choice as a bolus can be given prior to transfer of the patient to a thrombectomy centre.

The major criteria for thrombolysis are:

- Age: no restriction in current guidelines (previously 18–80).
- Within 4.5 hours of stroke onset.
- Between 4.5 and 9 hours of known onset, or within 9 hours of the midpoint of sleep when they have woken with symptoms, AND there is evidence from CT/MR perfusion (core-perfusion mismatch) or MRI (DWI-FLAIR mismatch) of the potential to salvage brain tissue.
- Haemorrhagic stroke excluded on CT.
- Patients with strokes of all severity should be assessed clinically for thrombolysis: previously, patients with an NIHSS score of 5–25 were eligible, excluding very minor and very major strokes.
- No surgery or trauma within the last 14 days.
- No stroke within the preceding 3 months.
- BP <185/110 (higher BP is lowered, e.g. with labetalol).
- Not on anticoagulation with warfarin or DOAC (prior aspirin and clopidogrel OK).
- A range of serious illnesses with haemorrhagic potential are potential contraindications.
- Consent/assent/best interests.

About 11% of stroke patients currently get thrombolysis. Suitable patients should have thrombolysis, irrespective of whether they have an LVO and might benefit from MT.

Mechanical thrombectomy

NHS England commissioned MT for ACiS in 2018. If the patient is eligible for thrombolysis, this is given first, but for patients with LVOs where recanalisation may not occur or those with contraindications to thrombolysis (such as the concurrent use of oral anticoagulants at the time of stroke or recent surgery), MT should be offered. If the patient is not for thrombolysis because they are out of the time window or it is contraindicated, aspirin is given whether or not they are for MT. This is limited by the availability of specialist neuroradiologists, and there is a postcode lottery. One strategy to improve availability is 'drip and ship' – give thrombolysis and send the patient on to a specialist thrombectomy hub.

Clinically, the patients who are most likely to benefit from MT are:

- Those with an occlusion of an internal carotid or proximal middle cerebral artery (MCA – M1 segment),
- Who were previously independent – a premorbid modified Rankin score (mRS) of 2 or less. The mRS is used to measure functional outcome and ranges from 0 (no symptoms) to 6 (dead; see Appendix).

There is no age restriction, but studies are looking at premorbid frailty – rather than an mRS score – and outcome. Patients who do not

have a proximal intracranial LVO are excluded from the guidelines, but trials are underway to determine if patients with more distal MCA clots (M2 or even M3 segments) benefit from MT.

Various scores have been developed to quantify the pattern and extent of ischaemic damage on a CT head scan to guide the use of MT. The ASPECTS score has been widely used (with a cut point of ≥6 for considering MT), but in recent trials, even those with ASPECTS scores <6 may stand to benefit. This is an area in which artificial intelligence is contributing. Because of the lack of neuroradiologists AI tools such as Brainomix are being used to help clinicians. In the East of England, all the DGHs have Brainomix up and running. The Brainomix 360 Mobile app, supported by the Brainomix 360 Cloud, allows physicians to quickly and securely access, review and share images, and data across a network, send messages, make calls, and flag patients eligible for thrombectomy – all designed to optimise workflow, facilitating faster transfer and treatment decisions.

Mechanical clot retrieval involves using a device to remove the occluding arterial blood clot, restore blood flow and minimise ischaemic brain damage.

- MT can be carried out with LA, sedation or full GA.
- A catheter is inserted into the femoral artery and fed intravascularly to the site of the clot.
- The clot is then physically pulled out through the catheter.

In ACiS, MT performed within 6 hours of onset time is highly effective in reducing progression to severe disability without increasing total mortality figures when used with thrombolysis and specialist stroke unit care. The absolute chance of patients being able to function independently at 90 days after stroke was improved by 20% (19–22%) among those undergoing MT compared with controls (NNT 5 for functional independence and 3 for reduction in disability at 90 days). As with thrombolysis, 'time is neurone'; the HERMES study found that the absolute chance of being functionally independent 90 days after thrombectomy diminishes by 3.4% with each hour of delay to starting the procedure. Further trials have shown that patients with LVO treated at later time points – sometimes guided by CT perfusion imaging – may still benefit from MT. In the future, it is likely that any patient with an acute LVO will be considered for MT.

The national target is that 10% of all strokes should get MT. So far, only the London area has achieved this. 1,825 thrombectomies were performed in England, Wales, and Northern Ireland from April 2022 to March 2023.

- 48% had received thrombolysis.
- 54% were transferred to a hub.
- A quarter of patients were over 80, with a small number aged 90+.

The median NIHSS on arrival was 17. The most common complication was distal clot migration/embolisation. 32% were discharged with an mRS of 0–2, but this worsened from before the stroke to discharge by 2 or more levels in 71% of patients.

Decompressive hemicraniectomy

In 2–8% of patients with ACiS (due to occlusion of the internal carotid, MCA, ACA, or a combination), large-volume brain infarction causes space-occupying brain swelling, which, untreated, has a mortality rate of about 80%.

- Hemicraniectomy (neurosurgical removal of part of the skull to reduce intracerebral pressure) is lifesaving.
- There is also functional benefit for those under 60, particularly if surgery is performed within 48 hours of onset, but most survivors have major disabilities.

Hemicraniectomy was only considered for patients under 60, but following a review by NICE in 2019, older patients can be offered hemicraniectomy as there is a survival benefit, but functional improvement is even more limited. At all ages, there must be extensive discussion with the family, considering the patient's known wishes and making it clear that there is certainty of significant disability if surgery is performed. Hemicraniectomy rates are falling with the advent of MT.

Stroke audits

Stroke is an area of medicine where evidence-based protocols and audits are embedded in routine practice.

- **SITS**: Safe Implementation of Treatments in Stroke is a non-profit, research-driven, independent, international collaboration that started as a registry for IV thrombolysis with alteplase. It is coordinated by the Karolinska Institute. This has proved very useful in showing that the benefits seen in RCTs could be translated into protocol-based clinical practice.
- **SSNAP**: The Sentinel Stroke National Audit Programme monitors the delivery of stroke care in England, Wales, and Northern Ireland. Annual reports document all aspects of care against goals.

Early care on the stroke unit

Many patients presenting with acute strokes will have other problems that need management.

- 10% have at least three comorbidities.
- Frailty is an independent predictor of poor outcomes.

Remember, most stroke patients do not receive thrombolysis or thrombectomy, either because they fall outside the relevant time window or because of a contraindication.

- Patients should be admitted directly to a *stroke unit*. However, performance has worsened in this respect – in 2022/23, only 40% of patients were directly admitted to a stroke unit within 4 hours, and only 73% spent at least 90% of their stay on a stroke unit.
- Initially, patients are *closely monitored* – strict neurological observation is needed because of the risk of intracerebral bleeding, raised intracranial pressures and airway compromise. A cardiac monitor is used to look for important arrhythmias, such as AF.
- The patient should be managed in the most *comfortable position* (flat or propped up) except after MT, when patients should lie flat for the first 12–24 hours (HeadPoST trial).
- The aim is to maintain *normal physiological parameters*, including oxygen saturation, hydration, temperature, and blood glucose levels (aim 5–15 mmol/L). Oxygen is only given if saturation falls below 95%, or a suitable target in COPD. A sudden drop suggests aspiration or, at a later stage, pulmonary embolus and more gradual deterioration may be due to pneumonia, which occurs in around 10% of stroke patients in hospital and is associated with worse outcomes.
- *The prevention of further complications* is essential. The drowsy patient will need attentive nursing care and expert moving and handling to avoid aspiration, shoulder subluxation on the hemiparetic side, pressure damage and contractures. Good mouth care with an electric toothbrush and antibacterial oral gel may reduce pneumonia.
- *Swallowing* should be screened within 4 hours, before being given any food or fluid by mouth. If swallowing appears unsafe, IV fluids should be started, and a full swallowing assessment should be arranged. Nasogastric feeding should be considered within 24 hours (see later).
- If not already administered, *aspirin* 300 mg should be given to patients with disabling ischaemic stroke within 24 hours orally, or rectally/ by

enteral tube if dysphagic. Aspirin 300 mg is continued for 2 weeks or discharge, when long-term antiplatelet treatment is started.
- Although subcutaneous low-molecular-weight heparin reduces deaths from *VTE*, haemorrhagic deaths are increased. Low-molecular-weight heparin or graduated compression stockings are not used routinely. Intermittent pneumatic compression is recommended, starting within 3 days and continuing for 30 days if needed.
- In the case of ischaemic stroke, *hypertension* should only be treated in the acute phase to enable thrombolysis or if it is likely to produce its own complications, such as hypertensive encephalopathy. Studies have shown that BP lowering in the context of acute stroke is associated with poorer outcomes. Hypertension is treated more aggressively in intracranial haemorrhage (see later).
- Stroke units should have programmes to promote *continence*. Active toileting regimes work if there are enough staff to implement them.
- Effective *communication* is particularly important in stroke because of the sudden and often devastating nature of the condition, with a significant risk of early death or survival with long-term disability. The future of the spouse, as well as that of the patient, may also be completely changed in an instant.
  ○ If a patient has had a devastating stroke, particularly if they were already living with severe frailty, initiate early discussion with the family about the patient's prior views and which interventions are not likely to be of benefit. Ask whether the patient has a health and welfare attorney or an advance decision.
  ○ Discussions might include the use of IV antibiotics, whether CPR should be attempted, feeding, which is usually addressed by a formal MDT, and when to move to end-of-life care (see Chapter 22).
  ○ Ensure that all members of MDT are up to date with the clinical situation and plans as they evolve. Patients may have long admissions; families talk to many members of the team and become frustrated and upset by mixed messages.

Hydration and nutrition

Post-stroke swallowing difficulty is seen in up to half of acute presentations. It is associated with the risk of aspiration pneumonia, an increased length of stay, and mortality. On admission, the patient should be 'nil by mouth' while a bedside swallowing assessment is undertaken. A trained nurse or speech and language therapist assesses the ability to swallow fluids by sitting the patient up and observing the ability to swallow a teaspoon of fluid, followed by a tablespoon, and finally 50–100 mL of water. Pooling of fluid in the mouth, choking, coughing, a 'wet' voice, or delayed swallowing are noted. It is apparent if there is obvious aspiration, but a significant number of individuals will aspirate 'silently'; monitoring oxygen saturation may be helpful.

- Initially, IV fluids are given to those who cannot swallow safely.
- A decision on whether to 'artificially' feed a patient is usually taken within the first 24–36 hours of admission, influenced by the type of stroke and perceived progress of the patient. This is usually done via a fine-bore nasogastric (NG) tube. NG tubes that are not secured (bridled) are easily dislodged, and it is important to remember that NG feeding does not completely remove aspiration risk, nor does it protect the airway. Great care should be taken to confirm the correct placement before starting every feed. Early tube feeding is associated with improved survival after stroke, but at the risk of increasing the proportion of patients with a poor functional outcome (also see Chapter 21).
- Percutaneous endoscopic gastrostomy (PEG) placement will be considered for patients whose swallow does not recover. Referral to the feeding issues MDT (FIMDT) should be made at 4 weeks if the patient is still reliant on NG feeding.

The decision-making process is complex and involves obtaining information from the family/patient's representative or their attorney about what the patient would have wanted and discussion with team members, including speech therapists, dieticians, and gastroenterologists. The FIMDT will consider the practical and ethical implications of PEG insertion. PEG feeding is a more secure way of providing nutrition and medications. However, it requires an invasive procedure, which increases the risk of complications and is associated with an overall mortality rate of up to 4% (higher morbidity and mortality in the very frail). In older people, the combination of dementia and a stroke is usually a contraindication for PEG.

The patient now begins a journey that encompasses a daily multidisciplinary approach involving stroke physicians, nurses, dieticians, speech and language specialists, therapy teams, clinical psychologists, pharmacists, and social services.

- Time spent educating willing friends and relatives on how to help with rehab tasks can be highly effective.
- Patients and families benefit from signposting to the Stroke Association for information and educational materials.
- Compared with a general ward, the NNT in a specialist stroke unit is 18 (95% CI 12–32) to prevent dependency or death.

It is unclear which component of stroke unit care leads to improved outcomes, but stroke units have been the most important advance in stroke in the past 40 years (despite the high profile of hyperacute treatments).

Clinical problems

- **Dysphagia**: common initially (see management of hydration and nutrition). Dysphagia can occur because of a specific neuronal pathway disruption or in an unconscious or drowsy patient. By 3 months, around 75% of patients who initially had dysphagia have recovered. Persistent dysphagia is a marker of a severe disabling stroke and/or a brain stem stroke, e.g. in lateral medullary syndrome, where dysphagia is often the most disabling feature but eventually recovers.
- **Delirium**: occurs in over 10% of patients in the first week, predicted by pre-existing cognitive impairment, right hemisphere stroke, large lesion, and post-stroke infection. Delirium is known to increase all-cause hospital mortality and length of stay. Delirium may contribute to or worsen dementia. The stroke damage itself may lead to cognitive decline (see vascular dementia in Chapter 8).
- **Depression**: occurs in about a third of patients, both initially and after discharge, when the elation of getting home is tempered by the reality of the residual handicap. In half, presentation occurs at 3–6 months, which is one of the drivers for the recommended 6-month review. Clinical psychology input is now mandated. Individuals with post-stroke depression are more at risk of suboptimal recovery, poor quality of life, recurrent vascular events, and mortality. The pathophysiology requires further evaluation but may involve inflammation, cerebrovascular deregulation, and disruption of glutamate neurotransmission. There is debate as to whether the location of the stroke is pertinent. Motivational interviewing may be considered, but an antidepressant is often needed. No one drug class has been found to be superior for post-stroke depression, but an SSRI is usually used. As always, the response (or not) to treatment should be monitored. In the FOCUS trial, fluoxetine given orally for 6 months after acute stroke 'prophylactically' did reduce the occurrence of depression but did not improve functional outcomes, and more patients sustained fractures.
- **Dysphasia**: a disorder of language affecting some right-handed patients with left-hemisphere lesions. It is the second most common major impairment after stroke. It can disrupt the production and comprehension of speech, as well as reading and writing.
  - **Anterior dysphasia**: non-fluent, impaired naming.
  - **Posterior dysphasia**: often fluent, jargon-type, receptive dysphasia. Fluent dysphasia is often confused with acute confusion. In left-handers, two-thirds have left-sided speech dominance; those who have right-sided dominance may/may not develop dysphasia, irrespective of the side of the lesion.
- **Dysarthria**: affects articulation but not the content of the speech. This can be due to unilateral VII palsy but otherwise suggests bilateral disease (or pathology in the cerebellum or basal ganglia).
- **Dyspraxia**: inability to perform purposeful movement despite adequate comprehension and motor function. Varieties include dressing apraxia.
- **Sensory neglect**: this is a neuropsychological disorder of attention in which patients fail to report or respond to sensory stimuli from the opposite side of the brain damage, even though the specific sensory pathways are intact. It is most common with right parietal damage.
  - **Visual**: the most common form - exclude hemianopia first. Line bisection or line cancellation (Albert's test). Milder cases often improve.
  - **Tactile or personal hemineglect**: if gross, includes loss of body image and denial of the problem.
- **Visuospatial perception**: non-dominant hemisphere lesion – bedside tests include asking the patient to draw simple objects such as a house, face, or clock face.
- **Executive function difficulties**: trail-making B, a timed join-the-dots test with attentional switching 1 to A to 2 to B, etc. may help predict driving ability.
- **Weakness of limbs**: usually with increased tone; prolonged flaccidity and marked 'clasp-knife' spasticity are both adverse signs.
- **Sensory loss**: any modality; gross position sense loss is a very adverse finding.
- **Hemianopia**: this does not recover. It is important to screen for it, as it affects the return to driving. Bedside testing includes checking the fields to confrontation. Hemianopia tends to sharply obey the vertical meridian, unlike neglect, where there is a gradient of inattention that may overlap into the ipsilateral hemispace. Patients, families, and non-specialist staff will not understand the effect of a typical homonymous hemianopia and benefit from an explanation. Remember that if a patient with left hemiparesis has homonymous hemianopia, it will be to the left. At first, approach the patient from the side they can see to. Later in rehab, approaching from the 'blind' side and calling their name encourages head turning. Hemianopia is a major handicap unless the patient is aware and able to compensate by turning their head. Screening by an orthoptist is now recommended. Prisms may be helpful to broaden the field of view and for diplopia.
- **Hearing loss**: there may be a central component if the temporal lobe is involved. Patients often report deterioration, so hearing should be assessed and referrals made, e.g. for new hearing aids.
- **Thalamic pain**: try an antidepressant or anticonvulsant.
- **Shoulder pain**: a very disabling and painful syndrome with multifactorial causes – neurological and musculoskeletal. Subluxation may follow traction on the weak arm, e.g. from poor manual handling, and early good positioning is important. Stroke units should develop pathways for the management of shoulder pain, including intraarticular injections to reduce pain and specific physiotherapy techniques; more trials are needed on functional electrical stimulation.
- **Fatigue**: a big problem for patients; it often develops between 3 and 6 months and impairs rehab. It is sometimes linked to depression. An assessment of fatigue should be made with a validated scale and an explanation of symptoms given to patients and families with the positive news that the fatigue will usually lift between 9 and 12 months.

Rehabilitation

Rehabilitation for stroke follows general principles and should be driven by stroke-specific goals that are important to the individual across a range of areas, including education, social participation, psychological well-being, and functional improvement. Services are becoming 'needs-led' rather than 'time limited', based on achievable goals identified between the team and patient. This may be called a 'rehab prescription'. Rehab usually starts in the stroke unit and continues in a community hospital or at home.

Early, structured mobilisation reduces the risk of long-term immobility and increases the chances of functional recovery. However, some evidence suggests that mobilisation attempts should not be made too hastily.

- An international randomised trial (AVERT Trial Collaboration Group, 2015) highlighted that, when compared to usual care, very early mobilisation (<24 hours post-symptom onset) was associated with worse functional outcomes at 3 months.
- The current recommendations from the RCP therefore suggest frequent, short periods of daily activity (sitting out of bed, transferring from bed to chair, standing) carried out by appropriately trained staff beginning between 24 and 48 hours after stroke onset.
- Those who need little help from the onset should continue to mobilise as able.
- Chest physiotherapy may be needed especially if patients cannot sit out or pneumonia develops.

After the first 2 weeks, people with motor recovery goals following stroke should receive at least 3 hours a day of therapy (physiotherapist-delivered or supervised) on at least 5 days in 7 and should be supported to remain active for up to 6 hours a day. Older people have been shown to cope with this. For people with some upper limb movement or impaired mobility or balance after stroke, repetitive task practice is the principal rehab approach.

Most stroke units use a mix of group therapy sessions and individual sessions with the use of iPad-delivered/telerehab therapy to get the overall 'dose' up.

Occupational therapists initially focus on promoting self-care using both restorative strategies, e.g. encouraging people with hemisensory inattention to attend to the neglected side, and compensatory strategies, e.g. training people to dress one-handed using aids. A range of aids and appliances may support independence.

Speech and language therapists may have to focus more on swallowing than communication if provision is limited, but should assess people with communication difficulties, supervise treatment programmes and coach carers. Patients with aphasia and dysarthria should have individualised therapy, and communication aids may be needed. There is renewed interest in the use of music therapy for speech problems stemming from the classic observation that some patients with non-fluent aphasia may still be able to sing – a right hemisphere function. Melody, rhythm, eye contact and synchronisation may have a role and multiple mechanisms may be involved, from improved mood and concentration to neuroplasticity and mirror neurons. Improved breathing, voicing and articulation may help with dysarthria.

Progression through the sequence of sitting, transferring, standing, and walking may take a couple of months if the initial hemiparesis is severe. In general, proximal movements recover better than distal, and lower limbs recover more than upper.

An interesting recent approach is the use of 'mirror therapy' (Figure 9.5), which exploits the brain's preference for visual feedback and may act through the mirror neurone system. There is moderate evidence that, in combination with traditional therapy and considerable practice, it helps with upper limb function. Small gains in hand and finger movement can markedly improve function. Another approach that is not established but is generating considerable research interest is the use of robotic arm interventions. The paretic arm is supported by an exoskeleton attached to a computer, and activities such as playing computer games provide a fun method of carrying out repetitive tasks (see the Stroke Foundation clip in the references).

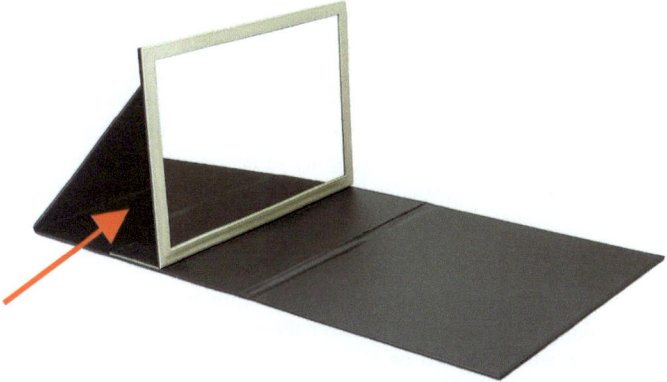

Figure 9.5 Equipment for mirror therapy. The patient sits with their paretic arm in the box (arrow) and focuses on the reflection of the unaffected hand in the mirror, performing movements (e.g. pronation and supination or touching the thumb to the fingertips) as if it were the affected hand.

Discharge from hospital

'Early supported discharge' (ESD) is an intervention for adults after a stroke that allows their care to be transferred from a hospital to a community setting at an earlier stage than would otherwise be possible because of the provision of a dedicated community stroke rehab team. It is now universal in England.

The expertise of the team and intensity of the rehab should be the same as on a stroke unit. Systems where staff rotate between the ESD team and hospital stroke unit work well.

- Suitability is assessed by the hospital MDT; it is appropriate for around 40% of stroke patients who can transfer with minimum assistance.
- The nurse in the ESD team is of invaluable help with medication and continence.
- ESD reduces the length of hospital stay and the risk of dependency.

Telerehab is attractive for organisations looking after stroke patients at home in rural areas. It suits some patients who have adequate technology and internet access. Trials are heterogeneous, but in comparison with in-person rehab, clinically important psychological harms were found, including depression. However, virtual reality games and other software may make stroke rehab more fun. A mixed approach is best.

Patients with moderate to severe disabilities need considerable input from the hospital MDT to discharge them home, including the provision of equipment and a care package. Whether this is possible depends on the patient's home environment, family support and resources. Funding for major changes such as a wet room or stair lift is limited, and people are expected to live downstairs and make do with a strip wash. Long-term 'maintenance' therapy is not provided, and deterioration is common.

Around 8% of stroke survivors leaving hospital in the UK are discharged to care homes. The stroke unit should provide advice on feeding, positioning, continence, and seating; this is an area where improvement is needed.

Haemorrhagic stroke

Haemorrhage accounts for 15% of all strokes in the UK and is caused by arterial rupture into the intraparenchymal, subarachnoid, and/or intraventricular space. ICH (intracerebral haemorrhage) refers to those who have bled into the brain parenchyma.

Haemorrhagic and ischaemic strokes are clinically indistinguishable, but the incidence of headache, vomiting, coma, and seizure activity is greater in haemorrhagic strokes. Between 3% and 17% of these patients will have a seizure in the first 2 weeks, but prophylactic antiepileptic medication is not recommended. CT brain imaging is the first investigation, but CT or MR angiography may be needed to delineate any underlying lesions, such as aneurysms or mass lesions.

Management of ICH due to hypertension

When hypertension is the cause, bleeding commonly arises from small penetrating arteries that originate from the main brain arteries. Patients presenting acutely should be given blood pressure-lowering therapy, aiming for a systolic blood pressure target of 130–139 mmHg within 1 hour. Beta-blockers or calcium channel blockers can be used for this purpose. Intravenous labetalol should be considered in those with systolic blood pressures >200 mmHg to achieve a more rapid response. Care must be taken to avoid cerebral hypoperfusion because of iatrogenic hypotension. Rapid BP lowering should not be considered in those who have an underlying structural cause or in those with an expected poor prognosis.

Anticoagulants should be stopped or reversed, if possible. Placement of a caval filter should be considered in such patients who then develop venous thromboembolism (for which they are at high risk).

Neurosurgery

Neurosurgical intervention is considered in non-frail patients whose intracerebral haematoma is expanding, causing raised intracranial pressure (ICP). Intracerebral haematomas may continue to expand up to 12 hours, with associated cerebral oedema and subsequent raised intracranial pressures. Ventricular compression may lead to hydrocephalus. Those being considered for neurosurgical intervention should be managed in a neuro-intensive care setting where raised ICP can be addressed using mannitol, hyperventilation techniques and careful patient positioning. Neurosurgical techniques include intraventricular drains, decompressive craniotomy, and the evacuation of haematomas. Evacuation of the haematoma is indicated in those with cerebellar haemorrhage and hydrocephalus or brainstem compression. Patients with cerebellar haemorrhages >3 cm in diameter will have better outcomes with surgery. Other techniques currently under trial-level scrutiny include stereotactic evacuation.

Cerebral amyloid angiopathy

CAA is an important cause of intracerebral haemorrhage in older patients. This condition is characterised by amyloid B peptide deposition in small arterial vessels, causing cerebral 'microbleeds' that are often missed by CT imaging (but seen on MRI). They tend to occur mainly in peripheral cortical and subcortical locations, in contrast with deeper hypertensive bleeds. Patients can present with transient focal neurological episodes (imaginatively referred to as 'amyloid spells'), which can mimic both positive seizure-like or negative TIA-like episodes. However, lobar cortical haemorrhage can occur. Multiple areas of haemorrhage on imaging or an area of haemorrhage and evidence of previous microbleeds support this diagnosis (see Figure 9.2). Treatment options for CAA are limited, although antiepileptics may be considered for those experiencing amyloid spells (clinical data, no RCT).

Secondary prevention after ICH

- Recommend increased physical activity, a healthy diet, a reduction in alcohol consumption, stopping smoking, and cessation of cocaine/amphetamine use if relevant.
- Aim for tight BP control: <130/80 mmHg if tolerated.

- Specialist advice should be sought in those with ICH and AF, and hence a risk of future embolic stroke. Other options, e.g. left atrial appendage closure, may be possible.
- There is no role for statins unless they are indicated for other reasons, e.g. for IHD.

Posterior circulation stroke

Posterior circulation stroke (PCS) is due to impaired perfusion of the brainstem, cerebellum, thalamus, and/or occipitoparietal lobe due to occlusion of, or haemorrhage from, the vertebrobasilar system. It is less common than anterior circulation stroke (ACS), accounting for 20% of all strokes (corresponding to around 20% brain blood flow being from the vertebral arteries). As would be expected, proximal basilar artery occlusion carries the worst prognosis, with mortality in some series as high as 80%.

Diagnosis

The diagnosis of PCS is more difficult than ACS.

- The presentation is often stuttering or progressive.
- The anatomy of the vessels, and hence the clinical effects, is more variable than the anterior circulation.
- The deficits are confusing. They may be non-lateralising, or crossed as the corticospinal pathways decussate in the medulla (ipsilateral LMN cranial nerve signs with contralateral UMN motor or sensory deficits).
- The plethora of named syndromes in the literature can be counterproductive – the classic forms are rare; what matters is the recognition of a stroke.
- The most common symptom, dizziness, is a feature of common labyrinthine disorders.

A useful mnemonic to make you consider PCS is the 5Ds/3Ns.

If your patient has some of:	5 Ds	3 Ns
1	Dizziness and ataxia	Nystagmus
2	Diplopia or field defect	Nausea/vomiting
3	Dysarthria or dysphonia	Numbness
4	Dysphagia	
5	Drop attacks	
Could it be a posterior circulation stroke?		

Some common symptoms, such as unilateral limb weakness and dysarthria, will suggest stroke, but others – headache and nausea or vomiting – are common in a variety of acute illnesses and non-specific. If PCS is a possibility, a careful neurological examination is needed. Around 95% of people with PCS will have neurological signs, but they may be subtle. Pay particular attention to the eyes (Horner's, nystagmus, which changes direction – patient looks to right, fast component or 'beats' to the right, looks to left, 'beats' to left – field defects, gaze palsies), palatal movement, pain and temperature over face and limbs, look for limb or truncal ataxia, and check gait.

The HINTs examination (described in detail in Chapter 11) can be used to distinguish between peripheral and central vertigo but needs practice.

Differential diagnosis of PCS

This includes:

- **Benign positional paroxysmal vertigo (BPPV):** brief episodes of intense vertigo, precipitated by a change in position, usually looking up.

- **Ménière's disease**: simultaneous vertigo, partial hearing loss and tinnitus.
- **Migrainous vertigo**: features of migraine, normal neurological exam.
- **Vestibular neuritis**: crescendo onset, marked nausea, unidirectional nystagmus (regardless of where the patient looks) accentuated when looking away from the affected ear; may be unsteady but no ataxia or other neurological signs.
- **Labyrinthitis**: thought to be the same disease process as vestibular neuritis (viral), with the additional involvement of the auditory system (hearing loss and tinnitus)
- **Multiple sclerosis**: acute demyelination.

Imaging

Non-contrast CT scanning is done to exclude haemorrhage. It does not visualise the posterior fossa well, as the thick skull base degrades the quality of the image, so CT angiogram or MRI are then the modalities of choice.

Acute treatment

Acute management of PCiS is similar to ACiS with intravenous thrombolysis and, more recently, consideration of MT. Only 5% of LVOs are in the posterior circulation. Posterior circulation anatomy is more variable, the vertebral arteries are smaller than the carotids, the procedure is more technically demanding, and intracranial atherosclerotic stenosis is more common. Early trials of MT were not encouraging (partly attributed to study design), but more recent trials and registry data suggest benefit. It is being used for basilar and posterior cerebral artery LVOs if an MRI of the brainstem does not show irreversible damage. More data is needed.

Causes of deterioration

Progressive basilar artery thrombosis may lead to stuttering deterioration, and eventual coma. Cerebellar infarcts (or haematomas) can lead to dangerous cerebral oedema within the posterior fossa where compression of the fourth ventricle can cause hydrocephalus. Cerebral oedema in this area can also compress the brainstem, leading to fatal herniation.

Rehab and secondary prevention are similar to anterior circulation strokes, but carotid Doppler studies are not relevant.

Outcomes following stroke

This is dependent on the aetiology, brain volume, and anatomical location affected. Haemorrhagic strokes have a worse outcome than ischaemic strokes. Although case fatality has fallen since Bamford's work, the pattern of outcome according to the type of stroke remains similar. As with most acute illnesses, underlying frailty, co-morbidity, and age are also relevant.

During the first decade of the twenty-first century, stroke mortality rates in England halved. This was due to an overall fall in stroke event rates (by about 20%) and a more dramatic fall in case fatality (by about 40%). However, for people aged 85+, both have similar importance. These impressive statistics have been attributed to better prevention and education, access to faster imaging and intervention, and stroke unit care.

In the UK, 30-day mortality after admission to hospital for ischaemic stroke has continued to fall, from 18% in 2007 to 12% in 2020, and for haemorrhagic stroke, from 37% in 2008 to 30% in 2020 (NICE-CKS, 2023). However, care must be taken to look behind the summary figures as the event rate for stroke in younger people (who have a lower case fatality) is increasing.

Despite these achievements, at 6 months after a stroke:

- Up to 30% of patients have died.
- 20–30% have moderate to severe disability.
- 20–30% have mild to moderate disability.
- 20–30% are without deficits.

Figures vary depending on the population, but this gives an overall estimate and shows the need for ongoing support.

Living with a stroke

Everyone should receive a 6 month review by a member of the stroke MDT. This is an opportunity to:

- Review progress and reassess ongoing rehab goals.
- Check secondary prevention and that referrals, e.g. optometry or hearing aids, have taken place.
- Encourage advance care planning, particularly for frail patients or those with significant disabilities.
- Facilitate engagement with community support.

There is qualitative evidence for the benefits of community participation, so systems should encourage patients and families to explore local options and participate in groups. Patients and their families may have been given information shortly after their stroke but have been too overwhelmed to engage. Patients with minor strokes who make a good physical recovery need comprehensive information to enable them to participate in active secondary prevention, recover from the psychological effects, and move forward. Those with ongoing disabilities need encouragement to continue with long-term rehab and may need support with a variety of issues. The Stroke Association and Carers UK are good places to start.

The Stroke Association provides a huge amount of information, e.g. on benefits and equipment, and educational resources – e.g. see the material on visual problems. It hosts a website of other third-sector organisations that provide community stroke support. The range available is wide but depends on the locality. Groups include social meetings, exercise classes, dance, art therapy, music therapy, etc. and support for carers. Transport is often an issue for older people. Some can use the online options; others appreciate a weekly phone call.

Driving advice

After a TIA or stroke of any severity, the patient must not drive for a month and should inform their insurance company. Driving may be resumed after 1 month if there is no residual deficit; if there is a deficit, the Driver and Vehicle Licensing Authority (DVLA) must be informed, and a formal assessment may be required (see Chapter 21). Cognitive and visual problems are more of a challenge than physical limitations, which can be managed by adapting the car.

Other stroke syndromes

Subarachnoid haemorrhage

Subarachnoid haemorrhage (SAH) is a bleed from a cerebral blood vessel, an aneurysm (85% of cases) or vascular malformation, into the subarachnoid space (i.e. the space surrounding the brain where blood vessels lie between the arachnoid and pial layers). SAH accounts for about 5% of strokes. The worldwide incidence of aneurysmal SAH is falling, in parallel with the prevalence of smoking and hypertension. There is geographical variation, with a higher incidence in Finland and Japan. The mean age of aneurysmal SAH is 50–55 years old; however, 10% of patients are older than 75. Older patients have a worse prognosis, with more complications such as intraventricular haemorrhage and hydrocephalus.

The patient classically presents with a severe sudden-onset (thunderclap) headache, often with vomiting and neck stiffness, with or without neurological signs. Older patients can also present in a comatose state or with seizures. About 25% of people die within the first 24 hours, and the overall survival rate is about 70%, half of whom will have residual disability.

CT brain imaging should be obtained urgently. If CT does not confirm the diagnosis, a lumbar puncture should be performed after 12 hours to look for xanthochromia. If the diagnosis is confirmed, oral nimodipine is started; supportive measures are similar for a stroke, with opiate analgesia as required. Discuss the patient urgently with a neurosurgeon and request CT angiography to identify the cause and appropriate treatment. Recent data show better outcomes with endovascular coiling performed by specialist interventional radiologists, but a ruptured aneurysm may be clipped or ablated neurosurgically if coiling is not possible. A decision about treatment will be taken after discussion between the neurosurgeons and interventional radiologists. Tranexamic acid may be considered to reduce the risk of rebleeding if there is a delay in surgical treatment. Treatable complications include secondary hydrocephalus, which may require a surgical drain.

If there is a family history of SAH or polycystic renal disease, genetic counselling is needed. Long-term BP control must be strict, and patients should stop smoking. NICE guidance suggests that treatment with antiplatelet drugs or anticoagulants should not be withheld solely because of an aneurysmal SAH if the culprit aneurysm has been secured by coiling or clipping. Specialist advice should be sought before re-instigating these medications.

Cervical artery dissection

A small proportion of patients with acute ischaemic stroke will have a carotid or vertebral dissection. Patients tend to be younger and may have had neck trauma. CT or MR angiography is needed for diagnosis. This is not a contraindication to acute thrombolysis, and longer-term, antiplatelets or anticoagulants are used.

Central venous thrombosis

Cerebral venous thrombosis is a rare cause of stroke in young adults (mean age 33 years, predominantly female) caused by complete or partial occlusion of the major cerebral venous sinuses (cerebral venous sinus thrombosis) or the smaller feeding cortical veins (cortical vein thrombosis). This may present like a stroke, but there is often a history of headache and fits. It is more common if there is a prothrombotic tendency, e.g. disseminated malignancy or sinus infection. The wide range of clinical findings may be a result of highly variable deep venous system drainage. The damage does not align with an arterial territory. Fewer than 10% cases occur in the over 65s, in whom an underlying cancer, drowsiness and delirium are common, and prognosis is poor. MR venography is often needed for diagnosis. Although there is a risk of bleeding into the brain, the treatment is to anticoagulate. Deteriorating patients can be considered for endovascular procedures. There is no conclusive evidence to support the use of corticosteroids.

Spinal cord infarction

An ischaemic stroke within the arteries supplying the spinal cord is often caused by atherosclerosis or a space-occupying lesion. Spinal strokes account for less than 1% of total strokes. This causes sudden or rapidly progressive paraplegic or quadriplegic symptoms, depending on the site of the lesion. Other symptoms include sensory disturbance, back pain, and incontinence. Patients can describe similar aching pain in their legs (neurogenic claudication) to those suffering from peripheral vascular disease.

Complications can be severe, including infection and pressure sores; however, several (small) studies have suggested that long-term mortality is lower for spinal strokes than for cerebral infarction. This is thought to be related to the lower incidence of other vascular diseases at presentation.

The mainstay of treatment is prompt and determined attempts at physical and psychological rehab, consideration of lifestyle modifications/equipment, and addressing reversible cardiovascular risk factors.

📖 REFERENCES AND FURTHER READING

UK Parliament Hansard Volume 828: (2023) *Stroke Rehabilitation and Community Services* https://hansard.parliament.uk/Lords/2023-03-22/debates/2CF1DE3C-65AF-4444-AC41-C7F47FC899E/StrokeRehabilitationAndCommunityServices See page 1,751

NICE Guideline 128 (updated 2022) *Stroke and transient ischaemic attack in over 16s: diagnosis and initial management.* www.nice.org.uk/guidance/ng128

NICE CKS (2023). *Stroke and TIA.* https://cks.nice.org.uk/topics/stroke-tia.

Canadian stroke best practices – *a useful compilation of recommendations from a transatlantic perspective* https://www.strokebestpractices.ca/resources.

National Clinical Guideline for stroke for the United Kingdom and Ireland 2023 edition London: *Intercollegiate Stroke Working Party;* 2023 *May 4.* Available at: www.strokeguideline.org https://www.strokeguideline.org/contents/?_gl=1*947vkp*_up*MQ..*_ga*MTc3MTA2NDE5LjE3MDExMjY1MTQ.*_ga_EE3BZMVLRT*MTcwMTEyNjUxMy4xLjEuMTcwMTEyNjYyNi4wLjAuMA.

Bamford J, Sandercock P, Dennis M, et al. (1991). Classification and natural history of clinically identifiable subtypes of cerebral infarction. *The Lancet* 337:1521–1526. doi: 10.1016/0140-6736(91)93206-O

Wilbers J, Sondag L, Mulder S et al. (2020). Cancer prevalence higher in stroke patients than in the general population: the Dutch String-of-Pearls Institute (PSI) stroke study. *European Journal of Neurology* 27: 85–91, doi: https://doi.org/10.1111/ene.14037.

Turner M, Murchie P, Derby S et al. (2022). Is stroke incidence increased in survivors of adult cancers? A systematic review and meta-analysis. *Journal of Cancer Survivorship* 16: 1414–1448, doi: 10.1007/s11764-021-01122-7.

Rioux B, Touma L, Nehme A et al. (2021). Frequency and predictors of occult cancer in ischemic stroke: a systematic review and meta-analysis. *International Journal of Stroke* 16: 12–19. DOI: 10.1177/1747493020971104.

NICE Interventional Procedures Guidance 777 (2023) *Percutaneous transarterial carotid artery stent placement for asymptomatic extracranial carotid stenosis.* www.nice.org.uk/guidance/ipg777/chapter/2-The-condition-current-treatments-and-procedure

NICE CKS Scenario: *Secondary prevention following stroke and TIA* (revised 2023) https://cks.nice.org.uk/topics/stroke-tia/management/secondary-prevention-following-stroke-tia

Okumura K, Akao M, Yoshida T et al. for the ELDERCARE-AF group (2020). Low-dose edoxaban in very elderly patients with atrial fibrillation. *NEJM* 383: 1735–1745, https://doi.org/10.1056/NEJMoa2012883.

Evans NR, Tarkin JM, Chowdhury MM et al. (2020). Dual-tracer PET for identification of culprit carotid plaques and pathophysiology in vivo. *Circulation: Cardiovascular Imaging* 13: e009539, doi: 10.1161/CIRCIMAGING.119.009539.

Luengo-Fernandez R, Li L, Silver L et al. (2022) Long-term impact of urgent secondary prevention after transient ischemic attack and minor stroke: ten-year follow-up of the EXPRESS study. *Stroke* 53: 488–496. DOI: 10.1161/STROKEAHA.121.034279.

Flynn D, Ford GA, Rodgers H et al. (2014). A time series evaluation of the FAST National Stroke Awareness Campaign in England. *PLoS One* 9: e104289, doi: https://doi.org/10.1371/journal.pone.0104289

NHS England (2023). Stroke survivors and their 'savers' call on people to act F.A.S.T. as part of NHS campaign https://www.england.nhs.uk/2023/03/stroke-survivors-and-their-savers-call-on-people-to-act-f-a-s-t-as-part-of-nhs-campaign

Potla N, Ganti L (2022). Tenecteplase vs. alteplase for acute ischemic stroke: a systematic review. *International Journal of Emergency Medicine* 15: 1. https://doi.org/10.1186/s12245-021-00399-w.

Pego PM, Nunes AP, Ferreira P et al. (2016). Thrombolysis in patients aged over 80 years is equally effective and safe. *Journal of Stroke Cerebrovascular Diseases* 25: 1532–1538, doi: 10.1016/j.jstrokecerebrovasdis.2016.03.007

Kilic İD, Hakeem A, Marmagkiolis K et al. (2019). Endovascular therapy for acute ischemic stroke: a comprehensive review of current status. *Cardiovascular Revascularization Medicine* 20: 424–431, doi: https://doi.org/10.1016/j.carrev.2018.07.010.

NHS England (2019). Clinical Commissioning Policy: Mechanical thrombectomy for acute ischaemic stroke (all ages) NHS England Reference: 170033P https://www.england.nhs.uk/wp-content/uploads/2019/05/Mechanical-thrombectomy-for-acute-ischaemic-stroke-ERRATA-29-05-19.pdf

Saver JL, Goyal M, van der Lugt A et al. for HERMES Collaborators (2016). Time to treatment with endovascular thrombectomy and outcomes from ischemic stroke: a meta-analysis. *JAMA* 316: 1279–88, doi: https://doi.org/10.1001/jama.2016.13647.

Brainomix (n.d.) https://www.brainomix.com/stroke

NICE Guideline 128 (2019) Evidence reviews for decompressive hemicraniectomy. https://www.ncbi.nlm.nih.gov/books/NBK577869

Sentinel Stroke National Audit Programme SSNAP https://www.strokeaudit.org

SSNAP National results (2023) https://www.strokeaudit.org/Results2/Clinical-audit/National-Results.aspx

Anderson CS, Arima H, Lavados P et al. for HeadPoST investigators (2017) Cluster-randomized, crossover trial of head positioning in acute stroke. *NEJM* 376: 2437–2447. doi: 10.1056/NEJMoa1615715.

Dennis M for the FOCUS collaborators (2019). Effects of fluoxetine on functional outcomes after acute stroke (FOCUS): a pragmatic, double-blind, randomised, controlled trial. *The Lancet* 933: 265–274. https://www.thelancet.com/action/showPdf?pii=S0140-6736%2818%2932823-X.

Shughoury A, Mackay D, Singh S (2023). Visual Neglect. American Academy of Ophthalmology EyeWiki https://eyewiki.aao.org/Visual_Neglect

NICE Guideline 236 (2023) Stroke rehabilitation in adults. www.nice.org.uk/guidance/ng236

Langhorne P, Wu O, Rodgers H et al. (2017). A very early rehabilitation trial after stroke (AVERT): a phase III, multicentre, randomised controlled trial. *Health Technology Assessment* 54: 1–120, doi: 10.3310/hta21540.

The Stroke Foundation. https://thestrokefoundation.org/robotic-arm-helps-in-rehabilitating-arm-use-after-stroke

Langhorne P, Baylan S; Early Supported Discharge Trialists (2017). Early supported discharge services for people with acute stroke. *Cochrane Database of Systematic Reviews* 7: CD000443, doi: 10.1002/14651858.CD000443.pub4.

Krishnamurthi RV, Ikeda T, Feigin VL (2020). Global, regional and country-specific burden of ischaemic stroke, intracerebral haemorrhage and subarachnoid haemorrhage: a systematic analysis of the global burden of disease study 2017. *Neuroepidemiology* 54: 171–179. https://doi.org/10.1159/000506396.

Singh B, Lavezo J, Gavito-Higueroa J et al. (2022). Updated outlook of cerebral amyloid angiopathy and inflammatory subtypes: pathophysiology, clinical manifestations. Diagnosis and management. *Journal of Alzheimer's Disease* 18(6): 627–639, doi: 10.3233/ADR-220055.

Kuhn J, Sharman T (2023) Cerebral Amyloid Angiopathy. StatPearls [Internet]. https://www.ncbi.nlm.nih.gov/books/NBK556105

Schneider AM, Neuhaus AA, Hadley G et al. (2023). Posterior circulation ischaemic stroke diagnosis and management. *Clinical Medicine* 23: 219–227, doi: https://doi.org/10.7861/clinmed.2022-0499.

Seminog OO, Scarborough P, Wright FL et al. (2019). Determinants of the decline in mortality from acute stroke in England: linked national database study of 795 869 adults. *BMJ* 365: l1778, doi: 10.1136/bmj.l1778.

NICE Guideline 228 (2022) Subarachnoid haemorrhage caused by a ruptured aneurysm: diagnosis and management www.nice.org.uk/guidance/ng228

To look at future developments. Clinical Trials.gov is a place to learn about worldwide clinical studies https://clinicaltrials.gov/search?cond=Stroke

INFORMATION FOR PATIENTS AND FAMILIES

Aphasia support: https://aphasiasupport.org

Carers UK: https://www.carersuk.org

Information about visual problems: www.stroke.org.uk/vision_problems_after_stroke_guide.pdf

Stroke Association: www.stroke.org.uk

All websites were accessed in August 2024.

10

Musculoskeletal

Bone metabolism

The skeleton is essential for locomotion, breathing, protection of internal organs, haematopoiesis, and calcium metabolism. Bone is not static; it changes throughout life due to remodelling. About 1% of the skeleton is turned over each day; the skeleton is said to be replaced every 10 years. There is a delicate balance between bone formation and resorption. Bone homeostasis ensures the maintenance of bone integrity, the repair of micro-damage, the replacement of brittle older bone, and the adaptation of bone to mechanical and metabolic demands. It involves a complex interplay between bone cells (osteoblasts, osteocytes, and osteoclasts), hormones, and environmental factors.

Osteoblasts build bone. They sit on the bone surface, make new osteoid, and mineralise this using calcium and phosphate released by bone resorption. Osteoblasts also secrete proteins, including Receptor Activator of Nuclear Factor Kappa-B ligand (RANKL) and osteoprotegerin (OPG). These have opposing effects.

- RANKL has a role in osteoclast formation, function, and survival, promoting bone resorption.
- OPG is soluble and binds RANKL, preventing osteoclast action and protecting against bone loss.

As new bone is made, up to 20% of the osteoblasts become entrapped in the bone and differentiate into osteocytes.

Osteocytes, the most numerous cells in bone, develop long dendritic cell processes to form a neuron-like network through the bone. Osteocytes are important for maintaining bone mineralisation. They also detect mechanical loading and play a critical role in bone remodelling through the secretion of paracrine factors regulating the differentiation and activity of osteoblasts and osteoclasts. Sclerostin is a key osteocyte-derived factor that suppresses bone formation by inhibiting a pathway known as Wnt.

Osteoclasts break down bone. Osteoclast precursors also sit on the bone surface, and when they are activated, they fuse to produce multinucleated giant cells. They move to areas of microfracture and start to reabsorb bone, so active osteoclasts are found in pits on the bone surface. Osteoclast precursors and mature osteoclasts have RANK receptors. When RANKL binds to RANK receptors on several mononucleate osteoclast precursors, it stimulates them to fuse into multinucleate osteoclasts. RANKL activates osteoclasts to secrete enzymes including collagenase, which break down the osteoid (a collagen protein matrix), and acid to break down crystals of hydroxyapatite into its constituent calcium and phosphate.

Factors affecting bone remodelling

- Several genes affect how bone is laid down and remodelled.
- Weight-bearing exercise and mechanical stress on bones stimulate osteoblastic activity.
- Adequate calcium and phosphate levels are essential for bone mineralisation.
- Parathyroid hormone (PTH) stimulates osteoclasts, releasing calcium into the blood stream.
- Calcitonin inhibits osteoclasts, promoting calcium deposition in the bone.
- The ratio of RANKL to OPG plays a vital role.
- Cytokines and growth factors also regulate the balance between osteoclast and osteoblast activity. Interleukins 1 and 6 influence osteoclasts and, thus, bone resorption. Bone morphogenetic proteins such as transforming growth factor beta (TGF-β) stimulate bone formation.

Bone ageing

1 Adipose tissue accumulates in the bone marrow, and there is loss of mesenchymal stem cells, which leads to a decline in osteoblast numbers.
2 Bone is lost because resorption by osteoclasts exceeds production by osteoblasts.
3 Oestrogen inhibits osteoclasts, promotes osteoblasts, limits RANKL production, and promotes OPG production. When oestrogen levels fall at the menopause, changes in all these factors favour bone resorption.
4 Testosterone, which also promotes bone formation, decreases gradually as men age, but declining bioavailable oestrogen levels in men may be more important later in life.
5 Most older people exercise less.
6 Inflammation increases with ageing, and pro-inflammatory cytokines such as IL-6 stimulate osteoclasts.
7 Vitamin D deficiency is more common and impairs calcium absorption and bone mineralisation.
8 Bone loss per year is 0.2% of the total from the age of 35 years. This rate of loss increases to 1% after menopause in women. Therefore, on average, by the age of 80, a woman will have lost 30% of her bone mass, whilst a man of the same age will have lost 10%. Peak bone mass is generally higher in men, so they have a greater reserve.
9 Ageing affects trabecular bone more than cortical bone. The shape of long bones also changes with increasing age; the internal cavity increases in diameter, the outer cortical layer becomes thinner, and the total bone diameter is expanded. These changes result in weaker bones.

Geriatric Medicine and Elderly Care: Lecture Notes, Ninth Edition. Claire G. Nicholl, K. Jane Wilson, and Shaun D'Souza.
© 2025 John Wiley & Sons Ltd. Published 2025 by John Wiley & Sons Ltd.
Companion website: www.wiley.com/go/lecturenotesgeriatricmedicine9e

Osteoporosis

Osteoporosis is a disease characterised by low bone mass and structural deterioration of bone tissue, with a consequent increase in bone fragility and susceptibility to fracture (see Figure 10.1). It is defined by the WHO as a bone mineral density (BMD) of 2.5 standard deviations below the mean peak mass (average of young, healthy adults) as measured by dual-energy x-ray absorptiometry (DXA) applied to the femoral neck and reported as a T-score. However, BMD measurement does not assess bone structure, and most osteoporotic fractures occur in women who do not have a T-score $\leq$–2.5. The molecular composition of osteoporotic bone is similar to normal bone, but the micro-architecture is disorganised so that the bone is fragile and at increased risk of fracturing from low-energy trauma, e.g. falling from standing or even a twisting movement.

Epidemiology

- In women, the incidence of osteoporosis increases markedly, from around 2% at 50 years old to almost 50% at 80 years old.
- In England and Wales, more than two million women have osteoporosis.
- White women and men are at increased risk of fragility fracture compared with other ethnic groups.
- Around one in two women and one in five men will sustain one or more osteoporotic fractures in their lifetime.

Financial burden

- There are 549,000 fragility fractures per year in the UK (National Osteoporosis Guidelines Group, NOGG 2021).
- This costs the NHS £5.4 billion per year (2.4% of total healthcare spend, 2019).
- 25% of UK orthopaedic beds are occupied by patients with fractured hips. Patients admitted with osteoporotic fractures account for over one million bed days annually in the NHS.

Classification

Osteoporosis may be primary (which includes age-related and postmenopausal osteoporosis) or secondary where there is a clearly defined cause. Older women usually have age-related and postmenopausal bone loss, with a variable contribution from lifestyle factors and comorbidities. Secondary osteoporosis is more common in men, especially in younger men, where over half of cases may be secondary (alcohol abuse, glucocorticoid excess and hypogonadism being the most common).

Risk factors

- Age > 65.
- Female sex: the fall in oestrogen at menopause causes a marked acceleration of bone loss, as described earlier.
- Failure to achieve good peak bone mass by early adulthood because of poor nutrition or low oestrogen, e.g. secondary to anorexia nervosa.
- Family history, especially maternal hip fracture.
- Previous fragility fractures double the fracture risk.
- Lifestyle:
  - Low BMI (<20 kg/m²).
  - Vegan diet.
  - Smoking (inhibits calcium absorption, causes chronic inflammation, reduces blood supply to bone, toxic effect on bone cells, and impairs collagen synthesis).
  - Alcohol excess (dose-dependent; also increases falls risk).
  - Lack of exercise (weight-bearing activity is particularly important for maintaining BMD).
  - High caffeine intake increases calcium excretion and reduces calcium, increasing PTH levels.
- Coexisting diseases:
  Their effects are usually multifactorial and may include direct endocrine effects, chronic inflammation where inflammatory molecules and cells accelerate bone loss, drug effects, low activity levels and limited sun exposure with vitamin D deficiency.
- Endocrine disorders:
  - Type 1 and 2 diabetes.
  - Hypogonadism, including untreated premature menopause.
  - Hyperthyroidism (accelerated bone resorption, lower bone density and increased fracture risk, especially in younger people).
  - Primary and secondary hyperparathyroidism.
  - Cushing's syndrome.
- Malabsorption leading to reduced levels of calcium and vitamin D, e.g. due to:
  - Coeliac disease.
  - Chronic pancreatitis.
  - Crohn's disease (plus may be taking oral steroids).
  - Gastric surgery.
- Drugs:
  - Steroids: 30–50% of patients on long-term glucocorticoids will have a fracture.
  - Antiepileptics, especially phenytoin, decrease the absorption of vitamin D.
  - Hormone-blocking treatments, e.g. for breast cancer (tamoxifen) or prostate cancer (goserelin).

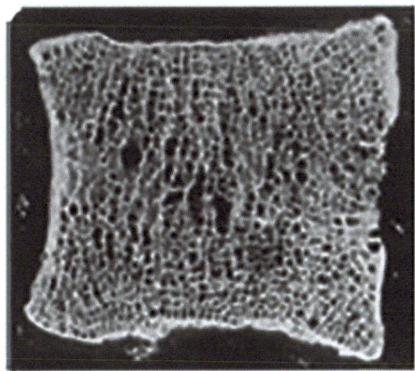

Normal bone

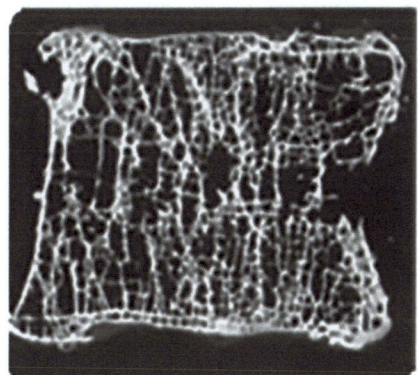

Osteoporotic bone

Figure 10.1 Bone from a healthy 37-year-old male on the left and bone from a 75-year-old woman with osteoporosis on the right. *Source*: Turner Biomechanics Laboratory/Wikimedia Commons/Public domain.

- o SSRIs.
- o Proton pump inhibitors (PPIs).
- o Thiazolidinediones.
- Inflammatory conditions:
  - o Rheumatoid arthritis (RA) increases the risk of osteoporosis, independent of BMD.
- Chronic diseases:
  - o Chronic kidney disease (CKD), liver disease, COPD, and CHF.
  - o Parkinson's disease, recently recognised as a secondary risk factor (via reduced physical activity, chronic inflammation, and endocrine effects).
  - o Stroke

Falls are not a cause of osteoporosis but are strongly predictive of osteoporotic fractures. There is some confounding, as frequent fallers are not likely to exercise and may have other conditions that do cause osteoporosis.

Clinical features

Osteoporosis is asymptomatic until there is a fracture.

- A Colles' wrist fracture in women aged 50–65 is often the first presentation.
- Vertebral fractures may present with back pain, loss of height and dorsal kyphosis and cause considerable morbidity.
- Hip fractures have the highest mortality and are the commonest reason for urgent surgery in older people. Figure 10.2 shows a comminuted fracture of the left hip.
- Other fractures associated with osteoporosis include the neck of the humerus, pelvis, sacrum (difficult to see on a plain x-ray), and distal tibia/fibula.
- Fractures result in pain, reduced mobility, reduction in quality of life, loss of independence, an increased risk of being admitted to a care home, and increased mortality.

Fractured hip

A hip fracture or fractured neck of a femur is a fracture of the femur proximal to 5 cm below the lesser trochanter. Hip fracture incidence has stabilised or even reduced in many countries in recent years, but this reduction is insufficient to offset the increase as the global population

ages. There are now over 75,000 cases each year in the UK – 75% of whom are aged over 75. The number predicted worldwide in 2050 is 6.26 million. A hip fracture presents with pain in the hip and an inability to weight bear after falling. However, if the fracture is impacted, the patient may still be able to walk. The affected leg is shortened because the hip is flexed and externally rotated. If there is clinical suspicion but no fracture is seen on x-ray, ask for a CT hip.

National hip fracture database

There has been a national drive to improve outcomes for patients with hip fractures, led by the collaboration of the BGS and the British Orthopaedic Association (BOA) and the creation of the National Hip Fracture Database. All NHS trusts enter data about every patient admitted with a hip fracture. Enhanced clinical auditing with benchmarking and research has led to the identification of areas for service improvement and driven this through the development of best practice tariffs. There is a long history of individual geriatricians working in this area, but this has led to the national acceptance of orthogeriatrics as a major clinical subspecialty of geriatric medicine.

Management

The best outcomes are seen where there is close working between orthopaedic surgeons, anaesthetists, orthogeriatricians – geriatricians with a specialist interest in fragility fractures, working with a dedicated multidisciplinary team and fracture liaison service. Best practice includes:

- A pain score and nerve block in the ED, IV fluids and transfer to an orthopaedic ward within 4 hr.
- Rapid assessment by an orthogeriatrician, including a falls assessment. Review by an orthogeriatrician can reduce the cost per patient by £529 and reduce the odds ratio of mortality at 365 days to 0.8.
- Initial assessment of cognition and risk of delirium.
- Good nursing and medical management include effective analgesia, VTE prophylaxis, and rapid optimisation of medical conditions without delaying surgery unless essential, pressure area care, avoidance of routine catheterisation, avoiding prolonged nil-by-mouth, liaising with the family, identifying barriers to discharge, etc.
- Surgery within 36 hr on a planned daytime trauma list. Delay leads to a longer length of stay with a higher risk of nosocomial adverse events.
- Good therapy management includes mobilisation within a day of surgery and daily thereafter, including at weekends. More patients regain their premorbid mobility if they are mobilised early. Weekend physiotherapy (PT) can reduce the length of stay by 2.32 days and reduce the cost by £676. Occupational therapy (OT) input expedites discharge, particularly for frailer patients, to their own homes.
- Continued attention to measures to reduce delirium and maximise recovery: good nutrition, bowel care, etc.
- Plan for secondary prevention of osteoporosis. Some centres are pragmatically giving IV zoledronate before discharge if the vitamin D is >40 nmol/L and the creatinine clearance is >30–35 mL/min, recognising that the frailest patients may be too frail to return for an infusion and may not live long enough to need a second dose.

Surgical fixation

The type of surgery depends on the fracture and the patient (see Figure 10.3), but the aim is to allow full weight bearing in the immediate post-operative period. Surgery can also be a palliative measure to control pain in very frail people with a life expectancy of days to a few weeks.

- A femoral neck fracture is also known as sub-capital or intracapsular. In intracapsular fractures, the blood supply to the femoral head is damaged, so there is more likelihood of non-union and avascular necrosis of the femoral head, particularly with the simplest procedure,

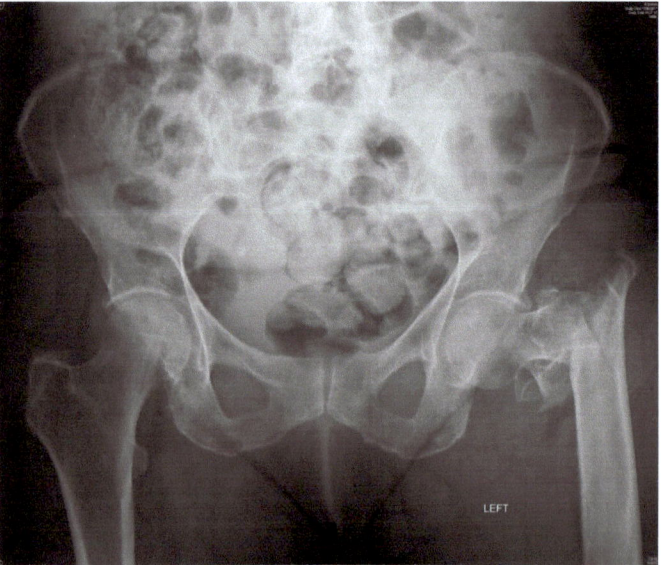

Figure 10.2 Radiograph of a comminuted intertrochanteric fracture of the left hip.

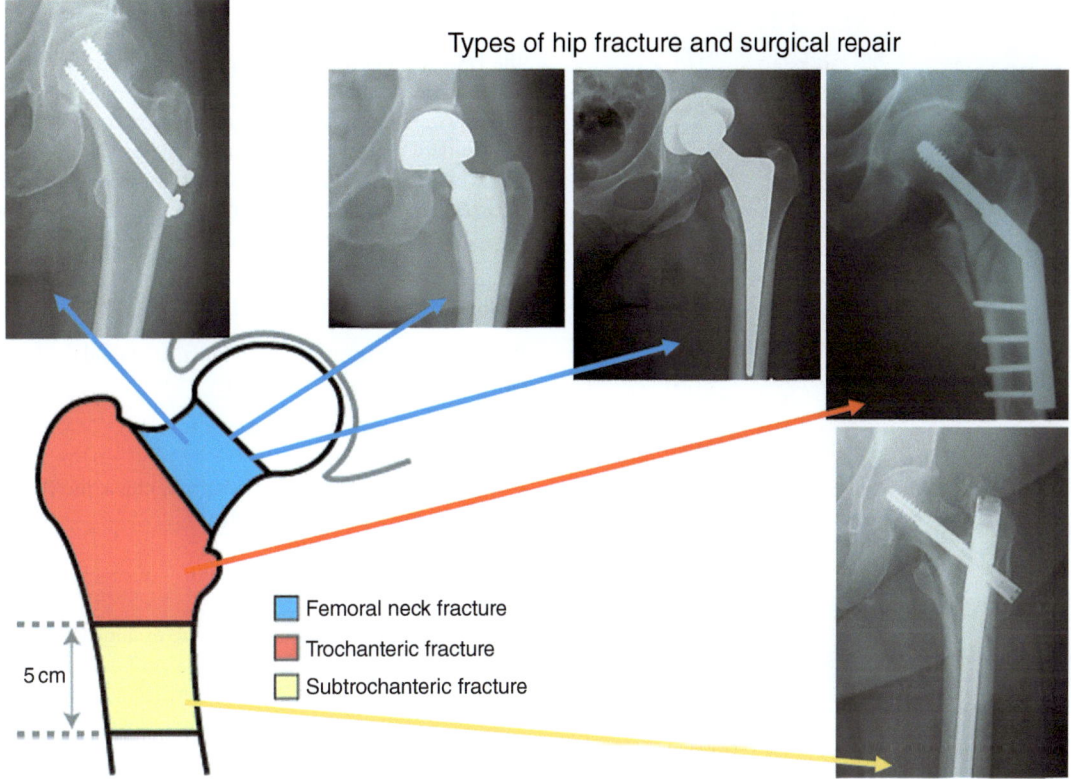

Types of hip fracture and surgical repair

Femoral neck fracture
Trochanteric fracture
Subtrochanteric fracture

5 cm

Figure 10.3 A simplified outline of the types of hip fractures and the usual approach to surgery.

which is reduction and internal fixation with cancellous screws. Femoral head replacement is preferred. In hemiarthroplasty, only the head and neck are replaced. The addition of an acetabular cup results in a total hip replacement or total hip arthroplasty (the biggest operation so only considered for those able to walk outdoors before their fracture, with a good prognosis for independence). Confusingly, hemiarthroplasty can be unipolar (fixed) or bipolar, which has an acetabular cup that fits into the existing acetabulum but is not fixed to it.

- Intertrochanteric and subtrochanteric fractures are subcapsular (extracapsular).

  Trochanteric fractures: sliding hip screws, e.g. dynamic hip screws.
  Subtrochanteric fractures: intramedullary nail.

Outcomes

- The mortality rate at 1 month after a hip fracture is around 6% in England.
- At the end of 1 year, the mortality rate is 26%.
- 70% of people with hip fractures return to their original residence.
- 40% never regain their full premorbid function.
- The cost per person is currently £14,700.
- 50% of patients admitted with hip fractures have had a previous fracture, but only 12% are taking bone protection, i.e. there has been a missed opportunity for secondary prevention.

Pelvic fractures

Fractures commonly occur in the pubic rami (see Figure 10.4); as the pelvis is a ring, it is likely to fracture in two places, so always look for a second fracture.

- Often caused by trivial trauma after falling.
- Produces severe groin pain that is worse when getting up from sitting and walking.
- Treatment is conservative: appropriate analgesia and early mobilisation.

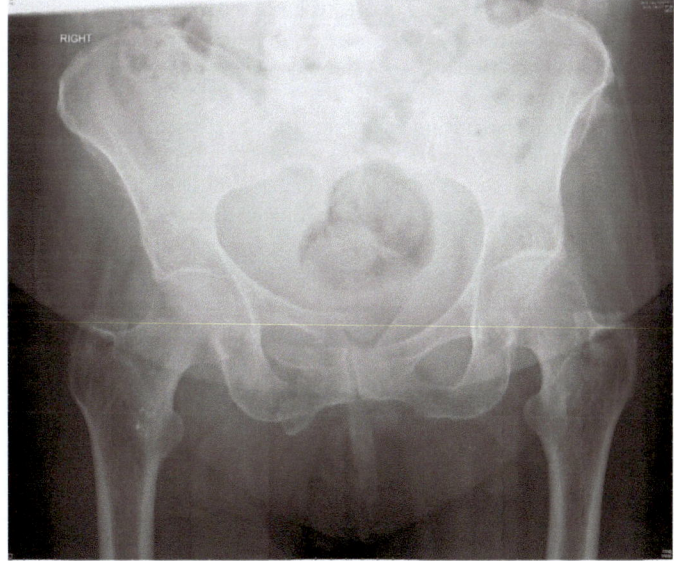

Figure 10.4 X-ray of fractured right inferior pubic ramus.

- Most heal within 6–8 weeks.
- The mortality rate at 1 year is 15–20%.
- Remember to start secondary prevention of osteoporosis.

Vertebral fractures

These are common in postmenopausal women and are underdiagnosed and therefore undertreated. They may be noted on CT scans performed for other reasons (Figure 10.5), but even when present, may not be reported.

- Vertebral fractures may present with severe mid-thoracic or low back pain, often with no history of trauma, and may be misdiagnosed as 'muscular' pain.

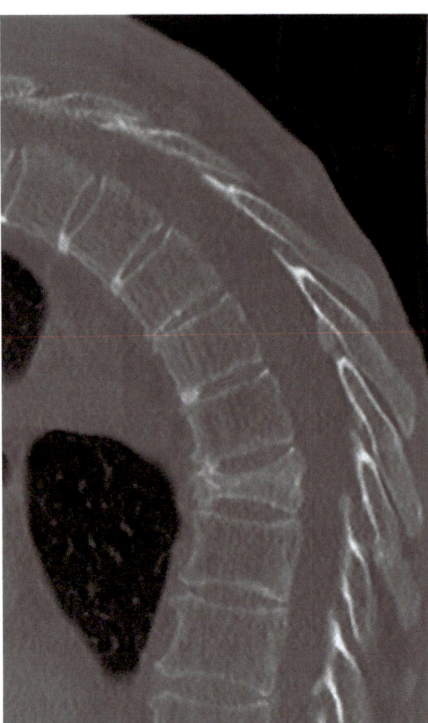

Figure 10.5 CT scan shows a fracture of the T8 vertebral body contributing to marked dorsal kyphosis.

- A loss of >4 cm in height suggests at least one vertebral fracture. More marked loss of height and dorsal kyphosis occur if there are multiple vertebral fractures.
- Diagnosis should lead to the full assessment of bone density and treatment for osteoporosis.
- Serious sequelae include chronic pain, decreased mobility, and reduced quality of life.
- Dorsal kyphosis results in increased lumbar lordosis and a protuberant abdomen. There may be contact between the ribs and iliac crests. Both can cause abdominal discomfort. Severe kyphosis carries great social stigma, makes dressing, eating, and walking difficult, and may reduce chest wall mobility sufficiently to lead to type 2 respiratory failure.
- Cord compression is a rare complication of osteoporotic vertebral collapse.

Assessing the risk of osteoporosis

- All patients with a fragility fracture should be assessed for osteoporosis and secondary prevention.
- As the first clinical sign of osteoporosis is a fracture, efforts are made to identify asymptomatic, high-risk individuals so that they can be offered primary prevention. NICE recommends assessing:
  - All women aged 65 years and over, and all men aged 75 years and over.
  - All women aged 50–64 years and all men aged 50–74 years with a major risk factor.

Use an online risk calculator to collate clinical information and risk factors, either QFracture' (preferred by NICE, CKS, and SIGN) or the WHO FRAX' tool (preferred by NOGG), which can include BMD. These tools provide an estimation of the 10-year probability of a hip fracture or a major osteoporotic fracture (spine, wrist, hip, or shoulder). If treatment is being considered, a DXA scan is preferred as a baseline to monitor treatment, but if scan availability is limited, NICE recommends treating women aged 75+ with a prior fragility fracture. FRAX gives an intervention threshold that can be used to recommend treatment if DXA is not feasible. Both tools are included in the Appendix.

DXA scanning

The DXA scanner measures bone density, usually at the proximal femur and lumbar vertebrae (because these are clinically important sites for fragility fractures). As noted earlier, osteoporosis is defined as a BMD less than 2.5 standard deviations below that of a normal pre-menopausal woman and is expressed as a T score (i.e. T – 2.5 or below). Osteopenia describes a decrease in BMD below normal reference values, yet not low enough to meet the diagnostic criteria for osteoporosis, i.e. a T score of –1 to –2.5.

Investigations for secondary osteoporosis

Basic biochemistry and thyroid function should be checked in everyone. Other tests are done if indicated.

- Liver and renal function tests.
- Bone function tests.
- If serum or urine calcium is raised, check the PTH level to exclude primary hyperparathyroidism.
- Thyroid function tests.
- Testosterone: in men with suspected hypogonadotropic hypogonadism.
- Dexamethasone suppression test to exclude Cushing's disease.
- Tissue transglutaminase (tTG-IgA) antibodies to exclude coeliac disease (see Gastroenterology chapter 14).
- ESR, serum immunoglobulins, light chains or urinary Bence–Jones protein to exclude myeloma.

Management
Prevention

These measures should be discussed with people with osteopenia and osteoporosis to help minimise deterioration.

- Adequate nutrition, especially protein and calcium (minimum of 700 mg) – found in dairy and fish.
- Exercise should be regular and weight-bearing, e.g. brisk walking, upper body resistance exercises, Tai Chi. There is no evidence that a higher level of exercise works better.
- Stop smoking and reduce alcohol intake (≤2 units a day).
- Maintain levels of vitamin D greater than 75 nmol/L. NHS guidelines are for all adults to take 400 IU (10 µg) daily from October to March in the UK as sunshine is limited, or year-round if frail.
- Hormone replacement therapy is most useful for women in early menopause.
- Offer bisphosphonates to those treated with ≥7.5 mg of prednisolone for three or more months.
- Refer to a falls prevention programme, if appropriate.

General measures for osteoporosis

- Educate the patient and their family about osteoporosis.
- Provide information about patient support groups.
- Treat the causes of secondary osteoporosis.
- Effective pain control is essential for all osteoporotic fractures to promote early remobilisation.
- Consider a PT referral for advice about a suitable exercise programme.
- Prescribe appropriate medication. Concordance with oral medication for this long-term condition is extremely poor, even 3 months after it is first prescribed. Good explanations may help. There are different preparations of vitamin D and calcium, including soluble and capsule forms as well as the familiar chalky tablets, so work with each patient to find the most palatable option for them. Consider yearly zoledronate or 6 monthly denosumab injections; they are expensive but are cheaper than hospital admission for fractures.

Drug treatment

Calcium and vitamin D

The debate about the use of calcium and vitamin D continues, including the efficacy of each element, the optimum dose, and possible harms. Calcium and vitamin D reduce hip fractures in frail care home residents, but there is controversy about their use in older people living in the community. There is limited evidence that calcium supplements improve BMD or reduce fractures, and they may increase renal stones and the risk of vascular events. The rapid rise in blood calcium after taking a tablet (as opposed to absorbing calcium from food) could be a factor in calcifying the coronary arteries. Vitamin D has benefits for people who are deficient but not otherwise.

The Scientific Advisory Committee on Nutrition is undertaking a new review of this controversial area. Pragmatically, if a patient has a good dietary calcium intake, give vitamin D alone; otherwise, use a combination. However, all the trials demonstrating the efficacy of bisphosphonates and teriparatide co-prescribed a calcium and vitamin D combination.

Specific drugs

Drugs for osteoporosis are divided into those that limit bone resorption and those that build bone (see Table 10.1). Bisphosphonates and denosumab can be used for primary and secondary prevention in women and men. The other options are restricted to secondary prevention.

Antiresorptive agents

Bisphosphonates

- Bisphosphonates, e.g. alendronate, risedronate, and zoledronate, are anti-resorptive. They are analogues of pyrophosphate and attach to hydroxyapatite binding sites on the bone. As osteoclasts resorb bone, the bisphosphonate is released and impairs the osteoclast's ability to adhere and continue bone resorption.
- Effects are seen in the first 6–12 months of use.
- They are proven to increase bone mass in the spine and hips and reduce fractures.
- Alendronate or risedronate, given weekly, are first-line medications in primary care. They must be taken on an empty stomach with a glass of plain water to ensure absorption, prevent the formation of complexes with calcium, and reduce the risk of oesophagitis. Thus, patients only need to miss their early morning cup of tea once a week! The patient also must remain upright (sitting is OK) for 30 min to reduce the risk of oesophageal ulceration.
- Gastrointestinal side effects are most common.
- IV zoledronate is given annually. The infusion is usually given in hospitals because a few patients developed atrial fibrillation in the drug trials. More common side effects include flu-like symptoms, fever, headache, diarrhoea, and vomiting. Zoledronate is more potent than the other bisphosphonates. It is useful if adherence to oral drugs is problematic.
- Bisphosphonates can cause hypocalcaemia and hypophosphatemia.
- Osteonecrosis of the jaw is a rare complication, affecting 1 in 100,000. It is more likely in patients on high-dose bisphosphonates for cancer, but advise patients to inform their dentists if they are planning any invasive dental treatment.
- Another rare complication is an atypical stress fracture below the neck of the femur which produces a characteristic 'beak' appearance on the radiograph of the fracture site or a clean snap.
- Contraindicated in hypocalcaemia and oesophageal abnormalities and avoided if creatinine clearance is less than 30–35 mL/min.
- Current advice is to reassess the patient's risk–benefit ratio after 5 years of treatment and consider stopping the bisphosphonate. Some protection persists.

Denosumab

Denosumab is a human monoclonal antibody to RANK ligand.

- It is given by subcutaneous injections 6 monthly to postmenopausal women. The mechanism of action is shown in Figure 10.6.
- Side effects include hypocalcaemia, infections such as cellulitis and cystitis, skin problems such as eczema and dermatitis, musculoskeletal pain affecting areas including the back and extremities, and a few reports of osteonecrosis of the jaw and atypical fractures. Severe allergic reactions are rare.
- Denosumab must not be given without correcting calcium and vitamin D levels.
- If creatinine clearance is less than 30 mL/minute, monitor for hypocalcaemia.

Table 10.1 Summary of types of treatment for osteoporosis.

Antiresorptive agents	Anabolic agents
Bisphosphonates: alendronate, risedronate orally, weekly zoledronate IV infusion, annually	**PTH analogue:** Teriparatide SC injection, daily
MAb to RANKL: Denosumab SC injection, 6 monthly	**MAb to sclerostin:** Romosozumab SC injection, monthly
Selective oestrogen receptor modulator: raloxifene orally, daily	

IV, intravenous; SC, subcutaneous; IM, intramuscular; MAb monoclonal antibody; RANKL, RANK ligand; PTH, parathyroid hormone.

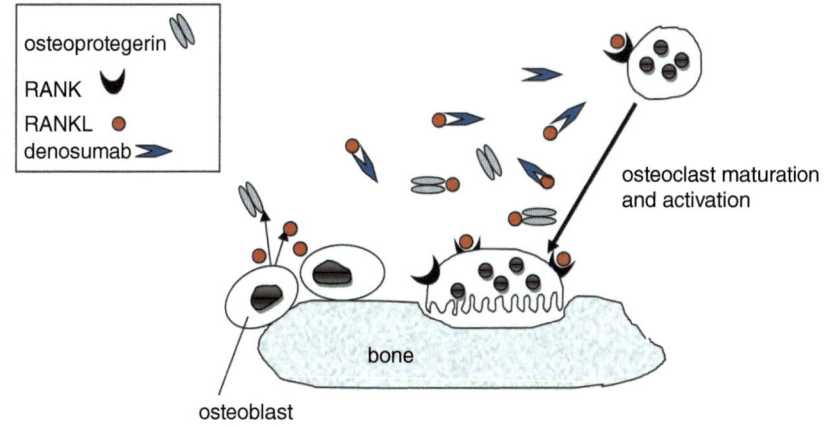

Figure 10.6 The mechanism of action of denosumab. Osteoblasts build bone and have a role in bone resorption by producing RANK ligand (RANKL) and osteoprotegerin. RANKL binds to its receptor RANK and mediates osteoclast differentiation, activation, and survival. The protein osteoprotegerin binds to RANKL and functions as an endogenous inhibitor of this pathway. Denosumab is a monoclonal antibody to RANKL and functions like osteoprotegerin, mopping up RANKL, reducing osteoclast activity, and decreasing bone resorption.

- When it is discontinued, the patient must be treated with another preparation, e.g. IV zoledronate, or there is profound rebound bone resorption, and multiple vertebral fractures may occur.

Anabolic agents
Teriparatide

Teriparatide is a recombinant fragment of the terminal 1–34N amino acids of PTH. Given intermittently, PTH is anabolic and stimulates osteoblast activity, contrary to the effect of continuous endogenous PTH, which is catabolic.

- It is usually self-administered by daily subcutaneous injection for a maximum of 24 months.
- Restricted to patients with severe disease (particularly in the vertebra) who have not tolerated or responded to other treatments because of cost.
- When the course is completed, IV zoledronate is usually given to avoid losing the new bone.
- Side effects include gastrointestinal upset, hypercalcaemia, and hypercalciuria, with an increased risk of renal stones and gout.
- Caution in moderate renal impairment; avoid if severe.

Romosozumab

Romosozumab is a humanised monoclonal antibody that binds to sclerostin. It stimulates osteoblasts and reduces bone resorption by osteoclasts, leading to rapid bone formation.

- Highly effective in vertebral osteoporosis.
- NICE guidelines restrict its use to postmenopausal women who have already sustained a fracture and are deemed to have a substantial risk of further fractures, because of cost. It is administered by monthly subcutaneous injection (two injections at different sites) for 1 year.
- When the course is completed, another treatment must be given, or all the new bone will be lost.
- Contraindicated in patients with hypocalcaemia, heart attack or stroke within the last year.
- Can be used in severe renal failure or dialysis if calcium is monitored.

Selective oestrogen receptor modulators

Selective oestrogen receptor modulators (SERMs), e.g. raloxifene, act as oestrogen agonists in the bone and liver but as oestrogen antagonists in the breast and uterus. They therefore increase bone density without increasing the risk of breast or uterine cancer. Only the risk of vertebral fractures is reduced. Raloxifene is NO LONGER recommended for primary prevention but can be used for secondary prevention if other treatments are contraindicated or not tolerated.

- Contraindicated in premenopausal women.
- Common side effects are hot flushes, leg cramps, and peripheral oedema.
- Rare but serious side effects include an increased risk of venous thromboembolism and stroke.
- Caution in mild to moderate renal impairment and avoid, if severe.

Strontium

Withdrawn from the UK in 2017 because of cardiac concerns and a fall in market share, it returned in 2019 as an option for severe osteoporosis when other drugs are contraindicated.

Calcitonin

Withdrawn for treatment of osteoporosis in Europe and the UK in 2012 because of concern about the increase in cancer, but still available for short-term use in Paget's disease of the bone (PDB) and hypercalcaemia of malignancy.

Vertebral augmentation

Two similar procedures can physically restore the shape of a wedged osteoporotic vertebra.

- In **vertebroplasty**, a needle is inserted into the collapsed vertebra, and methyl methacrylate (bone cement) is injected under high pressure to expand the vertebra.
- In **kyphoplasty**, a balloon is inflated in the vertebra to expand the vertebra by creating a cavity, which is then filled with bone cement at low pressure.

Both improve pain and quality of life in the short term, but studies using a sham procedure suggest that the effect is due to a placebo response rather than the vertebral augmentation. In 2013, NICE approved the procedures for severe ongoing pain after a recent vertebral fracture, despite optimal pain management. This is quoted by the private clinics that offer these procedures. However, recent Cochrane reviews found vertebroplasty has no important benefit in terms of pain, disability, or quality of life compared with a sham procedure. Kyphoplasty has not been compared to a sham procedure, but head-to-head results are similar to vertebroplasty. Numerous serious adverse events have been observed following vertebroplasty. However, these procedures are still recommended by the Royal Osteoporosis Society.

Osteomalacia

This is impaired mineralisation of the osteoid matrix due to vitamin D deficiency. The amount of bone is normal, but it is soft and weak compared with normal bone. In children, this leads to rickets.

Prevalence

This is uncertain and depends on the population studied.

- Average UK population: 0.1%. It is increasing.
- Post-mortem study of older patients: 12%.
- Biopsies of the bone of patients with hip fractures: 25%.

Causes
Reduced vitamin D availability

- Deficient diet (inadequate D_2 and D_3).
- Reduced sun exposure: most common in Muslim and Hindu cultures (where women cover their heads) and home-bound older people, but also seen in those who adhere strictly to sun avoidance and use high SPF sunscreen to reduce melanoma risk. Ultraviolet light converts 7-dehydrocholesterol to a pre-vitamin D_3 and then to vitamin D_3 (cholecalciferol). Ten to fifteen minutes exposure to sunlight in the UK summer is sufficient to replenish the body's stores. Vitamin D-binding protein carries D_2 and D_3 to the liver, which converts them to 25-hydroxyvitamin D. Then 1-alpha-hydroxylase in the proximal tubule of the kidney converts it to 1, 25-dihydroxycholecalciferol.
- Malabsorption of vitamin D from food and supplements occurs in coeliac disease, diverticular disease of the small bowel, postgastrectomy, and pancreatic insufficiency.

Impaired vitamin D metabolism

- CKD (reduced activity of 1-hydroxylation).
- Drugs that induce liver enzymes, e.g. phenytoin and carbamazepine.

Clinical features

- Pain in the axial skeleton (spine, shoulders, ribs, and pelvis).
- Muscle weakness, usually proximal, leads to a waddling gait and difficulty standing from sitting.
- Fragility fractures.

Investigations

- X-rays may show insufficiency fractures or Looser's zones.
- Bone scintigram may show 'hungry bones', so-called because the bones take up the isotope so readily that they are very bright, and the kidneys may not be visible.
- Blood tests: raised alkaline phosphatase (ALP), low corrected calcium, low phosphate, and raised PTH.
- Serum 25-hydroxyvitamin D_3 is low.
- A bone biopsy will clinch the diagnosis where there is doubt.

Treatment

- Oral vitamin D supplements: there is a lack of clarity about the loading dose for severe deficiency; up to 50,000 international units may be given once a week for 6 weeks. Note: 1 µg of vitamin D is the same as 40 IU. Long term maintenance is then be given (400 IU daily).
- In renal disease, give a hydroxylated preparation, i.e. alfacalcidol or calcitriol.
- Watch for hypercalcaemia.

Paget's disease of the bone

Paget's disease of the bone (PDB) is a localised abnormality of bone due to increased numbers and activity of osteoclasts, leading to marked bone resorption. The osteoclasts are abnormally large and contain more nuclei, which have inclusion bodies. Bone resorption is followed by increased osteoblast activity, producing bone with an abnormal matrix that is expanded but weak and more likely to deform and fracture.

PDB most frequently affects the pelvis (70%), femur (55%), lumbar and thoracic spine (53%), skull (42%), and tibia (32%), but it can occur in any bone. A single bone is affected in 10% of cases.

Epidemiology

The incidence increases with age. There is a slight male preponderance. PDB has a striking geographical distribution. It is more common in the UK, especially Northwest England (fascinatingly, 15% of the 14th-century skeletons from Norton Priory in Cheshire had extensive Paget-like disease), Northern Europe apart from Scandinavia and Ireland, and people of European descent living in Australia and New Zealand, but much less common in Asian and African countries. The age-adjusted incidence has been falling steadily since the second half of the 20th century. Current figures are not available, but the prevalence among those aged ≥85 is probably now less than 5%.

Aetiology

This remains unknown, but the epidemiology supports both a genetic basis and a strong environmental trigger.

Familial cases of PDB have been linked to multiple mutations in the sequestosome 1 gene (*SQSTM1*), which can increase activation of RANKL, which may explain the focal nature of the abnormal bone.

Reduced exposure to viruses, including measles and respiratory syncytial virus, or environmental toxins, such as heavy metals, have been postulated to explain the falling incidence of PDB, but neither has been proven.

Clinical features

PDB is usually asymptomatic and diagnosed incidentally because of an isolated raised ALP or on imaging.

- Pain affects 40% of cases and may be localised to the affected bone (microfractures are common) or secondary to nerve entrapment, including radiculopathy.
- Deformity is present in 30% of cases, e.g. enlargement of the skull, anterior bowing of the tibia, or lateral bowing of the femur.
- The skin overlying the affected bone may be hot to the touch due to the increased blood supply.

Complications

- Fractures of abnormal bone, usually the femur or tibia.
- Secondary osteoarthritis (OA) of adjacent joints.
- Neurological: compression of the cranial nerves as they exit the skull most commonly affects the eighth nerve but can also affect the second and the fifth. Hydrocephalus due to brainstem compression and paraplegia due to spinal cord compression are very rare.
- The increased vascularity of the affected bone can cause bleeding during orthopaedic surgery, but high-output heart failure is rare.
- The development of malignant tumours is also rare, e.g. osteosarcoma incidence <1%.

Investigations

- Raised serum ALP.
- Raised urinary hydroxyproline suggests active disease.
- Serum calcium is raised in patients who are immobile. (Hyperparathyroidism is a much more common cause of hypercalcaemia.)
- Check the vitamin D level, both to rule out other causes of raised ALP and to ensure levels are sufficiently high to give IV bisphosphonate.
- X-rays show affected bones to be enlarged, abnormally dense and distorted, e.g. the cottonwool appearance of the skull, bowing of long bones, and the picture frame appearance of vertebrae.
- Bone scintigraphy demonstrates the extent of the disease.

Treatment

The aim is to treat pain and prevent deformities and fractures.

- The current mainstay of treatment is a single dose of IV zoledronate. This reduces osteoclast activity (mirrored by a fall in serum ALP and urinary hydroxyproline) and encourages osteoblasts to produce normal bone. Pain is reduced within days of starting treatment. Follow-up studies show no recurrence for up to 6 years.
- Zoledronate leads to remission in 90% of patients.
- Dental work should be completed before treatment to reduce the risk of osteonecrosis of the jaw.
- Alternatives to zoledronate include oral risedronate for 2 months or calcitonin injections.
- Treatment can be repeated if necessary.

Primary hyperparathyroidism

Excess PTH is secreted autonomously by one or more of the parathyroid glands. In 80% of cases, there is an adenoma in a single gland. Less commonly, two or more glands are adenomatous or hyperplastic. Parathyroid cancer is very rare.

Epidemiology

- Common, affecting 1 in 500 women and 1 in 2000 men per year.
- Occurs worldwide.
- 55% are women over 70 years of age.
- The familial forms, e.g. multiple endocrine neoplasia, usually present in young adults.
- Consider in any patient with hypercalcaemia, normal renal function, and no history of malignancy.

Clinical features

- Most older people affected (up to 80%) are asymptomatic, and an unexpectedly high calcium level is found on biochemical testing done for other reasons.
- In resource-poor countries, presentation with symptoms (fatigue, myalgia, anorexia, constipation, depression, cognitive impairment, thirst, and polyuria) or complications is more common.
- Check the PTH level and serum calcium. Serum phosphate may be low.
- Asymptomatic patients should simply be observed, and their biochemistry monitored.
- However, 12% of cases with hypercalcaemia will have had documented episodes of confusion and dehydration and merit treatment unless there are other major co-morbidities.
- Severe cases can lead to kidney stones, bone pain and fractures (due to overstimulation of bone resorption, especially of cortical bone).
- Replace vitamin D if low; there is no role for restricting dietary calcium.
- Imaging usually includes neck ultrasound.
- Sestamibi scan: technetium[99] is preferentially taken up by an overactive parathyroid gland and is used to demonstrate anatomy prior to surgery.
- Minimally invasive parathyroidectomy has reliable results and short hospital stays.

Hypercalcaemia

There are many causes of hypercalcaemia. In practice, the following are the main groups affecting older people:

- Primary hyperparathyroidism, as mentioned earlier.
- Hypercalcaemia in malignancy may be due to bone metastases but also to non-metastatic manifestations of malignant disease. PTH is suppressed in this context. Check PTHrP.
- Myeloma (see Chapter 14). Myeloma activates RANK and thus osteoclasts but not osteoblasts, explaining why there are only lytic lesions. Calcium is raised, but not ALP.
- Drug-induced: thiazide diuretics, lithium, and vitamin D; calcium co-prescribed with antacids.
- CKD (see Chapter 13).
- Sarcoidosis, hyperthyroidism, and Addison's disease are all rare causes in this age group.

Emergency treatment: rehydration with IV normal saline. If the patient is fluid-overloaded, loop diuretics are useful for the urinary excretion of calcium. IV pamidronate or zoledronate are effective, especially in malignancy.

Osteomyelitis

Osteomyelitis is an inflammatory bone disease that is caused by an infecting micro-organism, leading to progressive bone destruction and loss. If the periosteum becomes involved, necrosis occurs. The infection reaches bone in two ways:

1 Haematogenous spread from a remote source, e.g. an abscess or infected urinary catheter. In older people, haematogenous infection often affects the vertebrae, long bones, and any prosthetic material. Discitis and involvement of adjacent vertebrae (vertebral osteomyelitis) may be stages of the same disease process.

2 Contiguous (direct) spread from infected tissue, e.g. after trauma. In older people, this is often from chronic cellulitis under areas of ulceration. Common scenarios are stage III/IV sacral pressure ulcers which erode the sacrum, or deep foot and leg ulcers, due to peripheral vascular disease and diabetes.

- Inflammatory markers, e.g. CRP, will be high and an ESR may be greater than 100 mm. Blood cultures are essential. Culture any pus; wound swabs often grow contaminants but may show MRSA.
- Plain x-rays are not helpful early on, but bone scintigrams may show hot spots. MRI is the most sensitive.
- Acute osteomyelitis (i.e. of less than 6 weeks duration) may respond to appropriate antibiotics, usually given IV at high doses. *Staphylococcus aureus* is the most common pathogen.
- Treat with flucloxacillin, clindamycin or vancomycin if MRSA is positive, but seek microbiology advice; diabetics may need treatment for Pseudomonas or anaerobes, and sacral osteomyelitis may need cover for bowel organisms.
- Chronic osteomyelitis (lasting more than 6 weeks) is more likely to need surgical intervention/debridement and extended courses of antibiotics, ideally under the care of the bone infection MDT or diabetic foot team.
- A frail older person with osteomyelitis and an infected joint replacement has a poor prognosis.

Joints

Ageing changes

1 There are changes in the cartilage: thinning of the subchondral bone, reduction in the lubricating effect of synovial fluid, changes in the ligaments so that joints become stiffer, and range of movement decreases with age.

2 Many people accept joint problems as a part of growing older, and arthritis is very common but not universal. The type of arthritis should be diagnosed so that management is appropriate.

Osteoarthritis

OA, the most common joint disorder, is a disorder of synovial joints that occurs when damage (repeated excessive loading or injury) triggers a repair process that leads to structural changes within the joint. The incidence increases with increasing age. Around 80% of 80-year-olds will have some x-ray evidence of OA, but not necessarily symptoms.

Risk factors

These tend to interact and include:

- Genetic predisposition: over 100 DNA variants have been associated with an increased risk of developing OA. Examples include growth differentiation factor 5 (*GDF5*), which is involved in joint development and maintenance; frizzled related protein (*FRZB*), which is important in cartilage development; collagen type II alpha 1 chain (*COL2A1*) gene mutations that cause early-onset OA; and DOT1-like

Table 10.2 Patient consulting rate per 1000 persons (by age in years) for patients with joint diseases.

	Consulting rate for joint diseases				
All ages	0–14	15–44	45–64	65–74	75
34	2	14	62	105	114

histone lysine methyltransferase (*DOT1-L*), which has been associated with an increased risk of OA hip.

- Increasing age (Table 10.2).
- Female gender.
- Obesity.
- Anatomical factors.
- Muscle weakness.
- Joint injury, especially if the articular surface is damaged, e.g. occupational damage due to kneeling, squatting and heavy lifting in agriculture and construction workers, sports injuries, and trauma, e.g. road traffic accidents.
- Secondary to other conditions:
  o Inflammatory arthritis, including gout and RA, and burnt-out RA may be difficult to differentiate from generalised OA in old age.
  o Avascular necrosis, especially of the hip.
  o Endocrine diseases, e.g. myxoedema and acromegaly.
  o Neuropathy, e.g. diabetic, and therefore painless.
  o Hereditary disease, e.g. haemophilia and hypermobility syndromes.
  o Metabolic disease, e.g. Wilson's disease, haemochromatosis, and homocystinuria.

Pathophysiology

Current understanding is that wear and tear combined with the loss of normal homeostasis in cartilage initiates an inflammatory response (secondary to the release of metalloproteases IL-6 and TNF-alpha), which leads to degradation of the matrix of the cartilage. Water makes up 80% of the normal cartilage matrix. This is reduced to 60% in damaged cartilage. Early in the disease, the cartilage is expanded, but as time goes by, it softens and loses elasticity. Eventually, the edges of the cartilage are weakened and become fibrillated. This exposes the subchondral bone, which then articulates with the bone on the other side of the joint. The subchondral bone becomes more cellular and may develop cysts. Abnormal new bone formation produces osteophytes. Mild synovitis is common.

Symptoms

- Pain: gradual in onset, intermittent, worse on movement and relieved by rest.
- Sleep may be disturbed in severe cases.
- Early-morning stiffness should last no longer than 30 min.
- Joints most often affected are DIPs, PIPs, the base of the thumb (painless but unsightly), hips, knees, and the cervical and lumbar spine.
- Hip pain is worse in the anterior groin and may radiate into the buttock or thigh.
- Knee pain is worse in the anterior knee and patellofemoral joint but may be referred to the hip.
- Functional problems include difficulty bending down to put on shoes, getting out of a chair, and walking long distances, which eventually lead to immobility.

Signs

- Tenderness and bony enlargement of the joint are secondary to osteophytes and swelling due to effusion.
- Painful, reduced range of movement of the affected joint.
- In OA of the hip, the leg may be shortened because the hip is flexed and externally rotated, and there may be marked quadriceps wasting.
- Crepitus.
- Heberden's nodes: swelling of DIP joints.
- Squaring at the base of the thumb, i.e. the first CMC joint.
- Eventually, the joint may become deformed, e.g. genu valgus (knock knees), varus (bow knees), and hallux valgus (bunion).
- Gait may be antalgic, i.e. less time is spent with weight on the affected side.

Radiological features

- Loss of joint space secondary to loss of cartilage (see Figure 10.7).
- Osteophytes.
- Subchondral erosions and cysts.
- The radiological appearance does not correlate well with the severity of the symptoms.

Management

The goals of treatment are to reduce pain and functional loss and, therefore, improve quality of life.

General measures

- Patient education to encourage sustained lifestyle changes is paramount. Minor changes may produce big improvements in symptoms and quality of life.
- Weight loss relieves the strain on the joints (especially knees and hips): the NICE guidelines advise aiming for 10%, but even 5% is beneficial.
- PT is aimed at improving the range of movement and strengthening the muscles surrounding the joint, thus stabilising it and reducing pain, e.g. reversing quadriceps wasting to protect the knee.
- Encourage older people to exercise regularly; swimming is good because it unloads the joints.
- Using a stick in the opposite hand or a frame can reduce the load on an affected hip or knee by 50%, reducing pain.
- Hot and cold packs for temporary relief of pain.

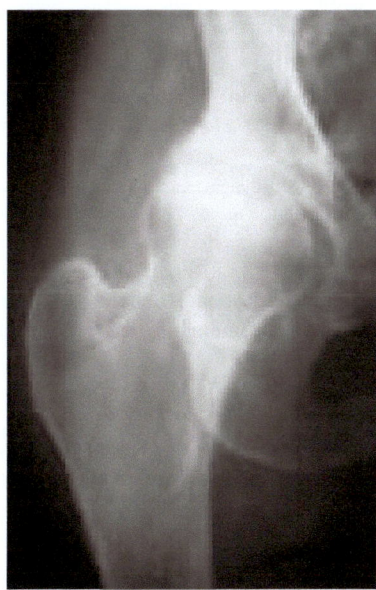

Figure 10.7 Radiograph of the right hip showing a severe loss of joint space.

- Correcting the malalignment of joints with a knee brace or orthotics. There is evidence from two small trials to support knee-taping in OA to improve proprioception and reduce knee pain.
- There is no proven benefit from acupuncture, TENS, or ultrasound therapy.

Drugs

- Topical NSAIDs, such as ibuprofen gel, may be highly effective, as the patient perceives improvement from direct application to the affected joint, and there are fewer side effects than with oral NSAIDs.
- NSAIDs should be reserved for flare-ups because of the side effects. COX-2 inhibitors, e.g. celecoxib, are avoided in older patients.
- Simple analgesia, such as paracetamol, can be taken as needed. There is no evidence that it is enough to control pain.
- Capsaicin, derived from chilli peppers, can be applied topically, which can give good pain relief.
- An intra-articular steroid injection can produce pain relief for a period of 2–4 weeks, sufficient to allow a patient to enjoy a special occasion, but is not indicated for long-term treatment.
- The only novel approach, tanezumab, a MAb targeting nerve growth factor to reduce pain, has been withdrawn as some patients developed rapidly-progressing OA.
- There is some evidence that combined glucosamine and chondroitin supplements can reduce knee pain due to OA. (Subgroup analysis of the GAIT trial and MOVES).
- The active compound of turmeric, curcumin, has anti-inflammatory properties; one study suggests it is as effective as ibuprofen.

Joint replacements

Joint replacement is reserved for severe cases when conservative measures are ineffective. OA is the cause in over 90% of procedures and knee and hip replacements make up over 90%. In England in 2018/19 there were around 94,000 knee and 81,000 hip replacements. Both are performed more often in women (about 60%), and half are done in the over 70s. Most patients report good outcomes, especially for hip surgery. Unfortunately, the waits for surgery on the NHS are very long and worse than the data suggests, as patients often struggle to see a GP initially and may spend a lengthy period being referred to physiotherapy, etc. before they finally see an orthopaedic surgeon.

The ideal patient for a joint replacement

- Refractory pain in a single joint or only one severely affected joint.
- Physically fit with preservation of muscles around the joint.
- Well-motivated.
- Mentally alert and orientated.
- Well-nourished, but not obese.
- Unlikely to place unreasonable demands on the new joint, i.e. normal mobility anticipated post-operatively and not excessive activity.
- Of sufficient age so that the patient is unlikely to outlive the new joint. About one-quarter of replacement hips need revision after 10 years.

Complications of joint replacement

- Infection affects about 1% of hip replacements. Usually, prophylactic antibiotics are given. The most common infection is a simple wound infection. Deeper infection may be more difficult to diagnose; a gallium scan can be helpful.
- DVT: subcutaneous low molecular weight heparin, or a DOAC or LMWH, followed by aspirin, is routinely given as prophylaxis, as per the 2018 NICE guidelines.
- Loosening of prosthesis: an x-ray or bone scan may demonstrate this.
- Fracture of adjacent bone: visible on x-ray.

- The patient outlives the prosthesis, and a second operation is needed.
- Increased mobility unmasks an additional pathology, e.g. angina, from the increased activity.

Rheumatoid arthritis

Rheumatoid arthritis (RA) is a systemic auto-immune, chronic inflammatory disorder leading to destructive, symmetrical synovitis. The peak age of incidence in the UK for both men and women is the 70s. It is thought that this is due to immunosenescence. The prevalence is about 2% worldwide among older people. It is commoner in women of all ages, but the female preponderance is less in late-onset RA. There is no consistency in the literature about what constitutes 'late-onset' RA, but there seem to be several patterns of disease:

- *Inactive disease*: an episode in earlier life that has burned itself out but left deformities and disabilities, sometimes presenting as a mixture of old RA and more recent OA. Deformities such as z thumbs, swan necking, ulnar deviation, and subluxation at the MCP joints (as seen in Figure 10.8) are increasingly rare due to the effectiveness of conventional disease-modifying anti-rheumatic drugs (cDMARDS) and biological DMARDs.
- *Classical RA*: likely to be rheumatoid factor (RF) positive and anti-cyclic citrullinated peptide antibody (anti-CCP) positive; higher frequency of acute onset with constitutional symptoms (anaemia, fatigue, fever, and weight loss); more frequently affects large joints, especially the knee, ankle, and shoulder.
- *PMR-like disease*: can be difficult to differentiate from PMR. Both present with severe early-morning stiffness, shoulder, and hip involvement and produce a raised ESR. Both may respond briskly to steroids. It is important not to miss RA so that patients can be offered DMARDs where appropriate to prevent joint deformities. A positive anti-CCP can clinch the diagnosis, but if this is negative, synovitis on ultrasound or MRI suggests RA.
- *RS3PE*: Remitting seronegative symmetrical synovitis with pitting (o) edema is a rare condition that is thought to be a variant of RA (usually RhF-negative) with the addition of marked pitting oedema of the hands (and sometimes feet). It responds briskly to prednisolone 15 mg daily. The important thing to remember is that it can be a non-metastatic manifestation of malignancy.

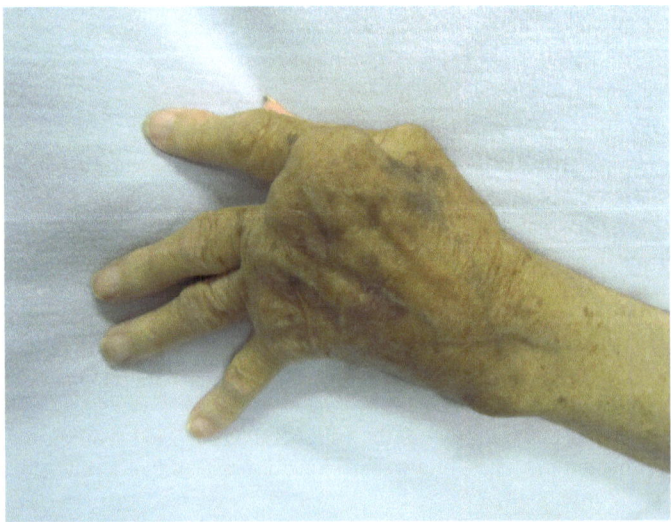

Figure 10.8 Severe rheumatoid arthritis of the left hand. Note ulnar deviation of the fingers, swelling of the metacarpophalangeal joints and over the ulna styloid process, and subluxation of the proximal phalanges on the MCP joints. *Source*: James Heilman/Wikimedia Commons/CC BY SA 3.0.

Investigations

- Rheumatoid factor (an autoantibody contributing to inflammation) is found in many patients with RA, but false positives increase with age.
- Anti-cyclic citrullinated (anti-CCP) peptide antibodies are more specific to RA than rheumatoid factor and can be associated with more severe disease outcomes.
- CRP and ESR are elevated due to the inflammation.
- X-rays, e.g. looking for soft tissue swelling around affected joints and erosions around the joint margins.
- Ultrasound and MRI can detect earlier changes, map disease progression/response to treatment, and detect non-articular manifestations.

Management

The aim is to reduce disease activity and inflammation, prevent joint damage and maximise quality of life.

General measures

New-onset patients should be referred to rheumatology unless they are living with severe frailty.

- Lifestyle advice: try to prevent muscle wasting with, e.g. swimming, static bike work, walking.
- The Mediterranean diet has been linked with reduced inflammation and better joint outcomes
- PT and OT have much to offer; severe upper-limb problems and other disorders will hinder a patient's ability to participate fully in an intensive PT programme, but a wide variety of aids can help maintain functional independence (see Chapter 4).
- Monitoring is also needed for non-articular manifestations of RA, including:
  - Normocytic anaemia (may be due to anaemia of chronic disease, iron deficiency if taking NSAIDs or steroids, or side effects of DMARDS),
  - Eye problems: dry eyes, episcleritis, scleritis, cataracts, and uveitis,
  - Sjogren's syndrome,
  - Pericarditis/myocarditis,
  - Pulmonary fibrosis/rheumatoid nodules in the lungs.

Drugs

Drug treatment is challenging because of the increased risk of side effects in older adults due to comorbidities and the use of other medications. However, drugs can control disease, reduce pain and deformity, and maintain mobility and independence. Frailty is more important than age in making treatment decisions.

- NSAIDS reduce pain and inflammation but are contraindicated for most older patients because of renal impairment, the risk of fluid overload, and GI bleeds.
- Rapid symptom relief may be the best way to preserve mobility and independence; therefore, steroids (despite their disadvantages) may be used earlier than in younger patients. Remember the usual precautions of PPIs and bisphosphonates.
- DMARDs need 2–3 months to take effect. Age and pathological changes in other systems increase the likelihood of side effects, e.g. renal impairment worsened by penicillamine and gold and visual impairment potentiated by chloroquine. Methotrexate is an effective once-weekly monotherapy. Folic acid is prescribed with it to reduce liver and gastrointestinal toxicity. Careful monitoring of blood counts, creatinine, aminotransferases, and chest symptoms is essential to detect toxic side effects early. The patient must be educated to take methotrexate once a *week* only. Consider giving *m*ethotrexate on *M*ondays and *f*olic acid on *F*ridays!

- Biologics may be considered for refractory cases. Examples include TNF-alpha inhibitors (e.g. etanercept and adalimumab), IL-6 receptor inhibitors, (e.g. tocilizumab), and CD20 inhibitors (e.g. rituximab).
- Careful monitoring for side effects is needed.

Polymyalgia rheumatica

Polymyalgia rheumatica (PMR) is a chronic, systemic inflammatory disorder that presents with generalised pain and tenderness, usually affecting the shoulder girdle, and then the pelvic girdle with marked stiffness.

- The pain is due to bursitis and synovitis.
- There is an association with HLA-DR4.
- A rise in IL-6 is thought to cause the constitutional symptoms of fatigue, malaise, anorexia, weight loss and mild fever.
- PMR does not affect the muscles; creatine kinase, muscle biopsy and EMG are all normal.
- It is likely to be part of the spectrum of giant-cell arteritis.
- It is usually idiopathic but may be triggered by a viral infection or indicate an underlying malignancy.

Epidemiology

- Most common in people aged 70–80.
- Female to male ratio is 2:1.
- Incidence is 20/100,000 per annum.
- PMR is the most common reason older people are prescribed steroids.

Diagnostic criteria

- Bilateral, symmetrical shoulder pain and/or neck stiffness.
- Onset of illness of less than 2 weeks.
- Initial ESR greater than 40.
- Duration of morning stiffness of more than 1 hr.
- Age greater than 65 years.
- Depression and/or weight loss.
- Bilateral tenderness in upper arms.

Three positives are suggestive of PMR. Those features higher in the list are most strongly predictive. A successful therapeutic trial with steroids will confirm the diagnosis: the response is often dramatic and within 3 days.

Complications of untreated PMR

- Chronic disability and impaired mobility.
- Normochromic anaemia.
- Hepatitis with raised ALP.
- Progression to giant-cell arteritis with major-vessel occlusion, leading to blindness, stroke, or myocardial infarction.

Treatment

- Steroids: 15 mg prednisolone daily is sufficient for PMR. Rapid improvement in symptoms supports the diagnosis. If the patient is not sure that they are better, then the diagnosis is not PMR.
- It is essential to warn the patient to report any symptoms suggestive of giant cell arteritis (GCA) as higher doses of steroids are necessary (see Chapter 9).
- Dosage should be monitored according to symptoms and level of ESR. Once symptoms are controlled and ESR has fallen to normal, reduce the dose slowly as per the NICE 2023 guidelines.

- Give the patient a blue steroid card to alert the healthcare team if an intercurrent illness develops.
- Bone protection and a PPI should be prescribed.
- Treatment may be necessary for 2 years or more.
- Symptoms may recur and require a further course of steroids.
- However, some patients are reluctant to stop steroids, which must be weaned if there is no evidence of disease activity.
- Methotrexate is a useful alternative to steroids.
- NICE permits 1 year of treatment with tocilizumab (anti-IL-6) for refractory cases.

Differential diagnosis for a single painful joint

An older person presenting for the first time with severe joint pain may have any of the following:

1 Trauma: the patient may not remember the index event if they blacked out or have cognitive impairment, so it is essential to examine all joints carefully.
2 Crystal arthropathy: the first attack of gout affects only one joint in 80% of cases.
3 Septic arthritis: this usually affects a single joint.
4 Osteoarthritis.
5 Rheumatoid disease can present initially with one joint.
6 Mechanical derangements of tendons and ligaments.

Crystal arthropathies

These are acute inflammatory joint disorders triggered by the accumulation of microcrystals in and around the joint. The two common types are gout and pseudogout. Both cause sudden onset, severe pain, joint swelling, erythema, a reduced range of movement, and tend to recur. They are more common with increasing age, and in older people, both sexes are affected equally; at a younger age, gout occurs more often in men, and the sex ratio in pseudogout varies in different studies.

- Note that both gout and pseudogout may be confused with acute joint sepsis. Aspiration for pus versus crystals is the best technique for differentiation.
- The differences between gout and pseudogout are detailed in Table 10.3.

Gout

Gout is a syndrome characterised by hyperuricaemia and the deposition of urate crystals, causing attacks of acute inflammatory arthritis, tophi around the joints, possible joint destruction, renal damage, and urolithiasis. There has been an increased interest in gout because:

- The incidence is rising.
- It is potentially curable but undertreated.
- It markedly reduces quality of life.
- Treatment reduces the progression of CKD.
- It is associated with an increase in all-cause mortality.

The central themes are to improve patient education and, therefore, concordance and treatment to target lower serum uric acid levels.

Management

Treatment of the first attack or flare

Advise the patient to rest, elevate the affected joint, and apply an ice pack.

Table 10.3 Table of clinical features, precipitating factors, and treatment of crystal arthropathies.

	Gout	Pseudogout
Type of crystal	Urate	Calcium pyrophosphate
Appearance under polarised light	Negatively birefringent needle-shaped crystals	Positively birefringent rhomboid crystals
Joints most affected	MTP joint of the great toe (podagra), ankle, and PIP joints of fingers	Large joints, most commonly knees, but occasionally the wrist or hand. Involvement of the neck causes 'crowned dens syndrome'.
Precipitating factors	Diuretics, overindulgence, fasting, uric acid-containing foods such as strawberries, acute illness, surgery, tumour lysis syndrome – chemo for blood cancers	A precipitant may not be identified, but acute illness or surgery is often responsible due to dehydration.
Extra-articular features	Tophi may be present around the affected joint or on the pinna; urolithiasis, worsening renal function.	None
Serum uric acid	May be raised or normal in an acute attack	Normal
X-ray appearance	Punched-out erosions (a longstanding disease)	Linear opacification of articular cartilage (also seen in OA)
Treatment of acute episode	Rest, elevation, and icepack to the affected joint; consideration of NSAIDs, colchicine, steroids – oral, IA or IM (see later)	Rest, elevation, and ice pack for the affected joint; consideration of NSAIDs, colchicine, steroids – oral or IA
Prevention	Allopurinol (febuxostat in CKD)	Avoid dehydration when ill. No drugs
Associated conditions	Obesity, type 2 diabetes, hypertension, IHD, CKD, dyslipidaemia	Diabetes, myxoedema, hyperparathyroidism
Family history	Common	Less common

IHD, ischaemic heart disease; CKD, chronic kidney disease; IA, intraarticular; IM, intramuscular; OA, osteoarthritis; PIP, proximal interphalangeal; MTP, metatarsophalangeal.

The choice of drugs can be challenging for older people:

- NSAIDs are usually avoided because of all the side effects.
- Colchicine (which disrupts neutrophil-endothelial interaction) is associated with GI side effects; the consensus is that 500 µg bd to qds is well-tolerated. Reduce the dose in moderate renal impairment.
- Oral steroids: NICE guidelines recommend 30–35 mg for 3–5 days and then stop. Watch for delirium (do not forget to co-prescribe a PPI).
- Consider an intra-articular or intramuscular steroid injection if the above treatments are contraindicated or not working.
- If there is no improvement, refer to rheumatology for consideration of IL-1 inhibitors, e.g. anakinra and canakinumab.

Prevention of further flares

Recommend a normal, healthy diet; advise against weight gain and to moderate alcohol intake.

- 4–6 weeks after the first episode or a flare, measure serum urate.
- Consider the risk of further episodes and comorbidities. In patients with recurrent flares or CKD 3–5, on diuretics, with tophi or chronic

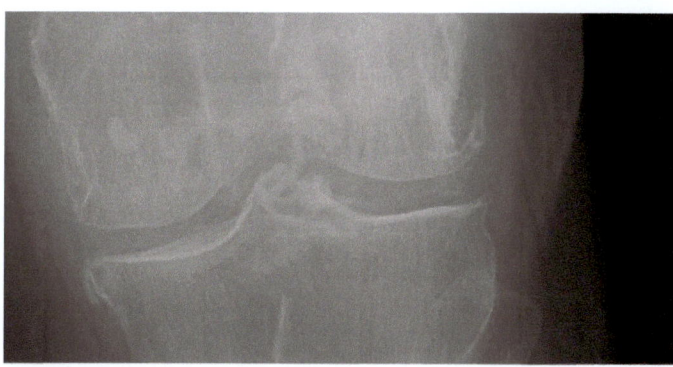

Figure 10.9 X-ray of the left knee showing chondrocalcinosis in the medial and lateral joint spaces.

gouty arthritis, discuss the benefits of taking urate-lowering therapy (ULT) to get the urate level below 300 acutely or 360 μmol/L long-term.
- The most commonly used drug is the xanthine oxidase inhibitor allopurinol. Start with 50–100 mg allopurinol daily and increase monthly if needed to achieve the target.
- Colchicine can be given to prevent acute flares when commencing/increasing the dose of prophylaxis.
- In CKD or when the maximum dose of allopurinol is insufficient, use febuxostat 80–120 mg daily instead.
- Febuxostat is more expensive than allopurinol, but there is no evidence of better outcomes except in patients with CKD and severe tophaceous gout.
- Monitor the serum urate level annually.

Pseudogout

This is acute inflammation of the synovium due to calcium pyrophosphate deposition disease (CPPD).

- Associated with chondrocalcinosis, which is the appearance of calcification in the cartilage in joint spaces, as in Figure 10.9.
- Pseudogout presents with one or more red, hot, swollen joints.
- The knee is the most common site, followed by the wrist, elbow, ankle, toe, shoulder, and hip.
- Crowned dens is a rare presentation of CPPD caused by calcification of the cruciform ligament around the odontoid process. This can be the explanation for a patient presenting with severe neck pain, fever, neck stiffness and markedly raised inflammatory markers who is clinically well.
- Pseudogout can occur spontaneously or due to acute infection, trauma, or surgery.
- Can be a cause of rising fever and inflammatory markers in a patient previously responding to antibiotics for sepsis.
- Large joint effusions can be aspirated – send for crystals to confirm the diagnosis.
- Can take longer to respond to treatment than gout (up to 3 months).

Septic arthritis

This is infection within a joint space, usually due to haematogenous spread from systemic infection. It should always be considered when a single joint is painful. It is a particular risk in prosthetic joints as it is extremely hard to eliminate. It is a musculoskeletal emergency because complications include joint destruction, chronic pain, loss of mobility, osteomyelitis, and death secondary to sepsis.

- Risk factors include older age, pre-existing arthritis, especially RA, recent joint surgery, urinary catheters, diabetes, and immunosuppression.

- The classical presentation is the acute onset of a hot, tender, and swollen joint with a reduced range of movement, plus fever and malaise. However, systemic toxic effects may be blunted in older people.
- Concurrent treatments may mask the problem, e.g. steroids, analgesics, and antibiotics for other infections.
- It may be difficult to diagnose in the presence of old joint deformities.
- Joint aspiration is essential to look for raised white cell count and Gram stain plus culture and look for crystals to exclude gout or pseudogout.
- Do not aspirate a hot prosthetic joint; refer to the orthopaedics team.
- Raised serum inflammatory markers confirm sepsis, i.e. WCC, CRP and ESR. There is no evidence that serum procalcitonin adds anything.
- Take multiple blood cultures.
- Common pathogens include *S. aureus, Streptococcus pneumoniae*, and Gram-negative organisms in older people. A more indolent presentation might suggest Mycobacterium.
- Radiology is not helpful in the acute phase.
- Treatment is with IV antibiotics appropriate for common pathogens whilst awaiting culture results: flucloxacillin for 2 weeks IV and then oral for 4 weeks; clindamycin for penicillin allergy; or vancomycin if MRSA positive.
- Needle aspiration is sufficient to drain small joints (as much fluid as possible should be drained), but larger joints, including joint replacements, will require orthopaedic washouts. When the infection is deep seated, the patient will need multiple interventions and is best managed by the bone infection MDT.

Back pain

The most common cause in older people is multilevel degenerative disease, but due to ageing and comorbidities, a serious underlying condition is more likely than in younger people (see Table 10.4). These must be considered to make the correct diagnosis and inform treatment.

Muscles

Ageing changes

1 Muscle bulk decreases with increasing age.
2 Type I (slow twitch) muscle fibres are relatively preserved; the major change is the decline in size of Type II (fast twitch) fibres.
3 The number of stem cells falls.
4 Muscle fibres are replaced by fat and fibrous tissue, and there is increased deposition of lipochrome pigment.
5 Falling oestrogen at the menopause reduces the proliferation of skeletal muscle cells and increases inflammation.
6 Complex biochemical changes include reduced muscle protein synthesis and changes in calcium flux and mitochondria.
7 Nerve damage that occurs with age may contribute to the changes seen in muscle.
8 Even in extreme old age, muscle bulk can still be increased by regular exercise.

Sarcopenia

The term 'sarcopenia' was coined in 1989 to describe 'age-related loss of muscle', and the two terms are sometimes still used synonymously. Loss of muscle mass and strength is important in the development of frailty

Table 10.4 Back pain in older people.

Cause	Example	Diagnostic pointers	Investigations
Vertebral fracture	40% of people over 80 years have vertebral fractures radiologically	Known osteoporosis. Sudden-onset severe pain. History of falling. Loss of height, kyphosis	X-ray spine for diagnosis. DXA for risk assessment. Noticed on CT scans done for trauma and other reasons
Infection	Discitis – limited to the disc (10 times more common in older people), Osteomyelitis (infection of the disc and vertebra)	Fever, Infection elsewhere, Worsening pain, especially at night	Raised inflammatory markers, Blood cultures, CT-guided aspiration
Inflammatory	Rheumatoid arthritis	Neck pain Morning stiffness lasting more than 30 min Pain improves with exercise	Raised ESR, Positive rheumatoid factor, anti-CCP
	New-onset ankylosing spondylitis is rare in older adults		
Tumours	Myeloma	Unexplained weight loss, Constant progressive pain, No relief from analgesia	Hypercalcaemia, M band, CT scan, Bone scintigram
	Metastases from other sources		MRI spine
Cauda equina	Due to central disc prolapse, spinal tumour	Sudden onset of pain, bowel, or bladder dysfunction, Saddle anaesthesia	
Non-spinal causes	Ruptured AAA, gall stones, urinary tract stones	Pulsatile abdominal mass, Tenderness (RUQ) or flanks	CT scan of the abdomen

Anti-CCP, anti-cyclic citrullinated peptide; AAA, abdominal aortic aneurysm; RUQ, right upper quadrant; M band, monoclonal band.

and loss of function. The European Working Group on Sarcopenia in Older People 2 (EWGSOP2), 2019, views sarcopenia as a muscle disease. It defines severe sarcopenia as 'low muscle strength, low muscle quantity or quality, and low physical performance'. The muscle changes include those listed earlier but are not exclusively due to ageing. They reflect a sedentary lifestyle and factors including a genetic predisposition, childhood development, and a host of comorbidities (see Figure 10.10). There are parallels to osteopenia and osteoporosis.

- The prevalence is rising because of demographic change, but estimates depend markedly on the definition used and the population studied (age, sex, and particularly whether they are living independently or in a care setting).
- There is an overlap with cachexia in cancer, which also results in the loss of fat.
- These factors explain the wide range of prevalence figures ranging from 5% to 75%!

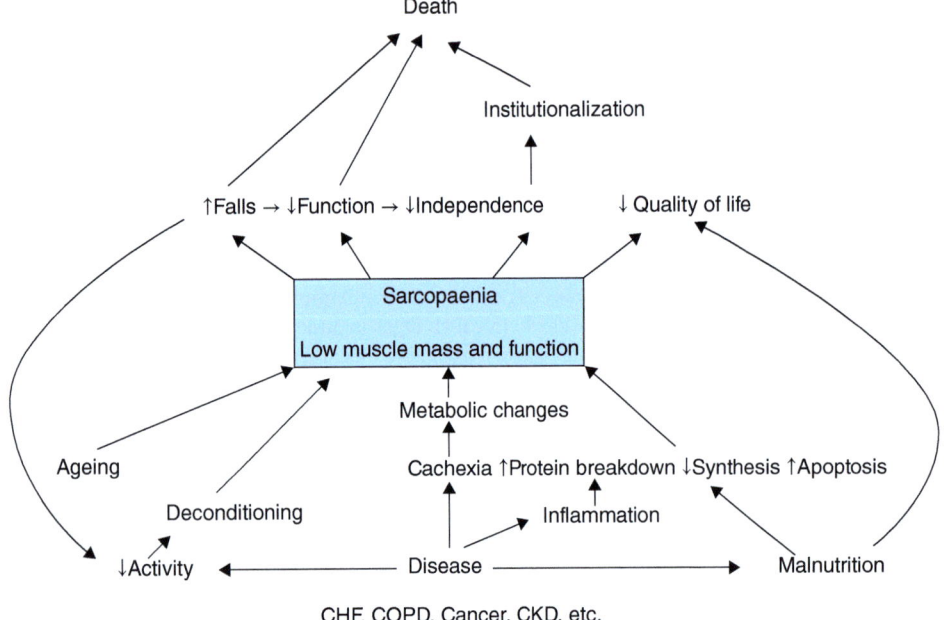

Figure 10.10 Pathogenesis and consequences of sarcopenia. CHF, chronic heart failure, COPD chronic obstructive pulmonary disease; CKD, chronic kidney disease.

- Risk factors include physical inactivity, malnutrition, smoking, extremes of sleep duration, diabetes, organ failure, arthritis, depression, and neurological deficits.

Sequelae of sarcopenia

- Increasing physical disability: loss of function such as getting out of a chair and climbing stairs.
- Reduced quality of life.
- Increased risk of falling over and fracturing.
- Doubled health care costs compared with people without sarcopenia.
- Increased risk of hospitalisation.
- Increased mortality.

Assessment

Researchers in falls assessment and prevention are frustrated with the lack of quantification of sarcopenia in clinical practice. EWGSOP2 recommends clinical assessment using the SARC-F questionnaire (see Appendix), and if this is positive, assess grip strength and the chair stand test. If these are also positive, assess further parameters such as gait speed, Timed Up and Go and 400 m walk (see EWGSOP2).

There is no universally accepted diagnostic tool, but using DXA to measure lean muscle mass has the advantages of wide availability, insignificant radiation exposure and being cheaper than CT or MRI scanning.

Management

- Evidence shows that the mainstay of treatment is resistance exercise, i.e. using weights/resistance bands. Resistance training should involve both the upper and lower body and be delivered twice weekly to achieve benefit. Exercise must be sustained over time, and there must be a systematic but gradual increase in intensity to maintain improvement. Additional advantages of resistance exercise are improvement in bone strength, reducing the risk of falls, and increasing social contact.
- The use of hormones to treat sarcopenia remains controversial. There is some evidence to suggest that replacing oestradiol at the perimenopause may enhance muscle health, but not long-term. Testosterone does increase muscle mass, but it has many side effects.
- Angiotensin converting enzyme 1 is implicated in processes such as oxidative stress, glucose metabolism, and inflammation. The potential of ACE inhibitors to reduce muscle mitochondrial decline, reduce inflammation, and improve endothelial function to prevent/reverse sarcopenia is an active research area.

Myopathies

Myopathies are muscle diseases that are not due to any abnormality of the innervation or the neuromuscular junction. There is usually symmetrical proximal muscle weakness without tenderness. There are a wide range of causes. Inherited (congenital) causes are not discussed further here, but always ask about a family history and the duration of symptoms, as some conditions present in adulthood or even old age. Symptoms are more profound if several causes coexist. Treat the underlying cause if possible.

Causes of acquired myopathy

- Endocrine causes: Cushing's disease, thyrotoxicosis, hypothyroidism, and Addison's disease.

- Drugs and toxins: e.g. statins, steroids, ciprofloxacin, colchicine, immune checkpoint inhibitors and alcohol. (There is no evidence to suggest an increased incidence of statin myopathy with age.)
- Metabolic: usually due to hypokalaemia (endocrine or drug-induced).
- Vitamin D deficiency (part of osteomalacia).
- Infectious: all types of infectious organisms can be responsible, but many viral infections cause transient inflammatory myopathy.
- Critical illness myopathy (a common multifactorial sequel to a long ICU admission).
- Inflammatory: see later.

Myositis

Myositis or idiopathic inflammatory myopathies are rare chronic diseases of skeletal muscle in which there is proximal muscle weakness, usually with muscle pain, and the muscle biopsy shows inflammation.

There are three main groups:

1. Polymyositis

Weakness develops over days (rare), weeks or months and usually affects getting out of a chair, walking, and lifting the arms, but can progress to distal muscles, especially the fingers and affect the voice, swallowing and occasionally the heart.

2. Dermatomyositis

Weakness is like PM, but skin signs may precede the weakness and include Gottron's papules (pink papules on the knuckles) and a heliotrope rash (patchy red/purple rash on the eyelids and neck).

Both polymyositis (PM) and dermatomyositis (DM) can occur at any age, but more females are affected than males. There may be systemic symptoms such as fever, weight loss, depression, and Raynaud's. They are autoimmune and may overlap with other conditions, such as systemic lupus and scleroderma. Muscle creatine kinase (CK) is usually extremely high; EMG demonstrates spiky polyphasic muscle action potentials and occasional spontaneous fibrillation; and biopsy shows muscle necrosis, muscle fibre regeneration and diffuse infiltration by CD8+ T lymphocytes. Both PM and DM may be associated with malignancy, particularly DM, but this is still rare. Both may be associated with antisynthetase antibodies (to aminoacyl tRNA), the most common of which is anti-Jo-1. Most cases respond to exercise, steroids and immunosuppressants.

3. Inclusion body myositis

Inclusion body myositis (IBM) is the most common acquired muscle disease in the over-50s, and occurs more often in men, but is still rare. It can present like PM, with which it is often confused, but often progresses slowly from distal to proximal muscles. CK is often normal or mildly raised. A biopsy shows characteristic inclusion bodies in the muscle fibres with an inflammatory infiltrate between the fibres. There is usually no response to steroids or immunosuppression (suggesting that the pathogenesis might be in part degenerative rather than primarily autoimmune), and this is often when the correct diagnosis is made. PT can be very helpful.

Myasthenia gravis

Myasthenia gravis is a chronic autoimmune disease that causes painless weakness that worsens when the muscles are used. The Eaton–Lambert (myasthenic) syndrome may present in a similar way and is often associated with malignancy (see Chapter 7).

📖 REFERENCES AND FURTHER READING

National Osteoporosis Guideline Group – UK (2021) *Clinical Guideline for the prevention and treatment of osteoporosis.* www.nogg.org.uk/full-guideline

NICE *A list of all products on osteoporosis.* www.nice.org.uk/guidance/conditions-and-diseases/diabetes-and-other-endocrinal--nutritional-and-metabolic-conditions/osteoporosis

NICE CKS (2023) *Osteoporosis – prevention of fragility fractures.* https://cks.nice.org.uk/topics/osteoporosis-prevention-of-fragility-fractures

The National Hip Fracture Database (look up your trust's performance live) www.nhfd.co.uk

The National Hip Fracture Database website: *Report on* 2021. www.nhfd.co.uk/2022report

Royal Osteoporosis Society (2019) Clinical *standards for fracture liaison services.* https://theros.org.uk/media/1eubz33w/ros-clinical-standards-for-fracture-liaison-services-august-2019.pdf

Baji P, Patel R, Judge A, et al. (2023) Organisational factors associated with hospital costs and patient mortality in the 365 days following hip fracture in England and Wales (REDUCE): a Record-Linkage Cohort Study. *Lancet.* doi: 10.1016/S2666-7568 (23)00086-7.

Poole K, Treece, G, Parson R, et al. (2022) Romosozumab enhances vertebral bone structure in women with low bone density. *J. Bone Mineral Res.* 37:256–264. doi: 10.1002/jbmr.4465.

NICE Technology appraisal guidance [TA279] (2013) *Percutaneous vertebroplasty and percutaneous balloon kyphoplasty for treating osteoporotic vertebral compression fractures* www.nice.org.uk/guidance/ta279

Buchbinder R, Johnston RV, Rischin KJ, et al. (2018) Percutaneous vertebroplasty for osteoporotic vertebral compression fracture. *Cochrane Database Syst. Rev.* 11:CD006349. doi: 10.1002/14651858. CD006349.pub4.

Arboleya L, Braña I, Pardo E, et al. (2023) Osteomalacia in adults: a practical insight for clinicians. *J. Clin. Med.* 12:2714. doi: 10.3390/jcm12072714.

Shaw B, Burrell CL, Green D, et al. (2019) Molecular insights into an ancient form of Paget's disease of bone. *Proc. Natl. Acad. Sci. U.S.A.* 116:10463–10472. https://www.ncbi.nlm.nih.gov/pmc/articles/PMC6535003.

Banaganapalli B, Fallatah I, Alsubhi F, et al. (2023) Paget's disease: a review of the epidemiology, etiology, genetics, and treatment. *Front. Genet.* 14:1131182. doi: 10.3389/fgene.2023.1131182

NICE CKS *Hypercalcaemia* (2019) https://cks.nice.org.uk/topics/hypercalcaemia

Lim W, Barras CD, Zadow S (2021) Radiologic mimics of osteomyelitis and septic arthritis: a pictorial essay. *Radiol. Res. Pract.* doi: 10.1155/2021/9912257.

Aubourg G, Rice SJ, Bruce-Wootton P, et al. (2022) Genetics of osteoarthritis. *Osteoarthritis Cartilage* 30:636–649. doi: 10.1016/j.joca.2021.03.002.

Kolasinski S, Neogi T, Hochberg M, et al. (2020) American College of Rheumatology/Arthritis Foundation Guidelines for the Management of Osteoarthritis of the hand, hip and knee. *Arthritis Rheumatol.* 72:220–233. https://assets.contentstack.io/v3/assets/bltee37abb6b278ab2c/blt6aa092f0134cac9a/63320f4750c8e90e3bf512c2/osteoarthritis-guideline-2019.pdf.

NICE guideline NG 226 (2022) *Osteoarthritis in over 16s: diagnosis and management.* www.nice.org.uk/guidance/ng226/chapter/Recommendations#diagnosis

NHS Digital (2020) Finalised patient reported outcome measures (PROMS) in England for hip and knee replacements https://digital.nhs.uk/data-and-information/publications/statistical/patient-reported-outcome-measures-proms/finalised-hip--knee-replacements-april-2018---march-2019/patient-profile

Serhal L, Lwin MN, Holroyd C (2020) Rheumatoid arthritis in the elderly: characteristics and treatment considerations. *Autoimmun. Rev.* 19:102528. doi: 10.1016/j.autrev.2020.102528.

Wu J, Yang F, Ma X, et al. (2023) Elderly-onset rheumatoid arthritis vs. polymyalgia rheumatica: differences in pathogenesis. *Front. Med. (Lausanne)* 9:1083879. doi: 10.3389/fmed.2022.1083879.

Morsley K, Kilner T, Steuer A (2015) Biologics prescribing for rheumatoid arthritis in older patients: a single-center retrospective cross-sectional study. *Rheumatol. Ther.* 2:165–172. doi: 10.1007/s40744-015-0021-z.

NICE CKS Polymyalgia rheumatica (2023) https://cks.nice.org.uk/topics/polymyalgia-rheumatica

NICE guideline [NG210] (2022) Gout: diagnosis and management www.nice.org.uk/guidance/ng219

Hui M, Carr A, Cameron S, et al. for the BSR Standards, Audit and Guidelines Working Group (2017). The British Society for Rheumatology guideline for the Management of Gout. *Rheumatology* 56:e1–e20. doi: 10.1093/rheumatology/kex156.

BMJ Best Practice (2024) *Septic arthritis* https://bestpractice.bmj.com/topics/en-gb/3000116

Walter N, Rupp M, Baertl S, et al. (2022) The role of multidisciplinary teams in musculoskeletal infection. *Bone Joint Res.* 11:6–7. doi: 10.1302/2046-3758.111.BJR-2021-0498

Cruz-Jentoft A, Bahat G, Bauer J, et al. Writing Group for the European Working Group on Sarcopenia in Older People 2 (EWGSOP2), and the Extended Group for EWGSOP2 (2019) Sarcopenia: revised European consensus on definition and diagnosis. *Age Ageing* 48: 16–31. doi: 10.1093/ageing/afy169.

Yuan S, Larsson SC (2023) Epidemiology of sarcopenia: prevalence, risk factors, and consequences. *Metabolism* 144:155533. doi: 10.1016/j.metabol.2023.155533.

Hurst C, Robinson SM, Witham MD, et al. (2022) Resistance exercise as a treatment for sarcopenia: prescription and delivery. *Age Ageing* 51:afac003. doi: 10.1093/ageing/afac003.

Geraci A, Calvani R, Ferri E, et al. (2021) Sarcopenia and menopause: the role of estradiol. *Front. Endocrinol. (Lausanne)* 12:682012. doi: 10.3389/fendo.2021.682012.

Cruz-Jentoft AJ (2021) Diagnosing sarcopenia: turn your eyes back on patients. *Age Ageing* 50:1904–1905. doi: 10.1093/ageing/afab184.

Iwere RB, Hewitt J (2015) Myopathy in older people receiving statin therapy: a systematic review and meta-analysis. *Br. J. Clin. Pharmacol.* 80:363–71. doi: 10.1111/bcp.12687.

Morren JA, Li Y (2023) Myasthenia gravis: frequently asked questions. *Cleveland Clin. J. Med.* 90:103–113. doi: 10.3949/ccjm.90a.22017.

INFORMATION FOR PATIENTS AND FAMILIES

NOGG: Information for patients and the public https://www.nogg.org.uk/

Royal Osteoporosis Society: https://theros.org.uk/information-and-support

NHS RightCare Susan's Story: https://gettingitrightfirsttime.co.uk/wp-content/uploads/2024/07/rightcare-susans-story-app1.pdf

Osteoarthritis: https://www.nhs.uk/conditions/osteoarthritis/treatment

Rheumatoid arthritis: https://patient.info/bones-joints-muscles/rheumatoid-arthritis-leaflet

Polymyalgia and Giant Cell Arteritis: https://pmrgca.org.uk

Patient information website Septic Arthritis: https://patient.info/bones-joints-muscles/arthritis/septic-arthritis

Paget's Association: Pagets Disease Home | http://paget.org.uk

Gout: https://patient.info/foot-care/gout-leaflet

Pseudogout: https://patient.info/bones-joints-muscles/calcium-pyrophosphate-deposition-pseudogout

All websites were accessed in February 2024.

11

Falls and immobility

Falls

Ageing changes

Ageing changes in a number of systems make people more likely to fall.

Sensory

- Eye changes: presbyopia, reduced depth perception and contrast sensitivity, and slower dark adaptation all increase the risk of falling (see Chapter 20).
- Balance impairment is secondary to the loss of labyrinthine hair cells, vestibular ganglion cells and nerve fibres, reducing vestibular input (see Chapter 20).
- Age-related hearing impairment is associated with a 1.7-fold increased risk of falling, but it is not clear whether it is an independent risk factor or reflects vestibular ageing.
- Reduced proprioception in the lower limbs.

CNS

- Age-related loss of neurons and neurotransmitters such as dopamine within the basal ganglia.
- Cerebrovascular changes contribute to cognitive impairment.
- Slower reaction time.

Musculoskeletal

- Sarcopenia: the loss of muscle mass and strength and increased fatigability (see Chapter 10).
- Increased prevalence of osteoporosis (leading to a kyphotic posture, so that the patient's centre of gravity is pushed forward, contributing to poor balance).
- Increased body sway. Women tend to sway more than men.
- Reduced walking speed with a shorter broad-based or more irregular gait pattern, a less effective heel strike, and more time spent in double support (i.e. both feet on the ground at the same time).

Overlap between falls, TLoC, syncope, and dizziness

These conditions overlap and can cause diagnostic confusion.

- A fall is 'an event which causes a person to, unintentionally, come to rest on the ground or lower level and is not a result of a major intrinsic event (such as a stroke) or overwhelming hazard.'
- Transient loss of consciousness (TLoC) is defined as 'a state of real or apparent LoC with loss of awareness, characterized by amnesia for the period of unconsciousness, abnormal motor control, loss of responsiveness, and a short duration.'
- Syncope is defined as 'a transient loss of consciousness (TLoC) due to transient global cerebral hypoperfusion characterized by rapid onset, short duration and spontaneous, complete recovery.'
- Many patients cannot recall falling, so causes of TLoC (in the absence of head trauma, principally syncope and epileptic seizures) need to be considered as part of a falls assessment.
- Patients who experience falls or presyncope use various descriptions of how they feel, often including dizziness, so this is discussed in this chapter.
- Note that in TIAs, there are focal neurological symptoms and signs. In carotid TIAs, consciousness is not lost. There may be LoC in vertebrobasilar TIAs, but there will always be abnormal neurological findings.

Epidemiology of falls

Falls are important because they are common and have serious consequences, including a reduction in quality of life and increased mortality.

- A third of people in the community aged over 65, and half of people aged over 80 fall at least once a year.
- 50% of these have multiple falls.
- Up to 25% of frequent fallers die within 1 year of presentation, not directly due to injuries but because of the underlying causes of the falls.
- Women fall more than men of the same age – they tend to be frailer.
- Frail older people living in residential homes fall most often (people who are bedbound in nursing homes tend to fall less often).
- Falls in people aged 65+ led to >223,000 emergency hospital admissions in 2021/2022 in England (many fallers do not seek help, and many are assessed at home by paramedics and not taken to the ED).
- Falls are the leading cause of injury-related deaths at 65+: 5,850 deaths in England and Wales in 2022.
- Falls are now recognised as an increasing global health issue; worldwide more people die from falls than from malaria, and there has been a WHO review for the first time.
- Falls are not an inevitable part of ageing, but the number of risk factors increases with age.

A geriatric syndrome

Falls are the epitome of a geriatric syndrome because they are due to the complex interplay of internal risk factors such as ageing changes, multimorbidity, medications and being unable to compensate for external environmental challenges to stability. An older person slipping on a wet floor cannot compensate quickly enough to save themselves, lands heavily and is more likely to sustain a fracture because of osteoporosis.

- Falls can be difficult to sort out because of the multiple components. Doctors are commonly trained to manage single problems.
- We must support patients in making choices about balancing risks, e.g. the risk of falling due to postural hypotension versus the risk of a stroke due to supine hypertension.
- Falls are an active, not a passive, process. Geriatricians are passionate about avoiding the terms 'mechanical fall' and 'unwitnessed fall' to encourage healthcare professionals to look for and address all reversible risk factors. Only 15% of falls are caused by circumstances that would cause anyone to fall, i.e. a true mechanical fall.
- Because of the above, falls are best managed using the principles of Comprehensive Geriatric Assessment followed by multi-agency interventions.

Assessing why a patient has fallen

It is essential to recognise the risks of falling at the first presentation and intervene, as a third of older people discharged from the ED after falling re-present within 3 months with a hip fracture or serious head injury. NICE advocates asking older patients if they have fallen every time they have contact with a health care practitioner.

A mnemonic for the main causes of falls

DAME (reminds you that women fall more often than men):

- **D**rugs (fall-risk-increasing drugs [FRIDS], polypharmacy, alcohol).
- **A**ge-related changes (as above: gait, balance, sarcopaenia, sensory impairment).
- **M**edical (musculoskeletal problems, heart disease, neurological disease, incontinence).
- **E**nvironmental (obstacles, trailing wires, poor lighting, etc.).

Alternatively, think about how one stands up – and deficits in all those mechanisms allow falls:

- Sensory inputs (eyes, labyrinths and hearing, proprioception, and afferent nerves).
- Central connections (especially the cortex, basal ganglia, and cerebellum).
- Motor output (efferent nerves, bones, muscles, joints).
- Blood supply to the brain (pump, patent arteries, and oxygenated blood).
- Drugs and alcohol.
- Environment.

History

A careful history may distinguish between a fall and a blackout. It is key to the detective work needed to identify all the risk factors for falling to trigger multifactorial interventions to reduce the risk of future falls.

Collateral history

A witness report is very helpful. The patient may play down the number and severity of the falls out of fear of consequences, e.g. being persuaded not to go out alone, to do less for themselves, or even to move to institutional care. They may not remember blacking out, especially briefly.

- The witness can give information about the duration of unconsciousness, whether the patient was standing/sitting, whether they were pale/sweaty, and whether there were tonic–clonic movements and post-ictal drowsiness, helping to differentiate syncope from epilepsy.

- Research shows that even cognitively intact older people living in the community do not remember details about a fall after 3 months.
- If there is a history of dementia or current delirium, information from the patient will be limited. Both conditions increase falls risk. People with dementia are eight times more likely to fall than their cognitively intact peers due to factors including:
  - Impulsivity/inappropriate risk-taking.
  - Abnormal gait/balance due to impaired central processing.
  - Orthostatic hypotension, e.g. in Lewy body dementia.
  - Visuo-spatial abnormalities due to strokes in vascular dementia.
  - Carotid sinus hypersensitivity may be secondary to atheroma and might be an early indicator of vascular dementia.
  - A treatable risk factor, e.g. cataracts, may be overlooked as the patient does not report difficulties.
  - Extrapyramidal side effects of antipsychotic drugs.
  - Sedation, e.g. secondary to benzodiazepines.

An aid to remembering what to ask about falls: SPLATT!

- **S**ymptoms: light-headedness, vertigo, chest pain or palpitations prior to falling, or TLoC.
- **P**revious falls: a first fall suggests an acute event, recurrent falls suggest frailty or chronic disease.
- **L**ocation: the further the patient is from their bedroom when they fall, the fitter the patient.
- **A**ctivity provoking the event: exertion, postural change, neck movement, coughing/straining/passing urine?
- **T**ime: getting out of bed, at night, after taking tablets, after a meal?
- **T**rauma sustained? Were they able to get off the floor on their own?

Symptoms

Ask about symptoms around the event and of underlying conditions that predispose to falls/TLoC.

- Do you ever feel dizzy or light-headed? Dizziness is usually multifactorial.
- Do you get the sensation of the world spinning around you? This suggests vertigo, as discussed below.
- Did you get palpitations? Were they regular/irregular, fast or slow? This suggests an arrhythmia.
- Did you have any chest pain/shortness of breath?
- Do you think you blacked out? How long for? How did you feel afterwards? A transient blackout suggests syncope. If the patient says, 'I must have tripped', it still may be syncope. Unless they had a blackout, the person usually recalls hitting the floor.
- Did you bite your tongue? Did you lose bladder control? Were you confused afterwards? Positive replies suggest seizures, especially if there was a prodrome, e.g. an abnormal smell in temporal lobe epilepsy, a longer period of LoC, and a slow recovery.
- Ask about stiff and painful joints.
- Have you noticed changes in your eyesight? Visual impairment (cataracts, glaucoma and inappropriate or dirty glasses) makes detection of hazards difficult. Slowed dark adaptation increases falls at night.
- Difficulty getting going, turning over in bed, or freezing in doorways suggests Parkinson's disease (PD).
- Numb feet or fingers suggest peripheral neuropathy. Common causes are diabetes, B_{12} deficiency and alcoholism.
- Ask about all the medications the patient is taking; remember over the counter medications (see later).
- Take a full alcohol history. Drinking more than 14 units of alcohol per week increases the risk of falling.

- Ask about the fear of falling, which is thought to affect 55% of older people and is more common in women. It can lead to activity avoidance, deconditioning, immobility and sometimes institutionalisation.

Previous falls

A history of falls is highly predictive of future falls.

- If this is the index fall, there may be an acute problem causing hypotension, e.g. an MI, GI bleed, pneumonia, or an acute episode of multifactorial delirium.
- Recurrent falls are more likely to be due to frailty, chronic disease, and dementia.

Location

- Patients who fall outside are fitter than their housebound peers and have a better prognosis.
- Falls in the bathroom may be due to a slippery floor, worsened by incontinence or emollients.

Activity

Finding out exactly what the patient was doing when they fell gives many clues.

- Postural dizziness, getting out of bed, suggests orthostatic hypotension.
- Situational syncope, e.g. blacking out after eating (post-prandial syncope), when passing urine (micturition syncope).
- Falling after turning the head to one side might suggest carotid sinus hypersensitivity or vertebrobasilar syndrome. Hanging clothes on a washing line and going to the hairdresser are risky activities!

Timing

- Falling in the morning when getting up suggests orthostatic hypotension.
- Falling at night may be secondary to nocturia due to prostatic hypertrophy in combination with postural hypotension, poor lighting in the hallway, and drowsiness secondary to hypnotics.
- How long were they on the ground? (before they were found and whilst waiting for the ambulance).

Trauma sustained

Older people falling from standing height now represent a high proportion of patients presenting to the ED with major trauma (Trauma Audit & Research Network report, 2017).

- The nature of the trauma may suggest the mechanism. If the patient fractured their wrist, they had time to try to save themselves, but if they sustained a facial injury, it is more likely they blacked out.
- 30% of falls lead to a hospital admission.
- Minor soft tissue injury occurs in 40–60% of falls: haematoma, skin tear, laceration.
- More serious soft tissue injury is seen in 5% of falls: this would include subdural haematomas (see Figure 11.1) and large haematomas requiring blood transfusion.
- 10% of falls lead to a fracture: most commonly, the wrist, humerus, vertebral, pelvis, and hip (2% of falls).

Other consequences of falls

- Superficial but painful friction burns from carpets.
- Burns needing grafting (secondary to falling against a fire or radiator and being unable to move away because of loss of consciousness or paralysis).

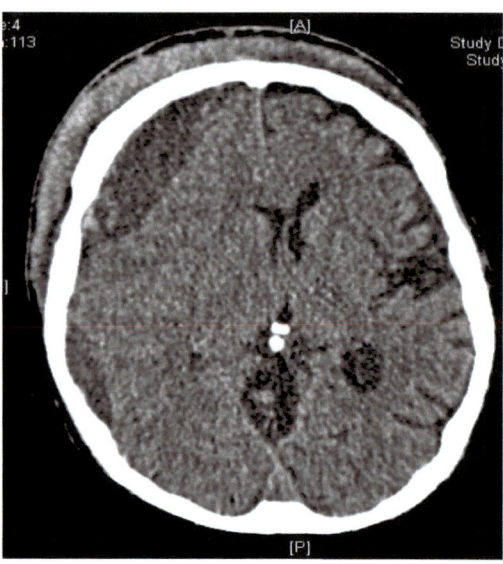

Figure 11.1 CT of the head shows an acute-to-chronic subdural haematoma. Note subcutaneous haematoma over the right side of the forehead, old darker subdural blood, brighter blood from new subdural haematoma, and midline shift.

- Quadriplegia due to a central cord lesion in a patient with a spinal cord compromised by spondylosis (fortunately rare).
- Anxiety/depression about the future.
- Anxiety in carers (formal and informal) may become intolerable, leading to the potential for elder abuse.
- The need to move to safer surroundings may separate the faller from their support network. Well-meaning families may move their parents away from where they have been based for many years.

Consequences of a long lie

A long lie is defined as remaining on the floor for 1 hr or more after falling.

- Pressure ulcers (see Chapter 19).
- Hypothermia may result if the patient falls in a cold environment, e.g. outside or in an unheated room (see Chapter 16).
- Hypostatic pneumonia.
- Rhabdomyolysis leading to with a high creatine kinase may cause an AKI.
- Crucially, 50% of patients who lie on the floor for >1 hr after falling are dead within 6 months, even if no injury was sustained from the fall (due to physical and social vulnerability).

Examination

- Core temperature, oxygen saturation and pressure areas after a long lie.
- Does the patient look ill? If so, consider acute problems such as an MI, PE or GI bleed and examine accordingly.

Thorough examination is needed, but pay particular attention to the following:

- Pulse rate and rhythm.
- Look at the JVP: what is the patient's fluid status?
- Check for postural hypotension (see below).
- Does the patient have anaemia or myxoedema?
- Listen for murmurs, especially aortic stenosis, and carotid bruits.
- Assess the CNS and look for lateralizing signs.

- Look for signs of PD: mask facies, tremors, rigidity, and bradykinesia. Examine the gait: shuffling, retropulsion and festination.
- Check for peripheral neuropathy.
- Check vision. A borrowed newspaper is more likely to be available than a Snellen chart or print and use the RCP screen. Ask the patient if they have had a recent eye test. Cataracts are easily treated.
- Bifocal and varifocal lenses increase falls risk; the view ahead in the lower part of the lens may be blurred, impairing depth perception and contrast sensitivity. This makes it difficult to negotiate steps and uneven pavements safely.
- Does the patient have hearing impairment? Are the hearing aids correctly inserted? There is evidence that wearing hearing aids reduces the risk of falling.
- Examine the neck movements. Does this cause dizziness?

Assessing the gait

Watch the patient walk and turn. The gait pattern may reveal an underlying condition.

- **Frontal-related gait pattern:** common in cerebrovascular disease, vascular dementia, and Alzheimer's disease. The gait is wide-based and apraxic, and the patient may freeze. There is an increased risk of falling when the patient turns or if they are distracted, as they cannot dual-task.
- **Normal pressure hydrocephalus:** a wide-based ataxic gait, associated with urinary incontinence and cognitive impairment. Head CT shows dilated ventricles.
- **Hemiplegic gait:** steps are slower and shorter, and the gait is less smooth because the affected leg is circumducted, i.e. the forefoot scrapes the floor in an arc.
- **Spastic paraparesis:** e.g. secondary to cervical myelopathy, bilateral scissoring of stiff legs.
- **Cerebellar disease:** an irregular, wide-based, unsteady gait.
- **Sensory ataxia:** e.g. peripheral neuropathy secondary to diabetes, the patient watches the ground and their feet rather than looking ahead. Romberg's test is positive. The patient may stamp their feet.
- **Vestibular ataxia:** think of this if the patient complains of nausea, vomiting and vertigo.
- **Parkinsonian gait:** hypokinetic, festinant, shuffling gait with reduced arm swing.
- **Antalgic gait:** e.g. secondary to osteoarthritis (OA), asymmetrical because the patient puts their weight through the side with the painful joint as briefly as possible.
- **Waddling gait:** weakness of the hip girdle muscles and difficulty getting out of a chair caused by proximal myopathy, e.g. secondary to steroids and osteomalacia.
- **Trendelenburg gait:** weakness of the gluteus medius on the affected side of the pelvis causes dipping when the patient stands on the contralateral leg. To compensate, the patient moves their trunk laterally, producing the characteristic lateral sway.
- **Foot drop:** high-stepping, foot-slapping gait, e.g. secondary to common peroneal nerve palsy caused by compression from a tight lower leg plaster cast.

Investigations

The range of investigations is wide and will be directed by the history and examination and whether the patient is well and attending a community falls clinic, has been admitted via ED after falling in the context of an acute illness, or has recurrent unexplained falls.

- **Basic screen:** may include FBC, U&E, LFTs, calcium, CRP, TSH, HbA1c, B$_{12}$, Vitamin D, and ECG.
- **Septic screen:** if there is suspicion of an infective precipitant: blood cultures, urine dip and culture, CXR.

- **Long lie:** check CK.
- **Imaging:** bone radiography if suspicion of fracture; CT or magnetic resonance imaging (MRI); head if new focal neurology; head trauma; or fluctuating GCS.
- **Cardiac investigations:** troponin, 24-hour tape, external or internal loop recorder, echocardiogram.
- **Further investigations for postural hypotension:** 24-hour BP monitoring, short Synacthen test.
- **Investigations for neurally medicated syncope:** tilt table test (TTT), carotid sinus massage (CSM).
- **Further investigations for neuropathy:** monoclonal bands, autoantibodies, nerve conduction studies.

Functional tests

These rapid tests can be done at baseline and after interventions. They are often done by a physio but can be done by any trained team member and are useful to monitor progress.

1 **Timed Up and Go (TUG):** time how long it takes for the patient to stand up from a chair, walk 3 metres, turn around, walk back to the chair, and sit down again. A longer time indicates a greater risk of falling (see Appendix).
2 **The Berg balance scale:** assesses the patient's ability to maintain equilibrium during various tasks, such as standing with eyes closed, reaching, and turning. Lower scores indicate a higher risk of falling.
3 **The functional reach test:** how far forward can the patient reach whilst standing in a fixed position to check dynamic balance and stability?
4 **The 6-min walking test:** how far can the patient walk in 6 min?

Interventions to reduce the risks of falling

Falls reduction requires a multidisciplinary and multi-agency approach. Many hospitals and community providers run falls prevention clinics. If the patient agrees, involve a family member to help ensure plans are carried out.

- The evidence is clear that management should be tailored to each patient.
- Identify and treat *all* reversible contributing causes and risk factors.
- Stop unnecessary FRIDs; the strongest evidence is the risk reduction achieved by stopping antipsychotics.
- Remember osteoporosis prevention and treatment; see Chapter 10 and vitamin D for all.
- Ask those with impaired vision/hearing to arrange a review with an optician/audiologist.
- Refer patients with significant bradycardia, heart block and cardioinhibitory syncope for pacing.
- Refer patients with significant aortic stenosis for cardiological evaluation.
- Refer people with PD to your local specialist service.
- Provide information on footwear:

   Bare feet and stocking feet are high-risk. Slippers are well-named, and high heels impair balance. Shoes should have a rigid toe box to protect the toes from trauma and compression, should fit well, have good padding, a small heel to encourage a clear heel strike, and the sole should be light, thin enough to allow proprioception, and have grooves to reduce slipping. Several suppliers sell shoes for swollen/deformed feet (e.g. Cosyfeet – not cheap, but patients may be VAT exempt).
- The physio will prescribe exercises and advise on transfer/walking aids.
- The OT will advise on equipment to optimise function and safety modifications to the home. A stair lift or living downstairs may be less disruptive than moving. Home hazard reduction is not evidence-based but is pragmatic.

Exercise prescription

Evidence shows that individually tailored exercise plans that incorporate strength, balance, flexibility, and endurance training prevent future falls. Examples include the Otago exercise plan and the FaME (Fitness and Mobility Exercise) programme.

- Exercise can reduce falls rates by 38% when it includes high-level strength and balance classes if:
  - The dose of exercise is correct. 2–3 times weekly (up to a total of 50 hr),
  - The duration is correct, usually 12 weeks.
  - The exercises get harder with time.
- Follow up at the end of the treatment programme with advice to engage in ongoing exercise, e.g. Tai Chi.
- Ensure the correct prescription and use of walking aids. For example, people with PD do better with rollator frames than Zimmer frames, which disrupt the flow of walking. See Table 11.5.
- Improve gait pattern, e.g. encourage people with PD to take longer steps and to stand straighter.
- Teach the patient how to get up from the floor.

Extrinsic risk factors for falling

- Older people tend to live in older housing, which may need repairs.
- Poor lighting, especially near doorways, steps, and stairs.
- A lifetime's clutter, especially if the patient has Diogenes' syndrome and has narrow 'corridors' between stacks of newspapers, etc.
- Pets underfoot.
- Trailing electrical cables.
- Slippery floors with loose rugs.
- Bathroom with a low toilet and a lack of grab rails by the bath or shower.
- Incorrect use of walking aids/inappropriate walking aids.
- Unfamiliar environment, e.g. hospital or a new care home.
- Wet, icy, or uneven pavements. The local council should ensure good maintenance of paving and lighting, especially outside warden-assisted flats, and arrange early gritting of pavements in freezing weather.

Role of technology

- Smartphones are increasingly being studied as a means of detecting falls and preventing further falls. Many older people have them; they are portable, and they usually include an accelerometer. However, if the phone is not being carried, falls will be missed.
- Increasing use of smart watches improves detection rates, and those that include an ECG can pick up atrial fibrillation.
- A variety of apps are available to guide those at risk of falls.
- Development teams need to involve older people to ensure that these devices are user-friendly, are suitable for assessing the physiology of older people, and improve outcomes.

Mitigating the consequences of falling

If falls cannot be prevented, their consequences can be reduced.

- Maintain an adequate environmental temperature.
- Soften floor coverings, i.e. carpet rooms.
- Remove obstacles and dangers, e.g. guard fires.
- Place emergency blankets where they can be reached from the floor, e.g. on the back of the sofa.
- Arrange for a personally worn alarm system or for frequent visitors.
- Educate the patient and their relatives about safety in the home and the risk of falls. Age UK produces helpful leaflets.

Common conditions presenting as falls

Syncope

Syncope describes an episode of loss of consciousness and postural tone due to transient global cerebral hypoperfusion.

- The incidence of syncope in over 60-year-olds is 6% (probably a gross underestimate owing to underdiagnosis).
- The 2-year recurrence rate is 30%.
- Syncope must be considered in all patients with recurrent, unexplained falls (see Table 11.1).
- Cerebral blood flow is about 50 mL/100 g/min in older people but is lower in those with hypertension or atherosclerosis.
- Symptoms of cerebral ischaemia occur when the blood flow is reduced to 25–30 mL/100 g/min.
- There are two major categories of syncope:
  1 Neurally mediated/reflex syncope (NMS)
  2 Cardiac syncope
- NMS is the most common and is due to an inappropriate autonomic reflex in response to a trigger, but the proportion of episodes caused by cardiac syncope increases with age.
- Syncope during exercise or when lying flat is suggestive of an arrhythmia or structural heart disease.
- Chest pain prior to syncope is suggestive of ischaemic heart disease.
- NMS has a better short-term prognosis; some patients have serious underlying conditions, but most do not need admission for urgent investigations of the collapse.

1. Neurally-mediated syncope

Uncomplicated vasovagal syncope

Anyone can faint – think of the 'three Ps', although NMS is most frequent in young people.

- **i Provoking factors:** having blood taken, pain, high emotion.
- **ii Prodrome:** feeling hot, sweaty, nauseous, and looking pale (often less prominent in older people)
- **iii Posture:** remaining upright (standing or even sitting up), e.g. in church because of embarrassment.

Advise people to be aware of their triggers, ensure good hydration and watch for and act on prodromal symptoms.

Orthostatic (postural) hypotension

This is common, occurring in about 20% of community-dwelling older people and, in some case series, up to 50% of care home residents.

- Reduced baroreceptor responsiveness and reduced arterial compliance increase the risk. It is more common among people with coexisting disorders, especially hypertension.
- Any drop in BP on standing up is poorly tolerated in older people because cerebral autoregulation is often defective, especially in those with a history of hypertension.
- Orthostatic hypotension is defined as a drop of >10 mmHg diastolic or >20 mmHg systolic provoked by standing up and accompanied by symptoms. Note whether there is compensatory tachycardia.
- A postural drop in BP may be an incidental finding and is only clinically relevant if there is a good correlation with symptoms on standing.
- Some centres use a systolic drop of 30 mmHg if the patient has a history of hypertension.
- Symptoms include dizziness, presyncope, syncope, falls, and visual disturbance. It is most common when getting out of bed first thing in the morning or standing after sitting for a long period.
- Ask about parkinsonian symptoms.
- Take a careful drug history.

Table 11.1 Causes, investigations, and management of types of syncope.

Cause	Subtypes	Diagnosis	Management
Neurally mediated			
Orthostatic hypotension	Primary autonomic failure, MSA, Parkinson's plus syndromes, Parkinson's disease	A drop in BP provoked by standing is associated with symptoms	Patient education Drugs: see below
	Secondary autonomic impairment: diabetes, amyloid, drugs		
Carotid sinus hypersensitivity	Cardio-inhibitory	CSM causes an asystolic pause	Pacemaker
	Vasodepressor	CSM causes a drop in BP	Lifestyle advice
	Mixed	CSM causes both	Pacemaker and lifestyle advice
Recurrent vasovagal syncope	Cardio-inhibitory	Bradycardia provoked by HUT	Pacemaker
	Vasodepressor	Hypotension on HUT	Advice about optimum fluid intake; consider extra salt and caffeine; recruit muscles if experiencing presyncope
	Mixed	Bradycardia and hypotension on HUT	Pacemaker and the above advice
Simple vasovagal syncope	Mixed	Provoking factor, prodrome and posture	Advice
Situational syncope	Cough	Good history	Avoid situations where practical. NB: DVLA is strict about patients with cough syncope not being able to drive
	Micturition/Defaecation	Good history	Suggest men sit to urinate and avoid constipation
	Swallowing	Good history	Suggest small mouthfuls
	Post-prandial	Note the delayed onset	Eat little and often
Cardiac syncope			
Cardiac ischaemia		ECG changes, troponin rises	See Chapter 12
Arrhythmias	Bradycardia/pauses	24-hour tape, external or internal loop recorder	Pacemaker (see Figure 11.2)
	Tachycardia		Antiarrhythmic drugs
	Tachybrady syndrome		'Pace and block'
Structural heart disease	Aortic stenosis	Echocardiogram	TAVI, or valve replacement
	HCM	Echocardiogram	ACEi
Severe heart failure	Any aetiology, reduced cardiac output, exacerbated by drugs and cardiac cachexia	Echocardiogram	Adjust medication
Subclavian steal syndrome	Syncope with ataxia, finger necrosis more likely to affect left side	An angiogram may show stenosis	Good management of cardiovascular risk factors

CSM, carotid sinus massage; HUT, head-up tilt; MSA, multiple system atrophy; HCM, hypertrophic cardiomyopathy; ACEi, ACE inhibitor.

Measuring the blood pressure

Measure the lying and standing BP and document the heart rate, especially first thing in the morning and after meals. Use a manual sphygmomanometer. Document standing BP immediately on standing and ideally using beat-to-beat monitoring for greater accuracy every 30 sec for 3 min.

If the heart rate goes up, this suggests volume loss. The absence of compensatory tachycardia is suggestive of autonomic failure.

Causes
- **Neurodegenerative disorders:** pure autonomic failure, multiple system atrophy, dementia with Lewy bodies, and longstanding PD.
- **Peripheral neuropathies with autonomic neuropathy:** diabetic neuropathy, amyloid neuropathy.
- **Drugs:** diuretics, alpha- and beta-blockers, calcium channel blockers, phenothiazines, antidepressants, levodopa, and vasodilators including alcohol, opiates, and nitrates.
- **Pump failure:** cardiac impairment of any cause.

- **Volume depletion:** a GI bleed, diarrhoea, Addison's disease.
- **Vasodilation:** fever.
- **Decreased autonomic function due to ageing and physiological stress:** post-prandial, post-exercise, deconditioning.

Management
- Correct any cause identified.
- Advise about sensible precautions (sit on the edge of the bed, 'march' on the spot, drink a large glass of cold water before standing, take a warm rather than hot bath or shower; see advice from Syncope UK).
- Stop drugs that may be contributing if possible or consider alternatives, e.g. nicorandil for angina instead of nitrates, which cause more venous vasodilatation.
- Prescribe compression stockings or tights, but these are difficult to put on and take off and must not be used if arterial supply to the feet is poor. An abdominal binder may be as effective and, surprisingly, easier to manage.

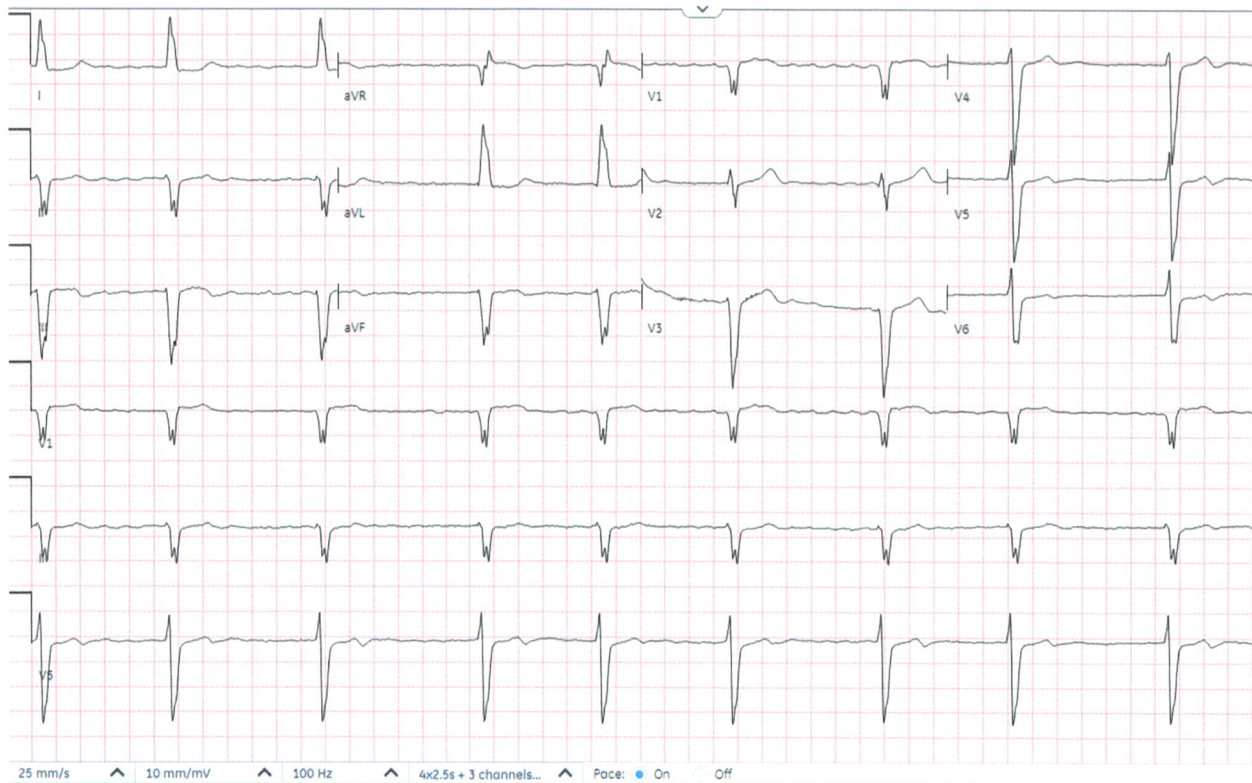

Figure 11.2 ECG shows atrial fibrillation, left axis deviation and left bundle block leading to bradycardia and causing recurrent syncope. The patient stopped 'falling' after pacemaker insertion.

- Medication
  - Fludrocortisone (a mineralocorticoid) that causes salt and water retention can be helpful, but its use is limited by leg oedema and hypokalaemia.
  - Midodrine, a peripheral alpha-agonist that causes arterial and venous constriction, is now licensed in the UK for treating orthostatic hypotension and has few side effects. Start with a low dose in the morning, then use bd, then tds and titrate up the dose; avoid after 18.00 to minimise supine hypertension. Avoid in patients with ischaemic heart disease.
- Head-up tilt to bed (10°) to promote salt retention and reduce nocturnal diuresis.
- When a patient presents after falling, it is important to inform them of the driving restrictions that may apply if the diagnosis is syncope or seizure. See DVLA guidance on medical fitness to drive.

Postprandial hypotension

This is a symptomatic drop in BP of 20 mmHg or more, or lower than 90 mmHg, within 2 hr of starting a meal (typically large, carbohydrate-rich). It is due to splanchnic pooling, and the risk factors are like those for orthostatic hypotension, which often coexists. It is missed unless it is considered, as it happens *after* the provoking meal. It is managed by eating small, frequent meals.

Investigations for neurally mediated syncope

Tilt table testing
A head-up TTT is used to investigate suspected NMS if the person has recurrent episodes of TLoC that adversely affect their quality of life or carry a substantial risk of injury, and to assess whether the syncope is accompanied by a severe cardioinhibitory response (usually asystole).

It can confirm suspected orthostatic hypotension. Cardiac causes of syncope should be excluded first. Most centres are moving to the Fast Italian protocol.

The patient lies on the table and the finger cuff, ECG leads, and blood pressure cuff are all put in place. After letting the patient relax for 5 min, an active stand is performed to measure lying and standing blood pressure. If this is normal, proceed to CSM, starting on the right-hand side. Exclude patients with TIAs or strokes within the past 3 months or concerns about carotid artery disease. If negative, the patient is strapped to the table, and the table is tilted to 70°. CSM is performed again, starting on the right and then the left. If there are still no abnormal findings, the patient remains passively at 70° for 10 min and then is given 300–400 μg sublingual GTN spray (if the patient has not experienced syncope) and a further 20 min at 70° (see Table 11.2).

- There is limited specificity, sensitivity, and reproducibility, i.e. depending on the operator, protocol and whether the patient can tolerate the procedure.
- The haemodynamic response to tilt testing may differ from the mechanism of spontaneous syncopal episodes, so an implantable loop recorder may be preferable.
- A positive test for vasovagal syncope is characterised by the development of syncope in association with a cardioinhibitory and/or vasodepressor response.

  Cardioinhibitory: parasympathetic predominance with bradycardia or asystole.

  Vasodepressor: insufficient sympathetic vasoconstriction results in hypotension.

Carotid sinus massage
In unexplained TLoC >60 years where carotid sinus syndrome (CSS) may be a possibility, CSM is offered as a first-line investigation (in a

Table 11.2 Types of response to tilt-testing.

Response/ Diagnosis	Characteristics
Vasodepressor syncope	SBP falls to <60 mmHg. HR during syncope does not fall by >10% peak.
Cardioinhibitory syncope without asystole	HR decreases <40 bpm, for more than 10 sec; without asystole >3 sec. BP falls before HR.
Cardioinhibitory syncope with asystole	Asystole >3 sec; decrease in HR precedes or coincides with BP fall.
Mixed syncope	HR decreases during syncope but does not reach <40 bpm, or reaches <40 bpm for <10 sec, with or without asystole <3 sec. BP falls before HR.
Classic orthostatic hypotension	A decrease in systolic BP ≥20 mmHg and diastolic BP ≥10 mmHg during the first 3 min, after standing. (You can also see initial or delayed responses.)
POTS (postural orthostatic tachycardia syndrome)	An increase in HR >30 bpm or HR >120 bpm after tilting is accompanied by symptoms and BP variability. Rare in old age.
Negative TTT	Syncope, orthostatic hypotension, or POTS are not provoked. The test may be *suggestive* of reflex syncope if reflex hypotension/bradycardia is induced without causing syncope.

Source: Adapted from European Society of Cardiology, 2015. SBP, systolic blood pressure; HR, heart rate; POTS, postural orthostatic tachycardia syndrome; TTT, tilt table test.

controlled environment with ECG recording and resuscitation equipment available), often as part of a TTT. CSM is contraindicated if there has been a stroke, TIA or myocardial infarction in the previous 3 months. The presence of a carotid bruit does not correlate well with carotid stenosis. Arrange carotid Dopplers first if concerned (the risk of neurological sequelae is quoted at 0.14%).

Diagnose CSS if CSM reproduces syncope due to marked bradycardia/asystole and/or marked hypotension.

2. Cardiac syncope

Causes of cardiac syncope are discussed in Chapter 12, but in brief:

i   High probability of arrhythmic syncope if the ECG shows:
   - Persistent sinus bradycardia.
   - Mobitz II, second and third AV blocks.
   - Alternating LBBB and RBBB.
   - VT, or rapid SVT.
   - Non-sustained VT.
   - Pacemaker malfunction.
ii Ischaemic cardiac syncope when the ECG shows evidence of an acute MI.
iii Suspect cardiopulmonary syncope when there is evidence of severe aortic stenosis, or PE.

Fall-risk-increasing drugs (FRIDS)

Around 50 per cent of over-75-year-olds have three or more comorbidities and are on multiple drugs. The more medications, the greater the risk of interactions and adverse events, including falls (see Table 11.3).

- 60% of over 60-year-olds taking four or more medications will fall in a year (but this group has chronic disease).
- There is a lack of evidence that reducing medications as a lone strategy reduces falls, but drug use is one of the most modifiable risk factors for an individual, and judicious deprescribing may have other benefits.
- Tools such as STOPP 2 and the anticholinergic burden (ACB) calculator to assess cholinergic burden are useful starting points.
- There are a variety of mechanisms by which drugs increase the risk of falling (hypotension, bradycardia, electrolyte disturbance) and a single drug may have several effects.
- All drugs that cause drowsiness or confusion will increase falls.
- Remember to discuss with the patient and their family why you feel it is useful to stop medications; otherwise, you may meet more resistance than you expected.

Dizziness

This can be a heart sink symptom because there are many and varied causes, but use it as an opportunity to employ your detective skills! Dizziness is a syndrome, i.e. there are multiple causes.

Causes

There are four main categories:

1 **Vertigo (perception of motion in the absence of motion):** peripheral (inner ear and vestibulocochlear nerve) or central (cerebellum or brain stem).
2 **Presyncope (sensation of feeling faint):** often cardiac or postural hypotension.
3 **Disequilibrium (the feeling of being off-balance or wobbly):** often impaired vision and proprioception.
4 **Light-headedness (sensation of giddiness, muzziness, feeling disconnected from the environment):** often anxiety-related, but may be early presyncope!

The illusion of rotation or movement in vertigo and the sensation of an impending blackout are usually more clearly described than the other sensations.

One approach is to consider which factors might affect each system, as in Table 11.4.

Benign Positional Paroxysmal Vertigo

1 in 2 people who fall have vestibular dysfunction.

- Benign positional paroxysmal vertigo (BPPV) is increasingly common with age, affecting 10% of over-70-year-olds.
- In some series, BPPV accounts for 25% of cases of dizziness presenting to the ED.
- It is characterised by a sudden, short-lasting (usually less than 1 min) illusion of movement accompanied by nausea, imbalance, and disequilibrium, triggered by movement, e.g. turning over in bed.
- Some patients develop chronic symptoms, which they learn to cope with, e.g. by sleeping with 4–5 pillows and avoiding extending the neck to look up.
- A third of cases of BPPV resolve spontaneously, especially if the patient is male, has sufficient vitamin D, and has normal bone density.
- BPPV can occur following an earlier fall that dislodged the otoconia (calcium carbonate crystals) from the utricle into a semicircular canal.
- There are several types, depending on where the otoconia drift to:
  ○ Posterior canal, accounts for 80% (due to gravity as it is the lowest part of the inner ear), brought on by rolling over.
  ○ Horizontal canal – the patient gets vertigo when moving their head in the horizontal plane.
  ○ Anterior canal, least common, and brought on by straight head hanging.
  ○ Multi-canal disease, due to otoconia landing in more than one canal, causes mixed symptoms.

Table 11.3 Common fall-risk-increasing drugs.

Drug	Examples	Mechanism	Management strategy
Cardiovascular drugs	Diuretics, calcium channel blockers Beta-blockers	Postural hypotension. Beta-blockers and non-dihydropyridine calcium channel blockers, e.g. diltiazem, may also worsen bradycardia secondary to conduction disorders	Regularly check BP, lying, and standing and pulse. Consider ambulatory blood pressure to exclude white-coat hypertension or overtreatment of hypertension
Opiate analgesics	Codeine, morphine, oxycodone	Cross the blood–brain barrier, slow central processing, and cause drowsiness	'Start low, go slow'
Long-acting hypoglycaemic agents	Glimepiride	Hypoglycaemia	Choose short-acting agents, e.g. glipizide or switch to metformin
Antipsychotics	Haloperidol, chlorpromazine, risperidone	Extrapyramidal side effects	Use non-pharmacological methods to reduce delirium/agitation. If antipsychotics are essential, use atypical agents and 'Start low, go slow'; reassess ongoing needs regularly and aim to stop
Hypnotics	Benzodiazepines and Z-drugs (Those with shorter half-lives tend to have fewer residual effects but higher risks of withdrawal)	Slow central processing. Drowsiness persisting the following morning	Avoid; if not possible, restrict to short-term use. Abrupt discontinuation may lead to withdrawal syndrome, so switch to diazepam and wean slowly as per BNF guidelines
Antidepressants	Tricyclics are more strongly associated with falls than SSRIs and SNRIs	Slow central processing. Risk factor for hyponatraemia, which causes delirium associated with a high risk of falls. Long QT syndrome: amitriptyline, citalopram	Tailor treatment to the patient; if there is a history of hyponatraemia, avoid SSRIs, especially citalopram; consider mirtazapine. Check electrolytes regularly. ECG before beginning the drug, and then again after
Anti-epileptics	Phenytoin, carbamazepine	Associated with dizziness and cerebellar dysfunction. Narrow therapeutic window. Effect on vitamin D metabolism	Consult neurology – is there a better drug? Check drug levels, as dizziness might be a sign of toxicity. Ensure the patient is treated with calcium and vitamin D, plus anti-resorptives where appropriate
Drugs for an overactive bladder	Oxybutynin	Anticholinergic	Is it effective? Consider alternatives.
Alcohol	Greater than 1 unit per day	Acute intoxication. Chronic subdural haematoma. Cerebellar disease. Wernicke–Korsakoff syndrome. Withdrawal	Get an accurate alcohol history. Ensure thiamine and magnesium levels are replete. Refer to support services. Prescribe chlordiazepoxide
OTC medicines	Dextromethorphan, e.g. 'Night Nurse' Codeine	Drowsiness	Educate patients and carers that just because a drug does not need to be prescribed, it does not mean it is safe

OTC, over the counter drugs; SNRIs, serotonin and noradrenergic reuptake inhibitors; SSRIs, serotonin reuptake inhibitors; TCA, tricyclic antidepressants; Z drugs, zopiclone family.

Diagnosis

BPPV is diagnosed using the **Dix-Hallpike manoeuvre**. There are many good videos on YouTube. Sit the patient on the bed and turn their head 45° towards the side producing the most symptoms. Then help them to lie down quickly until their neck is extended by 20°. The test is positive if there is rotational nystagmus towards the floor.

There is evidence that there is no need to rush to lie the patient down – if you have to go slowly, hold the position longer whilst looking for nystagmus. There is no need to extend the head over the end of the bed.

A pillow behind the chest is kind to people with COPD, kyphosis and back pain. (NB: if the patient is taking a vestibular sedative, the nystagmus may be blunted and more difficult to see.)

Treatment

Treat using the **Epley manoeuvre** to reposition the otoliths to the utricle. The patient sits on the bed with their head turned to 45° on the positive side. They then lie flat, keeping the head turned for 30 sec. Next, they turn their heads 90° again, holding the position for 30 sec. They roll

Table 11.4 Causes of dizziness.

Type	Disease	Symptoms	Diagnosis	Treatment
Labyrinth	Benign Positional Paroxysmal Vertigo (BPPV)	Recurrent brief episodes of a sensation of rotation, lasting <5 min, provoked by a change in head position.	Hallpike–Dix manoeuvre (reproduces symptoms and nystagmus)	Epley/Semont manoeuvre, see text
VIII (vestibulocochlear) nerve lesion	Vestibular schwannoma (acoustic neuroma)	Gradual onset and slow progression of unilateral hearing loss, tinnitus, and vertigo	ENT clinic. MRI internal auditory meatus	Surgical excision, where appropriate
Labyrinth and Cochlea	Ménière's disease	Recurrent episodic attacks (few min – 24 hr) of the triad of vertigo, hearing impairment and tinnitus, often unilateral	History. ENT clinic	Short-course prochlorperazine or cyclizine in the episode. Betahistine may reduce attacks
The vestibular branch of the vestibulocochlear nerve	Vestibular neuronitis	Sudden onset, severe vertigo, poor balance, and nausea for more than 24 hr.	History – often following a viral URTI.	Usually resolves in a few days to a couple of weeks. Short course prochlorperazine or cyclizine.
The vestibular *and* cochlear branches/the labyrinth	Labyrinthitis (both usually viral)	The addition of hearing loss/ tinnitus (usually unilateral) indicates labyrinthitis	Sudden hearing loss warrants an emergency ENT/ED referral	Short course of steroids for sudden hearing loss
External auditory meatus	Ear wax presses on the tympanic membrane	Vertigo, tinnitus, and mild nausea	Otoscopy	Drops to soften wax and remove by micro-suction.
CNS	Vertebrobasilar syndrome (posterior circulation TIAs)	Symptoms are variable but include vertigo, diplopia, ataxia, and sudden falls (loss of tone in the lower limbs)	History may be provoked by turning the head. Examination. CTA or MRA	See Chapter 9
	Cerebellar diseases: stroke	Depends on the artery but typically include vertigo, nausea, ataxia, and headache.	HINTS (see text) MRI head	See Chapter 9
	Tumour	Progressive symptoms		Surgery, radiotherapy, symptom control
Peripheral nerves	Neuropathy, e.g. diabetic, B_{12} deficiency, hypothyroidismv	Reduced proprioception in toes and ankles may be associated cognitive decline and autonomic neuropathy	HbA1c, B_{12}, folate, and TSH	Improve diabetic control, check feet, replace haematinics, levothyroxine
Cardiovascular causes of presyncope and syncope and orthostatic hypotension of all causes – see Table 11.1				
Metabolic	Hypoglycaemia	Dizziness after not eating	Low BM	Sugary drink, Hypostop, review diabetes drugs
	Hypothyroid	Cold intolerance, weight gain	High TSH, low T4	Oral levothyroxine replacement
	Addison's disease: primary adrenal failure, usually autoimmune	Lightheadedness, weight loss, fatigue	Synacthen® test, hyponatraemia, and hyperkalaemia	Replace glucocorticoid and mineralocorticoid
Psychiatric	Anxiety/depression	Constant, unrelieved dizziness. Other symptoms of low mood anhedonia, poor sleep, anxiety	Exclude organic causes determine whether depression or anxiety is the most prominent disease	See Chapter 8
Other	Anaemia	Insidious blood loss, e.g. secondary to a colonic tumour, may present with dizziness	FBC, haematinics, gastroscopy, CT abdomen, colonoscopy, as indicated	Treat cause
	Carbon monoxide toxicity	Headaches and dizziness	COHb level	High-flow oxygen, via a face mask. See Chapter 13

BPPV, benign paroxysmal positional vertigo; MRI, magnetic resonance image; HbA1c, glycosylated haemoglobin; COHb, carboxyhaemoglobin level; ENT, ear nose and throat.

onto the side they are facing for 30 more seconds and then sit up, still with the head turned, for 30 sec more. This process should be repeated three times. Warn the patient that it might provoke nausea and vertigo.

Some authorities report that the **Semont manoeuvre** is easier and as effective as the Epley manoeuvre. The patient sits on the edge of the bed with their head turned 45° towards the unaffected side. The clinician helps them lie down quickly on the affected side with their head still turned to 45° so that they end up with their head slightly off the edge of the bed at 30° below the horizontal. This position is held for 1–2 min to allow the dislodged otoconia in the posterior semicircular canal to reposition within the vestibular system. The clinician then helps the patient quickly sit up with their head still turned to 45°.

Acute central vertigo

Acute vestibular syndrome – vertigo, nausea or vomiting, nystagmus, and gait unsteadiness – is common, and it can be difficult to differentiate a posterior circulation stroke from a peripheral cause. The HINTS examination (Head-Impulse, Nystagmus, Test of Skew) is a clinical test used to help rule out a posterior circulation stroke. A video on YouTube by P. John shows how to do the tests, and normal and abnormal results.

1 **Head-Impulse test:** in peripheral disorders such as BPPV, the eye saccades are in the direction opposite to the head turn to compensate. Central disorders **do not** produce corrective saccades.
2 **Nystagmus:** in peripheral disorders, nystagmus typically has a unidirectional torsional or horizontal pattern. In central disorders, the nystagmus can be bidirectional or vertical and may persist in any gaze direction.
3 **Test of Skew:** vertical misalignment of the eyes suggests a central lesion.

If any one of these three oculomotor signs suggests a central cause; contact the stroke team for a full assessment and arrange an urgent MRI, although a very early MRI may be negative.

Falls in hospital

- Patients frequently fall in hospital: 2–7 per 1,000 patient days. The majority of these are recurrent falls.
- 11% of falls occur within 24 hr of admission, and 50% occur within the first 2 weeks.
- This suggests a first peak due to the acute illness and the unfamiliar environment, with a second peak owing to dementia and chronic instability.
- Falls in hospitals are strongly associated with cognitive impairment/acute delirium.
- Hospitals are unfamiliar surroundings with different routines, noise, and light at night, all of which lead to disturbed sleep and drowsiness the following morning when the physiotherapist arrives.
- In hospital, patients are encouraged to take all their medications. They may have (wisely) been omitting their diuretics and antihypertensives, so they become profoundly hypotensive when given them all together!
- Remember sick day rules for patients presenting with dehydration, diarrhoea, and sepsis. Omit their antihypertensives and watch the BP. Remember to double the dose of steroids for patients with inflammatory conditions such as rheumatoid arthritis.
- Various risk assessment tools have been tried to identify those at high risk, e.g. STRATIFY, but current experience is that all older people should be considered high-risk and managed as such.
- Ensure that there are no ongoing, reversible medical problems.
- There will always be a balance between the risk of falls and the benefits of encouraging rehabilitation.

Consequences of inpatient falls

- Loss of confidence in mobilising, increasing the risk of deconditioning.
- Recovery time is longer, even if minimal injury is sustained.
- Soft-tissue injuries and fractures, the majority of which are minor, but fractured hips (see Figure 11.3) and subdural haematomas, can be fatal.
- 80% of inpatient hip fractures happen on the first fall, i.e. one chance to get it (prevention) right.
- Unsurprisingly, most hip fractures occur on medical wards or admission units.
  Outcomes for inpatient hip fractures are worse than for the majority of hip fractures.
  ○ Higher mortality 30 days after fracture,
  ○ Longer length of stay,

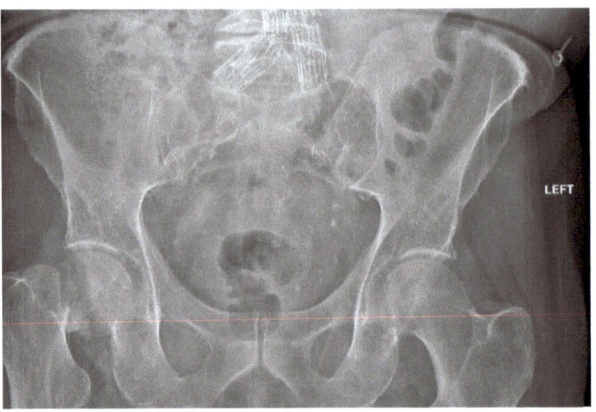

Figure 11.3 X-ray showing partially displaced fracture of the right neck of the femur sustained by a patient falling in hospital; note previous endovascular aneurysm repair and constipation reflecting multimorbidity.

  ○ Increased risk of nosocomial infections,
  ○ Less likely to return to their own homes,
  ○ Distress to families and ward staff.
- Overall costs to hospitals are £630 million per year in England.
- Legal action against hospital trusts.
- The deaths of patients who have fallen in hospital are often referred to the coroner. This may lead to the coroner writing a Prevention of Future Deaths Report, usually regarding failures, e.g. to perform falls risk assessments, communicate or document findings, or act on findings.

National audit of inpatient falls

The national audit of inpatient falls (NAIF) is a continuous national audit of all falls leading to a hip or femoral fracture in NHS trusts in England and Wales. Key advice arising from this:

- All patients 65-year-old or older should have a high-quality multifactorial falls risk assessment (MFRA) on admission.
- This must be followed up by the development of an individualised prevention plan for each patient.
- Use quality improvement to increase the proportion of patients having a MFRA and appropriate interventions.
- All patients should have lying and standing blood pressures checked.
- All patients should have an assessment of their vision – see the RCP bedside 'cat/fish' vision check tool.
- Education: there is an excellent eLearning package for nurses and trainee doctors: https://portal.e-lfh.org.uk/Component/Details/392168
- When a patient falls in hospital, they should see a doctor within 1 hr.
- Analgesia should be prescribed promptly.
- A CT head should be arranged if the patient has hit their head, is anticoagulated, or the fall is not witnessed.
- Remember to use a flat lifting device to prevent worsening injuries if there is a concern about a possible hip fracture or spinal injury.

Immobility

Epidemiology

Immobility is defined as 'the loss of ability to move independently around one's environment'.

It is multifactorial and due to the interplay of physical, psychological, and socio-economic risk factors.

- Reduced mobility ranges from not being able to drive to being housebound or wheelchair-dependent.

- Immobility increases with increasing age, and at its most severe, a bed-bound patient is unable to reposition themselves in bed.
- More than 50% of over-75-year-olds find it difficult to get around their own homes.
- Among ambulant people aged over 80, at least 25% need a walking aid such as a stick or frame.
- Around 20% of those over 80 are housebound, but NHS England does not record this data!
- Many older people find it difficult to get onto a bus, and if they do manage it, there are other pitfalls: getting up from the seat, walking down a crowded aisle possibly whilst the bus is still in motion, and worrying about identifying the correct stop and moving fast enough to get off.
- This coincides with the time that people are no longer able to drive because of failing vision, cognitive impairment, recurrent syncope, etc.

Causes

The most common reasons for reduced mobility are pain and stiffness in the joints and muscles, painful feet (Figure 11.4), and weakness due to neurological conditions or generalised systemic disease (see Table 11.5).

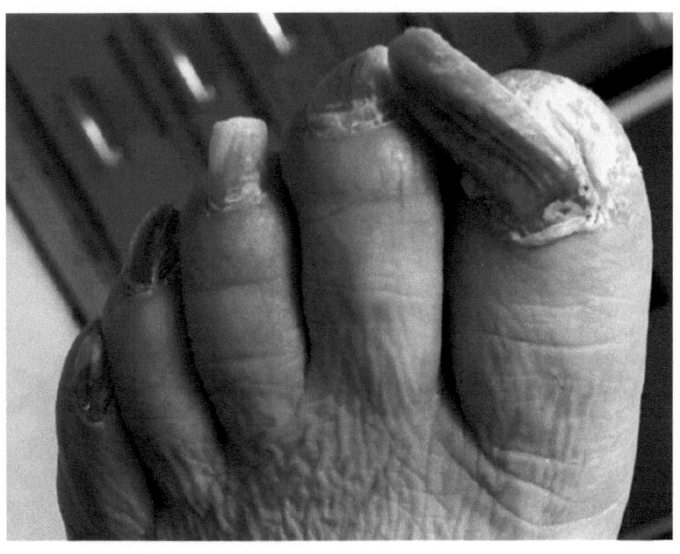

Figure 11.4 Onychogryphosis.

Table 11.5 Causes of reduced mobility.

	System affected	Examples	Mechanisms
Physical	Musculoskeletal	Chronic disease: Sarcopenia Osteoporosis Osteomalacia OA RA PMR	Pain and stiffness, fixed joints, leg length discrepancy. Muscle weakness Extreme frailty
		Acute disease: Fractures Gout flare Pseudogout Septic arthritis	Acute pain, swelling
	Neurological	Stroke PD Advanced dementia Neuropathies Paraplegias MND Severe visual impairment	Weakness, unsteadiness, spasticity, and navigational difficulty
	CVS and pulmonary	Heart failure Severe IHD Severe aortic stenosis Severe PAD Severe COPD	Fatigue, cachexia, breathlessness, and chest pain
	Foot problems	Onychogryphosis Diabetic ulcers Corns Flat feet Inappropriate footwear	Painful feet
	Medications	Opiates Anti-psychotics	Sedation, delirium Extrapyramidal side effects
	Iatrogenic	Sedation Unsuccessful orthopaedic procedures Amputations	
	Cancer	Metastatic disease	Pain (especially bone pain), breathlessness, fatigue, and cachexia

(Continued)

Table 11.5 (Continued)

	System affected	Examples	Mechanisms
	End of life	All causes	
Psychological	Depression Anxiety Poor motivation		
	Fear of further falls	After falling, especially in hospital	
Environmental	Inappropriate or out-of-reach walking aids Inappropriate use of bedrails Inappropriate use of fall alarms Stairs with only one rail Clutter Poor lighting Lack of ramps, grab rails, wheelchairs, and stairlifts		
Socio-economic	Social isolation Loneliness Caregiver burden Inadequate footwear Poor nutrition		

OA, osteoarthritis; RA, rheumatoid arthritis; PMR, polymyalgia rheumatica; PD, Parkinson's disease; MND, motor neuron disease; IHD, ischaemic heart disease; PAD, peripheral arterial disease; COPD, chronic obstructive pulmonary disease.

Exacerbating factors include:

- Visual impairment leading to anxiety about mobilising, especially in an unfamiliar environment like a new warden-assisted flat or hospital ward.
- Breathlessness on minimal exertion secondary to advanced pulmonary and cardiac disease.
- Psychological problems including fear of falling, anxiety, and depression.
- Deconditioning due to reduced activity during any acute illness.

Once we have learned to walk as toddlers, walking becomes automatic. There is often a period of reduced mobility after hospital admission, with an acute illness. Many older people need 'reablement' to get back to their previous level of function. Bed rest can have catastrophic consequences. Patients with advanced dementia who become immobile may not regain the ability to walk or transfer, even with considerable physiotherapy (physio); they can no longer sequence the complex series of movements required. In these patients, every effort should be made to maintain mobility during an admission even, for example, for an MI. Explaining that mobility may not be regained helps families understand that this is a risk, despite diligent care.

Complications

Physical

- The downward spiral into deconditioning (see Figure 11.5).
- Muscle wasting.
- Muscle contractures.
- Osteoporosis.
- Pressure ulcers.
- Hypothermia
- Hypostatic pneumonia.
- Constipation.
- Incontinence, both urinary and faecal.
- Deep-venous thrombosis.

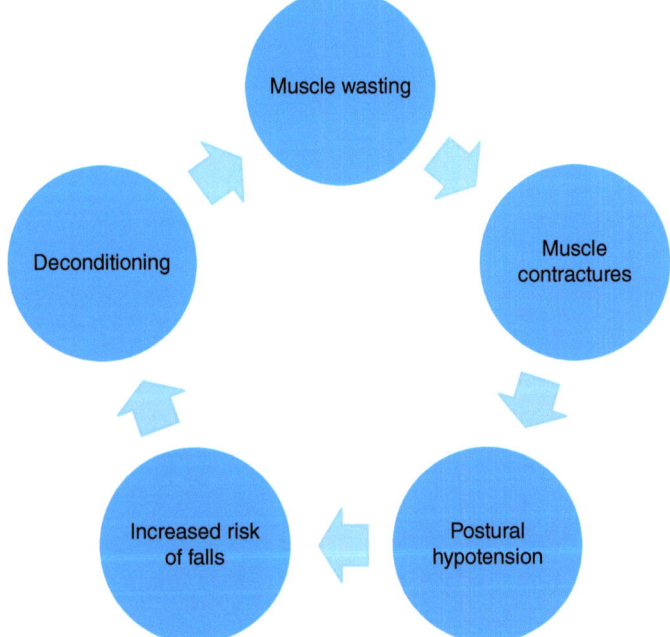

Figure 11.5 Downward cycle of deconditioning.

Psychological

- Depression.
- Loss of confidence.

Social

- Isolation.
- Increased risk of institutionalisation.

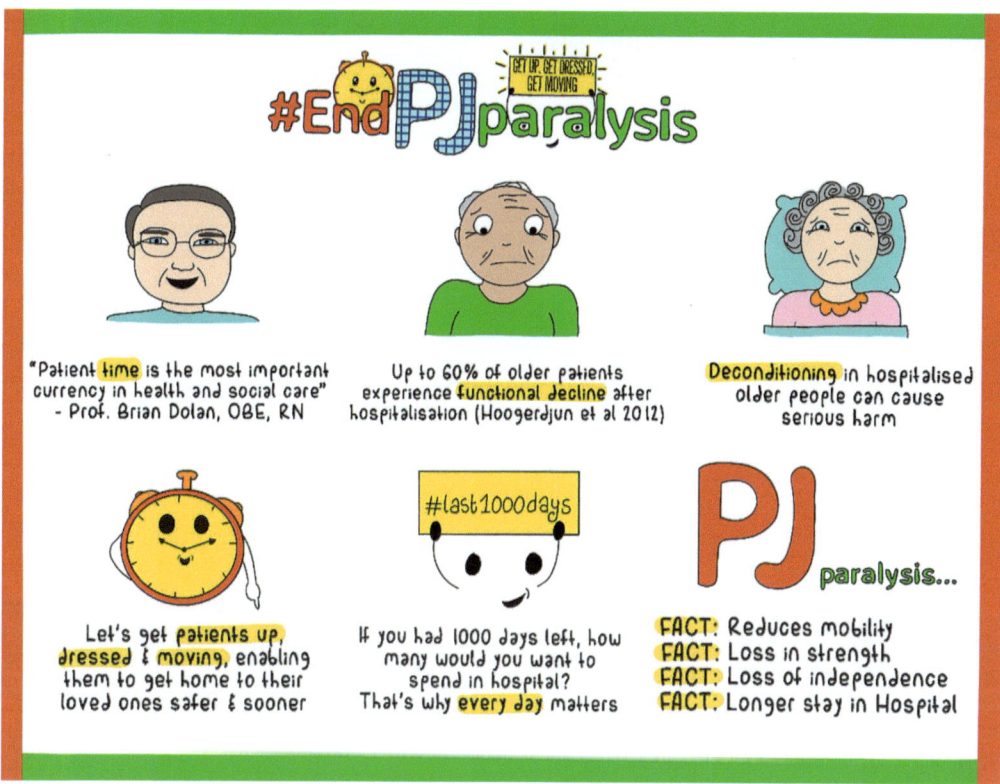

Figure 11.6 End PJ Paralysis https://endpjparalysis.org/downloads

Management

Personalised, multicomponent interventions comprising nutritional support and exercises including aerobic, strength, balance and flexibility components can reduce the risk of immobility by 22% over 3 years.

- Treat reversible medical problems.
- Ensure there are no missed fractures (especially vertebral) or/cauda equina syndrome.
- Optimise analgesia for painful joints/back.
- Look for and treat delirium, depression, and, if possible, dementia.
- Review medication to ensure the patient is not oversedated or parkinsonian secondary to psychotropic medication or prochlorperazine.
- Prescribe VTE prophylaxis.
- If the patient is likely to remain immobile, even for a brief period, ensure assessment for pressure-relieving equipment on the bed and chair. Monitor skin conditions and nutrition.
- Check that the seat has arms and is the correct height so that the patient's feet are on the floor.
- Encourage patients to sit out and walk as soon as possible, as advocated by 'End PJ paralysis' (see Figure 11.6).
- Refer to physio/OT for a review of posture, the use of correct mobility aids (see Table 11.6), and gait practice.
- Foot care remains a neglected area and deteriorated markedly during the COVID-19 lockdowns. Even in hospital, it is often impossible to get podiatrist input for painful in-growing toenails, onychogryphosis (Figure 11.4), bunions, corns, etc.
- Encourage older people to arrange regular podiatry; what the NHS funds depends on local commissioning and most only covers people with diabetes and circulatory problems. Routine nail cutting may be provided by AgeUK, and there may be a low-cost local community footcare scheme. Sessions cost £20–30.
- Refer fit patients with severe OA of the hips or knees for joint replacement.

Walking and transfer aids

A broad range of aids is available, mostly on the NHS. The right aid used correctly can improve a person's mobility, and transfer aids enable immobile patients to sit out of bed, use a wheelchair and proper toilet, and protect professional and family carers from injuring themselves.

Wheelchairs

These improve the patient's independence and quality of life.

- Patients are assessed for the most appropriate wheelchair by the physio team.
- Usually, non-specialist equipment is provided by the hospital, but specialist equipment is ordered from NHS wheelchair services.
- If the patient has sufficient upper-limb strength and stamina, provide them with a self-propelling wheelchair (big wheels).
- If not, an attendant-propelled wheelchair (small wheels and better handles, often with brakes on the handles) is appropriate. They can be borrowed from the British Red Cross for a deposit (donations are appreciated).
- Electric wheelchairs are ideal for cognitively intact but physically impaired patients with conditions such as multiple sclerosis and motor neuron disease.
- Specialist wheelchairs are needed for patients with no sitting balance, for example, after a stroke, or high BMI.
- The wheelchair assessment should include pressure-relieving cushioning.
- Outdoor buggies can improve the independence of cognitively intact, community-dwelling patients. Obtain one from Motability.
- Consider how the patient will transfer in and out of the chair.
- When the patient is being discharged home, it may be necessary to install a ramp up to the front door, and doorways and passages will need to be wide enough to accommodate the wheelchair.

Table 11.6 A comparison of types of walking and transfer aids.

Walking aid	Description	Use	Disadvantages
Stick	Wood or aluminium. The correct length is essential for functional gait pattern. Can be used singly or in pairs. Fisher grip: moulded hand grip may improve function.	Widens base of support and supports up to 25% of body weight. Use on same side for improving balance. Use on opposite side for weakness or painful/unstable joints.	Must be propped up/laid flat when not being used and becomes a trip hazard! Regularly check ferrules for wear.
Tripod/quadrupod	Aluminium with three or four feet.	Gives more support than a stick and stands up on its own. The wider the base of the device, the wider the base of support. Used on opposite side to hemiplegia.	Can be large and ungainly.
Elbow crutches	Aluminium crutches with forearm support. Used in pairs.	Can support 80% of body weight. Useful for non-weight-bearing on a lower limb, e.g. because of amputation or fracture.	Risk of tripping as above. Patient needs to have enough cognitive function to use them safely.
Axillary crutches	Crutches, which bear the weight under the arms.	More often used for younger patients. Can achieve speeds greater than normal walking!	Brachial nerve palsy if used too much.
Zimmer frame	Aluminium tubing with four rubber feet.	Offers maximum support to patients. A bag may be attached.	Patient must be able to learn new gait pattern: the frame is lifted up and forward, and the patient then steps into the frame. This can be especially difficult on carpet. Encourages poor posture, especially forward flexion.
Rollator	As above, but there are wheels on the two front legs.	Patients can push the frame continuously; which is especially useful for patients with PD.	Poor posture, slow gait, and difficulty using outdoors.
Gutter frame	Has support for the forearms.	Useful for patients with rheumatoid arthritis affecting their wrists and wrist injuries.	As above.
Delta frame	Usually a three-wheeled foldaway frame, often with a seat/space for shopping.	More robust, so can be used outside. The patient's feet should be in line with the back wheels when walking.	Heavy. Must be fully opened and locked for safety. Patients pay for their own equipment.

Table 11.6 (Continued)

Walking aid	Description	Use	Disadvantages
Rota stand	Consists of a frame with handles for the patient and carer and shin pads mounted on a turntable. Option for a sling to be used behind the patient's bottom.	Used to transfer patient from one seated position to another. Encourages the patient to participate actively. Can be used in patients' homes, care homes and hospitals. Lightweight and easy to transport. Cheaper than Sara Stedy	Proper training for patient and carers is needed. Max weight: 160 kg Patient must be strong enough to pull up on the handles. There is no seat. May cause trauma to patient's shins.
Sara Stedy transfer aid	Consists of a stable base with 4 wheels, a pivoting 2-part seat, kneepad, crossbar handle for the patient, and handles for the carer.	Allows patient to transfer from one seated position to another with a short transfer if needed, e.g. to another room. Easy to manoeuvre in small spaces. Intuitive to use.	Encourages the patient to be active during sit-to-stand transfers, but use instead of ongoing rehabilitation is detrimental to progress. Training needed. Max weight: 182 kg. Trauma to shins. Relatively expensive.
Full hoist	A mechanical device comprising of a track system mounted on the ceiling or on a free-standing frame with lift mechanism holding the sling that supports the patient.	Can be used to lift patients from seated or lying positions. High weight capacity. Broad base for safety. Reduces effort on carers.	Requires sufficient space for setup. Expensive. Can distress patients. May demotivate patients if used often. Requires regular maintenance.
Scoop hoist	Has a split design so that the team can place each half on either side of the patient without having to roll or lift them. Rigid to support the patient when lifting.	Used for lifting patients with suspected spinal injury off the floor to minimise risk of further injury. Radiolucent to permit imaging.	Mainly used in ambulances and emergency departments.

 ## REFERENCES AND FURTHER READING

UK Office for Health Improvement and Disparities (2022) *Falls – applying All Our Health.* https://www.gov.uk/government/publications/falls-applying-all-our-health/falls-applying-all-our-health

WHO (2021) *Step Safely: Strategies for preventing and managing falls across the life-course.* https://iris.who.int/bitstream/handle/10665/340962/9789240021914-eng.pdf?sequence=1

NICE CG161 (2013) *Falls in older people: assessing risk and prevention.* www.nice.org.uk/guidance/cg161

NICE QS86 (updated 2017) *Falls in older people.* www.nice.org.uk/guidance/qs86

Colón-Emeric CS, McDermott CL, Lee DS, et al. (2024) Risk assessment and prevention of falls in older community-dwelling adults: a review. *JAMA* 331:1397–1406. doi: 10.1001/jama.2024.1416.

Fisher JM, Bates C, Banerjee J (2017) The growing challenge of major trauma in older people: a role for comprehensive geriatric assessment? *Age Ageing* 46:709–712. https://academic.oup.com/ageing/article/46/5/709/3065037.

Sexton DJ, Canney M, O'Connell MDL, et al. (2017) Injurious falls and syncope in older community-dwelling adults meeting inclusion criteria for SPRINT. *JAMA Intern. Med.* 177:1385–1387. doi: 10.1001/jamainternmed.2017.2924.

Kubitza J, Schneider IT, Reuschenbach B (2023) Concept of the term long lie: a scoping review. *Eur. Rev. Aging Phys. Act.* 20:16. doi: 10.1186/s11556-023-00326-3.

RCP Guidelines (2023) *How to measure lying and standing blood pressure (BP) as part of a falls assessment.* www.rcplondon.ac.uk/file/5493/download#:~:text=Ask%20the%20patient%20to%20lie,Measure%20the%20BP.&text=Ask%20the%20patient%20to%20stand,standing%20in%20the%20first%20minute

RCP (2017) *Bedside vision check for falls prevention: assessment tool.* www.rcplondon.ac.uk/projects/outputs/bedside-vision-check-falls-prevention-assessment-tool

Lee J, Negm A, Peters R, et al. (2021) Deprescribing fall-risk increasing drugs (FRIDs) for the prevention of falls and fall-related complications: a systematic review and meta-analysis. *BMJ Open* 11:e035978. doi: 10.1136/bmjopen-2019-035978.

ACB (Anticholinergic burden) calculator https://www.acbcalc.com

Campos L, Prochazka A, Anderson M, et al. (2023) Consistent hearing aid use is associated with lower fall prevalence and risk in older adults with hearing loss. *J. Am. Geriatr. Soc.* 71:3163–3171. doi: 10.1111/jgs.18461.

Skelton DA, Rutherford OM, Dinan-Young S, et al. (2019) Effects of a falls exercise intervention on strength, power, functional ability, and bone in older frequent fallers: FaME (Falls Management Exercise) RCT secondary analysis. *J. Frailty Sarcopenia Falls* 4:11–19. doi: 10.22540/JFSF-04-011.

Bhanu C, Petersen I, Orlu M, et al. (2022) Incidence of postural hypotension recorded in UK general practice: an electronic health records study. *Br. J. Gen. Pract.* 73:e9–e15. doi: 10.3399/BJGP.2022.0111

DVLA (2018) Assessing fitness to drive: a guide for medical professionals:

- *Transient loss of consciousness ('blackouts') – or lost/altered awareness.*
- Cough syncope.
- Dizziness – liability to sudden and unprovoked or unprecipitated episodes of disabling dizziness. https://www.gov.uk/guidance/neurological-disorders-assessing-fitness-to-drive

Brignole M, Moya A, Lange F, et al. (2018) ESC Guidelines for the diagnosis and management of syncope. *Eur. Heart J.* 39:1883–1948. https://academic.oup.com/eurheartj/article/39/21/1883/4939241.

Russo V, Parente E, Tomaino M, et al. (2023) Short-duration head-up tilt test potentiated with sublingual nitroglycerin in suspected vasovagal syncope: the fast Italian protocol. *Eur. Heart J.* 44:2473–2479. doi: 10.1093/eurheartj/ehad322.

Simova I (2015) Role of tilt-table testing in syncope diagnosis and management. *e-J. Cardiol. Pract.*;13:35. https://www.escardio.org/Journals/E-Journal-of-Cardiology-Practice/Volume-13/role-of-tilt-table-testing-in-syncope-diagnosis-and-management.

Denfeld QE, Turrise S, MacLaughlin EJ, et al. (2022) Preventing and managing falls in adults with cardiovascular disease: a scientific statement from the American Heart Association. *Circulation* 15:e000108. doi: 10.1161/HCQ.0000000000000108.

Donovan J, De Silva L, Cox H, et al. (2023) Vestibular dysfunction in people who fall: a systemic review and meta-analysis. *Clin. Rehabil.* 7:1229–1247. doi: 10.1177/02692155231162423.

The HINTS examination. Dr Peter Johns, ED physician, the University of Ottawa. https://www.youtube.com/watch?v=1q-VTKPweuk

RCP *National Audit of Inpatient Falls (England and Wales)* www.rcplondon.ac.uk/projects/national-audit-inpatient-falls-naif

Morris ME, Webster K, Jones C, et al. (2022) Interventions to reduce falls in hospitals: a systematic review and meta-analysis. *Age Ageing* 51:afac077. doi: 10.1093/ageing/afac077.

Cameron ID, Dyer SM, Panagoda CE, et al. (2018) Interventions for preventing falls in older people in care facilities and hospitals. *Cochrane Database Syst. Rev.* 9:CD005465. doi: 10.1002/14651858.CD005465.pub4.

Bernabei R, Landi F, Calvani R, et al. (2022) Multicomponent intervention to prevent mobility disability in frail older adults: randomised controlled trial (SPRINTT project). *BMJ* 377:e068788. https://www.bmj.com/content/377/bmj-2021-068788.

INFORMATION FOR PATIENTS AND FAMILIES

Falls Prevention App by Safesteps: Preventing Falls in the Community with the Safe Steps Mobile App | Local Government Association

AGE UK falls leaflet: https://www.ageuk.org.uk/bp-assets/globalassets/waltham-forest/documents/advice-guides/falls-prevention-advice.pdf

Otago exercise plan video: https://www.youtube.com/watch?v=4iugjk9AbN8

RCP NAIF leaflet: Build your confidence after a fall in hospital: https://www.rcp.ac.uk/media/ookn3e4k/building-your-confidence-after-a-fall-in-hospital-naif-patient-resource-2023_0_0.pdf

Orthostatic hypotension: https://syncope.co.uk/postural-hypotension

Motability: www.motability.co.uk

Hertfordshire provides excellent information: https://www.hcpastopfalls.info

HCPC StopFalls App: StopFalls (http://hcpastopfalls.info)

The University of Nottingham App is designed for care homes but could be used by families as a checklist: https://play.google.com/store/apps/details?id=com.reacttofalls&gl=GB

All websites were accessed in April 2024.

12

Cardiovascular medicine

Ageing changes

1 Loss of cardiac myocytes secondary to apoptosis, with compensatory hypertrophy of remaining cells.
2 Accumulation of intracellular lipofuscin and extracellular amyloid.
3 Increased intercellular collagen leads to reduced left ventricular (LV) diastolic compliance.
4 Diastolic dysfunction secondary to prolonged LV relaxation means that filling pressure depends on atrial contraction.
5 Loss of pacemaker cells in the sino-atrial node, causing sinus bradycardia and predisposing to sick sinus syndrome.
6 Patchy fibrosis of the conduction system leads to an increased incidence of first-degree heart block and bundle branch block.
7 Reduced responsiveness of arteries to β adrenergic stimulation, which reduces the capacity for vasodilatation, plus reduced responsiveness of the myocardium, impairing relaxation.
8 Variable decline in stroke volume, cardiac output, maximum heart rate, and maximal oxygen consumption. Many of these changes can be reversed by regular exercise (for the average women aged 70–75 in the UK, walking at 5 km/h represents maximal aerobic exercise).
9 Lateral displacement of the apex beat is a common finding, and the cardiothoracic ratio on CXR is greater than 50% in 70% of women aged over 70, partly owing to chest distortion, e.g. kyphoscoliosis. This also means that murmurs may not be heard best or radiate in a 'classical' manner.
10 Calcification of aortic valve cusps and the mitral ring.
11 After years of pulsatile stretching, the arteries increase in length and diameter, leading to tortuosity of the aorta.
12 Changes including vascular endothelium dysfunction, elastin fragmentation, and collagen cross-linking lead to arterial and arteriolar wall stiffness and reduced compliance. This leads to an increase in systolic blood pressure (SBP), mean arterial pressure (MAP), and pulse pressure (PP), and a decreased ability to respond to abrupt hemodynamic changes.
13 Reduced baroreceptor sensitivity leads to an increased risk of orthostatic hypotension.

Prevalence of cardiovascular disease

Cardiovascular disease is extremely common in old age:

- 60% of >65-year-olds have hypertension.
- 7% of >65-year-olds have chronic stable angina.
- 20% of >80-year-olds have heart failure.
- 10% of >70-year-olds have atrial fibrillation rising to 28% at >85 years old.

Over 80% of all cardiac deaths in the UK occur in those aged over 65. Ischaemic heart disease is the most common cause of death for males in the UK.

Managing cardiovascular disease in older people

There is a huge body of research and guidelines on cardiovascular disease. However, guidelines for managing older people often contradict each other. There are several reasons for this:

- Historically, older people and women were under-represented in trials and registries of heart disease. Many studies considered those in their 60s as 'old' and people in their 70s as 'very old'!
- Older trial participants are usually not representative of their peers as they are extensively screened to exclude most co-morbidities.
- The underlying pathology in older people may differ from that commonly seen in younger patients (see discussion of Type 2 MI and heart failure with preserved ejection fraction).

Thus, many recommendations are extrapolated to older people without regard to whether the pathology is the same and without considering their other conditions, frailty, functional and cognitive abilities, not to mention pharmacological considerations. Evidence from trials in people in their 80s with a range of comorbidities is needed, and the recent trials of SGLT2 inhibitors in heart failure are good examples of this.

Presentations of heart disease

A wide range of pathologies can affect the heart, but the range of presentations is limited.

- Angina.
- Acute coronary syndromes: unstable angina and myocardial infarction.
- Heart failure.
- Arrhythmias.
- Sudden death.

Coronary artery disease

Coronary artery disease (CAD), or ischaemic heart disease (IHD), comprises a range of conditions in which atherosclerotic plaque formation in the coronary arteries limits blood flow to the heart muscle, causing

Geriatric Medicine and Elderly Care: Lecture Notes, Ninth Edition. Claire G. Nicholl, K. Jane Wilson, and Shaun D'Souza.
© 2025 John Wiley & Sons Ltd. Published 2025 by John Wiley & Sons Ltd.
Companion website: www.wiley.com/go/lecturenotesgeriatricmedicine9e

pain at times of increased demand or, if the plaque ruptures, thrombosis formation and an acute coronary syndrome. The sex incidence in old age is similar, unlike in younger age groups. The risk factors are the same as for cerebrovascular disease; see Chapter 9.

Chronic stable angina

Angina is pain secondary to ischaemia due to a mismatch between myocardial supply and demand. It is usually caused by IHD but can occur in other conditions such as hypertensive heart disease or aortic stenosis. Stable angina suggests stable plaque disease.

- The classical presentation is retrosternal pain radiating to the left arm and throat on exertion.
- The pain is reproducible by increased oxygen demand, e.g. on exertion and stress.
- The pain is not affected by inspiration, coughing, changing position or pressing on the chest wall.
- It is relieved by rest or sublingual glyceryl trinitrate (GTN) spray, usually in less than 5 min.
- Patients may deny pain but describe a heaviness or feeling of pressure across the chest.
- They may describe breathlessness on exertion, fatigue, or even faintness and these may be the only symptoms in older people.
- In older people, atherosclerosis is often diffuse throughout the coronary arteries, and co-existent heart failure is more likely.
- Chest pain that becomes more frequent, lasts longer or is more severe, suggests plaque rupture, i.e. an acute coronary syndrome (ACS).

Investigations:

- ECG: in angina the ECG may be normal or show signs of left ventricular hypertrophy or features of ischaemia, e.g. Q waves, ST and T wave flattening or inversion, or left bundle branch block (LBBB) from previous ischaemic events.
- CXR: likely to be normal but may show cardiomegaly or features of left ventricular failure (LVF). An echocardiogram would be indicated in this case.

Management:

This involves lifestyle advice, treating risk factors, GTN spray for episodes of angina, and anti-anginal medication to reduce the frequency of attacks. Most patients can be managed in this way, but if symptoms remain troublesome or escalate, revascularisation may be considered.

- Patient education: stop smoking, increase exercise, improve diet.
- For fit older people, consider lowering cholesterol, usually with simvastatin or atorvastatin.
- Address all risk factors (optimise diabetic control; treat anaemia, hypertension, and aortic valve disease).
- Aspirin 75 mg daily, or clopidogrel if aspirin not tolerated or with stroke/peripheral arterial disease.
- Offer as required GTN spray for when experiencing symptoms (suggest the patient tries a dose when well to familiarise themselves with the headache that commonly occurs).
- Commence anti-anginal treatment, for example:
  - Beta-blockers, e.g. bisoprolol, slow the heart rate, give more time for coronary perfusion, and are often used first.
  - Calcium antagonists, e.g. diltiazem and amlodipine (but watch out for ankle oedema), are alternative first-line treatment. Switch to a beta-blocker if not tolerated. If both are not tolerated, offer a second-line option. Only combine drugs if monotherapy is ineffective (avoid rate-limiting calcium channel blockers with beta-blockers).
  - Long-acting nitrates (ensure a nitrate-free period to prevent tachyphylaxis by giving isosorbide mononitrate modified release once daily or reminding the patient to take the patch off at night).
  - Nicorandil, a potassium channel opener, is a good choice for patients with low BP and symptoms of orthostatic hypotension secondary to other anti-anginal therapies. Avoid doses greater than 30 mg/d in older people because of the risk of large, painful mouth ulcers and occasionally anal ulcers, which may bleed.
  - Ranolazine is an add-on therapy for refractory angina. It inhibits the sodium current which occurs late in systole in ischaemic myocytes. It does not reduce the heart rate, or BP, during exercise. It does prolong the QT interval, but it does not seem to be pro-arrhythmogenic.
  - Ivabradine is a selective and specific blocker of the I_f channel of the sino-atrial node cells. Thus, the heart rate is reduced without lowering BP. It is most beneficial when patients cannot tolerate enough beta-blocker to slow the heart; use reduces hospital admissions.
- Stratification of fit older people for angiography and revascularization can be difficult. Exercise testing has a lower specificity and sensitivity in women and is not useful in LBBB. Older people are likely to have background calcification affecting CT calcium scoring. Therefore, a MIBI scan (technetium 99 2-methoxy isobutyl isonitrile) is often most useful.
- Angiography is appropriate for patients with severe symptoms or those being considered for vascular surgery, including aortic repair, femoral bypass, and carotid surgery.
- Appropriate older patients with complex multi-vessel disease and ongoing symptoms despite drug therapy should be considered for coronary artery bypass grafting. Decision making with regard to suitability is complex - NICE guidelines suggest that this is done in an MDT setting.

Acute coronary syndrome

ACS is divided into two broad groups:

1 ST-elevation myocardial infarct (STEMI)
2 Non-ST elevation ACS (NSTE-ACS), which includes non-ST elevation myocardial infarcts (NSTEMI) and unstable angina (UA).

STEMI and NSTEMI are often clinically indistinguishable, but they are managed differently and have different prognoses.

ST-elevation myocardial infarction (STEMI)

STEMI occurs because of coronary plaque rupture and the complete and persistent occlusion of one or more coronary arteries by thrombus, resulting in transmural ischaemia. The aim of treatment is very rapid dispersal of the thrombus to minimise myocyte death from ischaemia. Increasing evidence shows that older people with acute STEMI respond just as well to primary percutaneous coronary angiography and intervention (PCI) but are at higher risk of non-cardiac post-procedure morbidity, such as bleeding. This is a growing cohort; at least one in five patients who undergo PCI are aged 80+.

Reperfusion therapy with fibrinolytic drugs (thrombolysis) is increasingly rare as the gold standard treatment is PCI, which has better 30-day and 1-year mortality and a lower risk of cerebral haemorrhage than thrombolysis. Thrombolysis (e.g. with tenecteplase with a direct oral anticoagulant [DOAC] or IV heparin) can be offered if the patient presents within 12 hours of symptoms; PCI is not possible within 2 hours; and there are no major contraindications.

Historical reasons for the underuse of reperfusion strategies in older people

- Atypical presentation (see box entitled 'Clinical presentations of MI').
- Late presentation to medical help.
- Delay to the first ECG.
- Increased incidence of pre-existing bundle branch blocks.

- Multiplicity of co-morbidities and contraindications.
- Older people are more likely to be managed by non-cardiologists.

Examination

- The patient is usually severely unwell, clammy, and peripherally shut down.
- Monitor the pulse rate, rhythm, and blood pressure frequently – the patient should be managed in a monitored resuscitation area.

Investigations

- ECG changes: by definition, ST elevation (see Figure 12.1), new left bundle branch block.
- Serial troponin measurements demonstrate myocyte damage.
- The CXR may show cardiomegaly or signs of pulmonary oedema (see Figure 12.2).

Management:

Pre-hospital

- Give oxygen if needed to achieve a target of >94% or 88–92% in COPD.
- Treat pain with intravenous (IV) opiates (with antiemetic) to reduce sympathomimetic drive on the heart.
- Stat dose of 300 mg aspirin and 300 mg clopidogrel (75 mg if over 75).

Acute care

- Best practice is to admit to a specialist centre offering PCI. Angiography will demonstrate the nature of the lesion causing the ECG changes and will lead to appropriate intervention, including angioplasty or stenting.
- Dual antiplatelet therapy (DAPT) is given. Continue aspirin 75 mg (a cyclo-oxygenase inhibitor) plus a $P2Y_{12}$ receptor blocker (prasugrel, ticagrelor or clopidogrel). Prasugrel is most effective in terms of the relative risk reduction of further ischaemic events but is associated with a higher incidence of bleeding in older patients.

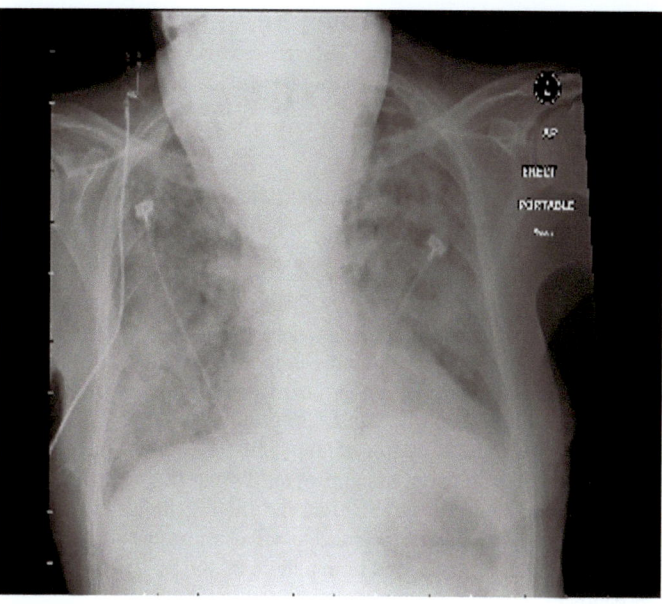

Figure 12.2 Chest radiograph demonstrating acute pulmonary oedema. Note: portable film with the head obscuring part of the chest suggesting the patient is sick; cardiomegaly even allowing for portable film; and (extensive pulmonary fluid).

- Radial rather than femoral puncture is preferred for PCI (lower incidence of bleeding and no relative delay in reperfusion time). Do not site an IV cannula near the right radial artery. Unfractionated heparin is given during the procedure.
- Drug-eluting stents are the preferred choice for amenable lesions as they are associated with reduced restenosis rates in comparison to bare metal stents. The placement of drug-eluting stents does,

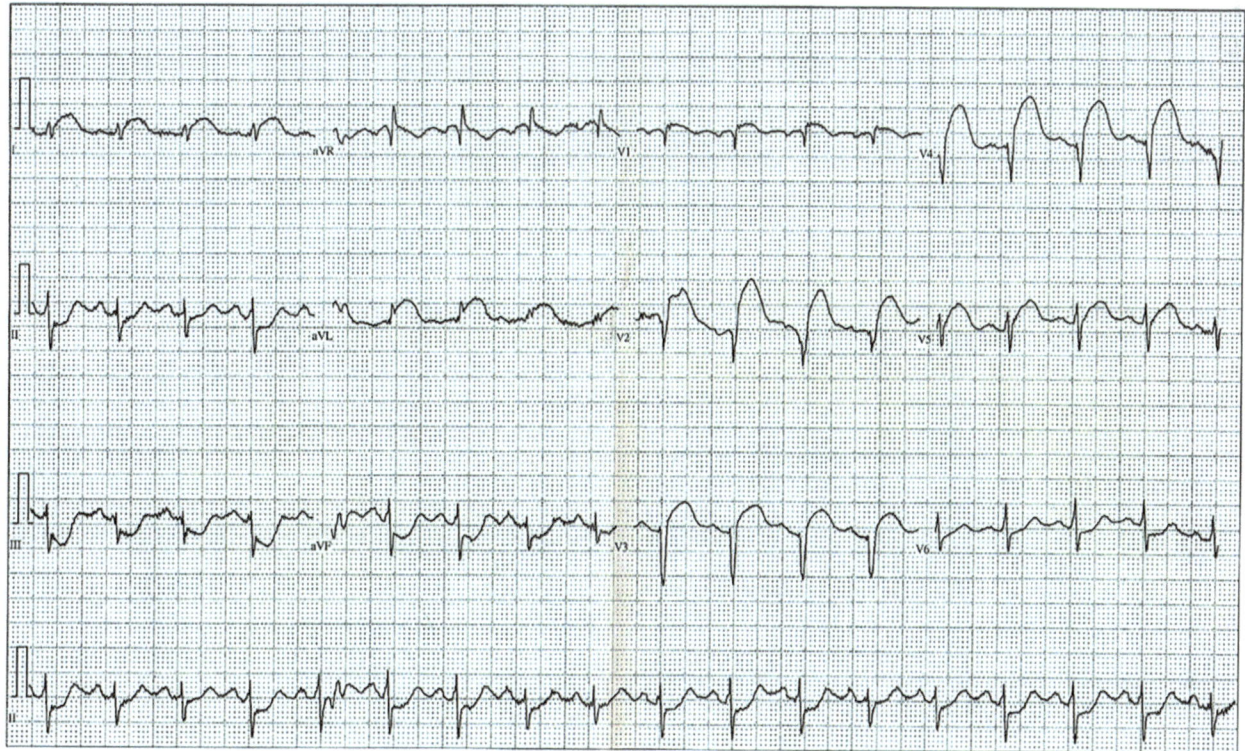

Figure 12.1 ECG shows acute STEMI. Note hyperacute 'tombstone' elevation of the anterior leads and tachycardia. From Wikimedia Commons (public domain).

however, necessitate the use of DAPT for at least a year post-procedure, a regimen that is associated with an increased risk of bleeding in older patients. The choice of stent must thus be considered on an individual patient basis.

Ongoing care

After acute management, the following drugs have been shown to be of long-term benefit and should be used long-term where appropriate:

- Beta-blockers (although a recent study suggests that after a small MI with a preserved EF > 50%, this may not be needed).
- ACE inhibitors (to reduce LV re-modelling) or ARBs if ACEi is not tolerated. Note that a considerable proportion of frail patients will not be able to tolerate the higher doses of ACEi that are associated with favourable outcomes in trials.
- High-dose statins (usually atorvastatin) help 'stabilise the plaques'.
- The default strategy after ACS is to give DAPT, preferably with prasugrel/ ticagrelor and aspirin for 12 months, and then continue the aspirin. If bleeding risk is a major concern, clopidogrel and aspirin can be used and given for a shorter period (a minimum of 30 days if possible) and clopidogrel monotherapy long-term.
- If a DOAC is also indicated, e.g. for AF, triple therapy is recommended for a week, and then continuing the DOAC with clopidogrel as the single oral antiplatelet agent long-term.
- Older patients on DAPT are usually given a PPI.
- Patients who develop cardiac failure will need a loop diuretic.

Non ST-elevation acute coronary syndromes (Please format correctly)

In NSTE-ACS, enlargement or rupture of an atherosclerotic plaque causes partial coronary artery occlusion and subendocardial ischaemia. The unstable plaque is profoundly thrombogenic, so treatment is aimed at reducing this. In NSTEMI, there is myocardial infarction (necrosis). In UA, there is 'no' necrosis (although this depends on the troponin assay and the cut point used), but without treatment, about half of patients would progress to infarction within 30 days. Features of UA include:

- Chest pain at rest or minimal exertion.
- Pain is not relieved by GTN.
- Pain lasting for more than 15 min.
- Crescendo angina on a chronic background.
- Angina of new-onset on minimal exertion.

Investigations

- Serial troponin measurements to assess myocyte damage. Also check U&Es, lipids, glucose, and FBC. Most patients with NSTE-ACS will have an elevated troponin, i.e. an NSTEMI.
- The ECG may show signs of IHD: LVH, Q waves from previous MI, and ST depression.
- The CXR may show cardiomegaly or signs of pulmonary oedema (see Figure 12.2).

Management

The pre-hospital management is as for STEMI (aspirin, clopidogrel, opiate, oxygen only if hypoxic). The ambulance service will usually take patients with NSTE-ACS to the nearest ED rather than a cardiac centre. Non-frail patients in their 80s should be admitted to the coronary care unit (CCU) but frail older patients with NSTEMI are often admitted to a geriatrics service.

- Admit to a monitored bed.
- Bed rest, but allow a bedside commode if possible.
- Continue 75 mg aspirin and offer a second antiplatelet drug, e.g. clopidogrel.

- GTN spray/tablet as required; IV GTN or opiate for ongoing pain.
- Give a beta-blocker unless contraindicated; metoprolol is short-acting and can be stopped if side effects develop.
- If the patient is not for immediate angiography, subcutaneous fondaparinux (an activated factor X inhibitor) can be given for 8 days or until discharge, if sooner. Unfractionated heparin is used if renal function is poor.
- Following acute management, address all risk factors and establish an oral medication regime as for STEMI.
- Further intervention in NSTEMI depends both on the risk of further events and the patient's frailty. The GRACE (Global Registry of Acute Coronary Events) score can help predict further events and 6-month mortality. Those at higher risk can be considered for prompt angiography and PCI. Those at lower risk can be managed medically in the first instance.
- If the patient is biologically fit, they should be considered for elective revascularization, either angioplasty or coronary bypass grafting.

Cardiac rehabilitation

All older patients with the capacity to benefit and who wish to take part should be offered a cardiac rehabilitation programme post-MI or as part of the management of heart failure.

Clinical presentations of MI

- Sudden death.
- Found collapsed, unconscious and hypotensive.
- 'Typical' chest pain (20%).
- Mild chest discomfort, sometimes attributed to indigestion.
- Middle/upper back pain (more common in women).
- Abdominal pain.
- 'Silent', i.e. ECG changes or rise in troponin levels with no chest pain (up to 45% in the longitudinal Framingham Heart Study 2004), in patients admitted after a fall or 'off legs'.
- Heart failure and shortness of breath.
- Arrhythmias.
- Functional decline or confusion.
- Stroke.
- Peripheral gangrene.
- Post-operative fever, tachycardia, and hypotension.

Type 1 and Type 2 myocardial infarction

Most patients presenting with MI have a 'type 1 MI' characterised by coronary plaque rupture and superimposed thrombosis. However, a sizable proportion, particularly older hospital inpatients, have 'a type 2 MI' characterised by an imbalance between myocardial oxygen supply and demand precipitated by a stressor such as anaemia, arrhythmias, hypertension, and hypotension in the absence of plaque erosion or rupture.

- Ageing changes in the heart, small vessel disease and processes like ventricular hypertrophy or chronic anaemia make the myocardium more vulnerable.
- Cardiac factors such as fast AF and non-cardiac factors such as pneumonia or a GI bleed may precipitate an infarction.

A definitive diagnosis is difficult.

- Atheroma is common, may coexist, and impair blood supply without thrombosis formation.
- The symptoms of type 1 MI are often absent, attenuated, or non-specific in older patients.
- Angiography is often not performed.

A type 2 MI should be considered in patients with a raised troponin level but no history of CAD, atypical symptoms, atypical ECG findings or evidence of factors that would lead to an increase in oxygen requirements or impaired oxygen delivery. The troponin is typically not as high as in a type 1 infarct. In a type 2 infarct, NT-proBNP and CRP tend to be higher, but there are no clear diagnostic criteria. As the distinction has only been recognised recently, there are no specific studies on treatment after a type 2 MI.

- Beta-blockers might be expected to be beneficial as they reduce myocardial oxygen demand.
- ACEi may help prevent ventricular remodelling following scarring from ischaemia of any cause.
- There is some evidence of benefit from cardiac rehabilitation.
- As thrombus is not part of the pathogenesis, antiplatelet drugs are not likely to play a key role.
- Likewise, statins might play a similar role to that in primary prevention.

The main message is that we lack evidence for what is beneficial, and all drugs have risks. In frail older people, it is always important to treat the individual. Rigid adherence to guidelines, e.g. for DAPT might do significant harm if the patient had a type 2 rather than a type 1 MI, so great caution is needed.

The significance of a raised troponin

The troponin (Tn) complex consists of three regulatory proteins that are integral to skeletal and cardiac muscle contraction:

1. TnC (binds calcium),
2. TnI (inhibits actomyosin) and
3. TnT (binds tropomyosin)

TnT and TnI have 'cardiac-specific' isoforms.

If the cardiac muscle is damaged by any insult, troponins leak into the circulation. High-sensitivity assays are available for TnT and TnI.

Troponin elevation is (generally) specific to myocardial injury, but this is not always due to plaque rupture. Other causes of high troponin include myocarditis, arrythmias, and cardiac trauma, which includes pacing and from non-cardiac causes, such as pulmonary embolus, sepsis, and stroke (possibly due to increased circulating catecholamines). Some of these acute stressors would now be recognised as causing a type 2 MI. Troponins are also elevated in acute and chronic renal failure due to cardiac damage **and** impaired excretion. Note also that cardiac TnT is not completely specific for the heart, as regenerating skeletal muscle (e.g. in severe myositis and renal failure) may re-express cardiac TnT. Be aware of which assay your trust uses and what the cut-off points are.

Heart failure

Heart failure (HF) is a complex clinical syndrome characterised by the heart's inability to pump blood effectively to meet the body's metabolic demands.

Classification

HF can be classified in several ways:

(a) **Time course**
   - Acute or chronic.
(b) **Symptomatic severity**, using the New York Heart Association (NYHA), functional classification:
   Class I: symptoms do not restrict daily activities.
   Class II: symptoms occur on moderate effort and slightly restrict daily activities.

Class III: symptoms occur on minimal effort. Significant restriction of activities.
Class IV: debilitating symptoms occur at rest.

(c) **Right or left-sided**
Traditionally, HF was classified according to the side of the heart thought to be most affected. The terms 'right heart failure', 'left heart failure', and 'congestive heart failure' are now discouraged by NICE as they can be misleading. However, they have been included, as your teachers may use these terms.
   - Simplistically, in left heart/ventricular failure, there is inadequate forward flow into the aorta and back pressure on the lungs, causing pulmonary oedema. A fall in cardiac output activates the renin-angiotensin-aldosterone system (RAAS). This leads to increased levels of angiotensin II and aldosterone, which cause vasoconstriction and sodium and water retention, initially restoring circulating volume but ultimately increasing cardiac workload and exacerbating heart failure. Sympathetic nervous system (SNS) activation leads to increased heart rate, contractility, and vasoconstriction, again of benefit initially but detrimental long-term. The heart releases natriuretic peptides in response to myocyte stretch. These have diuretic and vasodilatory effects and initially counterbalance the adverse effects of RAAS and SNS activation. Raised levels are used as a diagnostic test for heart failure.
   - In right heart/ventricular failure, there is compromised flow to the lungs and systemic back pressure, worsened by salt and water retention, leading to ankle oedema (sacral if bed-bound) and a raised JVP. Right heart/ventricular failure can be secondary to left heart failure or lung disease causing high pressure in the lungs, 'cor pulmonale' (heart disease secondary to lung disease). Failure of both ventricles was called biventricular failure or congestive heart failure.

(d) **According to the left ventricular ejection fraction**
Normal left ventricular ejection fraction (LVEF) as measured on echocardiogram is 50–70%. Heart failure may occur with a reduced, mildly reduced or preserved EF. The main differences are summarised in Table 12.1.
   - A reduced LVEF of 40% or less is HFrEF (heart failure with reduced ejection fraction).
   - A reduced LVEF of 41–49% is HFmrEF (heart failure with a mildly reduced ejection fraction).
   - Features of heart failure but with a LVEF of 50% or more is HFpEF (heart failure with preserved ejection fraction, pronounced 'hefpef'). This was previously known as diastolic heart failure.

Epidemiology

Heart failure is an extremely common cause of hospital admissions, readmissions, reduced function, and institutionalisation.

- One million UK residents (64 million worldwide) are living with a diagnosis of HF.
- HF is responsible for at least 5% of hospital admissions. Hence, alternative approaches are being tried for management of episodes of decompensation, including the use of 'virtual wards' and 'hospital at home'.
- The average age of men in England and Wales at first hospital admission with HF is 76 years, compared with 80 years for women in 2021/22 (HF audit data).
- Just under 56% of all patients had HFrEF, a reduction from 58% in 2020/21 and 62% in 2019/20.
- Overall in-hospital mortality for 2021/22 was 10.4% for those aged 75 or older. The all-age 30-day all-cause mortality was 14%, and the 1-year mortality rate was 32% (45% in those admitted to medicine for the elderly).

Table 12.1 Summary of the main differences between HFpEF and HFrEF.

	HFpEF	HFrEF
Ejection fraction	≥50%	≤40%
B-type natriuretic peptide (BNP)	Lower levels – may be below the cut point as the stiffer ventricle does not stretch as much	Higher levels – more likely to be released as the thinner wall is more stretched
Sex	F>M	M>F
Age	Older	Younger
Proportion of cases	Rising	Falling
Effect on the left ventricle	Impaired relaxation, concentric hypertrophy, and pressure overload	Impaired contraction, eccentric remodelling, chamber dilatation and volume overload
Outline pathogenesis	Chronic systemic inflammation, leading to early cardiac endothelial dysfunction, myocyte hypertrophy and interstitial fibrosis	Cardiomyocyte loss and inflammation are caused by local damage leading to late endothelial dysfunction. Patchy fibrosis in the scars after MI
Risk factors/comorbidities for both	HT, diabetes, kidney disease, AF, obesity (but higher prevalence in HFpEF)	
Particular risk factors	Systemic comorbidities, COPD, anaemia, liver disease, sleep apnoea, gout, and cancer	Myocardial infarction, myocarditis, cardiomyopathies
Drugs shown to reduce mortality, hospitalisation, and improve symptoms	None	ACEi/ARB/ARNI, β-blocker, MRA, SGLT2 inhibitor Ivabradine is in SR, and the rate is still ≥70bpm on β-B
Drugs that reduce hospitalisation and improve symptoms	SGLT2 inhibitor, some evidence for digoxin	
Drugs that improve symptoms (congestion)	Loop diuretic ± thiazide ± MRA	
Drugs to treat risk factors	According to the risk profile, as some people have intermediate EF (HFmrEF), drugs used for HFrEF are often used, e.g. ACEi for HT	
6-month mortality after hospitalisation with acute decompensation	Similar, around 15%	

HFpEF: heart failure with preserved ejection fraction.
HFrEF: heart failure with reduced ejection fraction.
HFmrEF: heart failure with a mildly reduced ejection fraction.
MI: myocardial infarction.
HT: hypertension.
AF: atrial fibrillation.
COPD: chronic obstructive pulmonary disease.
ACEi: angiotensin converting enzyme inhibitor.
ARB: angiotensin II receptor blocker.
ARNI: a combination of an ARB and a neprilysin inhibitor, e.g. sacubitril valsartan (neprilysin, an endopeptidase that cleaves peptides such as natriuretic peptides and bradykinin).
MRA: mineralocorticoid receptor antagonist.
SGLT2i: sodium-glucose cotransporter type 2 inhibitor.

Acute heart failure

This can be the first presentation of HF, usually after ACS, or an episode of decompensation in chronic, gradually progressive HF of any type, e.g. due to coexisting infection or fast AF.

Clinical features

- Severe breathlessness, orthopnoea, paroxysmal nocturnal dyspnoea.
- Frothy pink sputum.
- On examination, there may be tachycardia, a third heart sound, crackles at the lung bases, and signs of pleural effusion.

Investigations

- ECG may show evidence of an acute infarction, LV hypertrophy, tachycardia, or LBBB. Also, look for AF and other arrhythmias.

- Blood tests may show a rise in troponin. Iron deficiency should be excluded.
- In early failure, the CXR may show upper lobe blood diversion and fluid in the horizontal fissure or septal lines. With increasing pulmonary oedema, there may be perihilar shadowing and bilateral pleural effusions. If the effusion is unilateral, it is more likely to be on the right.

Management

- The patient is likely to be sitting bolt upright already but check as frail older patients slide down hospital beds!
- Give oxygen via a face mask to target saturation.
- IV loop diuretics, i.e. furosemide, either as a bolus or via 24-hour infusion.
- Treat precipitants, e.g. rate control for fast AF and antibiotics for pneumonia.

- GTN infusions are effective in offloading the right heart and reducing angina if present, but they are often poorly tolerated in older patients due to hypotension. Aim to keep systolic BP above 90 mmHg.
- Temporarily discontinue any ACEi/ARB to protect the kidneys before the blood pressure falls.
- Low-dose opiates (with an anti-emetic) can be useful, as they not only reduce anxiety and pain, therefore reducing oxygen demand, but also reduce pre-load.
- If there is evidence of an acute MI, treat as per the previous section.
- All patients with iron deficiency should receive intravenous iron replacement (this reduces the risk of further heart failure-related hospital admissions).

Chronic heart failure

Common features at all ages include breathlessness and oedema, but in older people, non-specific symptoms are frequent, including fatigue, functional decline, confusion, falls, and cachexia. Remember that ankle oedema is often non-cardiac: e.g. in the chair-bound, there is increased venous pressure due to gravity, loss of muscle-pump activity and pressure on thigh veins from the chair.

Causes of heart failure include

- Coronary artery disease (most common).
- Hypertension.
- Valvular heart disease.
- Cardiomyopathies.
- Arrhythmias, especially fast AF.
- Severe lung disease, especially massive pulmonary emboli.
- Amyloidosis.
- Myocarditis.
- Thyrotoxicosis.
- Severe anaemia.
- Drugs, including NSAIDs, that lead to fluid overload.

Investigations

NICE guidelines on heart failure recommend:

- Early transthoracic echo.
- Measure B-type natriuretic peptide (BNP) or N-terminal pro-B-type natriuretic peptide (NT-proBNP).
- High BNPs indicate a poor prognosis. (NB: also high in other conditions, including PE and may be low in obese patients, possibly because of the higher glomerular filtration rate and uptake by adipocytes).
- Baseline U&Es, eGFR, TSH, LFTs, fasting lipids, glucose/HbA1C, and FBC.
- CXR.
- Peak expiratory flow rate (PEFR) to exclude COPD.

Heart Failure with preserved Ejection Fraction

For people over 75 years of age, this accounts for over half of all patients with heart failure. Patients with HFpEF have signs and symptoms of heart failure but with a LVEF >50%. The European Society of Cardiology guidelines for diagnosis include elevated cardiac biomarkers (BNP and NT-proBNP) and echocardiographic features (LV hypertrophy or left atrial enlargement and/or diastolic dysfunction).

Risk factors include:

- Aged over 75.
- Female.
- Overweight.
- History of hypertension (leads to stiff arteries).

- Diabetes.
- CAD.
- AF.
- Chronic kidney disease.

The pathogenesis is complex but includes impaired LV relaxation (especially during exercise) owing to changes in cytoskeletal proteins of the myocardium and increased LV diastolic stiffness secondary to increased myocardial fibrosis. This leads to incomplete LV filling in diastole, which in turn increases diastolic pressures, causing pulmonary congestion and impaired ability to increase cardiac output.

- Flash pulmonary oedema may occur, precipitated by AF or fluid overload.
- The ECG may show LVH secondary to hypertension or a large left atrium (P mitrale).
- Echocardiography is essential for diagnosis: the LV ejection fraction should be above 50%, and the LV volumes should be normal with no significant valvular lesions.

Management
General measures

These apply to all HF patients.

- Education, the provision of literature and specific advice on when to ask for medical help.
- Lifestyle advice, e.g. smoking cessation, restricting alcohol.
- Control any risk factors (CAD, HT, DM, and lipids).
- Advice on reducing salt and fluid intake if there is hyponatraemia.
- Dietary advice depends on the stage, e.g. weight reduction or supplementation for cardiac cachexia.
- Encourage aerobic training, if able.
- Stop medication that may cause harm, e.g. NSAIDs and thiazolidinediones.
- Treat precipitating factors, e.g. control any abnormal rhythm, correct anaemia, optimise treatment of COPD, and refer for valve surgery if indicated.
- Loop diuretics to reduce overload (symptom relief). Care is needed not to overdiurese in HFpEF, as the stiffer heart needs a good filling pressure.
- Add thiazide to the diuretic regime for refractory oedema, but check urea and electrolytes (U&E) daily. If available, add metolazone starting with 2.5 mg once or twice a week.
- Anticoagulation is only indicated if there is a risk of thromboembolic disease or an echo suggests LV aneurysm or intracardiac thrombus.
- End-of-life care: opiates and oxygen as required.

Drugs that improve mortality in HFrEF

- ACE inhibitors, unless contraindicated by poor renal function, hypotension, or aortic valve disease (initiated in hospital in high-risk cases). Start low and titrate up.
- ARB if ACEi is not tolerated.
- There is an increasing role for beta-blockers such as carvedilol and bisoprolol in both acute and chronic heart failure (once fluid overload has been cleared by diuretics). Start low and titrate up.
- Mineralocorticoid receptor antagonists (MRAs), e.g. spironolactone, reduce morbidity and mortality and are often well tolerated in older people, but use caution in combination with ACEi or ARB. Check potassium frequently.
- Sodium-glucose cotransporter 2 inhibitors (SGLT2i), e.g. dapagliflozin, show benefit in T2DM patients with HF. Subsequent trials (see later) have confirmed significant benefits for non-diabetics, with a reduced risk of death and hospital admission (by as much as 25%).

- Patients with HFmrEF are an intermediate group, and drug trials had variable entry criteria, so if they tolerate them, they are often treated with drugs used in HFrEF.

Other measures

- The criteria for cardiac resynchronisation pacemaker therapy include symptoms of moderate HF, LVEF ≤35%, QRS of 150 ms or more, and optimal pharmacological treatment.
- An implantable cardioverter defibrillator (ICD) should be considered in all patients with symptomatic heart failure and an EF ≤35% who are expected to survive more than 1 year to reduce the risk of sudden cardiac death.

Drug treatment for HFpEF

Disappointingly, drugs have not been shown to improve survival.

- MRAs, e.g. spironolactone, reduce hospital admissions.
- SGLT2 inhibitors (2 trials: EMPEROR-preserved [empagliflozin] and DELIVER [dapagliflozin] and a meta-analysis) also reduced hospital admissions. This was seen in HFpEF as well as HFrEF. NICE UK guidelines therefore recommend either dapagliflozin or empagliflozin for all patients with HF who tolerate them, regardless of ejection fraction.
- If patients have comorbidities that could be treated with drugs used in HFrEF, these tend to be used, e.g. ACEi for hypertension and beta-blockers for rate control in AF.

Atrial fibrillation

Atrial fibrillation (AF) is a supraventricular tachyarrhythmia resulting from irregular, disorganised electrical activity and ineffective contraction of the atria. It is the most common arrhythmia.

- The prevalence increases with advancing age and increases markedly in those with heart failure and valvular heart disease. Rates are 5–15% for patients over 80. The lifetime risk is around 30%.
- The prevalence is increasing as detection has intensified, and opportunistic screening appears cost-effective in this cohort.
- Fibrotic changes in the myocardium of the left atrium predispose older people to AF. Rapidly firing foci commonly within the pulmonary vein lead to propagating wavelets, which may result in re-entrant circuits in an abnormal atrial myocardium. When the atrioventricular node receives more impulses than it can conduct, an irregular ventricular rhythm results.
- AF is often paroxysmal initially (PAF) and becomes permanent as the fibrosis progresses.
- The ventricular rate of untreated AF is often 160–180 beats per minute but is slower with age because of fibrosis of the conducting pathway and is less than 100 bpm in around a third of cases.
- AF is implicated in 20–30% of ischaemic strokes because the reduced contraction of the atria leads to reduced blood flow, allowing the development of mural thrombi specifically around the left atrial appendage which then embolise.
- Treatment aims are to reduce the risk of thromboembolic complications, reduce symptoms of AF by rate and/or rhythm control, and manage concomitant heart disease.

Common causes of AF

- Coronary artery disease.
- Long-standing hypertension.
- Biventricular heart failure from any cause.
- Valvular heart disease, especially mitral (30% of cases).
- Thyroid disease.

- PE.
- Pneumonia.
- Chronic alcohol excess.

Adverse outcomes associated with AF

AF is associated with increased mortality, and increased morbidity due to thromboembolism, and reduced cardiac output.

- Increased mortality is 1.5–3.5 times greater than age-matched controls not in AF.
- Stroke: risk increases threefold in nonvalvular AF and 17-fold in AF associated with mitral valve disease. See Chapter 9.
- Peripheral thromboembolic events.
- Heart failure (due to ineffective ventricular filling and tachycardia-induced cardiomyopathy).
- Increased risk of hospitalisation.
- Reduced quality of life.
- Reduced exercise capacity.
- Reduced cognitive function (association with vascular dementia).

History

- Establish whether AF is new-onset (not possible if AF is asymptomatic).
- Duration of symptoms.
- Frequency of episodes.
- Severity of symptoms.
- Risk factors for AF: CAD, HT, history of rheumatic fever.
- Complications of AF: heart failure, stroke.
- Ask about symptoms suggestive of hyperthyroidism, pneumonia, or pulmonary embolus.
- Check alcohol intake, drug history, and recreational drug use (cannabis, cocaine).

Examination

- Is the patient ill or well?
- Assess the radial and apical rates.
- Confirm the pulse is irregularly irregular.
- Check blood pressure.
- Look for signs of heart failure.
- Listen for murmurs.
- Listen for signs of pneumonia.
- Look for signs of thyrotoxicosis.

Investigations

- 12-lead ECG (with a rhythm strip of at least 30 sec) confirms the diagnosis of AF if there are no discernible repeating P waves and irregular RR intervals. Note the ventricular response rate, signs of acute or chronic ischaemia, and LV hypertrophy. Tachycardia and RV strain (S1Q3T3 is rare) suggest new PE.
- CXR: cardiac size, evidence of heart failure, pneumonia.
- Transthoracic echocardiogram: assess the valves, size of the left atrium, and LV ejection fraction.
- Consider Holter monitoring if symptoms occur 3–4 times per day, are paroxysmal or exercise-related, and AF has not as yet been identified on a resting ECG.
- Consider an event recorder if symptoms are less frequent.
- A transoesophageal echo may be useful to exclude a left atrial appendage or left atrial thrombus prior to cardioversion after 48 hours of symptoms.
- CT pulmonary angiogram (CTPA) if there is high suspicion of PE.
- Check TSH, FBC, U&Es, and LFTs.

Management

Remember education and general measures to reduce cardiovascular risk and improve fitness.

Rate control versus rhythm control

AF may revert spontaneously, especially if due to a reversible precipitant such as pneumonia, PE, or MI, but check that this is not PAF.

- Older people often have factors that make cardioversion unlikely to work:
  ○ Longstanding AF, or of uncertain duration.
  ○ Enlarged left atrium.
  ○ Previously failed cardioversion.
  ○ Mitral stenosis.
- Around half of older people revert to AF within a year of cardioversion anyway.

Rate control

Given the limitations of rhythm control, rate control is the most appropriate option for most older people with AF.

- Rate control is best achieved with a beta-blocker such as metoprolol or bisoprolol. A rate-limiting calcium channel blocker can be used if there is no heart failure (diltiazem is off-label but NICE-recommended and widely used, whereas verapamil, which is licensed, is usually avoided in older people as LV dysfunction is common and it is a potent antihypertensive). Digoxin monotherapy may be considered in non-paroxysmal AF in sedentary patients, those with heart failure (positive inotropic effect) or where there is concern about using the other drugs.
- If monotherapy is unsuccessful, consider two of the following: a beta-blocker, diltiazem, or digoxin.
- Amiodarone is not recommended for long-term rate control.
- The European Society of Cardiology Guidelines (2020) suggest aiming for a resting heart rate of <110 bpm. If aiming for tighter rate control (because of symptoms), repeat a Holter test to exclude bradyarrhythmias, AV block, and long pauses.
- If good rate control cannot be achieved with drugs alone, another option suitable for fitter older patients is pace and β block or 'pace and ablate'. A pacemaker is inserted to drive the ventricular rate, and AV ablation prevents rapid impulses from the atria from reaching the ventricles. Note that this procedure and pulmonary vein isolation (PVI) described later are both forms of 'catheter ablation'.

Rhythm control

This aims to restore and maintain sinus rhythm and is undertaken in selected older people.

New onset (less than 48 hours)

- If the patient is haemodynamically unstable, DC cardioversion is the most appropriate management.
- In the rare case of an older patient who is biologically fit with no history of CAD, structural heart disease, or echocardiographic evidence of failure, consider flecainide or amiodarone. Flecainide is contraindicated in CAD because of the risk of sudden cardiac death.
- Amiodarone can be given IV via a central line (to achieve prompt rhythm control) or oral loading regimen after baseline blood tests, including TFTs, LFTs, and U&E.
- If the patient is not anticoagulated, start low-molecular-weight heparin and continue this until a decision is made about long-term anticoagulation.

Beyond 48 hours

- If the plan is chemical or electrical cardioversion, arrange a transoesophageal echo, as mentioned earlier. If there are thrombi, the patient must be anticoagulated for 1 month prior to cardioversion.
- If sinus rhythm is achieved, continue with maintenance sotalol or amiodarone to prevent recurrence, remembering that older people are susceptible to the side effects of both drugs.
- Another method to restore sinus rhythm is PVI. This is a cardiac ablation procedure that uses heat or cold to create circumferential scars around the openings of the four pulmonary veins to block the abnormal electrical signals that initiate AF. It is a catheter procedure with a transseptal puncture to reach the left atrium. At 12 months, just over half of patients remain free of atrial arrhythmias off medication. It can also be used to maintain SR if there are frequent episodes of PAF. However, studies show that procedural complications and AF recurrence both increase with age.

Closure of the left atrial appendage

Left atrial appendage (LAA) is associated with thrombus formation and is an important source of thromboembolic events in those with nonvalvular AF. A variety of procedures (catheter-based or minimally invasive surgery) can be used to close the LAA in patients who have contraindications to anticoagulation.

Paroxysmal AF

Sotalol or amiodarone reduce the frequency of episodes of AF and the ventricular rate during them. Digoxin is avoided as it increases the tendency for the development of permanent AF. The risk of stroke remains high, so anticoagulate as for permanent AF.

Oral anticoagulation

In summary, AF and valvular heart disease confer an extremely high risk of thromboembolism, so anticoagulate unless there is a profound contraindication. For non-valvular AF, the CHA2DS2 VASc score, which is recommended by NICE, indicates that anticoagulation (DOACs are first line) should be offered if the age is ≥75. The risk of major bleeding with anticoagulation can be estimated by using the ORBIT scoring tool (see Chapter 9).

Atrial flutter

This is another supraventricular tachycardia, usually caused by a re-entry circuit in the right atrium, resulting in an atrial rate of around 300 bpm. The ventricular rate depends on the AV conduction ratio ('degree of AV block'). This is commonly 2:1, resulting in a ventricular rate of around 150 bpm. It may be paroxysmal or alternate with AF.

- The presentation is like AF, ranging from asymptomatic to syncope or heart failure.
- The ECG typically shows flutter waves, best seen in the inferior leads.
- Options for management are similar to AF and as the risk of stroke is also similar, most patients should be anticoagulated.

Cardiac pacemakers

Ageing leads to fibrosis of the conduction pathways in the heart; therefore, bradycardia and bradyarrhythmias are more common. Bradycardia is exacerbated by medications such as digoxin, beta-blockers, amiodarone, and calcium channel blockers, which should be stopped. Patients may present with recurrent unexplained falls, syncope, increasing angina and heart failure, or be asymptomatic.

If a pacemaker is needed, dual chamber pacemakers are used for most conditions except patients with persistent AF and the very frail, when single ventricular pacing with rate response (VVIR) is used.

Indications for pacemakers

These include:

- Complete heart block.
- Sick sinus syndrome.
- Tri-fascicular block, or lesser degree blocks with relevant symptoms.
- Cardio-inhibitory carotid sinus hypersensitivity and cardio-inhibitory vasodepression on tilting.
- Slow AF with sinus node dysfunction.
- 'Tachycardia-bradycardia syndrome' with a drug to prevent tachyarrhythmia.
- Cardiac resynchronisation therapy with pacing (CRT-P) for heart failure with a widened QRS. Three leads connect the pulse generator to the right atrium and both ventricles, which resynchronizes the contraction of the ventricles and improves the heart's pumping efficiency.

Valvular heart disease

Systolic murmurs are audible in 30–60% of older patients. The commonest cause is haemodynamically insignificant aortic sclerosis. Untreated valvular disease can result in heart failure.

Aortic stenosis

Aortic stenosis (AS) is the most common cardiovascular disease after hypertension and CAD. It is present in about 5% of those >65 years old. Degenerative fibrosis and calcification of a tri-leaflet valve account for nearly 80% of cases in Europe and the US, with stenosis of a congenital bicuspid valve accounting for most of the remainder. Rheumatic heart disease is now very uncommon, except in developing countries, where it remains prevalent.

- Inflammation of the valvular endocardium initiates fibrosis.
- Stenosis is slowly progressive with time and often follows aortic sclerosis (defined as aortic valve thickening without flow limitation).
- Pressure overload leads to concentric hypertrophy of the left ventricle, which eventually starts to fail. The average survival in symptomatic AS without treatment is 2–3 years.
- Risk factors are diabetes, hypertension, smoking, raised cholesterol, and a bicuspid valve.
- AF is poorly tolerated because the loss of atrial contraction plus rapid ventricular response reduces diastolic filling of the left ventricle.
- Symptoms include angina (30%), breathlessness (50%), and syncope or presyncope (15%).
- The slow-rising pulse may be absent because of the reduced elasticity of the carotid artery.
- The murmur (typically a harsh ejection systolic with radiation to the carotids) may be unimpressive.
- ECG may show LV hypertrophy. There may be conduction abnormalities, including RBBB and LBBB, secondary to calcification of the conduction pathway.
- Once the gradient across the valve is over 40 mmHg on echo or the aortic valve area is less than 1 cm², if symptoms are present and LV function is good, the patient should be considered for an aortic valve repair or replacement.
- Options for treatment include open valve replacement (the gold standard for patients able to tolerate major surgery) or transcatheter aortic valve implantation (TAVI).

- TAVI is useful for frailer patients. A balloon is fed via a catheter through the femoral vein into the heart and used to crush the native valve; a new valve is inserted in its root. TAVI avoids the need for a sternotomy or cardiopulmonary bypass and is performed without the need for a general anaesthetic. In randomised controlled trials, this procedure was associated with improved survival, a reduction in symptoms, and fewer hospital admissions when compared to standard medical therapy. Nonetheless, patients must be carefully triaged for suitability, often in a multidisciplinary setting. Co-morbidities associated with poorer outcomes include COPD, pulmonary hypertension, and dementia. The risks of embolic events such as stroke (up to 5%) or bowel ischaemia are similar to open surgical repair, although most subacute (1–30 days post-TAVI) events are related to new-onset AF.

Mitral regurgitation

Mitral regurgitation has a greater range of causes than aortic stenosis, and whereas aortic stenosis develops gradually, mitral regurgitation can be chronic and progressive, or acute if the mitral valve apparatus is damaged by a myocardial infarction.

- Chronic mitral regurgitation usually presents with dyspnoea on exertion and palpitations.
- The typical murmur is pansystolic, blowing and best heard at the apex with radiation to the axilla.
- Left ventricular failure eventually occurs due to volume overload.

Management options include open surgical repair or replacement and transcatheter mitral valve repair.

Common causes of mitral regurgitation in older people

- Calcification of the mitral ring.
- Dilatation of the LV and mitral ring.
- Mucoid (myxomatous) degeneration of cusps.
- Floppy mitral valve with prolapse of the posterior cusp.
- Papillary-muscle dysfunction – usually ischaemic.
- Rupture of chordae tendineae (often partial).
- Infective endocarditis.
- Rheumatic heart disease.

Infective endocarditis

Infective endocarditis (IE) is an infection of the endocardial surface of the heart. Pathogens such as *Staphylococcus aureus*, streptococci and enterococci adhere to proteins present on damaged valves and produce vegetations to hide in. Presentation is most commonly sub-acute.

- Left-sided endocarditis accounts for 95% of cases; aortic and mitral valves are affected equally (mitral incidence may increase with age).
- Despite advances, mortality remains 15–30%, with about 200 deaths in England and Wales each year. Most affected patients are aged 60 or older.
- The mortality rate is higher in older people because of co-morbidities and a lower likelihood of being fit enough for valve surgery. Other factors associated with increased mortality are multi-valvular disease, diabetes, renal impairment, history of intravenous drug use, and infection with enterococci.
- Risk factors include atheromatous and calcific valve disease, intracardiac devices, including prosthetic valves and pacemakers, exposure to nosocomial infections, and reduced host immunity.
- Published case series show that older people may be more often affected by gastrointestinal bacteria, including Group D streptococcus (*Streptococcus bovis*) and *Enterococcus faecalis*, compared with

younger people, who tend to have *Staphylococcus aureus* and Gram-negative organisms.

- This suggests that the portal of entry is more often colonic or urogenital than in younger people. A colonoscopy should be considered for those who are being treated for *S. bovis* IE.
- Antimicrobial prophylaxis with the aim of reducing the development of IE may be given to patients at 'high risk' from IE who are undergoing 'high-risk' procedures, but recommendations vary because of different judgements about antibiotic stewardship and small risks to individuals. High risk patients include those with prosthetic valves and previous IE and procedures include invasive dental work and some gastrointestinal and urological procedures, but UK guidance is unclear. Ask the patient's cardiologist.
- Patients with prosthetic heart valves merit scrupulous protection from nosocomial infections. Avoid all but essential urinary catheterisation.

Clinical features

IE often presents non-specifically, particularly in older patients.

Clinical suspicion of infectious endocarditis can be supported by using Duke's criteria, as in the box given later (updated in 2023 to include new microbiology diagnostics). Have a high index of suspicion in older people, as the response to infection may be attenuated, so that there may not be a fever or a leucocytosis.

Consider infective endocarditis in patients presenting with the following:

- Chronic, unexplained fever.
- Anorexia and weight loss.
- Malaise.
- Intermittent confusion.
- New or changing murmurs help clinch the diagnosis, but the absence of a murmur does not exclude it.
- Splinter haemorrhages at the nail base.
- Classical signs such as Janeway lesions (haemorrhagic macules, particularly on the palms and soles), Osler's nodes (small painful nodules in finger and toe pads), and Roth spots (oval pale retinal lesions surrounded by haemorrhage) are rare.

Modified Duke's criteria for diagnosis of infective endocarditis (*2023 modifications in italics*)

Major criteria

Multiple positive blood cultures.
Positive laboratory tests (such as PCR, immunofluorescence assays or immunoglobulin titres).
Positive findings on echocardiogram:
vegetations, abscesses, damage to the seating of a prosthetic valve.
New valvular regurgitation.
Positive findings on PET or CT scan.

Minor criteria

Predisposing heart disease or intravenous drug use.
Fever >38 °C.
Vascular phenomena: arterial emboli, septic infarcts, Janeway lesions.
Immunological phenomena: glomerulonephritis, Roth's spots, Osler's nodes.
Previous history of IE.
Endovascular intracardiac implantable device.
Definite diagnosis: 2 major or 1 major and 3 minor or 5 minor criteria
Likely diagnosis: 1 major and 1 minor or 3 minor criteria

Investigations

- Raised ESR and CRP.
- Mild–moderate normocytic normochromic anaemia.
- Three sets of blood cultures should be taken at least an hour apart from different sites. *Streptococcus viridans* is the organism most isolated.
- A urine dipstick may show haematuria and/or proteinuria (due to septic emboli).
- Transthoracic ECHO can miss endocarditis in older people because the vegetations are sometimes smaller.
- Transoesophageal echocardiography (TOE) can increase the diagnostic yield to 45%. It may also detect local complications such as valve ring abscesses.
- Formal dental review to look for the source of infection.

Management

- Ideally, your trust will have an IE multidisciplinary team (cardiologist with echocardiography expertise, cardiac surgeon, microbiologist or infectious diseases physician, and neurology input).
- Start empirical IV antibiotics, as guided by the local microbiology guidelines, until blood culture (taken before commencing antibiotics) results are available (e.g. penicillin/vancomycin and gentamycin) and a targeted approach can be undertaken. Empirical therapy should cover staphylococci, streptococci, and enterococci and will also depend on whether the treated valve is 'native' or 'prosthetic'.
- Antibiotic therapy duration will be at least 6 weeks in total but will depend on the site and specific pathogen. Serial echocardiography and blood cultures will help guide therapy. Once medically stable, ongoing antibiotic therapy could be considered via 'hospital at home' or 'virtual ward' pathways, often using a longer-dwelling peripherally inserted central catheter (PICC) line.
- If the valve is severely damaged, the organism is resistant, or if the patient is in refractory heart failure, refer for consideration of surgery.

Prevention

Guidelines differ.

- Advise the patient about the need for antibiotic prophylaxis for invasive dental procedures in the future (an episode of IE increases the risk of another episode).
- If the patient makes a good recovery, it may now be appropriate to look for an underlying colonic or urological tumour that may have allowed entry of the bacteria in the first place.

Syncope, transient loss of consciousness

Syncope is now defined as 'a transient loss of consciousness (T-LOC) due to transient global cerebral hypoperfusion characterised by rapid onset, short duration and spontaneous and complete recovery'. This is covered in Chapter 11 on falls; younger patients with syncope are likely to present to cardiology, but in older people, T-LOC is usually a differential of falls.

Hypertension

Definition

Hypertension is persistently raised arterial blood pressure (BP), and an arbitrary threshold is used to define the level of BP at which the benefit of treatment (lifestyle or pharmacological) has been clearly shown to outweigh the risk. Diastolic blood pressure (DBP) tends to increase up to the 50s due to the rise in arteriolar resistance. Large artery stiffening occurs later in life and contributes to a wider pulse pressure; in later life, isolated systolic hypertension (ISH) is most common.

The threshold for diagnosis is constantly being updated. Current NICE/British Hypertension Society Guidelines suggest a clinic BP of ≥140/90 mmHg under 80 years old and ≥150/90 mmHg over 80 years old. The thresholds for home BP monitoring or ambulatory BP monitoring are 5 mmHg lower. In people over 80 years, base the target on standing BP and use clinical judgement if there is frailty or multimorbidity. This is in line with the European guidelines. Isolated systolic hypertension implies that only the systolic pressure is elevated. The American College of Cardiology and American Heart Association are now advocating a systolic measurement of 140–145 and a diastolic of less than 90 for older people.

Prevalence

It is estimated that one in four adults in England has HT, rising to over 60% in people aged over 60 years.

Effects of hypertension

Hypertension is a major risk factor for atherosclerosis and, thus, stroke, coronary artery disease, heart failure, peripheral vascular disease, chronic kidney disease and vascular dementia.

Management

1 Try non-pharmacological therapies first: a low-salt, low-calorie, low-alcohol, high-exercise regime.
2 A calcium channel blocker is generally the first line for HT in people aged 55 or older, but drugs can be matched to other co-morbidities:
   - Calcium channel blockers are also indicated for AF and angina.
   - ACEi/ARBs and thiazide-like diuretics for patients with heart failure.
   - A combination of two, then three drugs from the drug groups mentioned earlier if monotherapy does not result in satisfactory reduction and the patient is taking the medication.
   - Alpha-blockers for men with BPH.
   - Beta-blockers are not first line for HT but are used when there is angina, heart failure, AF or after ACS.

Effects of treatment

Up to age 80, drug treatment produces considerable benefit in terms of total mortality and cardiovascular morbidity and mortality (the more benefit, the older the patient, as event rates are higher), but sometimes at the expense of making the patient feel worse.

The Hypertension in the Very Elderly Trial (HYVET) showed better outcomes from treating relatively fit older patients at older ages (mean age at baseline: 83.6 years), see Chapter 5. However, orthostatic hypotension is very prevalent in this age group, and the clinician must consider balancing the risk of cardiovascular events versus that of postural symptoms and falls. Frail and older hypertensive patients should be considered on an individual, case-by-case basis. This is particularly important for those with autonomic dysfunction, such as patients with Parkinson's disease. In those with a history of postural hypotension, base your target on the BP reading when standing.

Vascular disease

Arterial disease

Older people experience the range of arterial diseases seen in younger people, such as vasculitis, but atherosclerosis is the most common pathology.

Abdominal aortic aneurysm

An abdominal aortic aneurysm (AAA) is a pathological dilation of the abdominal aorta with a diameter over 1.5 times the expected anteroposterior diameter of that segment given the person's sex and body size; so, the usual threshold for diagnosis is an aortic diameter of 3.0 cm or greater. More than 90% originate below the renal arteries (infrarenal).

- AAA increases with age and is six times more common in men than women.
- Risk factors include smoking, hypertension, COPD, DM, and a strong association with family history.
- The prevalence of AAA peaked around 1997 and was already declining because of lower smoking and better treatment of hypertension when the UK screening programme was introduced between 2009 and 2013.
- Men are offered a screening ultrasound when they reach 65 years old. Men over 66 who missed screening can self-refer via the NHS website.
- The prevalence of AAA in the screening programme in England is now 1% (men aged 65).
- If the aortic diameter is over 3 cm, repeat US is offered. Over 5.5 cm, patients are referred to a vascular surgeon to discuss the risks and benefits of a procedure. Referral should be considered regardless of diameter if symptomatic.
- An AAA usually causes no symptoms, but if it ruptures, it is usually fatal (>80%). Symptoms of an impending rupture include a pulsating sensation in the abdomen, severe abdominal pain or back pain that radiates into the abdomen.
- Of those not operated on, 5% rupture per annum if the diameter is 5–6 cm; the rate rises exponentially if the aneurysm is larger.
- In 2019 there were around 3,000 deaths each year from ruptured AAA in men aged 65+ in England and Wales.

Management

- Medical management includes smoking cessation advice and tight management of hypertension, diabetes, and hyperlipidaemia.
- Aneurysm repair can be done via open surgery or laparoscopically. Open surgery involves a long general anaesthetic, and post-operative care is best managed in an intensive care unit.
- Infrarenal aneurysms that have not ruptured can be repaired by endovascular aneurysm repair (EVAR, Figure 12.3). A stent graft is inserted via a catheter in the femoral arteries. The stent graft is activated under x-ray guidance and positioned across the aneurysm. Further procedures may be necessary, including insertion of stents into the iliac arteries and femoro-femoral bypass grafts.
- EVAR has benefits when compared to open surgical repair, especially in men over 70 years old and women. The advantages of the EVAR are a shorter procedure under local anaesthetic, potentially leading to a shorter recovery time, less risk of major haemorrhage, and reduced post-operative pain. The disadvantage is the risk of small leaks ('endoleaks') at the edges of the stent graft, which are not always clinically obvious. EVAR patients also require post-procedure surveillance.

Peripheral arterial disease

This is most common in the lower limbs. Arterial disease is chronically progressive, eventually leading to peripheral vascular occlusion. It is often referred to as peripheral vascular disease (PVD). Risk factors mimic other atherosclerotic disease processes and include tobacco smoking, diabetes, hypertension, age, and hyperlipidaemia. Smoking is associated with the highest risk, with an odds ratio of 2.7.

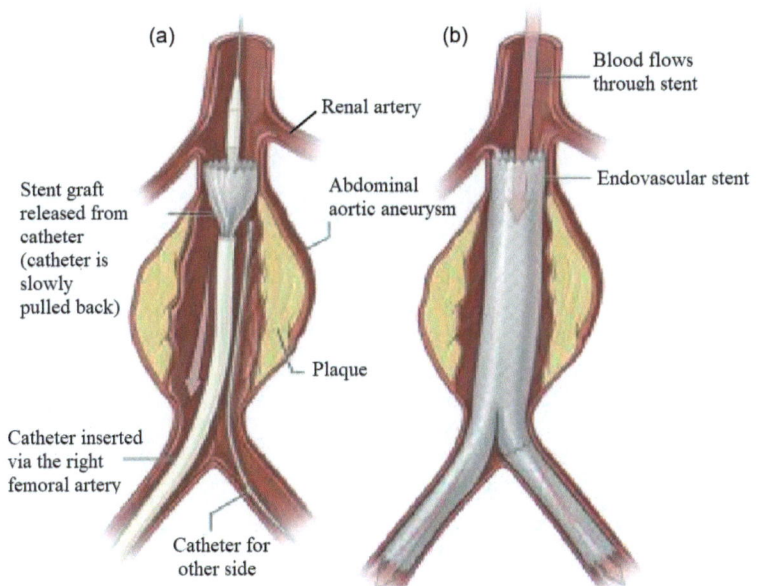

Figure 12.3 Placement of an EVAR stent in an infrarenal aneurysm. (a) Deployment via a catheter inserted into the right femoral artery. (b) The stent is released from the catheter, and the graft expands to allow blood to flow through it. *Source:* National Institutes of Health / https://www.nhlbi.nih.gov/health/aortic-aneurysm/treatment

Clinical features

- Intermittent claudication: pain usually in the back of both calves that comes on during exercise and is relieved by rest.
- Critical ischaemia may present as pain at rest, painful ulcers, and necrotic or septic skin lesions. This sometimes follows trauma or a haemodynamic crisis. Those with limited mobility may not give a history of previous claudication.
- Limb ischaemia due to progressive atheroma tends to be gradual, and symptoms may be less severe due to the development of collateral circulation. Presentation is usually with worsening claudication. Ischaemia due to embolic phenomenon tends to be acute in onset (acute limb ischaemia).
- On examination, affected extremities may be discoloured, with trophic changes in skin and nails (loss of hair on the legs is sensitive but extremely non-specific), cool and pulseless feet, and bruits over femoral, superficial femoral (frequent site of obstruction), or popliteal arteries.
- Elicit blanching on elevation, delayed hyperaemia, and venous filling on dependency.
- Embolic ischaemia may present with a limb that is painful and pale/white in colour (classically pain, pulseless, pallor, power loss, paraesthesia, and perishing with cold). Check for ulcers and gangrene (see Figure 12.4).

Investigations

Measure ankle systolic pressure with a Doppler probe; should be at least 0.8 of the brachial pressure.

Diagnosis is confirmed by visualisation of the vasculature and stenotic lesions by ultrasonography or contrast-enhanced CT imaging.

Management

Acute limb ischaemia is associated with a 20% mortality rate, and patients must be referred as an emergency to a vascular surgeon. In addition to pain relief, options include endovascular therapy, e.g. percutaneous mechanical thrombus extraction, thrombolysis or a revascularization procedure. Patients with critical ischaemia need urgent referral to surgery or interventional radiology (see Figure 12.5).

Medical

In more chronic situations, initial management comprises education, addressing cardiovascular risk, encouraging exercise to develop collaterals, and a limited role for drugs.

- Smoking cessation advice.
- Support with exercise regimes to improve the distance walked. Exercise improves claudication symptoms (although improvement in mortality has not been seen).

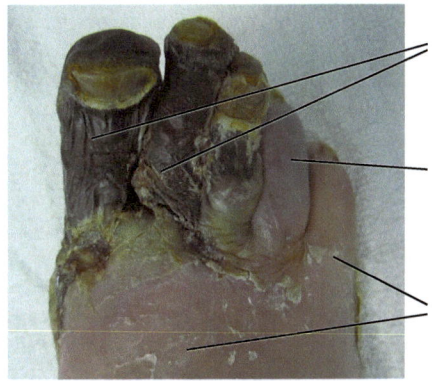

Dry gangrene - these toes would probably mummify

Blue/purple discoloration and swelling, more suggestive of wet gangrene that will spread

Red hyperaemic skin of just viable tissue

Figure 12.4 Gangrene of the toes in a diabetic. From: James Heilman/Wikimedia Commons/CC BY SA 3.0.

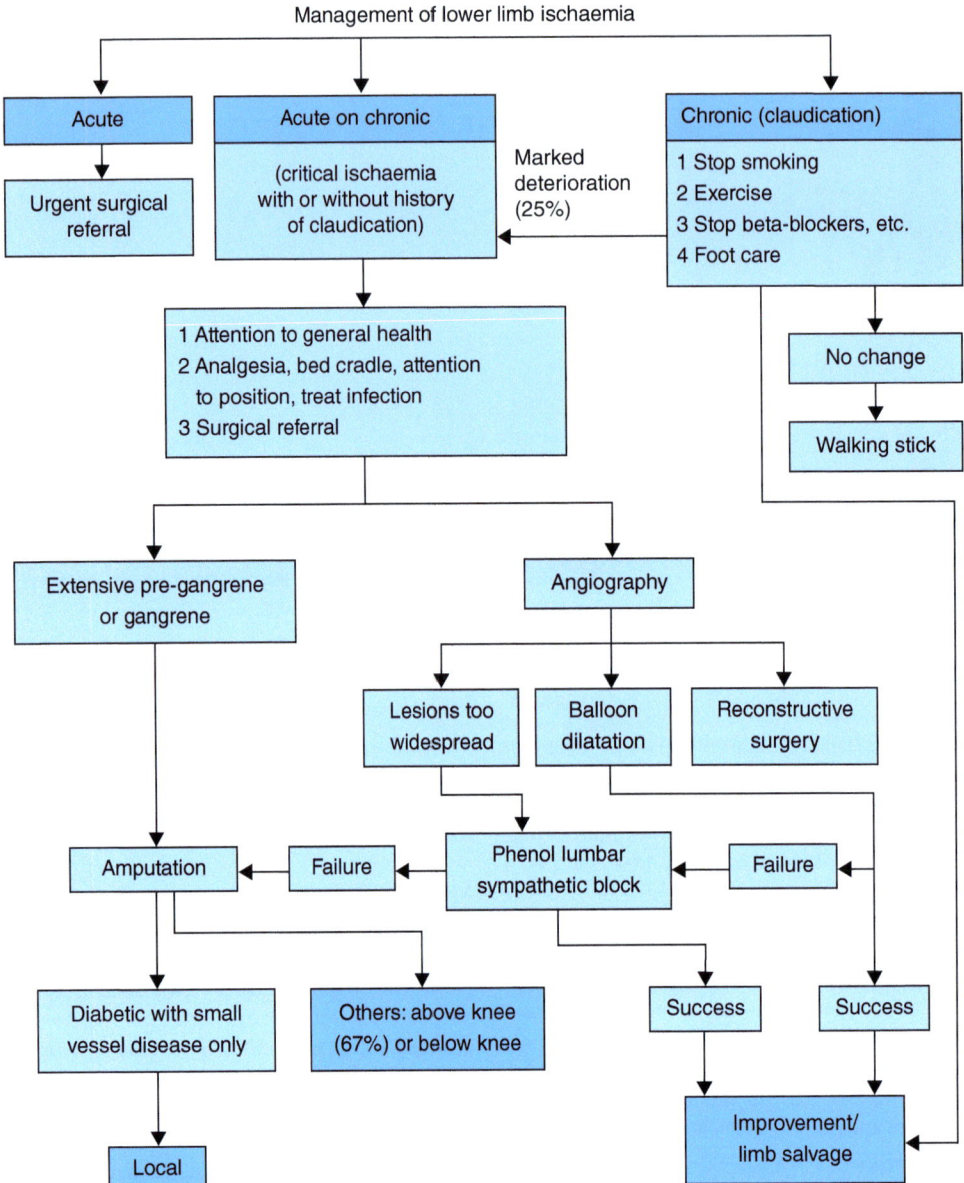

Figure 12.5 Management of lower limb ischaemia.

- Where relevant, treat with a statin, antihypertensives, and improve diabetes control.
- Daily clopidogrel or aspirin (no consensus about the dose of the latter).
- Naftidrofuryl (5-hydroxytryptamine-2-receptor antagonist) has limited evidence for an improvement in pain-free walking distance and is NICE-approved.
- Cilostazol (a phosphodiesterase inhibitor) has antiplatelet and vasodilator effects. Studies suggest limited improvement in exercise tolerance, and although it is not NICE-approved, it is sometimes used when there are no other options.
- Some pain clinics will perform lumbar sympathectomies for pain relief, initially with a local anaesthetic to assess the benefit and then with a destructive agent, such as phenol, but this is uncommon.

Revascularisation
Options for those with ongoing symptoms or critical ischaemia include endovascular stenting/balloon dilatation, and/or artery bypass grafting. The choice of procedure will be dependent on patient characteristics, site, and number of stenotic lesions.

Amputation
Amputation is the last resort for a gangrenous limb with no options for vascularization.

- In diabetes, ischaemic toes due to small vessel disease will often undergo mummification and may be left to auto-amputate. Limited surgery, e.g. ray amputation of the foot may be possible.
- In ascending wet gangrene, the options are end-of-life care or a major amputation.
- If the patient has capacity, plan ahead with the surgeon, as delirium is likely to develop, complicating decision making.
- Part of the skill of the vascular surgeon is deciding the level of amputation, preserving as much of the leg as possible, but producing a stump that will heal and not need a further procedure. Frail older people are most unlikely to manage the rehabilitation process associated with functional leg prostheses.
  - If a below-knee amputation will heal, this is the best option as the patient can manage sitting in a wheelchair with help to transfer, can see both knees, and a cosmetic prosthesis will give a near-normal appearance.

○ An above-knee amputation is more of a challenge to sitting balance and transfers; it needs greater psychological adjustment, and the thigh may be prone to lifting.

Arterial embolism

Other sites of arterial embolism are in the brain, Chapter 9 and mesenteric embolism, Chapter 14.

Venous disease

Chronic venous insufficiency

Chronic venous insufficiency, resulting from venous hypertension due to damage to the vein valves and calf muscle pump impairment is common, reduces quality of life, and may result in ulcers (see Chapter 19).

Superficial thrombophlebitis

A thrombus forms in a superficial vein, causing local inflammation. It usually presents a painful, warm, palpable cordlike vein in a patient with obvious varicose veins. Treat with an NSAID but have a low threshold for excluding deep vein thrombosis (DVT).

Venous thromboembolism

Venous thromboembolism (VTE) includes DVT and pulmonary embolus (PE). Classically, it excluded superficial thrombophlebitis, but reports of DVT and PE associated with superficial thrombophlebitis are increasing. Remember Virchow's triad for thrombus formation – vascular stasis, vascular wall damage and hypercoagulability. About two-thirds of all VTE events occur in patients over 70 years old.

Risk factors for VTE

- Increasing age.
- Immobility.
- Obesity.
- Smoking.
- Previous DVT (and current DVT for PE).
- Dehydration (especially in the context of inflammation).
- Surgery, especially abdominal.
- Fractures, especially the lower limb.
- Active cancer.
- Impaired venous return, e.g. right heart failure.
- Inflammatory conditions, e.g. acute infection (COVID-19), inflammatory bowel disease.
- Procoagulant states, e.g. antiphospholipid antibody syndrome, thrombocytosis.
- Drugs, including HRT, SERMs, tamoxifen, anastrozole and goserelin.

Deep-vein thrombosis

DVT is a thrombus (blood clot) in a deep vein that partially or completely obstructs blood flow. Thrombus formation is most common in the lower limb but can also occur in veins in the arm, abdomen, retina, and brain. DVTs in the leg or thigh are deep to the muscles and commonly cause asymmetrical leg swelling, unilateral leg pain, distension of superficial veins, and red or discoloured skin, but can be asymptomatic. Very rarely, a massive DVT causes severe swelling with oedema and can progress to venous gangrene.

Diagnosis

- This requires confirmation by an ultrasound scan of lower limb veins and, if negative but strongly suspected, CT (or MRI) venography.

- In older people, the most common differentials are cellulitis and a ruptured Baker's (popliteal) cyst. A bilateral DVT suggests a pelvic tumour.
- In older inpatients, investigation usually follows clinical suspicion (the Wells score [see Appendix] performs only slightly better than chance, and a D-dimer will often be raised).
- In ED, a Wells score may be used to classify the risk as 'DVT likely' (Wells score ≥ 2) or 'DVT unlikely' (Wells score < 2). A patient with a 'DVT likely' score needs a venous ultrasound; a 'DVT unlikely' score needs an age-adjusted D-dimer and an ultrasound if this is positive.

Management

- Patients with DVT who are otherwise well are treated as out-patients with treatment doses of DOACs such as apixaban, edoxaban or rivaroxaban. They are also first line for DVTs associated with cancer.
- Warfarin remains an alternative for those with significant renal impairment but takes several days to work, so low-molecular-weight heparin is required initially until the patient's international normalised ratio (INR) is greater than 2.
- The duration of treatment is usually 3 months, although a longer duration may be considered if the thrombosis is deemed 'unprovoked' (on the basis that an unprovoked DVT is more likely to recur).
- Around 5% of people with unprovoked DVT have occult cancer, so recheck the history and clinical examination to see if further blood tests are warranted.
- Prevention is always preferable to cure: prophylactic LMWH is given to high-risk hospitalised patients, which includes all older patients, those with underlying carcinoma, and those with reduced mobility.

Pulmonary Embolus

A potentially life-threatening condition caused by occlusion of the pulmonary arteries by emboli, most commonly thrombus from leg veins. There were 100,000 deaths worldwide from acute PE in 2018.

- Often underdiagnosed in older people because their presentation may be atypical.
- More than 40% of PEs found at post-mortem were not suspected in life.
- Increasingly common with increasing age.
- High morbidity and mortality, especially with high-risk features such as shock, tachyarrhythmia, and right heart failure.

Presenting features of PE

PE causes impaired gas exchange, pulmonary artery hypertension, lung inflammation, and infarction. A massive pulmonary embolus (usually a saddle embolus obstructing both pulmonary arteries) is a cause of sudden death. There may be a clinically apparent DVT.

Symptoms

- Breathlessness (50%).
- Pleuritic chest pain (40%).
- Cough (20%).
- Haemoptysis (10%).
- Syncope (8–20%).
- Feeling of impending doom.
- Retrosternal chest pain (right ventricular ischaemia).
- Palpitations.
- Confusion.
- Falls.
- Functional decline.

Signs

- Tachypnoea.
- Tachycardia.

- Hypotension.
- Fever.
- Raised JVP.
- Gallop.
- Pleural rub.
- Bronchospasm.
- Right heart failure.
- Pulmonary oedema.

Investigations

Have a high index of suspicion, as PEs can be asymptomatic or mistaken for other common cardiac and respiratory conditions.

- The ECG most commonly shows sinus tachycardia. Less commonly, there are signs of right heart strain or new AF. A classic 'S1Q3T3' pattern occurs in <20% of patients.
- CXR is often normal but may show a wedge-shaped infarction, segmental collapse, a raised hemidiaphragm or pleural effusion.
- Blood gases may be normal early on, but hypoxaemia and hypocapnia (secondary to hyperventilation) are suggestive of PE.
- D-dimer may give a false positive in inflammation. If it is used, then use an age-adjusted value in conjunction with the Wells Score for PE. A negative D-dimer in a patient with low clinical probability reliably excludes DVT/PE.
- CT pulmonary angiography (CTPA) is the diagnostic modality of choice, with a sensitivity of >80% and a specificity of 96% for PE. V/Q scans can be used in those in whom a contrast CT is contraindicated but are only helpful in those with a normal CXR appearance.
- An echocardiogram will identify those with right ventricular dysfunction who are therefore at higher risk.
- A troponin leak is associated with worse outcomes.

Management of PE

- Commence LMWH whilst confirming the diagnosis (do not wait for imaging if there is high clinical suspicion).
- Titrate oxygen to target saturations of 94–98% (or 88–92% for patients at risk of hypercapnic respiratory failure).
- Consider whether the patient is suitable for a DOAC. LMWH followed by warfarin remains an option. Once INR is within range, stop LMWH.
- Haemodynamically unstable patients with massive PE require an ABCDE approach and urgent reperfusion with thrombolysis.
  - Systemic thrombolysis (usually with t-PA) reduces the mortality rate to 2.5% (see Chapter 9 for complications associated with thrombolysis).
  - Catheter-directed thrombolysis is indicated in those with contraindications to or failed systemic thrombolysis, but in the UK, this is only available in specialist centres. The catheter used also delivers ultrasonic waves to aid clot dispersal.
  - If PE is the suspected cause of cardiac arrest, give thrombolysis and continue CPR for 90 min.
- Surgical pulmonary embolectomy is an option for those with massive/submassive PE who have an absolute contraindication to thrombolysis (such as previous intracranial haemorrhage or mass, or a stroke within the last 3 months), or who have failed to improve with thrombolytic therapy.

Duration of anticoagulation

- First idiopathic PE: 3 months.
- Older patients are at increased risk of haemorrhage with anticoagulation. Avoid concomitant use of aspirin unless required for coronary stenting or peripheral vascular disease. Those with a history of GI bleeding are most at risk.
- The risk–benefit of treating the ongoing risk of VTE versus bleeding must be assessed on an individual basis for those with recurrent PEs.

 REFERENCES AND FURTHER READING

Regnault V, Lacolley P, Laurent S (2024) Arterial stiffness: from basic primers to integrative physiology. *Annual Review of Physiology* 86:99–121, doi: 10.1146/annurev-physiol-042022-031925.

British Heart Foundation BHF (2024). Global heart and circulatory disease factsheet. www.bhf.org.uk/-/media/files/for-professionals/research/heart-statistics/bhf-cvd-statistics-global-factsheet.pdf?rev=f323972183254ca0a1043683a9707a01&hash=5AA21565EEE5D85691D37157B31E4AAA

BHF (2024). *UK Factsheet* www.bhf.org.uk/-/media/files/for-professionals/research/heart-statistics/bhf-cvd-statistics-uk-factsheet.pdf?rev=5c76af77f68e4c43b19f957890005bbe&hash=D31DB43089AAD361320212D15D4B70FB

NICE Clinical guidance CG126 (updated 2016) *Stable angina: management.* www.nice.org.uk/guidance/cg126/chapter/Introduction

Rousan TA, Thadani U (2019). Stable angina medical therapy management guidelines: a critical review of guidelines from the European Society of Cardiology and National Institute for Health and Care Excellence. *European Cardiology Review* 14:18–22, doi: 10.15420/ecr.2018.26.1.

Joshi PH, de Lemos JA (2021). Diagnosis and management of stable angina: a review. *JAMA* 25:1765–1778, doi: 10.1001/jama.2021.1527.

NICE Guidelines NG185 (2020) Acute coronary syndromes. www.nice.org.uk/guidance/conditions-and-diseases/cardiovascular-conditions/acute-coronary-syndromes

Byrne RA, Rossello X, Coughlan JJ et al. for the ESC Scientific Document Group (2023) ESC guidelines for the management of acute coronary syndromes: developed by the task force on the management of acute coronary syndromes of the European Society of Cardiology (ESC). *European Heart Journal* 44: 3720–3826, doi: 10.1093/eurheartj/ehad191.

Yndigegn T, Lindahl B, Mars K et al. for the REDUCE-AMI Investigators (2024). Beta-blockers after myocardial infarction and preserved ejection fraction. *NEJM*, doi: https://doi.org/10.1056/NEJMoa2401479.

Shanmugam VB, Harper R, Meredith I et al. (2015). An overview of PCI in the very elderly. *Journal of Geriatric Cardiology* 12:174–184, https://dx.doi.org/10.11909/j.issn.1671-5411.2015.02.012

Collinson P and Lindahl B (2016) Diagnosing Type 2 *Myocardial Infarction, American College of Cardiology - Expert Analysis.* https://www.acc.org/Latest-in-Cardiology/Articles/2016/05/18/13/58/Diagnosing-Type-2-Myocardial-Infarction

Putot A, Putot S, Chagué F (2022). New horizons in type 2 myocardial infarction: pathogenesis, assessment, and management of an emerging geriatric disease. *Age and Ageing* 51(4): afac085, doi: 10.1093/ageing/afac085.

NICE Clinical guideline CG187 (updated 2021) *Acute heart failure: diagnosis and management.* www.nice.org.uk/guidance/cg187

NICE guideline NG106 (2018) *Chronic heart failure in adults: diagnosis and management.* www.nice.org.uk/guidance/ng106

Simmonds SJ, Cuijpers I, Heymans S, et al. (2020). Cellular and molecular differences between HFpEF and HFrEF: a step ahead in an improved pathological understanding. *Cells* 18(9): 242, doi: 10.3390/cells9010242

McDonagh TA, Metra M, Adamo M, et al. (2021). ESC guidelines for the diagnosis and treatment of acute and chronic heart failure. *European Heart Journal* 42(36): 3599–3726. https://orbi.uliege.be/handle/2268/290864.

Jasinska-Piadlo A, Campbell P (2023). Management of patients with heart failure and preserved ejection fraction. *Heart* 109:874–883. https://heart.bmj.com/content/109/11/874

Kumbhani DJ (2023) *Empagliflozin Outcome Trial in Patients with Chronic Heart Failure with Preserved Ejection Fraction – EMPEROR-Preserved. Review for American Cardiology* Society. https://www.acc.

org/Latest-in-Cardiology/Clinical-Trials/2021/08/25/23/07/EMPEROR-Preserved

Kumbhani DJ (2023). *Dapagliflozin Evaluation to Improve the Lives of Patients with Preserved Ejection Fraction Heart Failure – DELIVER. Review for the American Cardiology Society.* https://www.acc.org/Latest-in-Cardiology/Clinical-Trials/2022/08/26/04/12/DELIVER

National Cardiac Audit Programme for England & Wales www.nicor.org.uk/national-cardiac-audit-programme. This hosts the 10 clinical audits in the national programme and is a useful resource.

NICE Guidelines NG196 (2021) Atrial fibrillation: diagnosis and management. www.nice.org.uk/guidance/ng196

NICE CKS (2023) *Atrial fibrillation.* https://cks.nice.org.uk/topics/atrial-fibrillation

Puette JP, Malek R, Ellison MB (2022) *Pacemaker.* Stat Pearls [Internet] https://www.ncbi.nlm.nih.gov/books/NBK526001

Rayner R, Adams H. (2023). Aortic stenosis and transcatheter aortic valve implantation in the elderly. *Australian Journal of General Practice*; 52(7), doi: https://doi.org/10.31128/AJGP-08-22-6527.

Muscente F, De Caterina R (2019). Risk of stroke after transcatheter aortic valve implant: the role of the new oral anticoagulants. *European Heart Journal Supplements* 21:B50–51, doi: 10.1093/eurheartj/suz016.

Scheggi V, Merilli I, Marcucci R et al. (2021). Predictors of mortality and adverse events in patients with infective endocarditis: a retrospective real world study in a surgical Centre. *BMC Cardiovascular Disorders* 21:28, doi: 10.1186/s12872-021-01853-6.

Fowler VG, Durack DT, Selton-Suty C et al. (2023). The 2023 Duke-International Society for Cardiovascular Infectious Diseases Criteria for infective endocarditis: updating the modified Duke criteria. *Clinical Infectious Diseases* 77:518–526, doi: 10.1093/cid/ciad271

NICE Guidelines NG136 (2023) *Hypertension in adults: diagnosis and management.* www.nice.org.uk/guidance/ng136

Mukhtar O and Jackson SHD (2012). The Hypertension in the Very Elderly Trial – latest data. *Br J Clin Pharmacol* 75:951–954. doi: 10.1111/j.1365-2125.2012.04427.x

NICE Guidelines NG156 (2020) *Abdominal aortic aneurysm: diagnosis and management.* www.nice.org.uk/guidance/ng156

Obara H, Matsubara K, Kitagawa Y (2018). Acute limb ischemia. *Annals of Vascular Diseases* 11:443–448, doi: /10.3400/avd.ra.18-00074

Vyas V, Goyal A (2022) *Acute Pulmonary Embolism.* StatPearls [Internet] https://www.ncbi.nlm.nih.gov/books/NBK560551

Howard LSGE, Barden S, Condliffe R (2018). British Thoracic Society guideline for the outpatient management of pulmonary embolism. *Thorax* 73:ii1–ii29, doi: 10.1136/thoraxjnl-2018-211539

NICE CKS (2023) *Management of deep vein thrombosis.* https://cks.nice.org.uk/topics/deep-vein-thrombosis/management/management#

Silveira PC, Ip IK, Goldhaber SZ et al. (2015). Performance of wells score for deep vein thrombosis in the inpatient setting. *JAMA Internal Medicine* 175(7):1112–1117, doi: 10.1001/jamainternmed.2015.1687.

INFORMATION FOR PATIENTS AND FAMILIES

American Heart Association: https://www.heart.org/en/health-topics

British Heart Foundation: www.bhf.org.uk/informationsupport

Patient UK: Heart disease: symptoms, types, and treatments https://patient.info/heart-health/heart-disease

All websites were accessed in December 2024.

13

Respiratory medicine

Age-related changes

Age-related changes affect all aspects of the respiratory system. Structural and functional changes occur, decreasing the efficiency of gas transfer. However, because the lungs have a huge reserve capacity, significant clinical issues only arise when an older person becomes sick, unless lung function has been progressively damaged by smoking or air pollution. Older people may have difficulty performing many lung function tests, but spirometry is usually possible.

1 Changes in the shape of the ribcage (especially if there is kyphosis) and diaphragmatic weakness make breathing less efficient.
2 Reduced lung elasticity and chest wall compliance lead to air trapping, a rise in residual volume and a fall in the forced vital capacity (FVC), forced expiratory volume in 1 sec (FEV_1), and peak expiratory flow, as shown in Figures 13.1 and 13.2. Some normal older people will have an FEV_1/FVC ratio of <0.7. Do not treat them (beyond smoking cessation advice) unless they are symptomatic.
3 An increase in airway size and a loss of alveolar surface decrease the lung volume available for gas exchange and increase dead space, reducing the efficiency of gas exchange. Premature closure of small airways results in ventilation–perfusion mismatching, contributing to an increase in the alveolar-arterial oxygen gradient. Arterial oxygen tension (PaO_2) falls from 12.7 kPa at age 30 to 10 kPa at age 60.
4 Oxygen delivery to tissues decreases due to age-related decreases in cardiac output and body muscle mass, as well as ventilation-perfusion mismatching and decreased alveolar volume.
5 Decreased sensitivity of respiratory centres to hypoxia or hypercapnia results in a diminished ventilatory response in heart failure or infection.
6 Mucociliary protection of the lower airway is impaired.
7 Complex changes in the alveoli lead to higher levels of basal inflammation and an impaired immune response.

Examination of the chest

Check the rate and pattern of respiration. Tachypnoea suggests a cardiorespiratory problem, which can be especially useful if the patient cannot give much history. Cheyne–Stokes respiration, in which the breathing becomes progressively shallower, sometimes culminating in an apnoeic episode before becoming progressively deeper again in a cyclical pattern, is more common in older people. It is often seen in strokes and at the end of life but may occur in normal individuals. Note the chest shape. Significant kyphosis is usually now due to osteoporosis or multilevel thoracic degenerative disc disease (previously TB). Look for thyroid and thoracotomy scars. The normal trachea may

deviate slightly to the right around an unfolded aorta. Many older patients have lung basal crackles that clear on coughing and have no clinical significance. Conversely, if the patient has poor air entry, an area of consolidation may appear silent. A silent chest is a danger sign in the context of airway obstruction.

Note any bruising or chest wall asymmetry in someone with a history of falls (rib fractures often lead to hypostatic pneumonia). Remember other systems associated with chest problems, e.g. aspiration in Parkinson's disease, and check for heart failure. Oxygen saturation, measured by a fingertip probe, is a useful bedside test. The admission CXR of an ill older patient is often difficult to interpret; usually taken AP (antero-posterior instead of the standard PA) or even supine (check for scapular lines), often with rotation (check relation of heads of clavicles to spinous processes), sometimes with the head in the chest, and with poor inspiration. A subtle diagnosis may require a repeat film when the patient is improving.

The burden of respiratory disease

Prior to the COVID-19 pandemic (see later) respiratory disease caused approximately 20% of all deaths. It was the second most common reason for emergency hospital attendance and attendance rates were rising at three times that of other conditions. Social inequality causes a higher proportion of respiratory deaths than any other disease. This is clearly shown in the atlas of variation for respiratory disease. Death rates increase steeply with age, and nearly 90% of respiratory deaths occur among people 65 years of age or older. Prior to COVID, the three main respiratory killers were lung cancer, pneumonia, and chronic obstructive pulmonary disease (COPD).

COPD causes about 90% of respiratory disability; 900,000 people have a formal diagnosis of COPD in the UK, with twice as many undiagnosed.

Upper respiratory tract infections

Coronavirus disease

Uncomplicated COVID-19 is an upper respiratory tract infection caused by the SARS-CoV-2 virus. Depending on the variant, the median incubation period is 5 days. Many have a flu-like illness, but symptoms vary depending on the individual and viral variant. Patients may be

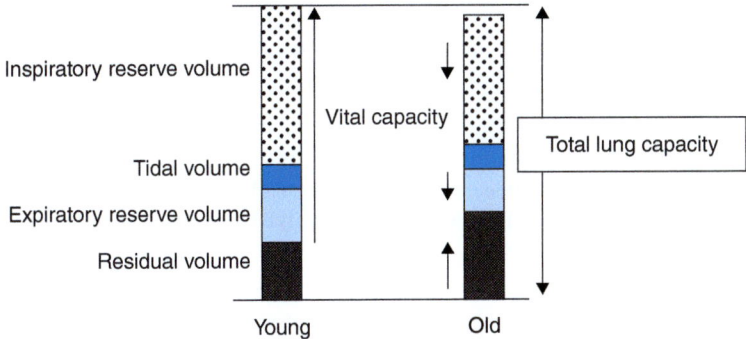

Figure 13.1 Changes in lung volumes with age.

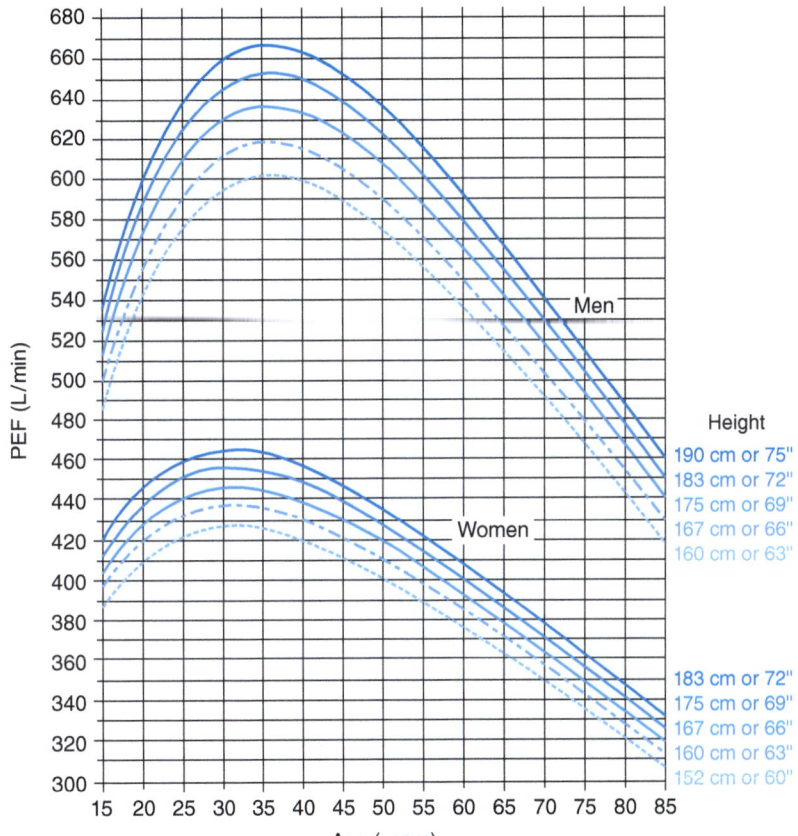

Figure 13.2 Normal values for peak expiratory flow (PEF) with age.

asymptomatic but still infectious. Several complications can occur. Pneumonia may develop with a massive inflammatory cytokine storm, which can be fatal. A proportion of patients, including some who had a mild initial illness, go on to develop a prolonged condition known as 'long COVID'.

This novel coronavirus (SARS-CoV-2), was first recognised in Hubei Province, China, in December 2019. The COVID-19 pandemic was declared in March 2020. COVID caused around seven million confirmed deaths worldwide between 2020 and April 2024 (Worldometer).

The pandemic changed many aspects of health care in the UK. During 2020 and 2021, COVID became the leading cause of death, overtaking dementia, ischaemic heart disease, stroke, and lung cancer. However, from January to June 2022, all-cause mortality fell and was lower than in any year since 2001, probably because vulnerable people had died prematurely in 2020 and 2021. COVID deaths have fallen overall since 2022 due to growing population immunity from vaccination and infection, less virulent strains of the virus circulating, and advances in our understanding and management. The virus is transitioning to an endemic phase, but challenges remain: anxiety about winter rises in admission rates, the possibility of new variants with higher case fatality and vaccine escape, the organisational cost of ongoing vaccination programmes, and the effects and costs of long-term COVID. Health inequalities and waiting lists were worsening before the pandemic, and the deterioration has continued. During the height of the pandemic, there was gratitude towards health services, but since then, the belief that the 'NHS will be there if you need it' has been damaged, perhaps irreparably. Globally, the pandemic did untold damage to financial markets and healthcare economies. The unprecedented social changes (lockdowns, social isolation, mask-wearing, home working and virtual meetings) have had marked ongoing effects on people of all ages.

The single greatest risk factor for death from COVID is age. The infection–fatality ratio (IFR) is the probability of an individual dying from pathogen-related disease complications once infected with a pathogen. Prior to vaccination, age-specific global estimates of IFR showed a J-shape curve with the lowest IFR at age 7, rising to 0.06% at 30 years and increasing exponentially to 1% at 60 and 20% at 90 years.

Other risk factors for poor outcomes include deprivation, ethnicity – especially Bangladeshi, Pakistani, or Black Caribbean heritage – and having one of a broad range of comorbidities (including dementia, diabetes, hypertension, chronic lung, heart and renal diseases, active cancer, immune suppression, and obesity).

Particular challenges for older people with COVID in the UK included:

- Greater likelihood of severe disease, with a higher rate of hospitalisation (1 in 5 of the people aged 80+ with COVID), need for intensive care, and a higher death rate.
- Atypical presentation, e.g. gastrointestinal symptoms and delirium in variants where cough and fever were predominant in younger people.
- Concern about ageist practice when resources were very limited and risked being overwhelmed (e.g. whether to admit to hospital or intensive care).
- Rapid discharge from hospital at the start of the pandemic, often without testing – which was not widely available at the time – to clear beds for the expected influx of patients. Infection was taken into care homes; one of the factors that led to high death rates there together with the frailty of the residents, the difficulty of isolating people with dementia, poor provision of PPE, and staff working in more than one facility.
- Visiting restrictions due to national lockdowns and institutional rules applied at all ages, but older people were least able to manage the electronic options for communication, and as they were most likely to die, they were the people that died without family support.
- Multidisciplinary, rehabilitation and community services were curtailed.
- As services focused on COVID, many other conditions were not diagnosed promptly or managed effectively, and older people were most likely to be affected. As well as the publicised delays in the diagnosis of cancer and heart disease, failure to manage other less obvious conditions had major effects on quality of life. People struggled to get their hearing aids fixed, went blind from macular degeneration that might have been treatable, and struggled with chronic pain from arthritic hips and knees.
- The risk of rapid cognitive deterioration due to a lack of stimulation appears to have been most marked in those already suffering from mild to moderate dementia in care homes due to a lack of contact with family, visitors, and restrictions on activities.
- The incidence of hip fractures increased in 2023, possibly because of the deconditioning effects of lockdowns.

Elsewhere, there were reports of scandals, such as old people being found dead after being abandoned in care homes. Once vaccination became available, as well as concern about the lack of global justice in distribution, there were reports (from the WHO) that older people were not prioritised for vaccination.

Investigations

Diagnostic tests use nasopharyngeal samples. RT-PCR tests which amplify viral RNA remain the gold standard and have 95% sensitivity and specificity. Tests for the antigen in the form of lateral flow tests became widely available during the pandemic and were distributed without charge in the UK. Sensitivity and specificity depend on the kit used, but specificity is usually very high. Testing for antibodies is a research tool, not a diagnostic test.

No single clinical, biochemical or haematology marker appears specific for COVID infection. However, look for lymphopaenia, high urea, high CRP, and infiltrates on CXR, typically peripheral and often bilateral. Chest CT should not be used as a screening test for COVID, although a CT pulmonary angiogram is indicated if a pulmonary embolism is suspected (seen in up to 8% of patients). Unsurprisingly, the most common complications are respiratory (acute respiratory distress syndrome [ARDS] in up to 30% of patients), but arrhythmias and acute kidney injury are also common.

Management of COVID-19

The NICE rapid guideline (updated May 2024) is shorter than previous versions but still runs to 80 pages. Long COVID has separate guidance.

In the community

Drugs are available in the community for adults who do not require supplemental oxygen but are at increased risk of progression to severe COVID. The list of conditions that are considered to increase risk includes many that are common in older people such as cancer and Parkinson's disease. Age itself is also now included as a significant risk factor, and by mid 2025, drugs will be available to everyone aged 70 years or over. Treatment is organised locally. People who think they may be at high risk should do a lateral flow test (one each day for 3 days if negative), and if they are positive, contact their GP or NHS 111. Treatment options whilst still at home include:

- **Nirmatrelvir plus ritonavir (Paxlovid):** for mild to moderate disease but at risk of disease progression, oral for 5 days.
- **Sotrovimab (Xevudy):** given as an IV infusion, so the patient must attend a suitable facility for a single dose.

Nirmatrelvir targets the main polyprotein protease of SARS-CoV-2 in the replication cycle, dramatically decreasing the viral load. Ritonavir is a protease inhibitor and a CYP3A4 antagonist, inhibiting nirmatrelvir breakdown and enhancing its pharmacokinetics. Sotrovimab (a monoclonal antibody that binds to the spike protein receptor and prevents viral cell entry) is second line if Paxlovid is not suitable.

Symptomatic management is like that for flu and includes:

- **Cough:** honey, codeine linctus (needs a prescription)
- **Fever:** adequate fluids, paracetamol, or ibuprofen

Clinical features of severe COVID

Symptoms of severe COVID include breathlessness at rest, haemoptysis, syncope, new confusion, and reduced urine output. Signs include cyanosis, mottled skin, and oxygen saturation below 91% (all less reliable in people with dark skin).

Discuss admission or options, if appropriate, such as a virtual ward or palliative care.

Management in hospital

Infection control should be considered in the choice of ward (see trust policy).

Start with an ABCD approach in a sick patient. Oxygen should be given to ensure saturations are >92% in those without a history of hypercapnic respiratory failure. High-flow nasal cannula (HFNC), non-invasive ventilation (NIV), and invasive mechanical ventilation (IMV) are widely used to support respiration. Empirical treatment is usually given for pneumonia. If oxygen saturation falls further, look for PE or heart failure.

Drugs options

- **Paxlovid** is recommended if *supplemental oxygen is not needed*, but there is an increased risk of progression to severe COVID with sotrovimab as the second line (see earlier).
- **Dexamethasone** 6 mg orally (or IV) once a day for 10 days is indicated for patients who *need supplemental oxygen* to meet their prescribed saturation, even if they cannot tolerate it (RECOVERY trial). Watch closely for steroid-induced hyperactive delirium (which restricted its use in clinical trials). Prednisolone, 40 mg a day, is an alternative.

- **Tocilizumab** (an IL-6 receptor blocker) is an option for patients on oxygen and dexamethasone to reduce the cytokine storm. Baricitinib (a JAK inhibitor) is an alternative.

COVID is very thrombogenic; prescribe a standard prophylactic dose of low molecular-weight heparin and continue after discharge for 7–14 days.

Maintaining euvolaemia reduces AKI.

Myocardial injury can raise troponins, so look for evolving ECG changes if ACS is suspected.

Positioning: nursing conscious older patients in a prone position is not generally helpful.

Treatment failure

In the initial stages of the pandemic, patients deteriorated rapidly, and the death rate was high. In a study of 7,000 patients in Italy who died from COVID, the median time from onset of symptoms to hospitalisation was 5 days, and the onset of symptoms to death was 9 days. In a report from 2020, over a quarter of all people needing hospitalisation with COVID died. Older patients were often assessed as unlikely to benefit from intensive care. If patients deteriorated in the ICU, the only further option was extracorporeal membrane oxygenation (ECMO), an extremely limited resource reserved for previously healthy young people.

The situation has changed with the availability of effective drugs, but frail older people with COVID will not always benefit from assisted or full ventilation and still have high mortality (see Figure 13.3)

It is important to consider the resuscitation status of the patient at an early stage, as clinical deterioration can be rapid. In the UK, the DHSC commissioned a review from the CQC into 'do not attempt cardiopulmonary resuscitation' (DNACPR) decisions during the pandemic. It found that decisions were made without involving the patient or family and were sometimes applied to groups of people (such as those in care homes). Planning for a range of eventualities with the patient if possible or the family, e.g. using the ReSPECT documentation (see Chapter 21), should take place as soon as possible after admission.

End-of-life care

A severe COVID infection still carries a 10% mortality risk for older hospital patients. If active treatment is no longer appropriate, end-of-life care is needed. Patients may experience rapidly escalating and distressing symptoms such as breathlessness, fever, and agitation. Experience early in the pandemic showed that the drugs in routine use for end-of-life care give effective symptom relief. Opiates are useful for helping with symptoms of breathlessness, and oxygen can be used if it provides comfort. Benzodiazepines can be used in combination with opiates to relieve severe anxiety. Nonpharmacological measures such as cool wipes may help, but a fan is not recommended due to the risk of particle dispersion. A nominated family member should be allowed to make an informed choice about whether they would wish to visit to provide additional comfort, and consideration should also be given to the use of multimedia (e.g. 'virtual' visits) to alleviate feelings of isolation.

Vaccination

The first COVID vaccine outside a clinical trial was administered on 8 December 2020, to a 90-year-old grandmother in Coventry, England. The vaccination of older people in the UK proceeded rapidly through the spring of 2021. In England, by mid-May 2021, >95% of people aged 65+ (and >77% of those aged 40+) had had at least one dose, and >83% aged 65+ had received two doses. Subsequent waves of infection have led to fewer patients needing hospital admission and far fewer deaths. A case-control study in the US among hospitalised patients during March–January 2022 found that vaccination was associated with a 90% reduction in the risk of severe outcomes, including mechanical ventilation and death. However, COVID has not gone away. People either forget how devastating COVID was or think they must be immune; the booster offered in England to those aged 75+ in spring 2023 was taken up by only 70%.

Long COVID

Most people who get COVID recover within a few days or weeks. However, some have symptoms that linger, and still others improve but then develop new symptoms. Symptoms continuing after 4 or 12 weeks (the period is not yet standardised) are now known as long COVID.

- Common symptoms include fatigue, 'brain fog', muscle aches, dyspnoea, anxiety, low mood, poor sleep, headache, and cough. Diabetes and postural orthostatic tachycardia syndrome may develop.
- In older people, chronic disorders such as heart failure, lung disease or dementia may worsen. If causation is proven, the implications for the long-term health of older people are serious.
- Long COVID appears to be most common in those aged 35–69, 4% of whom report ongoing symptoms for least 12 weeks after COVID. The comparable figure is 2% in those aged 70+.
- Many cases have similarities with myalgic encephalomyelitis/chronic fatigue, but long COVID is a syndrome, and multiple pathogenetic mechanisms have been proposed, including viral persistence, ongoing inflammation and fibrosis, reactivation of other viruses,

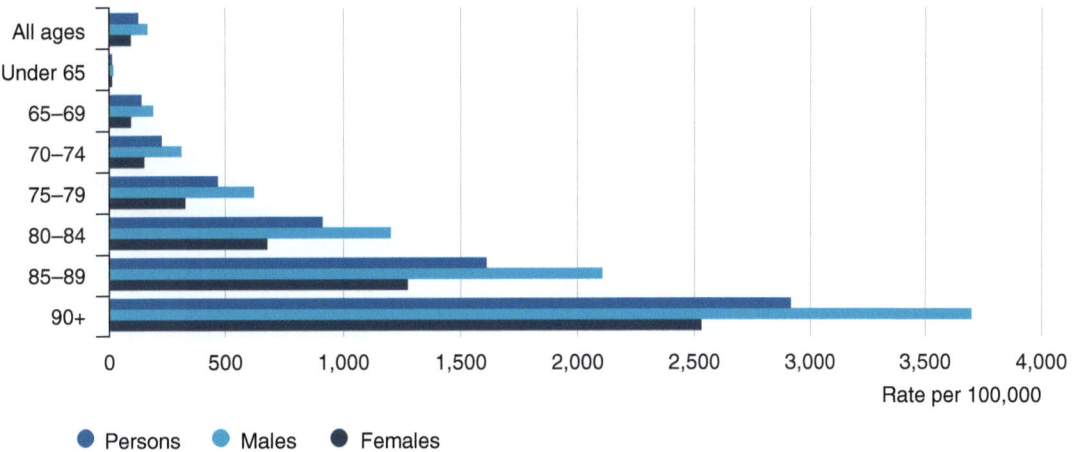

Figure 13.3 Age-standardised and age-specific mortality rates for deaths due to COVID-19 by sex and age group, per 100,000 people, England and Wales, 2020/Office for National Statistics/CC BY 3.0.

autoimmunity, changes in the gut microbiota, and microclot formation. Considerable research is ongoing.

- Vaccination reduces serious illness with COVID and is thought to reduce long COVID. The prevalence of long COVID appears to have been less with omicron (dominant in 2022) than earlier variants, including delta, the main variant in 2021, but new variants may increase the risk of long COVID.
- Treatment remains unsatisfactory; pacing appears more important than building up exercise tolerance.

Colds

Rhinoviruses (species of the genus *Enterovirus* from the *Picorna*virus family) and coronaviruses are the commonest causes of coryza, the common cold. This is a mild systemic upset with nasal symptoms, but older people, particularly smokers and those with preexisting chronic illnesses, may develop lower respiratory complications.

Influenza

Flu is usually debilitating in older people, particularly in the presence of chronic heart, chest, or renal disease, or diabetes and may be complicated by pneumonia, especially due to *Staphylococcus aureus*. Everyone aged over 65 years is offered immunisation for seasonal flu in October/November (in the UK). Influenza viruses are constantly altering their antigenic structure, so every year WHO recommends which strains should be included in the flu vaccine. The vaccine may cause a mild local reaction, and hypersensitivity to egg products is a contraindication. Immunity takes 2–4 weeks to develop and lasts 6–8 months. There is evidence that immunisation of staff is the best way to protect residents of institutions, and hospitals offer free vaccination to staff. The last flu pandemic in 2009, swine flu A (H1N1), was relatively mild.

Amid the concern about COVID, it is worth remembering that more people died from seasonal flu than COVID in winter 2022–2023; nearly 15,000 excess deaths associated with flu were recorded, the highest since the 2017–2018 flu season. The rise was thought to be due to the dominant circulating strain A (H3N2) being more severe in older people, lower population immunity after social distancing, and more testing. Vaccination cuts the risk of hospital admission by a quarter in people over 65.

Lower respiratory tract infections

Pneumonia

Pneumonia is an infection of the lung tissue in which the alveoli become filled with microorganisms, fluid, and inflammatory cells, affecting the function of the lungs.

Causative organisms

As in younger adults, the commonest organism is *Streptococcus pneumoniae*, followed by *Haemophilus influenza*. Other organisms include *Mycoplasma* in epidemic years, viruses, *Legionella*, *Chlamydia pneumoniae* and *S. aureus,* especially during outbreaks of influenza. Prevalent pathogens and their sensitivities vary from one locality to another. It is often difficult to identify the organism, as older patients tend to struggle to produce a sputum sample, but blood culture is sometimes positive. Urinary antigen testing is available for legionella and pneumococcus. The presentation may be typical or atypical, with tachypnoea and functional decline. Preexisting airway disease is almost certain to worsen.

Aspiration pneumonia is common in older patients with swallowing disorders or following an episode of unconsciousness.

Pneumococcal pneumonia has a mortality rate of around 15% in older individuals. Pneumococcal polysaccharide vaccine, an inactivated, 23-valent vaccine, is given to people when they reach 65.

Assessment of severity

The CURB-65 score predicts the likely outcome of community-acquired pneumonia in adults of all ages, and together with clinical judgement, it can help guide decision making:

- **C**onfusion of new onset (AMT of 8 or less).
- **U**rea > 7 mol/L.
- **R**espiratory rate of 30 breaths per minute or more.
- **B**lood pressure < 90 mmHg systolic or < 60 mmHg diastolic.
- **65** years or older.

Pneumonia with a CURB-65 score < 2 may be appropriate for management at home with oral antibiotics, whereas a higher CURB score (indicating a mortality rate > 13%) is likely to warrant hospital admission for intravenous antibiotics. In the community when blood urea is not available, the CRB-65 score can be used in a comparable way (score 0: consider home treatment, 1–2: consider hospital assessment, 3: arrange urgent admission).

Other features indicating life-threatening pneumonia include arterial $PO_2 < 8$ kPa, WBC $> 20 \times 10^9$/L or $< 4 \times 10^9$/L, multiple lobes affected on CXR, serum albumin < 35 g/L, or co-morbidity, e.g. diabetes, heart disease. CRP is generally high; > 100 mg/L makes pneumonia likely, whereas CRP < 20 mg/L with symptoms for more than 24 hours make pneumonia highly unlikely.

CXR appearances typically suggest consolidation (as the alveoli and bronchioles fill with pus), so look for obscuring of pulmonary vessels, and obliteration of normally visible outlines between lung fields and adjacent structures (see Figure 13.4). Conversely, do not exclude a lower respiratory tract infection based on a normal CXR; clinical assessment takes precedence when deciding whether antibiotic treatment is required.

Management

Antibiotics are traditionally given intravenously in the first instance to those with life-threatening features, as well as those unable to swallow, although there is little evidence of greater effectiveness by this route. Most hospitals have an antibiotics policy – be familiar with yours and see the BNF section 'Respiratory system infections, antibacterial therapy'. Antibiotic choice depends on whether the illness was acquired in the community or in hospital. The regime often begins with penicillin and a macrolide (for community-acquired pneumonia, CAP). If co-amoxiclav is used, there is usually no need to add flucloxacillin after influenza or metronidazole for aspiration. In penicillin allergy, doxycycline or clarithromycin is used for moderate-severity CAP and levofloxacin is an option for severe CAP. Levofloxacin has greater activity against pneumococci than ciprofloxacin, but all fluoroquinolones can cause tendon rupture. Vancomycin or linezolid (orally) can be used for MRSA.

Other measures include oxygen (same precautions as in airway obstruction), IV fluids, physiotherapy for retained secretions (mobilisation is often used), relief of bronchospasm if prominent, and nutritional supplements if cachectic.

A follow-up CXR is recommended at 6 weeks to check that the consolidation has resolved fully; persistent shadowing should prompt a chest CT scan to exclude cancer (Figure 13.4).

Pulmonary tuberculosis

Epidemiology

In 2021, people born outside the UK accounted for three-quarters of TB notifications in England, with the highest numbers coming from

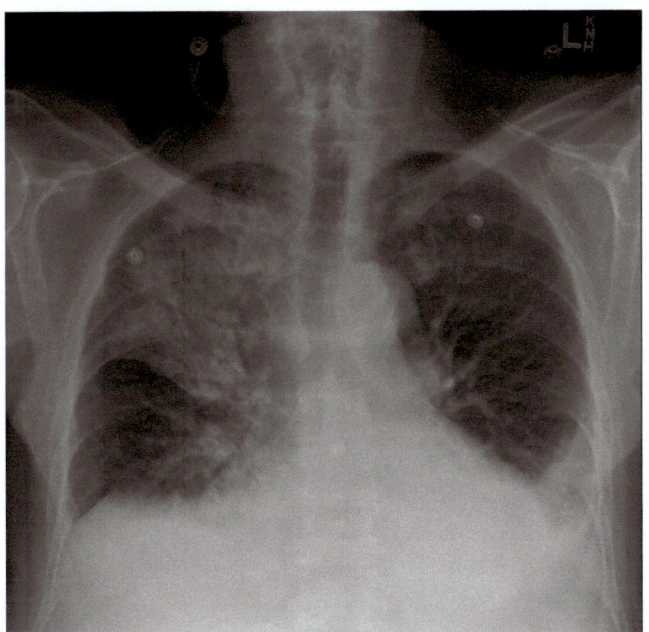

Figure 13.4 CXR shows right upper lobe and left lower lobe consolidation, suggestive of bilateral pneumonia.

India and Pakistan. TB is more common in men and conurbations, with Newham in London and Leicester City having the highest rates. There is a strong association with social deprivation. Just over half of all notified cases in England (53%) are pulmonary (so there are many cases of non-pulmonary TB). In UK-born people, nearly 20% of cases occur in those aged 65+. This is now in line with the proportion of people in this age group. Until a decade ago, incidence rates were higher in old age as TB survivors from the pre-drug era experienced reactivation as their immunity waned, but this cohort has now died. In non-UK-born people, most cases occur in young adults, but because rates are higher overall, more older people with TB were born elsewhere (see Figures 13.5a and 13.5b and note the different vertical scales).

So, remain alert to the possibility of TB, especially in older immigrants from the Indian subcontinent or Eastern Europe (consider multi-drug resistance) and in conurbations, especially London. TB mortality rates were the highest recorded for 10 years in 2021; vigilance is needed as TB should be treatable.

Clinical features

Pulmonary TB is usually the reactivation of a primary infection and typically presents with cough, haemoptysis, fever, drenching night sweats and weight loss. There may be a non-specific rapid decline in older people, especially if there is blood-borne military spread

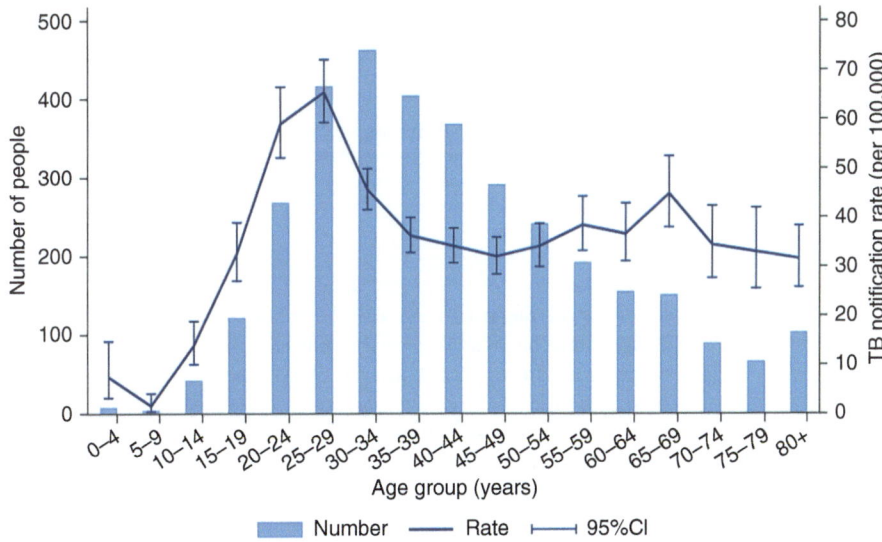

Figure 13.5a Non-UK-born TB case reports and rates by age. Source: UKHSA data 2021/Crown copyright/CC BY 3.0.

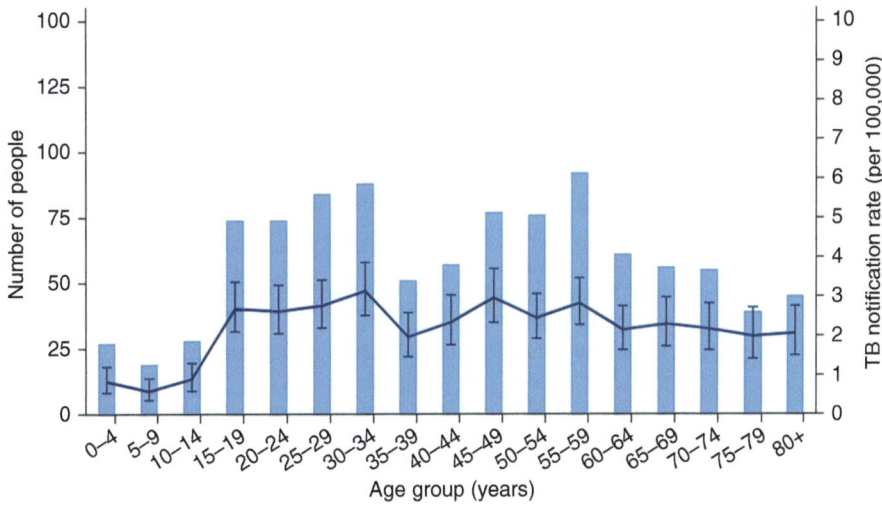

Figure 13.5b UK-born TB case reports and rates by age. Source: UKHSA data 2021/Crown copyright/CC BY 3.0.

(impaired cell-mediated immunity). Physical signs may be absent, there may be cachexia, lymphadenopathy, or focal chest findings.

Diagnosis

Isolate patients with suspected TB and a productive cough until the sputum smear microscopy has been found negative for alcohol-acid-fast bacilli (AAFB).

CXR may show apical calcification, upper lobe infiltrates, granulomas, mediastinal lymphadenopathy, pleural effusion or multiple 'rice grain' opacities of miliary disease. There may be cavitation or bronchiectasis. Haemoptysis may indicate the recrudescence of TB or a complication, such as the development of a fungus ball (aspergilloma) in an old cavity. Infections with atypical mycobacteria occur in damaged lungs and immunosuppressed patients.

Send three sputum samples for AAFB (microscopy and Ziehl-Neelsen stain), culture and molecular tests/drug sensitivity screening (e.g. Xpert Ultra, a cassette-based PCR system), depending on local protocols. Request a respiratory opinion and a CT chest.

Management

Respiratory colleagues may wish to start treatment without waiting for culture results if the patient has clinical signs and symptoms of TB and complete treatment even if culture results are negative. The standard regimen is a '6-month, four-drug initial regimen' of 2 months of isoniazid, rifampicin, pyrazinamide, and ethambutol, followed by 4 months of isoniazid and rifampicin. If your patient dies, alert the pathologist, and send autopsy samples for culture if respiratory TB is a possibility.

Bronchiectasis

Bronchiectasis is abnormal irreversible thickening and dilatation of the muscular and elastic walls of the bronchi, resulting in chronic infection. It affects over 1% of people aged over 70 years.

- It causes a chronic cough with the persistent production of mucopurulent sputum.
- In older people, it is usually post-infectious (measles, whooping cough, TB, or recurrent exacerbations of COPD) or associated with connective tissue disorders.
- The initial insult impairs mucociliary clearance and initiates an inflammatory cycle.
- A high-resolution CT (HRCT) scan is the diagnostic investigation of choice.
- The features and treatment overlap with recurrent chest infections and COPD; physiotherapy with airway clearance techniques and postural drainage are particularly important.
- Saline and bronchodilator nebulisers and then LAMA and LABA may be used (see later) but avoid inhaled corticosteroids unless there is coexisting asthma.
- As with all lung diseases causing breathlessness, pulmonary rehabilitation is useful.

The prognosis is worse once *Pseudomonas aeruginosa* colonisation occurs. Local guidelines and, preferably, sputum samples should guide antibiotic use. The use of carbocysteine, a mucolytic, is not evidence-based.

Airflow obstruction

Most cases are due to COPD (Chronic Obstructive Pulmonary Disease), but some patients have long-standing asthma, and late-onset asthma may be increasing. GOLD (the Global initiative for chronic Obstructive Lung Disease) 2023 defines COPD as a heterogeneous lung condition characterised by chronic respiratory symptoms (dyspnoea, cough, expectoration, and/or exacerbations) due to abnormalities of the airways (bronchitis, bronchiolitis) and/or alveoli (emphysema) that cause persistent, often progressive, airflow obstruction. Thus, COPD includes:

- Chronic bronchitis defined clinically as sputum production on most days for 3 months of two successive years, and
- Emphysema defined histologically as air space dilatation due to inflammation and destruction of alveolar walls, followed by increased sputum production, which further blocks airflow.

COPD causes progressive breathlessness and a reduction in exercise capacity. An estimated 1.2 million people in the UK have COPD; most are diagnosed over 50 yrs old, and many more are undiagnosed. There may be a reversible component, especially in asthmatics who have smoked. The presence of airflow obstruction should be confirmed by *post-bronchodilator* spirometry. About 15% of those dying from COPD have never smoked (as high as 70% of cases in LMICs), and air pollution/second-hand smoking is thought to be a significant factor.

Clinical features of a severe exacerbation

- Unable to cope at home.
- Already receiving long-term oxygen therapy (LTOT).
- Cannot complete sentences.
- Respiratory rate > 25/min.
- Pulse rate > 110 bpm. (unreliable in AF).
- Peak flow < 50% of the patient's normal or predicted.
- $SaO_2 < 90\%$.
- $PO_2 < 7\,kPa$, $PCO_2 > 6.7\,kPa$ on air.

Management of an acute severe exacerbation

- Admission is needed.
- Humidified oxygen: 24% or 28% to keep the SaO_2 within an individualised target range (usually 88–92% for an older COPD patient). Oxygen must be prescribed on the drug chart. If the patient is very ill or becomes drowsy, check arterial blood gases (ABGs) urgently for pCO_2 and pH.
- β_2-agonist (2.5 mg salbutamol) by nebuliser using humidified air (not oxygen) as the carrier. Be mindful that this may exacerbate any underlying cardiac arrhythmias.
- Antimuscarinic (ipratropium bromide, 500 mcg) by nebuliser.
- Antibiotics if evidence of infection (guided by sensitives if available or local formulary – often amoxicillin, doxycycline, or clarithromycin). GOLD recommends 5 days or less. Treat as pneumonia (e.g. with co-amoxiclav) if the sputum is purulent, the patient is ill or febrile, has a high WBC or CRP, or the CXR is suggestive.
- Prednisolone 30–40 mg daily for 5–7 days. 100 mg IV hydrocortisone is an alternative for those unable to take tablets, but remember that this only has a half-life of 6 hours and hence may need to be re-prescribed accordingly. Older patients may have problems with short courses of steroids, including steroid psychosis, fluid overload and the unmasking of diabetes (as well as the well-known long-term complications).
- Monitor temperature, pulse rate, and respiration, oxygen saturation, and peak flow.
- Chest physiotherapy (or mobilisation if able) if secretions are retained.
- DVT prophylaxis, unless contraindicated.
- Consider an aminophylline infusion if obstruction remains severe (not if already on oral theophylline unless levels are available). In practice, this step is used infrequently now due to the availability of NIV (see later).

If the patient is beginning to tire, CO_2 is rising and pH is <7.35, consider:

o Non-invasive ventilation (NIV). This is a good option for patients who are poor candidates for intubation because extubation may be difficult. NIV is the recognised gold standard treatment for acute decompensated respiratory failure and is proven to reduce mortality and intubation rates when compared to standard medical therapy.

o Intensive care for ventilation is needed if the measures mentioned earlier are ineffective. Find out about the patient's functional status prior to this illness and discuss their wishes before contacting the ICU to discuss admission.

General management of the post-acute/chronic phase

Unless the patient is very disabled, stopping smoking is still worthwhile. Patients need advice and information. Results are better with nicotine replacement therapy (many products available, including vapes), bupropion, or the selective nicotine receptor partial agonist varenicline; refer to a 'stop-smoking clinic'.

1 Education: Patients should receive education about all aspects of their condition to encourage effective self-management.
2 Optimise general health and other comorbidities, e.g. anaemia, heart failure.
3 Depression is common – consider an SSRI.
4 Pneumococcal, RSV and annual flu and COVID vaccines should be offered.
5 Pulmonary rehabilitation programme for those with respiratory disability (exercise and nutrition). The 'myCOPD' app can be used (while more evidence is generated to assess its value), to deliver pulmonary rehabilitation programmes for COPD patients who cannot have or do not want face-to-face pulmonary rehabilitation.
6 Consider supplying antibiotics and oral steroids for the patient to initiate self-treatment of an exacerbation (the so-called 'RESCUE pack' with clear instructions).
7 Domiciliary oxygen can be provided as short burst oxygen therapy (SBOT) for symptomatic relief of episodic severe breathlessness (cylinder) or as long-term oxygen therapy (LTOT) if the patient meets the criteria listed in the BNF (PaO_2 on air when stable <7.3 kPa) and will use oxygen for at least 15 hours a day; then LTOT via a concentrator improves life expectancy. A Home Oxygen Order Form (HOOF) can be completed by the hospital or GP/community respiratory nurse services. The patient must have stopped smoking (for obvious reasons).
8 There is increasing evidence that NIV can be used in the treatment of chronic hypercapnic respiratory failure.
9 Palliative care for end-stage chronic lung disease. In addition to oxygen, an opiate or benzodiazepine can relieve respiratory distress.

Table 13.1 GOLD groups guiding the treatment of COPD.

Group	Breathlessness	Symptom impact	Exacerbations in the past 12 months
A	Minimal mMRC dyspnoea score 0–1	Low CAT score < 10	0–1 moderate episode not leading to hospitalisation
B	Moderate mMRC ≥2	Moderate CAT score ≥10	0–1 moderate episode not leading to hospitalisation
E	Not scored		2 or more moderate exacerbations or 1 or more leading to hospitalisation

The modified MRC dyspnoea score ranges from 0 to 4.
The COPD Assessment Test (CAT) score ranges from 0 to 40.

Drug management for COPD

Inhaled drugs

These include:

- **SABA** (short-acting beta$_2$ agonists) – salbutamol, terbutaline.
- **SAMA** (short-acting muscarinic antagonists) – ipratropium.
- **LABA** (long-acting beta$_2$ agonists) – salmeterol, formoterol.
- **LAMA** (long-acting muscarinic antagonists) – tiotropium, glycopyrronium.
- **ICS** (inhaled corticosteroids) and ICS/LABA/LAMA combinations –
  o Budesonide/formoterol = Symbicort
  o Fluticasone/salmeterol = Seretide
  o Beclometasone/formoterol/glycopyrronium = Trimbow.

ICS has been shown to increase the incidence of pneumonia, but the benefit in terms of reducing exacerbations may be worth it. Recurrent exacerbations are associated with increasing morbidity and are a strong predictor of mortality. However, GOLD is recommending less use of ICS in COPD.

Several types of inhalers are available, requiring various levels of manual dexterity, cognition, and inspiratory flow. Ensure the inhaler and spacer device are understood by the patient.

The GOLD groups that guide treatment have been simplified to A, B and E (see Table 13.1) and the recommended initial management of COPD is shown in Figure 13.6.

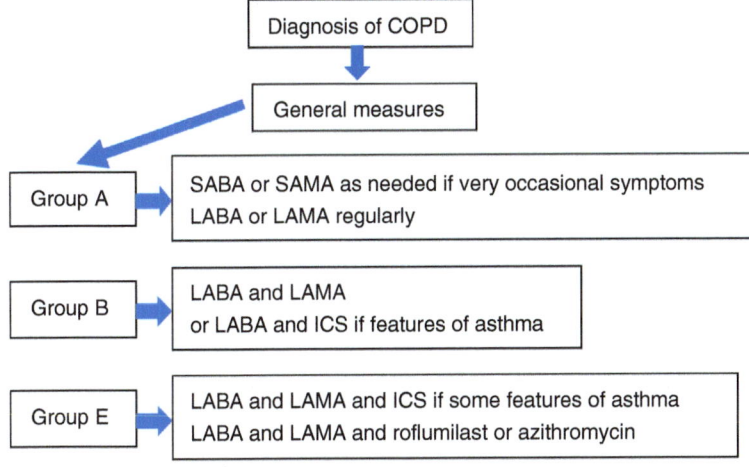

Figure 13.6 The initial management of COPD based on NICE and GOLD 2023. Source: Adapted from NICE and GOLD 2023.

Other drugs

- Mucolytics, e.g. carbocysteine, may be useful if sputum production is marked.
- Long-term corticosteroids should be avoided if possible – if frequent courses are given, remember osteoporosis prophylaxis.
- Prophylactic azithromycin can prevent exacerbations, particularly in older patients.
- Phosphodiesterase-4 inhibitors (theophylline, roflumilast – also anti-inflammatory) are usually only given once inhaled therapy is maximal and in the context of multiple exacerbations because of their narrow therapeutic index; caution with macrolides and fluoroquinolones, which increase levels. Suitable patients usually have an $FEV_1 < 50\%$ (grade 3 or 4).

Diseases of the pleura

Pleural effusion

A pleural effusion develops when the rate of fluid formation in the pleural space is greater than that of fluid removal. The fluid may be a transudate or an exudate depending on its cause and protein concentration (see later).

Clinical features

It is a common cause of breathlessness, cough, and pleuritic chest pain, an be diagnosed clinically with absent breath sounds, a stony dull percussion note with decreased vocal resonance, and is confirmed on CXR and then ultrasound.

Common causes

- Left ventricular failure (LVF) (transudate, but closer to an exudate after prolonged diuretics).
- Para-pneumonic effusion complicates 40% of cases of pneumonia: the fluid is an exudate and contains neutrophils. If the parapneumonic effusion becomes fibrinous and infected by a microorganism this is an empyema. The fluid looks like frank pus with neutrophils, decreased glucose, acidosis, and high lactate dehydrogenase (LDH). Culture is often negative; sensitivity is improved by using blood culture bottles for the aspirate. Older people are more at risk of empyema due to frailty, hospitalisation, and preexisting disease, e.g. bronchiectasis, diabetes, and alcoholism.
- Empyema can also complicate cardiothoracic surgery or result from penetrating trauma introducing organisms into the pleural space.
- Malignancy (1° or 2°), especially if 'white-out' on CXR (exudate, often bloody).
- Pulmonary embolism should be considered if there is no obvious cause for an effusion. Pleural effusions are seen on CTPA in around 30% of pulmonary emboli and are generally small, an exudate, and can be contralateral to the embolus.

Management

If LVF is likely, monitor the response to diuretics and only perform a pleural aspiration if features are atypical, or treatment fails, and the patient becomes distressed. Effusions are classified as an exudate (protein > 30 g/L) or a transudate, but this is often less clear-cut in an older patient with low serum albumin, so measure total protein and LDH in blood and pleural fluid. Diagnostic aspiration should be done with ultrasound guidance and is usually performed by 'pleural teams' often led by skilled specialist nurses. Pleural fluid is sent for:

- Protein (if pleural fluid protein divided by serum protein is >0.5 = exudate).
- LDH (if pleural fluid LDH divided by serum LDH is >0.6 = exudate).
- Gram stain.
- Microbiological culture (in blood culture bottles).
- Cytology (all the remaining sample).
- Additional tests only if specific indication.

If the diagnosis is still unclear, request a contrast-enhanced CT chest and a specialist opinion.

A sick patient with empyema needs a wide-bore (28-F) chest drain. If the fluid is multi-loculated, video-assisted thoracoscopic surgery (VATS) may be needed to break down the locules.

Therapeutic aspiration may be needed to relieve breathlessness from a huge effusion. Advice should be sought from the respiratory team for the management of symptomatic, recurrent malignant pleural effusions. For example, a talc slurry pleurodesis may be performed: fluid is removed to 'dryness' with a small-bore tube, and lidocaine and graded talc are introduced. An indwelling pleural drain, which can be managed in the community by specialist nurses, is an option to explore to prevent recurrent hospital admission. Patients with mesothelioma need prophylactic radiotherapy to prevent seeding if a large-bore chest drain is used; but this is not a complication of diagnostic aspiration.

Pleural plaques

Pleural plaques are discrete circumscribed areas of hyaline fibrosis, usually of the parietal pleura, and are a result of migrated, inhaled asbestos fibres. They are considered benign and usually asymptomatic, but they are the commonest manifestation of past exposure to asbestos (usually more than 10 years previously). A 2018 study of 2,000 asbestos-exposed workers found pleural plaques in 89% of the group. 20% of plaques calcify and are hence often picked up incidentally on CXR (see Figure 13.7). The discovery of pleural plaques should prompt exploration of the patient's occupational history and consideration of CT thorax contrast imaging if there are signs or symptoms of respiratory disease. Asbestos exposure increases the risk of lung cancer, so patients with plaques should be given extra support to stop smoking. In the UK, the presence of pleural plaques alone does not qualify for industrial injury benefits.

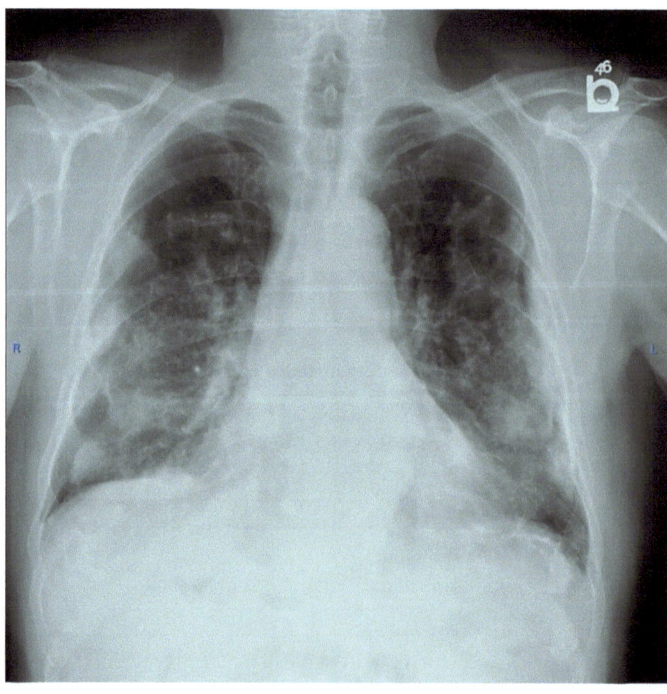

Figure 13.7 CXR with bilateral pleural plaques.

Mesothelioma

This malignancy arises in the pleura because of asbestos exposure and presents with chest pain, dyspnoea, and a bloody pleural effusion. Check for a history of industrial exposure – e.g. builders, shipyard workers, and the person who washed the overalls may also be at risk. The initial course may be indolent, and a high-resolution CT scan may be helpful, but diagnosis requires a pleural biopsy. Because of the association with asbestos and the long interval between exposure and presentation, the effect of strict industrial regulation will not be apparent for years. It is important to diagnose; although management is palliative, compensation may be available – seek specialist advice. All mesothelioma-related deaths must be discussed with a coroner before a death certificate is issued.

Lung cancer

This refers to tumours arising in the bronchus or lung parenchyma.

Epidemiology

Lung cancer is the third most common cause of cancer in the UK and the commonest cause of cancer death in the UK and worldwide. Over the last decade, overall lung cancer incidence rates have remained stable as rates in females have increased and rates in males have fallen. It is mainly a disease of old age (50% of deaths occur in those aged 75 and over, as shown in Figure 13.8) and has a strong association with social deprivation.

Classification

Lung cancers are classified into two main categories:

1 Small-cell lung cancers (SCLC), which account for approximately 20% of cases.
2 Non-small-cell lung cancers (NSCLC), which account for the other 80%. NSCLC includes squamous-cell carcinomas (35%), adenocarcinomas (27%), and large-cell carcinomas (10%).

50% of lung cancers in non-smokers are adenocarcinomas.

Clinical features

The presentation may be cough, haemoptysis, dyspnoea, or a slowly resolving infection. Less common chest presentations include:

- Pleural effusion (but not all effusions in patients with lung cancer are malignant).
- Superior vena cava syndrome usually due to a right upper lobe tumour with fixed dilated neck veins, facial plethora and oedema.
- Pancoast syndrome due to an apical tumour with shoulder pain.
- Horner's syndrome, wasting of the small muscles of the ipsilateral hand, and hoarse voice due to recurrent laryngeal nerve palsy, usually due to a left-sided tumour.

Late presentation is common, with symptoms relating to distant spread or non-metastatic metabolic complications.

Diagnosis

After CXR, a contrast 'staging' CT scan including the liver and adrenals is usually done before bronchoscopy for central lesions or transcutaneous biopsy for peripheral lesions. PET CT scanning is helpful in staging patients. Ideally, patients are managed by a multidisciplinary team that includes respiratory physicians, oncologists, and cancer nurse specialists. In practice, however, general physicians or geriatricians often supervise the initial diagnosis and ongoing care after discussion by the MDT, particularly if treatment options are limited.

Management

In early NSCLC, lobectomy (or more radical surgery) remains the treatment of choice. There is a 70% 5-year survival rate for T1N0M0 tumours if the patient is fit enough and lung function is adequate ($FEV_1 > 1.5L$). Surgical outcomes have improved; the perioperative mortality of pneumonectomy is around 6% (right pneumonectomy is riskier), but there is major morbidity in 30% of cases. Carefully selected older patients do as well as younger ones. In patients who are not suitable for surgery, stereotactic ablative radiotherapy (SABR) with intent to cure is used for primary lung tumours ≤5 cm in diameter without evidence of metastatic spread, unless the tumour is within 2 cm of the main airways. If SABR is contraindicated, conventional or hyperfractionated

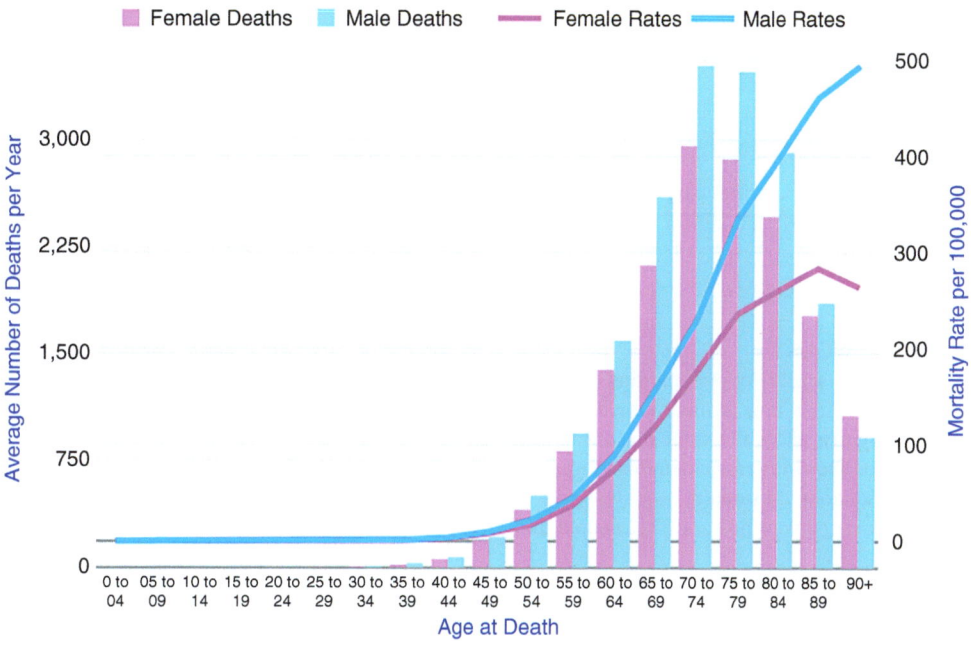

Figure 13.8 Average annual number of deaths from lung cancer and age-specific mortality UK, 2017–2019 Cancer Research UK.

radiotherapy is offered. Adjuvant chemotherapy may be used after surgery or radiotherapy.

Advanced NSCLC may be treated with a range of systemic options, depending on tumour histology and molecular genetics. These may offer worthwhile life extensions (a few months). The options include platinum-based chemotherapy, such as cisplatin and a taxane such as docetaxel; checkpoint inhibitors such as nintedanib; and in metastatic tumours expressing elevated levels of PDL-1 protein, monoclonal antibodies including pembrolizumab and nivolumab, which block PD-1; and atezolizumab, a PDL-1 inhibitor (see Chapter 18).

Radiotherapy offers useful palliation for superior mediastinal obstruction, chest pain, painful bony metastases, and haemoptysis.

SCLC has usually metastasized at presentation and is staged as limited or extensive disease. Unless the patient is too frail, multi-drug platinum-based chemotherapy is offered and continued for 4–6 cycles if there is a response. The 5-year survival rate is 27% if diagnosed at an early stage and treated; however, overall 5-year survival for SCLC is 5–10%. Involve palliative care services early.

Interstitial lung disease

Interstitial lung disease (ILD) affects the lung parenchyma (alveoli, alveolar ducts, and bronchioles). ILD describes a heterogeneous group of non-infectious, non-malignant processes of the lower respiratory tract characterised by the abnormal accumulation of cells and/or non-cellular material within the walls of the alveoli. This results in thickening and stiffness of the elastic tissues of the lung, so that patients breathe in a rapid and shallow manner. Alveolar thickening decreases the efficiency of oxygen transfer.

It is assumed that triggers, e.g. viruses, smoking, and pollution, in people with a genetic predisposition result in alveolar damage and then an inflammatory and fibrotic cycle. The conditions are loosely referred to as 'pulmonary fibrosis' but the relative amounts of fibrosis and inflammation depend on the aetiology. In general, inflammation is more amenable to treatment than fibrosis. Alveolar filling diseases present with similar symptoms and x-ray findings and are included as ILDs.

ILD is poorly understood (by most doctors as well as students).

- 'Rag bag' of conditions, many of which are very rare.
- Classification, particularly of the 'idiopathic' types, keeps changing.
- Names are cumbersome and overlap.
- Pathogenesis is poorly understood.

But it is important as:

- The incidence is increasing in the UK/US.
- The commonest idiopathic subgroup, pulmonary fibrosis (IPF), causes more deaths each year than ovarian cancer, lymphoma, or leukaemia.

Causes

- Granulomatous disease, e.g. sarcoidosis.
- Inhalational, e.g. asbestosis; hypersensitivity pneumonitis (extrinsic allergic alveolitis); e.g. pigeon fancier's lung; farmer's lung due to the mould *Thermoactinomyces vulgaris*; silicosis in stone masons; pneumoconiosis due to coal dust; berylliosis in aerospace industry workers (histology is granulomatous and looks like sarcoid).
- Connective tissue disease associated with ILD, e.g. rheumatoid and scleroderma.
- Systemic vasculitis associated with ILD, e.g. granulomatosis with polyangiitis, Churg–Strauss syndrome.
- Drug-induced, e.g. amiodarone, bleomycin.
- Post radiotherapy.

- Viral infection such as Epstein–Barr virus is a postulated cause but there is limited evidence. There is concern that COVID infection may lead to lung fibrosis. In a small study of hospitalised patients fibrotic-like appearances were seen on HRCT in 20% of non-ventilated and 72% of ventilated patients 4 months after hospitalisation. Larger, longer-term studies are needed.
- Association with obstructive sleep apnoea.
- Idiopathic interstitial pneumonias comprise around 40% of cases:
  - Idiopathic pulmonary fibrosis (IPF), previously 'cryptogenic fibrosing alveolitis'.
  - Non-IPF interstitial pneumonias:
    - Non-specific interstitial pneumonia (NSIP).
    - Acute interstitial pneumonia (AIP) idiopathic acute respiratory distress syndrome – mortality >50%.
    - Cryptogenic organising pneumonia (COP).
- Alveolar filling diseases, e.g. alveolar proteinosis.

Clinical features

Most patients present with insidious progressive breathlessness, and some have a troublesome dry cough, but other cases have an acute or episodic presentation. Fine 'Velcro' end-inspiratory crackles (bibasal in IPF) that do not disappear on coughing are typical, and clubbing may be found. Look for the features of any associated disease. Check for the loud P2 component of the second heart sound, a fixed split S2, a pan systolic tricuspid regurgitation murmur, raised JVP and pedal oedema of pulmonary hypertension with cor pulmonale. The course is progressive, but the rate is very variable depending on the aetiology and this was a major factor driving the recent classification.

Investigations

- Lung function tests typically show a restrictive defect with reduced lung volumes and reduced transfer factor for carbon monoxide (TLCO), also known as diffusing capacity for carbon monoxide (DLCO).
- ABGs / oxygen saturation – reduced oxygen level, usually with a normal carbon dioxide level
- 6-min walk test (6 MWT) – oxygen desaturation.
- HRCT chest – the most important for diagnosis.
- Bronchoscopy with bronchoalveolar lavage or biopsy may be used in difficult cases.
- ECHO – used to evaluate pulmonary hypertension.

  Serial spirometry and the 6 MWT are used to monitor progression.

Idiopathic pulmonary fibrosis

Idiopathic pulmonary fibrosis (IPF), the most common form of ILD, has a mean age at diagnosis of 74 years (SD 64–84 years). It is often picked up by geriatricians when basal crackles do not disappear with furosemide! It is more common in males and those with a smoking history. Only a few percent of cases are familial, but genetic associations are being discovered. It is thought that a trigger in a susceptible host leads to alveolar damage and that fibrosis results from aberrant healing; alveolar cells produce cytokines leading to mesenchymal proliferation and activation with the formation of myofibroblast and fibroblast foci. Impaired apoptosis is one of the factors leading to ongoing fibrosis, accumulation of extracellular matrix, and the destruction of lung tissue.

IPF is rapidly progressive, with median survival from diagnosis around 3–5 years.

- Pulmonary hypertension is frequent.
- Drugs slow progression, but there is no cure, and lung transplantation is offered to younger patients. Nintedanib and pirfenidone are

approved by NICE. Nintedanib, a tyrosine kinase inhibitor, inhibits profibrotic mediators including platelet-derived growth factor, fibroblast growth factor and transforming growth factor (TGF)-beta, as well as vascular endothelia growth factor (VEGF), reducing fibroblast activity. Pirfenidone limits the production of profibrotic growth factors, including TGF-beta, leading to reduced fibroblast proliferation.

- CXR shows basal peripheral reticular shadowing with volume loss and diagnosis is usually based on the clinical features and HRCT (reticular pattern, honeycombing, traction bronchiectasis and ground glass opacity).
- A biopsy is rarely required, but histology shows usual interstitial pneumonitis (UIP), patchy dense fibrosis with the destruction of lung architecture, and fibroblastic foci at the advancing edge.
- People with IPF are more susceptible to COVID and have more severe disease.

Non-specific interstitial pneumonia

Non-specific interstitial pneumonia (NSIP) is clinically indistinguishable from IPF but has a median survival of around 6 years. The histology of intra-alveolar septal fibrosis is more homogeneous and is seen in several ILDs, including connective tissue disorders, drug-induced fibrosis and following ARDS and COP. Treatment is directed at the underlying disease and can include a combination of immunosuppressive and cytotoxic drugs, including azathioprine, cyclophosphamide, mycophenolate, steroids, and rituximab, as well as antifibrosis drugs.

Cryptogenic organising pneumonia

Cryptogenic organising pneumonia (COP), previously known as bronchiolitis obliterans organising pneumonia (BOOP), presents with subacute breathlessness developing over a few weeks, cough with clear sputum, and constitutional symptoms. CXR often shows multifocal consolidation that cannot be distinguished from infection or malignancy. Bronchoscopy is often needed to exclude the former and for transbronchial biopsy. The prognosis is good, and unlike many ILDs, COP usually responds well to corticosteroids. Acute histology shows budding of fibro-proliferative tissue into alveolar spaces and chronically resembles NSIP.

Some elderly patients have documented pulmonary fibrosis for several years, usually NSIP.

Miscellaneous

Chest trauma

- Rib fracture: common after mild trauma, particularly if osteoporotic.
- Diagnosis: local tenderness and pain on springing the chest.
- Complications: shallow breathing and a reluctance to cough may cause sputum retention and segmental collapse, with subsequent pneumonia. A flail segment affects breathing the most. Pneumo- or haemothorax: refer for usual treatment.
- Treatment: adequate regular analgesia (e.g. paracetamol, an NSAID with gut protection if renal function is good, or tramadol/meptazinol), usually with physiotherapy, is essential to avoid infection. If associated with minor trauma, treat long-term for osteoporosis.

Carbon monoxide poisoning

Incidence

- Accounts for 40,000 emergency room attendances in the US per year.
- Causes the death of 40 people per year in the UK.

Clinical features

- Carbon monoxide (CO) reduces oxygen delivery to tissues by two effects: it has an affinity for haemoglobin 220 times greater than that of oxygen, and it shifts the oxyhaemoglobin dissociation curve to the left.
- CO also binds to intracellular proteins, causes the activation of neutrophils, leading to lipid peroxidation, and may cause apoptosis in the brain.
- Think about this possibility if an older couple present together with confusion.
- Patients are hypoxic but not cyanosed. The skin and mucous membranes may appear 'cherry red', but this is rare unless on the post-mortem slab.
- Mild exposure: carboxyhaemoglobin (COHb) < 30%: headache, lethargy, nausea, and vomiting.
- Moderate exposure: COHb 50–60%: tachycardia, tachypnoea, syncope, and fits.
- High exposure: COHb > 60%: cardiorespiratory failure and death.
- CNS tissue damage can progress for up to 80 days after exposure (lipid peroxidation causes delayed reversible demyelination), causing neuropsychiatric problems including parkinsonism, akinetic mutism, as well as acute confusion.

Causes

CO is produced by incomplete combustion of carbon-containing compounds with an inadequate supply of oxygen.

- Smoke inhalation, e.g. house fire.
- Faulty heating and cooking appliances, especially solid fuel, but oil, paraffin, and gas too.
- Poor ventilation of such appliances.
- Deliberate inhalation of car exhaust fumes is less common in older people.

Management and prevention

- The key is to think about the possibility of CO poisoning and to take an arterial sample to check the level of carboxyhaemoglobin (COHb).
- Give 100% oxygen via a face mask for up to 24 hours.
- Do not be misled by pulse oximeter readings: the oximeter cannot distinguish between COHb and HbO_2.
- Hyperbaric oxygen is not recommended in the UK.
- Treat seizures with IV benzodiazepines.
- Prevention is obviously important. CO alarms are readily available. In the UK, landlords are legally required to have all domestic gas appliances checked annually by an approved engineer and provide an alarm.

📖 REFERENCES AND FURTHER READING

Torrelles JB, Restrepo BI, Bai Y et al. (2022). The impact of aging on the lung alveolar environment, predetermining susceptibility to respiratory infections. *Frontiers Aging* 3:818700, doi: 10.3389/fragi.2022.818700.

Public Health England (2019). The 2nd Atlas of variation in risk factors and healthcare for respiratory disease in England. file:///C:/Users/Dell8930/Downloads/AllRespiratoryDisease.pdf

The King's Fund (updated 2022) Deaths from Covid-19 (coronavirus): how are they counted and what do they show? www.kingsfund.org.uk/publications/deaths-covid-19#conclusion

COVID-19 Forecasting Team (2022) Variation in the COVID-19 infection–fatality ratio by age, time, and geography during the pre-vaccine era: a systematic analysis. *The Lancet* 399:10334, 1469–1488, doi: 10.1016/S0140-6736(21)02867-1.

ONS *Deaths due to COVID-19, registered in England and Wales:2020.* www.ons.gov.uk/peoplepopulationandcommunity/birthsdeathsandmarriages/deaths/articles/deathsregisteredduetocovid19/2020

NICE (2023) COVID-19 rapid guideline: Managing COVID-19. Update to 2024 https://www.nice.org.uk/guidance/ng191/resources/covid19-rapid-guideline-managing-covid19-pdf-66142077109189

NICE Technology appraisal guidance [TA878] (2023) Casirivimab plus imdevimab, nirmatrelvir plus ritonavir, sotrovimab and tocilizumab for treating COVID-19. www.nice.org.uk/guidance/ta878

SIGN guidelines (2021) Presentations and management of COVID-19 in older people in acute care. www.sign.ac.uk/media/1826/presentations-and-management-of-covid-19-in-older-people-v2-final.pdf.

Zhu Y, Sharma L, Chang D (2023) Pathophysiology and clinical management of coronavirus disease (COVID-19): a mini-review. *Frontiers Immunology* 14:1116131, doi:10.3389/fimmu.2023.1116131

Ting R, Edmonds P, Higginson IJ et al. (2020) Palliative care for patients with severe covid-19. *BMJ* 370:m2710, doi: 10.1136/bmj.m2710.

Care Quality Commission (2021). Protect, respect, connect – decisions about living and dying well during COVID-19. www.cqc.org.uk/publications/themed-work/protect-respect-connect-decisions-about-living-dying-well-during-covid-19.

Tenforde MW, Self WH, Gaglani M et al. (2022). Effectiveness of mRNA vaccination in preventing COVID-19-associated invasive mechanical ventilation and death – United States, March 2021-January 2022. *Morbidity Mortality Weekly Report* 71(12): 459–465. https://www.ncbi.nlm.nih.gov/pmc/articles/PMC8956334

Public Health England Covid 19 vaccinations England 8th December 2020 to 16th May 2021 National Immunisation Management Service (NIMS). https://www.england.nhs.uk/statistics/statistical-work-areas/covid-19-vaccinations

Lloyd-Sherlock P, Kandiyil NM, McKee M et al. (2021). Pandemic lessons from India: inappropriate prioritisation for vaccination. *BMJ* 373:n1464, doi: 10.1136/bmj.n1464.

Davis HE, McCorkell L, Vogel JM et al. (2023). Long COVID: major findings, mechanisms, and recommendations. *Nature Reviews Microbiology* 21:133–146, doi: 10.1038/s41579-022-00846-2.

ONS Prevalence of ongoing symptoms following coronavirus (COVID-19) infection in the UK 30 March 2023 data set. www.ons.gov.uk/peoplepopulationandcommunity/healthandsocialcare/conditionsanddiseases/datasets/alldatarelatingtoprevalenceofongoingsymptomsfollowingcoronaviruscovid19infectionintheuk.

Lewthwaite H, Byrne A, Brew B et al. (2023). Treatable traits for long COVID. *Respirology*, doi: https://doi.org/10.1111/resp.14596.

Plummer AM, Matos YL, Lin HC et al. (2023). Gut-brain pathogenesis of post-acute COVID-19 neurocognitive symptoms. *Frontiers in Neuroscience* 17:1232480, doi: 10.3389/fnins.2023.1232480

George PM, Barratt SL, Condliffe R et al. (2020). Respiratory follow-up of patients with COVID-19 pneumonia. *Thorax* 75:1009–1016. https://thorax.bmj.com/content/thoraxjnl/75/11/1009.full.pdf.

Mahase E (2023). Flu deaths in UK hit five year high last winter. *BMJ* 381:1445, doi: https://doi.org/10.1136/bmj.p1445.

Brown NM, Goodman AL, Horner C et al. (2021). Treatment of methicillin-resistant Staphylococcus aureus (MRSA): updated guidelines from the UK. *JAC-Antimicrobial Resistance* 3, doi: 10.1093/jacamr/dlaa114.

Health Protection Agency Centre for Infections (2010) Tuberculosis in the UK: Annual report on tuberculosis surveillance in the UK, 2010. www.hpa.org.uk/web/HPAwebFile/HPAweb_C/1287143594275.

UK Health Security Agency TB incidence and epidemiology in England 2021 *(updated* 2023*)*. https://www.gov.uk/government/publications/tuberculosis-in-england-2022-report-data-up-to-end-of-2021/tb-incidence-and-epidemiology-in-england-2021#social-and-demographic-characteristics-of-people-with-tb-in-england

Agustí A, Celli BR, Gerard J. et al. (2023). Global initiative for chronic obstructive lung disease 2023 report: GOLD executive summary. *European Respiratory Journal* 61(4): 2300239, doi: 10.1183/13993003.00239-2023.

Cancer Research UK Lung cancer mortality by age. https://www.cancerresearchuk.org/health-professional/cancer-statistics/statistics-by-cancer-type/lung-cancer/mortality#heading-One.

NICE CKS (2021). Lung and pleural cancers – recognition and referral. https://cks.nice.org.uk/topics/lung-pleural-cancers-recognition-referral

NICE (updated 2023) Lung cancer: diagnosis and management. www.nice.org.uk/guidance/ng122.

Cottin V, Bonniaud P, Cadranel J et al. (2023). French practical guidelines for the diagnosis and management of idiopathic pulmonary fibrosis – 2021 update. *Respiratory Medicine and Research* 83:100948, doi: 10.1016/j.resmer.2022.100948.

British Thoracic Society *Management guidelines* https://www.brit-thoracic.org.uk/quality-improvement/guidelines

NICE: *Respiratory conditions with guidelines* www.nice.org.uk/guidance/conditions-and-diseases/respiratory-conditions

INFORMATION FOR PATIENTS AND FAMILIES

Asthma and Lung UK *Lung Conditions A-Z:* www.asthmaandlung.org.uk/conditions

Compensation and benefits for mesothelioma: Mesothelioma compensation claims | Macmillan Cancer Support https://www.macmillan.org.uk/cancer-information-and-support/impacts-of-cancer/mesothelioma-compensation

OpenMD is a useful website with links to a vast range of conditions: https://openmd.com

All websites were accessed in September 2024.

14

Gastroenterology

Gastrointestinal (GI) symptoms are common throughout life. Structural changes, such as hiatus hernia and diverticular disease, and functional changes such as bowel dysmotility, are more common with increasing age. Almost one-fifth of patients presenting to a geriatric outpatient clinic have GI problems.

Age-related changes

1 Impairment of taste due to reduced numbers of taste buds can further reduce poor appetite and lead to a less varied diet potentially causing reduced intake of micronutrients.
2 A reduction in the quantity and quality of saliva production causes dryness of the mouth.
3 Appetite may also be reduced due to changes in hormones. Cholecystokinin (CCK) levels are higher in older people and reduce gastric emptying, which leads to early satiety. Leptin is produced in fat cells. Levels are often higher in older people, again suppressing appetite. Insulin reinforces the leptin signals to the hypothalamus and suppresses ghrelin, a hormone that normally stimulates appetite.
4 Older people cannot open their mouths as wide and chew with less power than younger people because of the reduced range of movement of the temporomandibular joint and the reduced power of the masseter muscles.
5 Increased risk of tooth loss and/or poorly fitting dentures secondary to alveolar margin atrophy also impair mastication.
6 Tongue atrophy means older people can only manage smaller boluses of food.
7 Impaired coordination of swallowing and uncoordinated or reduced oesophageal peristalsis contribute to dysphagia. The term presbyoesophagus has fallen out of use due to our improved understanding of the multiple factors involved and the fact that not all are age-related.
8 Reduced pressure of the upper oesophageal sphincter and delayed relaxation after swallowing make the oesophageal phase of swallowing less effective.
9 Reduced oesophageal sensation due to a reduction in neurones in the myenteric plexus means that odynophagia occurs only in advanced disease.
10 Slower gastric emptying of fluids but not solids may contribute to early satiety when eating.
11 Reduced secretion of gastric acid can lead to bacterial overgrowth in the small bowel.
12 The volume of the liver is reduced by 20–40% in older age.
13 Liver blood flow is reduced by 35–50%.
14 Reduced activity of enzymes such as cytochrome P450 and superoxide dismutase leads to reduced metabolism of drugs that are cleared by the liver, which may lead to high plasma levels.
15 Reduced exocrine pancreatic function due to duct and parenchymatous changes may lead to malabsorption.
16 Reduced splanchnic blood flow.
17 Reduced small bowel surface area.
18 Changes in intestinal microflora, including a decrease in anaerobes and bifidobacteria and an increase in enterobacteria, reduce immunity to *Clostridioides difficile*.
19 Diverticula develop in the bowel.
20 Reduced large bowel motility predisposes to constipation.
21 Reduced rectal wall elasticity increases the risk of faecal incontinence.

Investigations for GI disease

X-rays

- Plain x-rays are still useful to diagnose perforation (and distinguish free air under the diaphragm from Chilaiditi syndrome, where a bowel loop is interposed between the liver and right hemidiaphragm), bowel obstruction, the extent of faecal loading in constipation, and may show colitis and opacities due to chronic pancreatitis and renal and biliary stones.
- Barium swallow may be used in dysphagia, but barium enema is rarely performed.

Endoscopy in older people

Diagnostic and therapeutic techniques have advanced over decades and age alone should not exclude older patients from endoscopic procedures. The literature suggests that older people are at a slightly higher risk of complications.

Oesophagogastroduodenoscopy

Oesophagogastroduodenoscopy (OGD) is generally safe and well tolerated, even by frail older people.

Sigmoidoscopy

Should pose no special issues, but ensure the preparation is adequate, or this is a waste of time.

Geriatric Medicine and Elderly Care: Lecture Notes, Ninth Edition. Claire G. Nicholl, K. Jane Wilson, and Shaun D'Souza.
© 2025 John Wiley & Sons Ltd. Published 2025 by John Wiley & Sons Ltd.
Companion website: www.wiley.com/go/lecturenotesgeriatricmedicine9e

Colonoscopy

Indications are common in old age.

- The procedure is safe if care is taken with selection, preparation, and sedation, especially for those over 80. (Do not use Picolax if there is any suspicion of bowel perforation.)
- Complete examination rates (i.e. reaching the ileo-caecal valve) may be reduced to 50–60% in the frailest.
- Abnormalities are common in the over-80s, at about 80%. Diverticular disease is the most common, but 11% reveal carcinoma, 25% have polyps, and 13% have multiple pathologies.
- It has both diagnostic and therapeutic potential, e.g. biopsy, polypectomy, and stent insertion.

CT abdomen and pelvis

- Usually done with IV contrast, the procedure is well tolerated by frail elderly patients. Modern machines take less than 15 min to produce the scan.
- CT has the advantage of demonstrating the bowel and other abdominal lesions causing extrinsic compression, as well as disease in other solid organs, bones, the aorta, and abnormal collections of fluid.

CT colonography

- Computers are used to produce two- and three-dimensional views of the bowel and abdomen: the 'virtual colonoscopy'. The procedure is superior to CT in showing the bowel lumen.
- The patient must be able to manage a 48-hour bowel preparation that includes a low-fibre diet and drinking Gastrografin which is a laxative as well as a contrast agent.
- The procedure involves insufflation of the bowel with CO_2 and patients must be able to retain this. Intravenous contrast and antispasmodics are given. The usual care must be taken with patients with CKD.
- The patient must be able to turn over because views are taken supine and prone; they must also be able to follow commands about taking deep breaths, etc.
- Radiation exposure from CT colonography is 8 mSv, compared with 5 mSv from an abdominal CT; annual background radiation is 1–3 mSv.

Abnormalities of the mouth

Lips

- **Herpes simplex** (cold sores) are red, painful vesicles or ulcers on the lips. As in younger patients, they may indicate systemic disease.
- **Angular stomatitis/cheilitis** is usually due to leakage of saliva due to poor lip closure. The corners of the mouth become red and sore, especially if complicated by a fungal (*Candida*) infection.
- **Venous lake/phlebectasis:** a small compressible purple/blue lump on usually the lower lip, more common in men and thought to be due to sun exposure. It is a benign vascular lesion that can be treated by surgical excision or a pulsed dye laser, if wanted, but not usually on the NHS.

Oral mucosa

- **Pemphigoid and pemphigus** produce blisters in the mouth (see Chapter 19).
- **Lichen planus** presents as white lacey patches or very bright red gums associated with autoimmune disease.
- *Candida* **infections** are white plaques on the tongue and oral mucosa that can be scraped off with a swab. *Candida albicans* accounts for 80% of oral thrush. It is more common in immunocompromised patients but also affects those taking oral or inhaled steroids and antibiotics, as well as people with diabetes or dentures.
- **Aphthous ulcers** are painful, round, shallow and well-circumscribed. They are usually self-limiting but can be caused by drugs such as nicorandil.
- **Leukoplakia:** thick white patches on the oral mucosa that cannot be wiped off. May be pre-cancerous and often related to heavy smoking or drinking alcohol.
- **Oral cancers:** usually squamous cell in origin and are strongly linked with smoking.

Tongue

- **Smooth and shiny:** due to atrophy of the filiform papillae, causes include iron deficiency.
- **Red and sore:** glossitis, e.g. vitamin B group deficiency.
- **Geographical/furred tongue:** this appearance is due to patchy loss of the papillae, causing areas of red with white borders. It is usually asymptomatic.
- **Black hairy tongue:** papillae grow long if people chew little because of poor intake and become discoloured due to smoking or poor oral hygiene. Treat by scraping with a soft toothbrush or tongue cleaner.
- **Injury to the lateral borders:** consider tongue-biting during seizures.
- **Ulceration:** consider malignancy, but trauma from jagged teeth is much more common.
- **Fasciculation:** the tongue looks like a 'bag of worms'; consider motor neuron disease (MND) (LMN type).
- **Asymmetrical protrusion of the tongue:** points to the side of weakness, e.g. a base of skull tumour.
- **Small spastic tongue:** pseudobulbar palsy (UMN lesion).

Teeth

- Tooth loss is not inevitable with ageing; it is mainly due to periodontal disease. This starts as gingivitis (gum inflammation) associated with bacterial plaque around the teeth and gums. Warning signs are bleeding gums, gum recession and bad breath. If plaque is not removed by effective brushing and flossing, the inflammation progresses and causes pockets between the tooth and gums, leading to pain and tooth loss.
- Risk factors for periodontal disease include smoking, diabetes, dry mouth, and compromised immunity.
- Regular dental review is important because, with age, the dental pulp atrophies, so caries cause less toothache.
- Older people with reduced dexterity, neurological deficits and dementia depend on others for their daily dental care. It is challenging to get immobile people to a dentist, even if an NHS dentist can be found.
- Teeth can also be damaged by excess acid from gastro-oesophageal reflux, acidic fizzy drinks, and fruit juice. This causes the loss of enamel, leading to dental sensitivity.
- Grinding of teeth (bruxism), especially at night, can also damage teeth and cause dental and TMJ pain; recommend the use of night guards to protect the surfaces of the teeth.
- Bruxism can also be caused by SSRIs.
- Psychotropic drugs can damage teeth by causing a double hit of reduced saliva and tardive dyskinesia.
- In the UK, 1.3% of people aged 65–74 have no natural teeth (i.e. are edentulous), rising to 7.5% at 80+.
- In the past, every effort was made to rescue remaining teeth. Modern dentists work more to preserve periodontal health as tooth implants are very effective but extremely expensive.
- 60% of patients are unhappy with their dentures, usually complaining of looseness.

Table 14.1 Summary of oral problems.

	Age-related	Common diseases	Drug-related	Other
Sore mouth		Periodontal disease Dental caries Trauma from dentures Aphthous ulcers Candidiasis HSV Crohn's disease	NSAIDs Nicorandil causes mouth ulcers Phenytoin causes gum hypertrophy	Mouth cancers: risk factors include smoking, alcohol, and HPV Lack of dental screening is leading to rising deaths in the UK
Dry mouth (xerostomia)	Reduced quantity and quality of salvia secretion	Sjogren's syndrome Diabetes	Anticholinergic drugs Tricyclic anti-depressants PD treatments Morphine	Post radiotherapy to head and neck cancer
Reduced or absent taste (dysgeusia and ageusia)		Zinc deficiency Bell's palsy Post-COVID	ACE inhibitors lithium clarithromycin metronidazole levodopa glipizide	Burning mouth syndrome

HSV, *Herpes simplex* virus; HPV, *Human papilloma* virus.

- Plaque builds up on dentures, so they need to be brushed with toothpaste.
- 12% of those provided with dentures never wear them.
- Edentulous people need to continue to go to a dentist to maintain the health of the alveolar ridges to ensure that the dentures continue to fit as well as possible.
- Dentures should only be supplied to those who are prepared to wear them.
- Dentures should be left in situ in a cardiac arrest unless they are obstructing the airway.
- Wearing well-fitting dentures preserve dignity, improve chewing, and help with normal speech.
- The presence of surviving teeth helps secure dental plates and improves the fit.
- New dentures are supplied labelled. Older dentures can be labelled using alcohol-based ink sealed with clear nail varnish to avoid loss if the owner is admitted to an institution.

See Table 14.1 for a summary of causes of dry mouth, sore mouth and reduced taste sensation.

Oesophageal disease

Dysphagia

Dysphagia is increasingly common in older adults affecting:

- 10% of older people admitted acutely to hospital.
- 50% of nursing home residents.
- Up to 60% of people post-stroke.

Patients with dysphagia have a worse 6-month mortality rate than those without. This is due to an increased risk of aspiration pneumonia, impaired nutrition, and dehydration.

There are three stages of swallowing, and dysfunction results from a combination of age-related problems and pathology.

Dysphagia can affect the oropharynx or oesophagus and be due to structural changes or neuromuscular disease (Table 14.2).

Table 14.2 Causes of dysphagia.

	Oropharyngeal	Oesophageal
Structural	Zenker's diverticulum, pharyngeal pouch	Peptic stricture, rings, or webs Severe oesophagitis
	Carcinoma of the palate or tongue Infection, abscess	Intrinsic oesophageal carcinoma Severe candidiasis Compression from extrinsic carcinoma, e.g. bronchial Vascular compression, e.g. aortic aneurysm Foreign body
Neuromuscular	Stroke Bulbar palsy, e.g. MND, pseudobulbar palsy PD	Achalasia Diffuse muscle spasms
		Motility disorder secondary to GORD
	MS	Motility disorder secondary to systemic diseases such as diabetes, CREST
	Brain stem lesions, including tumours Polymyositis, dermatomyositis Myasthenia gravis	

MND, motor neuron disease; PD, Parkinson's disease; MS, multiple sclerosis; GORD, gastro-oesophageal reflux disease.

Assessment

1 Is it new-onset or chronic?
2 Has there been weight loss?
3 Is it difficult to swallow liquids (suggests neurological problem), solids (suggests obstruction) or both?
4 Is there evidence of inflammation: indigestion, acid reflux?

5 Does the food stick at one level? Is it suprasternal (suggests pharyngeal pouch) or retrosternal (suggesting obstruction or compression in the thorax).

6 Does swallowing fatigue, or is there diplopia or dysphonia – suggests myasthenia gravis (see Chapter 7)?

Check dentition, fit of dentures, and look for candidiasis. Check neurology if relevant – are there features such as tongue fasciculations suggestive of MND, signs of stroke or Parkinson's disease (PD), ptosis or facial weakness?

Investigation

If there is concern that endoscopy may perforate the oesophagus, arrange a barium swallow first. This will show pathology such as a pharyngeal pouch, corkscrew contractions secondary to achalasia, or 'shouldering' characteristic of oesophageal carcinoma.

Gastroscopy allows the direct visualisation and biopsy of abnormal tissue. It also allows other interventions: cautery or clipping of actively bleeding vessels; dilatation of a benign stricture; or stenting of a malignant stricture.

Management

Specific management depends on the cause. The approach involves discussion between doctors, dieticians and speech and language therapists and is usually led by a gastroenterologist: the Feeding Issues Multidisciplinary Team (FIMDT).

Neuromuscular dysphagia

- Changes due to ageing of the oesophagus include reduced motility, peristalsis, and reduced efficacy of the upper and lower oesophageal sphincters.
- Pseudobulbar palsy is a bilateral upper motor neuron spastic weakness of muscles supplied by (V, VII), IX, X, and XII secondary to lesions of the corticobulbar tracts in the mid-pons, e.g. bilateral internal capsule strokes or multiple sclerosis (MS).
- Bulbar palsy is impairment of the function of the cranial nerves due to a lower motor lesion. A posterior inferior cerebellar artery infarct results in ipsilateral pharyngeal paralysis with contralateral paresis of the arm and leg (Wallenberg's syndrome).
- **PD:** akinesia impairs swallowing; up to half of PD patients have dysphagia. Levodopa and speech therapy may be helpful.
- Myasthenia gravis is rare but important because it responds well to anticholinesterases, e.g. pyridostigmine. Bulbar involvement is more common in late-onset MG.
- Achalasia is more common in younger patients, but symptoms may merge with ageing changes, and it is a risk factor for oesophageal cancer.

Options for tube feeding will be discussed later.

As with all soft tubular structures, narrowing of the oesophageal lumen can arise because of:

1 external compression,
2 lesions in the wall,
3 obstruction in the lumen.

Extrinsic pressure

- Pharyngeal pouches. All pouches become more common with increasing age. Zenker's diverticulum, through the posterior pharyngeal wall at the upper level of the cricopharyngeus, may result from uncoordinated contractions. When large and full, it may hinder the passage of a food bolus. Symptomatic pouches can be removed surgically, and endoscopic techniques allow operations on frailer patients. More rarely, pouches occur lower in the oesophagus.
- Superior mediastinal obstruction – malignancy (usually carcinoma of the bronchus).
- Dilated left atrium in severe heart disease. A CXR, in conjunction with clinical signs, will usually be sufficient to make the diagnosis.
- Aortic-arch dilatation.
- Posterior pressure from spinal osteophytes (rare).

Inflammatory disease

Oesophagitis due to reflux

Inflammation in the lower oesophagus is associated with hiatus hernia and acid reflux. The patient often describes a long history of indigestion. Chronic inflammation can lead to strictures. Endoscopy is the best diagnostic modality as biopsies can be taken (essential if there is any suspicion of malignant change), and Barrett's oesophagus may be noted. Symptoms respond to antacids, but proton-pump inhibitors – PPIs (e.g. omeprazole) or H2 antagonists (e.g. famotidine) are necessary for healing. Strictures can be dilated endoscopically.

Barrett's oesophagus

This is defined as the replacement of normal oesophageal squamous cells by metaplastic columnar epithelium, usually affecting the lower one-third of the oesophagus.

- Risk factors include being male, over 60, smoking and drinking alcohol. It usually develops in combination with hiatus hernia, low oesophageal tone, and duodenal reflux.
- It is premalignant and may progress to adenocarcinoma.
- Most older patients will die of other diseases, but fit older people without significant other pathologies should be offered regular surveillance.

Oesophageal candidiasis

Frail older people are at risk, especially if immunosuppressed, using steroid inhalers or after antibiotics. The typical white patches of thrush are often (but not always) present in the mouth. Endoscopy confirms oesophageal involvement. Oral fluconazole is the treatment of choice.

Pill oesophagitis

This is more common in older adults due to reduced oesophageal motility, polypharmacy, and not taking medications with sufficient water.

- Common culprits are NSAIDs, aspirin, iron, doxycycline, and bisphosphonates.
- Odynophagia is the most common symptom (pain when swallowing).
- It occurs more often in women and people with diabetes.

Carcinoma of the oesophagus

This commonly occurs in the sixth and seventh decades; it is 20 times more common in those aged over 65 than in the younger population. The UK incidence in men is 17.5 per 100,000 and 8.8 per 100,000 in women. There are two main types: adenocarcinoma and squamous cell carcinoma.

1 Adenocarcinoma is becoming more common in the West, is more common in men, affects slightly younger patients, and tends to affect the lower third of the oesophagus. The strongest risk factor is reflux. Barrett's oesophagus is a premalignant stage.
2 Squamous cell carcinoma is more common worldwide and is related to smoking, alcohol, and vitamin deficiencies. The increased incidence in China is attributed to riboflavin deficiency.

Clinical features

Symptoms: dysphagia, first for solids and then liquids. Weight loss is extremely common. Some patients experience retrosternal pain. Hoarseness suggests invasion of the left recurrent laryngeal nerve. Coughing and breathlessness may be due to aspiration or direct invasion of the bronchial tree. Examine for cervical lymph nodes.

Investigation

- A barium swallow may be used for the initial evaluation, and great care is needed during endoscopy to avoid perforation.
- Endoscopy allows biopsy.
- CT scanning is needed for staging.

Management

Curative treatment is rare; tumours are discovered late and have often already spread, so palliation is the aim.

- **Multidisciplinary approach:** patients should be discussed by an upper GI MDT to assess their performance status and frailty.
- **Oesophagectomy:** may be considered for lower oesophageal cancer on a case-by-case basis. Frail older patients with other comorbidities are unlikely to make a good recovery.
- **Combinations of chemotherapy and radiotherapy:** may be an option for biologically fit patients with high-performance status and localised disease.
- **Dysphagia:** can be reduced by debulking with endoluminal brachytherapy or photodynamic therapy.
- **Stent insertion:** the treatment of choice for obstructive symptoms when other measures are not justified; pain and complications are common. If the tumour blocks the stent, this can be debulked with a Yttrium Aluminium Garnet (YAG) laser or photodynamic therapy.
- **Patient support:** patients and their families should be given the support of a cancer nurse specialist and contact details for support networks (e.g. www.macmillan.org).
- **Nutrition:** do not forget to optimise a patient's oral intake by referring to the dietician for supplements.
- **Palliative care:** refer early for help with symptoms and further support (see Chapter 22).

Intraluminal obstruction

Impacted objects may include food (especially if not properly chewed), missing dentures and other foreign bodies that can be removed endoscopically. Cognitively impaired patients are particularly at risk.

Gastric disease

Dyspepsia

Indigestion is common at all ages (30% of the population); 2–3% of prescribed drugs are antacids. In many older patients, diagnosis is difficult as the symptoms are vague and non-specific, plus there may be several causes.

- Many drugs cause dyspepsia so a drug history, including over the counter preparations, is essential. Avoid NSAIDs, bisphosphonates and calcium channel blockers, and remember to co-prescribe PPIs with steroids.
- *Helicobacter pylori* infection rates rise with age (up to 60% of older people are infected) and should be treated if proven by biopsy, culture, breath test or serology.
- All pathologies potentially responsible for indigestion become more common in old age. See the list in the box provided later.

- A therapeutic trial may identify the responsible lesion, as many of the conditions that are commonly found may be incidental, e.g. 20% hiatus hernia and up to 50% gallstones are asymptomatic.
- Late-onset dyspepsia should be investigated. Endoscopy is the investigation of choice (except in the presence of dysphagia) and is acceptable for most elderly patients; extra care is needed with pre-medication in those with poor respiratory reserve. Ultrasound examination is the best technique for suspected gallbladder and pancreatic disease.
- Watch for side effects from medication used to treat GI symptoms, for example:
  - Metoclopramide may precipitate or worsen extrapyramidal syndromes.
  - Avoid aluminium salts in constipated patients and magnesium in those with diarrhoea.
  - Bile salts have proved disappointing for dissolving gallstones, and side effects, especially diarrhoea, can be troublesome.
  - PPIs can cause hyponatraemia, malabsorption of calcium (increasing fractures), magnesium, and vitamin B_{12}, diarrhoea, increase the risk of *Clostridioides difficile* and long-term use has been linked to an increased risk of gastric cancer.
  - Clopidogrel is an inactive prodrug that is activated by several cytochrome P450 enzymes, including CYP2C19. Lansoprazole causes less inhibition of CYP2C19 and therefore is less likely to reduce the effectiveness of clopidogrel (compared with omeprazole and esomeprazole, which are more potent inhibitors).
  - Patients with osteoporotic kyphosis are at increased risk of oesophageal perforation with bisphosphonates.

Lesions potentially responsible for 'indigestion'

- Hiatus hernia (affects 60% of over-70-year-olds).
- Gastritis (especially drug-induced).
- Peptic ulceration (found in 20% of over-70-year-olds).
- Carcinoma of the stomach.
- Gallstones (found in 38% of over-70-year-olds).
- Pancreatic disease.
- Mesenteric ischaemia.
- Carcinoma of the large bowel.

Gastro-oesophageal reflux disease

Gastro-oesophageal reflux disease (GORD) is the return of gastric contents into the oesophagus.

- Heartburn is common, but GORD may cause respiratory symptoms such as chronic cough or asthma and non-cardiac chest pain.
- Lifestyle changes should be tried first: weight loss, raising the head of the bed (if there are nocturnal symptoms), avoiding dietary triggers such as fatty food, spicy food, and caffeine, and stopping smoking.
- PPIs are the most successful treatment in combination with *H. pylori* eradication.
- Only endoscope if treatment does not relieve symptoms.
- Oesophagitis, strictures, Barrett's oesophagus, and adenocarcinoma are complications.

Gastric carcinoma

The incidence of gastric cancer has fallen over the past couple of decades, variously attributed to reduced salt intake, refrigeration, increased intake of fresh fruit and vegetables, and the eradication of *H. pylori*.

The rate for men is about twice that for women. Peak incidence is in the eighth decade, and most (>80%) have advanced disease at diagnosis, underlining the importance of investigating late-onset dyspepsia. Five-year survival for all new cases over 70 is 5–12%.

- The most common site is the gastro-oesophageal junction.
- Risk factors include genetic predisposition and an association with blood group A, smoking, atrophic gastritis, pernicious anaemia, previous gastric resection, and infection with *H. pylori*.
- There is considerable geographical variation in incidence and prognosis. It is prevalent in Japan, but the prognosis there is more favourable; earlier diagnosis, which 'improves' survival time, may account for some of this, but other factors are probably involved.
- Prolonged use of PPIs may predispose to malignant changes.
- Symptoms tend to reflect advanced disease, including weight loss, vomiting, haematemesis, melaena, and abdominal pain. Check for a left supraclavicular lymph node (Virchow).
- The general principles are as for oesophageal cancer.
- Diagnosis is usually made by endoscopic biopsy, followed by staging CT of the chest, abdomen, and pelvis.
- The prognosis is poor, and treatment is usually palliative. In early cases where the patient is biologically very fit, this may include gastrectomy, adjuvant chemotherapy (e.g. etoposide and 5-fluorouracil), radiotherapy or a bypass procedure.
- Once the cancer has metastasized, the prognosis is likely to be only a matter of months, so the focus should move to good symptom control (see Chapter 22).

Liver disease

Jaundice

- Surgical causes are common and must be identified rapidly before the condition becomes irremediable; ultrasound is the investigation of first choice.
- Medical causes of jaundice should be investigated and treated, as in younger patients.
- Primary biliary cholangitis (PBC) and chronic hepatitis are more common in older patients than appreciated. The prognosis in late life is often better than in younger patients.

Intrahepatic cholestasis

- Older patients in hospital often develop a cholestatic picture of raised liver function tests (i.e. raised alkaline phosphatase [ALP]) when they are being treated for sepsis, even when this does not affect the liver. The abnormal LFTs should resolve as the underlying infection is treated.
- Other causes of cholestasis that could occur at the same time include gallstones and the effects of drugs such as Augmentin and flucloxacillin.
- Back pressure due to heart failure is a non-hepatic cause of raised alkaline phosphatase.

Chronic liver disease

All forms of chronic liver disease are becoming more common in older people, with an increased number of deaths from liver disease. Some cases are detected by chance with routine blood tests. Only 6% of liver biopsies are performed in over 80-year-olds, but there is no evidence of increased risk. Diagnosis is important because of treatment options, e.g. anti-viral agents, immunosuppression, and lifestyle advice. Ascites can be managed with spironolactone or paracentesis.

Alcoholic liver disease

Dubbed the 'invisible epidemic' of older people, problem drinking has increased markedly and worsened during COVID-19 lockdowns. Most older risky drinkers have a longstanding alcohol problem, but around a third, particularly women, develop drinking problems in later life because of chronic limiting or painful physical conditions, depression, and social factors including increased isolation and bereavement. A longer life expectancy in old age gives more time for cirrhotic change to develop.

Older people have a reduced volume of distribution for alcohol and a less efficient alcohol metabolism due to a decline in alcohol dehydrogenase and aldehyde dehydrogenase.

- 28% of cases of alcoholic liver disease (ALD) are over 65.
- More common in men than women, but the gap is narrowing.
- May present very non-specifically. Most patients have a prolonged course of 20–30 years leading to cirrhosis, 10 years with cirrhotic changes, and 5 years of severe symptoms in the period prior to death.
- Jaundice and ascites are late features; 34% of older patients diagnosed with ALD are dead within 1 year.
- Consider alcohol withdrawal if patients develop new-onset delirium 1–2 days after admission to hospital.

Metabolic dysfunction-associated liver disease

Metabolic dysfunction-associated liver disease (MASLD) is the new name for non-alcoholic fatty liver disease. The incidence of this is rising with the increasing prevalence of obesity and type 2 diabetes. Fat accumulation and inflammation of the hepatocytes lead to liver fibrosis and eventually cirrhosis.

- MASLD is part of the metabolic syndrome with insulin resistance.
- The prevalence among over-65-year-olds is 35%.
- Ideally, it should be diagnosed early before irreversible fibrotic change occurs.
- Management is by lifestyle changes, i.e. weight reduction and increasing exercise by 5–10% can reduce fat accumulation by 40%. Metformin can be used to reduce insulin resistance. GLP-1 agonists offer future promise.

Viral hepatitis

Hepatitis C is the most significant cause. It is a blood-borne virus and was a risk from blood transfusions in the UK prior to blood screening in 1991. Worldwide, the reuse or inadequate sterilisation of medical equipment, especially syringes and needles, in healthcare settings is a major cause. Intravenous drug use is a less common cause in older people.

- It occurs in all WHO regions, with the highest prevalence in Eastern Europe (including Ukraine) and Central Asia.
- Depending on the genotype of the virus and the person's cirrhosis status, combinations of direct-acting antivirals (DAAs) such as sofosbuvir/velpatasvir have replaced treatment with interferon and ribavirin.

Autoimmune hepatitis

- Check blood for raised IgG and autoantibodies, including antinuclear antibodies, smooth muscle antibodies and type 1 liver–kidney microsomal antibodies.
- Treat with prednisolone plus or minus azathioprine.

Primary biliary cholangitis

Primary biliary cholangitis (PBC) is an autoimmune liver disease characterised by portal inflammation and immune-mediated destruction of the intrahepatic bile ducts, leading to cholestasis and occasionally to fibrosis and secondary biliary cirrhosis. Liver function tests show a cholestatic picture (i.e. raised ALP and gamma GT).

- Half of cases of PBC are among over-65-year-olds.
- It is much more common in women than in men.
- Antimitochondrial autoantibodies are present in 95% of cases.
- Ursodeoxycholic acid can slow disease progression.
- The itch can be reduced with cholestyramine.

Liver cancer

Primary liver cancer is most commonly hepatocellular carcinoma and is more common in cirrhosis due to alcohol, hepatitis B or C, and as with most cancers, the highest rates are in 85–89-year-olds. Surgery is often not possible, but a variety of other options such as chemoembolisation, radiofrequency ablation, radiotherapy, and targeted cancer drugs such as atezolizumab and bevacizumab may be useful. Liver secondaries are common, particularly from breast, bowel, lung and pancreatic cancers, and any treatment depends on the primary, performance state, and frailty of the patient. Symptom control and referral to palliative care are essential.

Biliary disease

Cholelithiasis

Gallstones are common in older people and are found in 38% of women and 22% of men by the age of 90. Increasing age is thought to cause increased viscosity of the bile and reduced motility of the gallbladder means that it does not contract fully leading to bile stasis, and a tendency for the common bile duct to become dilated. Other risk factors in later life include the metabolic syndrome, MASLD, HRT, and androgen suppression for prostate cancer.

Acute cholecystitis

This is due to gallstones in 90% of cases. Classically, inflammation of the gall bladder presents with severe right upper quadrant pain. However, older people may not present with classical symptoms, especially if they have diabetes. Look for a raised white cell count and raised CRP. The LFTs are usually normal, unless there are complications.

- Older people may also decompensate quickly with infections.
- Diagnosis is usually made by ultrasound.
- Supportive treatment includes IV fluids, analgesia, and IV antibiotics for frail or immunosuppressed older people.
- Emerging literature suggests that older people do better if they have cholecystectomy early, but this has not yet become clinical practice. Very frail patients are sometimes managed by percutaneous cholecystostomy: a drainage tube is inserted into the gallbladder under ultrasound guidance and left on free drainage for 2 weeks.

Choledocholithiasis is the presence of gallstones in the common bile duct. Magnetic resonance cholangiopancreatography (MRCP) is useful in showing the anatomy of the biliary tree and the site of impacted stones in frail patients. However, endoscopic retrograde cholangiopancreatography (ERCP) may still be needed for biopsies and treatment, e.g. to remove small biliary stones or insert stents. ERCP is said to have a 5–10% risk of pancreatitis.

Cholangiocarcinoma

This rare cancer develops in the bile ducts: extrahepatic and perihilar lesions present with obstructive jaundice, and itch, whilst the symptoms of intrahepatic cholangiocarcinoma tend to be non-specific with malaise, weight loss and abdominal pain. Extrahepatic lesions may be resectable, chemotherapy (e.g. gemcitabine and cisplatin) may be used, and pegaptanib may be offered if there are changes in the fibroblast growth factor receptor 2 (*FGFR2*) gene. Diagnosis is usually late, and palliative care and stenting are often used.

Pancreatic disease

Pancreatitis

The causes include gallstones blocking the pancreatic duct and alcohol.

- Serum amylase is raised.
- Treatment is supportive (IV fluids, nutrition, analgesia, and oxygen)
- Morbidity and mortality are higher in older patients.

Pancreatic insufficiency

Exocrine pancreatic insufficiency is often associated with chronic pancreatitis and previous upper GI surgery. Less commonly, it occurs in diabetes and coeliac disease.

- Presents with abdominal discomfort, loose, hard-to-flush stools, bloating, flatulence, and weight loss.
- Check faecal elastase.
- Treat by replacing the pancreatic enzymes with Creon with meals and vitamins A, D, E, and K if deficient.

Pancreatic carcinoma

The incidence of pancreatic cancer is increasing in most developed countries, although paradoxically, not in Japan. It is common in older men. Eight-five per cent of cases have already metastasized by the time of diagnosis, and the prognosis is poor (overall 20% 1-year survival).

- Aetiological factors include cigarette smoking, high alcohol intake, high dietary fat, and occupational exposure in the chemical and metal industries.
- Weight loss is usually striking.
- If there is abdominal pain, this radiates through to the back. Look for erythema ab igne on the epigastric skin from a hot water bottle used to ease pain.
- In most cases, the head of the pancreas is involved, leading to obstructive jaundice.
- An ultrasound scan may detect pancreatic cancer, but CT is needed for staging.
- Radical surgery is usually not an option because of frailty and comorbidities, but stenting procedures provide temporary relief from the symptoms secondary to biliary obstruction.
- Chemotherapy prolongs life by a few months in trials but does not improve quality of life.
- Depending on the mutation pattern in the cancer cells, small-molecule inhibitors and checkpoint inhibitors may be used.

Small bowel disease

Malabsorption

Small-bowel function declines with age, but nutritional deficiencies only occur when other factors intervene, e.g. a poor diet or ill health.

- Causes seen in younger patients also occur in old age, e.g. coeliac disease.
- Maldigestion is more common than malabsorption, e.g. due to pancreatic insufficiency.

- Bacterial change in the small-bowel lumen due to stasis or diverticular disease is common (10% of older people) and is often clinically significant.
- Ischaemia as a cause of malabsorption is rare, even in old age.
- Iatrogenic causes must always be considered, e.g. post-gastrectomy, alcohol, and some drugs, e.g. biguanides.

Indicators of malabsorption

- Weight loss (especially around the face) despite good dietary intake.
- Low serum albumin.
- Unexplained iron-deficiency anaemia (with negative faecal occult blood).
- Macrocytic anaemia.
- Osteomalacia, leading to falls and proximal muscle weakness.
- Abdominal distension secondary to gas.
- Frank steatorrhoea is uncommon.

Causes of malabsorption in old age

See Table 14.3.

Coeliac disease

Coeliac disease is an autoimmune gluten-sensitive enteropathy: the gliadin component causes an immunologically mediated inflammation of the lining of the small intestine, leading to subtotal villous atrophy. Enteropathy leads to maldigestion and malabsorption. Gluten is found in wheat, rye, and barley. Oats (that are not contaminated by wheat) are safe for most patients.

- The incidence is around 1% of the population, most common in temperate European countries, especially Ireland and Finland.
- 25% of newly diagnosed cases are aged over 60.
- Cases are diagnosed ever later in life; even in the ninth decade.

Table 14.3 Common causes, investigation, and treatment of malabsorption in older people.

Cause	Investigation	Treatment
Coeliac disease	Anti-tissue transglutaminase antibodies (tTG-IgA), low total IgA	Gluten-free diet
Bacterial overgrowth	Positive hydrogen breath test, serum red cell folate high	Course of antibiotics
Pancreatic insufficiency	Low faecal elastase	Creon capsules with every meal (including supplements) and snacks
Crohn's disease of the small bowel	Biopsy	Mesalazine, steroids
Atrophic gastritis, previous partial gastrectomy	Low B_{12}	Course of intramuscular hydroxocobalamin with 3 monthly top-ups
Lymphoma	Biopsy results	Depends on the type and grade of disease
Mesenteric ischaemia	Barium/CT appearance	Surgical in the fit patient, otherwise consider anticoagulation, and palliation for very frail patients
Drugs, e.g. biguanides, cholestyramine	From drug history	Stop culprit drugs wherever possible

- 95% of people with coeliac disease are positive for HLA DQ2 and the remaining 5% are positive for HLA DQ8.
- Associated autoimmune conditions include thyroid disease, type 1 diabetes, primary biliary cirrhosis and Sjogren's syndrome. There is also an association with epilepsy, ataxia, and dementia.

Clinical features

- GI symptoms include chronic or intermittent diarrhoea, steatorrhoea, flatulence, borborygmi, weight loss, abdominal bloating, and cramping, but older people may present with complications, e.g. progressive osteoporosis despite treatment.
- Features on examination might include evidence of weight loss, muscle wasting, oedema, cheilosis, and glossitis. Dermatitis herpetiformis is an exuberant, itchy erythematous rash often occurring on the extensor surfaces of the arms, legs, and buttocks, which usually (but not always) resolves if gluten is avoided.
- There are also non-GI manifestations (see Table 14.4).

Investigations

- Blood tests might show mixed or macrocytic anaemia, low ferritin and folate levels, hypocalcaemia, hypokalaemia, and low vitamin D. Coeliac disease is sometimes the underlying cause of persistently raised transaminase, with no other explanation.
- NICE recommends using IgA anti-tissue transglutaminase IgA antibodies (tTG-IgA) as the first line for diagnosis, as this is the most sensitive. If the result is equivocal, check for IgA anti-endomysial antibodies (EMAs). The EMA is the most specific test, but levels fall rapidly once gluten is removed from the diet. If both are negative, check total IgA levels to exclude IgA deficiency.
- NICE also recommends a duodenal biopsy (Figure 14.1) to confirm the serological diagnosis.

Management

- Treatment is a lifelong gluten-free diet. This is difficult as many surprising and cheaper foodstuffs contain wheat, e.g. as a thickener, and adherence requires obsessional checking of food labels. Gluten-free bread, rolls and flour are now the only foods available on prescription in some parts of the UK.
- Correct any vitamin deficiencies.
- Patients are more likely to adhere to their diet if they and their families receive education and support at diagnosis from a dietician and a support group such as Coeliac UK.
- Adherence to the gluten-free diet protects against malignant change, including lymphoma and adenocarcinoma of the gut. Worsening symptoms or blood tests may be due to poor dietary adherence or small intestinal malignancy – consider capsule endoscopy.

Table 14.4 Non-gastrointestinal manifestations of coeliac disease and cause.

Non-gastrointestinal manifestations	Due to reduced absorption of:
Anaemia and fatigue	Iron and folate (B_{12} less common)
Bleeding diathesis	Fat-soluble vitamin K
Osteomalacia and osteoporosis	Vitamin D
Neuropsychiatric	Calcium
Peripheral neuropathy	Folate
Dermatitis herpetiformis	Due to the immune effect

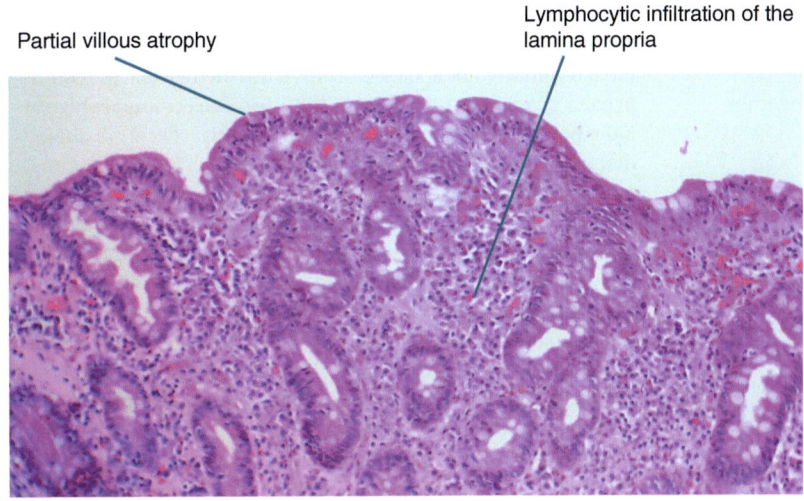

Partial villous atrophy

Lymphocytic infiltration of the lamina propria

Figure 14.1 Histology of Coeliac Disease. *Source*: Samir/ Wikimedia Commons/CC BY SA 3.0.

Large-bowel disease

Acute diarrhoea

There is an arbitrary cutoff of <2 weeks for 'acute' diarrhoea. The cause is usually obvious from the history.

Infective

Cultures must be taken, and patients must be isolated (if in hospital) whilst results are awaited.

- **Viral** most commonly Norovirus (also known as winter vomiting), which causes outbreaks, e.g. in hospitals, care homes and cruise ships. The incubation period is 12–48 hours. Symptoms usually last for 24–60 hours and include sudden-onset projectile vomiting, abdominal discomfort, and watery diarrhoea. Supportive measures are all that are usually needed. Transmission is mainly faeco-oral but also person-to-person, via fomites and airborne, as the highly contagious virus is easily aerosolized in the vomitus. Wash your hands – alcohol rubs are *not* effective as this RNA virus does not have a lipid envelope.
- **Bacterial** food poisoning: Organisms include *Salmonella, Escherichia coli, and Campylobacter*; antibiotics are only justified in severe disease, as in mild cases they may prolong symptoms and produce carrier states.

Clostridioides difficile-associated diarrhoea

Clostridioides difficile-associated diarrhoea (CDAD) is the most serious cause of antibiotic-associated diarrhoea and occurs when commensal bacteria in the gut flora have been wiped out by broad-spectrum antibiotics. *Clostridioides difficile* is a Gram-positive spore-forming bacillus. (The name was changed in 2016 when it was recognised that it is a different genus from *Clostridium butyricum*). *C. difficile* produces two distinct exotoxins, A (enterotoxin) and B (cytotoxin). These bind to the intestinal epithelial brush border and trigger the release of inflammatory mediators, resulting in increased fluid secretion and inflammation. Biopsies reveal patchy necrosis with an exudate of fibrin and neutrophils. In severe disease, extensive necrosis and ulceration may result in the development of a pseudo-membrane, which can be seen at sigmoidoscopy/colonoscopy.

Clinical features

The most common presentation is malaise, abdominal pain, nausea, anorexia, and very watery, foul-smelling diarrhoea after a course of broad-spectrum antibiotics. Worsening pain and diarrhoea may herald complications. Check for a low-grade fever and abdominal tenderness. Fever and severe abdominal tenderness are signs of impending complications (see Table 14.5).

Investigation

Nurses have long claimed that they can recognise CDAD by its characteristic smell; this may be due to the volatile fatty acids produced. White cell count and CRP are raised. The most widely used diagnostic test is the enzyme-linked immunosorbent assay (ELISA) for toxins A and/or B. AXR/CT of the abdomen is needed if complications are suspected, and sigmoidoscopy will visualise the pseudo-membrane.

Complications

Pseudomembranous colitis, toxic megacolon, and colonic perforation all have high mortality rates in older people. Relapses are common, and morbidity is high.

Management

- Isolate the patient as soon as the suspicion of *C. difficile* is raised.
- Stop any culprit antibiotic and PPI whenever possible.
- Replace fluid and electrolytes.
- First-line therapy is oral vancomycin, 125 mg q.d.s. The dose can be increased to 250 mg q.d.s. in resistant cases. As oral vancomycin is poorly absorbed, the risk of systemic side effects such as ototoxicity is minimal.

Table 14.5 Assessing the severity of *C. difficile* disease.

	Mild	Moderate	Severe	Life-threatening
WCC	Normal	<15× 10⁹/l	>15× 10⁹/l	>15× 10⁹/l
Number of loose motions	Fewer than 3 per 24 hr	3–5 episodes per 24 hr	Not a reliable indicator	Not a reliable indicator
Renal function	Normal	Normal	Cr raised by 50% above baseline	
Clinical signs of impending complications			Fever >38.5 C	Hypotension Ileus Toxic megacolon

WCC, white cell count; Cr, Creatinine.

- Second-line therapy is fidaxomicin, an antibiotic designed for the treatment of CDAD that works by inhibiting the release of toxins, thus reducing severity and reducing the risk of recurrence.
- Faecal microbiota transplant is being investigated as a treatment for recurrent CDAD.

Prevention

Prevention is extremely important. Considerable efforts have been made to educate hospital staff and visitors about handwashing with soap and water (alcohol gel is not effective against the spores). Hospitals have invested in deep cleaning strategies with misting and proper disinfection of contaminated surfaces. Antibiotic policies reduce the use of antibiotics most likely to lead to CDAD. Early studies suggested that probiotics reduced the risk of CDAD, but a large double-blind placebo-controlled trial showed no reduction in antibiotic-associated diarrhoea or CDAD, possibly because the prevalence had already fallen. Anti-peristaltic agents, PPIs, opiates, and anti-diarrhoea medications should be avoided.

Mandatory reporting

All acute trusts must report cases of CDAD to the Department of Health. There has been a national drive to reduce the number of cases per trust to reduce the high morbidity and mortality rates. Deaths peaked in 2007, and the number of cases fell steadily to 2014 but plateaued and may be increasing again (see Figure 14.2).

Chronic diarrhoea

This can be incapacitating in older age, especially if the patient is already disabled and immobile due to other pathologies. It may result in faecal incontinence which patients and carers find extremely difficult to manage at home.

A good history of the duration and associated features will indicate the likely diagnosis. Remember recurrence of *C. difficile,* especially if the patient lives in an institution or has been a recent in-patient. Lactose intolerance may follow diarrhoea of any cause so a period of avoiding milk products may help.

Causes of chronic diarrhoea

1 **Spurious:** i.e. obstruction with overflow must be excluded first by rectal examination and then by sigmoidoscopy if necessary. The cause may be simple, e.g. faecal impaction, or serious, e.g. carcinoma of the rectum. Patients and relatives need a clear explanation of the mechanism, particularly if they are to take laxatives whilst at home.
2 **Inflammatory:**
    (a) Up to a fifth of all new diagnoses of inflammatory bowel disease (IBD) are made after the age of 60. Crohn's disease is most common in older people and tends to be mainly colonic and inflammatory in nature. Ulcerative colitis tends to be primarily left-sided in older people. Diagnosis is made by colonoscopy and biopsy. Initial treatment is with steroids and mesalazine. It was thought that the course in older people was more benign, but rates of colectomy are high in older people with UC. It is unclear whether this reflects the disease or the reluctance to use immunosuppressants such as azathioprine and ciclosporin or biologicals like adalimumab in older people.
    (b) Microscopic colitis encompasses both collagenous and lymphocytic colitis. It causes watery, non-bloody diarrhoea and is increasingly common in older age. It can cause faecal incontinence and diarrhoea overnight. The mucosa looks normal at colonoscopy, but histology reveals an abnormal band of collagen above the basement membrane in collagenous colitis or lymphocytic infiltration in lymphocytic colitis. Smoking is a risk factor. Treatment includes stopping drugs that may be worsening the diarrhoea (aspirin, NSAIDs, PPIs, SSRIs), avoiding caffeine, looking for associated coeliac disease, loperamide, and a trial of budesonide.
3 **Metabolic:** uncommon but exclude thyrotoxicosis; some cases are secondary to diabetic neuropathy.
4 **Drugs:** antibiotic-associated diarrhoea is common, especially after cephalosporins and CDAD can be chronic. Consider purgative misuse. Other drugs causing diarrhoea include colchicine, PPIs, acetylcholinesterase inhibitors such as donepezil, metformin, magnesium-containing antacids, and iron.
5 **Iatrogenic:** a chronic complication of gastrectomy/vagotomy.
6 **Irritable bowel syndrome (IBS):** most often presents before the age of 50; if it develops later, malignancy must be ruled out.
7 **Rule out malabsorption:** see later.

Constipation

This is common, affecting 10% of older people living in the community and up to 75% of people living in nursing homes. Acute constipation develops in half of hospital inpatients aged over 65.

- Reduces the quality of life.
- Is a common and reversible cause of delirium.
- Other complications include obstruction, faecal impaction, overflow diarrhoea, and even perforation; megacolon predisposing to sigmoid volvulus and rectal prolapse; and urinary retention.
- Fear of becoming constipated is an aspect of old age that is more common than the genuine symptom. Seventy per cent of older people open their bowels once daily, 11% every other day, and 14% twice daily. Difficulty passing motions is of greater importance than frequency of defecation.

Causes of constipation

- **Poor bowel habits:** low-residue diet, poor fluid intake, lack of exercise and ignoring 'the call to stool'.
- **Poor appetite/oral intake:** leads to a reduced gastro-colic reflex but does **not** stop the bowels from working.
- **Immobility.**
- **Drugs:** opiate analgesics, anticholinergics, anti-Parkinson's medications, diuretics, calcium channel blockers, purgative abuse (cathartic colon), etc.
- **IBS**
- **Metabolic precipitants:** diabetes mellitus, hypothyroidism, hypercalcaemia, hypokalaemia, and hypomagnesaemia secondary to drugs, or bowel, endocrine or metabolic disease.
- **Psychiatric disorders:** depression, dementia.
- **Neurological causes:** PD, spinal cord injury, multiple sclerosis, and stroke disease.
- **Pain from peri-anal disease:** piles, fissures, and proctitis.

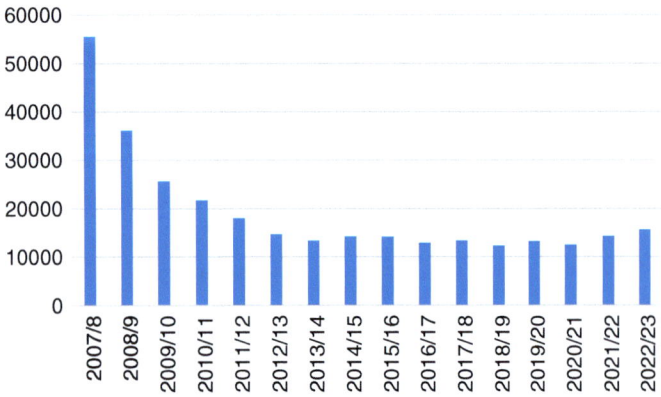

Figure 14.2 Number of *C. difficile* infections in acute trusts in England 2007–2023 (UK government).

History

Determine whether this is true constipation and whether it is acute or chronic. Exclude red flags: change in bowel habits, rectal bleeding with no anal symptoms, weight loss, family history of bowel cancer, and nocturnal bowel opening.

Ask the patient if they need to use 'digital manoeuvres' to help – this is under-reported because we do not ask about it.

Examination

Abdominal: scars from previous surgery, cachexia, palpable bowel, and distension.

Red flags include a rigid abdomen and a lack of bowel sounds.

Rectal examination: do not forget to take verbal consent and to have a chaperone and document their name and role.

Document perianal sensation, anal tone, piles, fissures, rectal masses, amount, and consistency of stool and whether there is any blood in or on the stool.

- Small, hard stools are often related to a low-fibre diet or dehydration; soft stools in a dilated rectum suggest chronic laxative abuse.
- Prostate size and texture in men.
- Document whether there is a rectal prolapse.

Investigation

FBC and haematinics to check for iron deficiency.

Progress to colonoscopy if there are red flags, including a positive faecal immunochemical test (FIT). Routine FIT tests are not offered after 74 years old, but the patient can request ongoing tests every 2 years.

Management

- Start with lifestyle advice: increase fluid intake, improve mobility, and increase fibre intake gradually to 30 g a day (difficult to achieve) to increase stool bulk to distend the colon and improve bowel motility. (1 serving of All-Bran contains 11 g of fibre, and a single carrot has 3 g of fibre.)
- Stop culprit drugs if possible.
- Encourage the patient to develop a regular time to empty the bowels, usually early in the morning or after breakfast. Recommend straining for no longer than 5 min. Suggest the patient lean forward and raise their feet on a stool 15 cm above the ground when sitting on the toilet to replicate a squatting position. This relaxes the puborectalis muscle and unkinks the rectum, thus reducing the strain needed to pass a motion.

The use of laxatives, suppositories and enemas is summarised in Table 14.6.

- If faecal impaction is imminent, prescribe enemas.
- If not impacted but a quick result is needed, prescribe a stimulant (senna); occasionally, an osmotic laxative (magnesium sulphate) will be needed in addition.
- For short-term treatment (associated with acute illness), ensure adequate fluid intake and mobilise as soon as possible. Prescribe senna if stools are bulky and soft. Opiates cause small and hard stools. Macrogols (Laxido) are often used for inpatients but take time for nurses to mix and administer.

Table 14.6 Summary of medication for constipation.

	Role	Onset of action	Side effects	Notes
Stimulant: E.g. Senna 15 mg	The first line for acute constipation and opioid-induced constipation	8–12 hr	Abdominal cramps, nausea. Yellow-brown discolouration of urine and melanosis coli with senna	Only licensed for short-term use. The syrup is unpalatable. Take it in the evening.
Co-danthramer and co-danthrusate	Palliative care			
Bulk-forming: E.g. ispaghula husk (also known as psyllium)	The first line for chronic constipation in less frail patients	2–3 days	Flatulence and bloating, allergic reactions	Must drink sufficient water. Do not take it just before bedtime. Avoid in opioid-induced constipation
Osmotic: E.g. macrogol	Second line for acute, chronic, and opioid-induced constipation, but often used first line in frail older people	2–3 days	Nausea, bloating, and abdominal cramps	Some people struggle to drink the prescribed volume. Avoid use with fluid thickeners for dysphagia, as they counteract the thickening,
Stool softener: Docusate is a surface-wetting agent (and a mild stimulant)	Useful in patients who find it hard to increase their fluid intake	1–2 days		
Prokinetic: Prucalopride	For intractable constipation		Headache, dizziness	Caution in ischaemic heart disease or arrhythmias
Stool softening suppository: glycerol	Rectum full of hard stools	15–60 min	Rectal irritation	Also, some stimulant effects
Stimulant enema: sodium citrate (Microlax)	Rectum full of soft stools	5–15 min		
Osmotic enema: phosphate	For hard, impacted stool	2–5 min		

- Faecal impaction in patients who are bedbound, e.g. due to spinal cord injury or following prolonged acute illness at home may require manual evacuation. A chaperone is needed. Sensible precautions include a plastic apron, two pairs of gloves, a lubricant such as KY jelly, plenty of wipes and a large clinical waste bag. Lignocaine gel will reduce pain if there is a skin tear. Surgical disimpaction under general anaesthetic is occasionally needed and may be lifesaving if caecal perforation is prevented.
- Review the need for laxatives once the patient has recovered from the acute illness. Only prescribe laxatives on discharge from hospital if the need continues, e.g. prior usage or continuing precipitant. Overuse of laxatives leads to diarrhoea with the risk of electrolyte abnormalities, especially low potassium, and faecal incontinence.
- For longer-term treatment where non-drug treatment fails or is impractical, prescribe a bulking agent in fitter mobile patients who will drink plenty of water, or macrogol.
- For intractable constipation, try a combination of treatments.
- The prokinetic prucalopride is a selective, high-affinity, serotonin [5-HT$_4$] receptor agonist which stimulates GI motility. NICE now recommends this if two laxatives from two different classes have been tried at the highest tolerated recommended doses for at least 6 months and invasive treatment is being considered. Prescribe a 4-week trial and review. The restriction 'for use in women' has been removed.
- Co-danthramer (dantron with poloxamer) and co-danthrusate (dantron and docusate), combinations of a stimulant and a softener, are restricted to palliative care because of carcinogenesis in rats.
- The high cost of lactulose (and increased flatus production) should restrict the use of this osmotic laxative to the prevention of hepatic encephalopathy.

Change in bowel habit

Alternating diarrhoea and constipation is always a worrying symptom. Carcinoma of the large bowel must be excluded, but diverticular disease, large bowel ischaemia and irritable colon are more common.

As described for the investigation of anaemia, abdominal CT with contrast and flexible sigmoidoscopy are often used in preference to colonoscopy in frail older people.

Faecal incontinence

This is common and distressing. The prevalence varies with age and where people live, affecting

1 7% of community-dwelling over 65-year-olds,
2 10–15% of those living in residential homes,
3 55% of those living in nursing homes. This is not surprising, as faecal incontinence is a common reason for older people moving/being moved to institutional care.
   The true prevalence is likely to be higher as faecal incontinence is under-reported; people are embarrassed or think it is a normal part

of ageing. Women with faecal incontinence post-partum develop compensatory mechanisms, but comorbidities affecting mobility or stool consistency cause the faecal incontinence to recur or become obvious in later life. Most cases are multifactorial (see Table 14.7).

- Take a good history, including food and fluid intake, history of GI and neurological disease, medications, and operations, especially obstetric and rectal procedures.
- Examine the abdomen, perform a digital examination of the rectum to assess anal tone and sensation, look for fissures or fistulae, and complete a full neurological assessment.
- Initial management involves a trial of simple measures. In patients with disinhibition and lack of insight, e.g. those with dementia, try bulking preparations, and regular toileting.
- The cost of managing faecal incontinence with pads is enormous, and although they are often used, they should be a last resort.
- Provide information, e.g. about Radar keys to access accessible toilets and Bladder and Bowel UK for advice.
- Treat the underlying cause where possible, e.g. surgery for rectal prolapse.
- Some frail older people do well with codeine phosphate to cause constipation and enemas at regular intervals to empty the bowel.
- Other available devices include anal plugs, which are placed in the rectum and swell up as they absorb fluid from the mucosa to block the rectum for several hours so that the patient can go out. Liaise with your local continence advisor.
- If these measures fail and the patient is appropriate for surgical treatment, consider further investigations. Anorectal physiology is assessed using a pressure balloon to measure the resting tone and active tone. An ultrasound probe can assess the integrity of the internal and external anal sphincters. This information can be used to decide whether the patient is best managed with a surgical technique or neuromodulation; see Table 14.7.

Diverticular disease

Diverticula are small mucosal herniations through the bowel wall at the sites of weakness caused by nutrient vessels. The sigmoid bowel is the most common site as bowel contents are under the highest pressure. Diverticulosis describes the condition of non-inflamed diverticula. The prevalence of diverticulosis is over 50% of older people, and up to 70% in the over 80s.

- Men and women are affected equally.
- Is said to be a disease of the Western world due to a low fibre diet, constipation, and obesity. Interestingly, Westernisation of the diet in Japan is leading to more cases there.
- Seventy-five per cent of people with diverticulosis remain asymptomatic and require no treatment.
- Of the 25% with symptoms, 75% develop diverticulitis (and 25% of these develop complications which may include a profuse haemorrhage).
- Diverticulitis occurs when faecal matter collects in a diverticulum and obstructs it. This leads to local inflammation with mucous secretion and bacterial overgrowth. This may compromise the vascular supply resulting in a microperforation.

Clinical features

- Mild diverticulitis may present with low-grade symptoms like those of IBS such as colic, bloating and flatulence. IBS coexists in 30% of patients. In the community, the antibiotics of choice are co-amoxiclav 500/125 tds or trimethoprim 200 mg bd WITH metronidazole 400 mg tds for 5 days. Patients with severe disease and signs of peritonism must be admitted.

Complications of faecal incontinence:

- **Skin issues:** perianal irritation, excoriation, and skin damage.
- **Psychological issues:** depression, anxiety, and poor self-image.
- **Social isolation:** reluctance to go out and mix with friends and family.
- **Financial issues:** cost of continence products (may not request help or given an inadequate supply)
- **Caregiver burden:** increased work, distress and cost.
- **Institutionalisation:** often results in a demand for nursing home placement.

Table 14.7 Causes, mechanisms, examples, and management of faecal incontinence.

Cause	Mechanism	Examples	Management
History of obstetric trauma with damage to the pelvic floor or sphincter	Third-degree tear Instrumental delivery	Large baby Forceps damage to the pudendal nerve	Physiotherapy and biofeedback Anterior sphincter repair Overlapping sphincteroplasty
Peri-anal surgery	Trauma from anal stretch	Treatment of fistulas, fissures, and piles	As mentioned earlier
Colorectal disease	Weakness of internal anal sphincter	Rectal prolapse	Delorme's procedure (mucosa of the prolapsed bowel is removed, and the muscle layer is folded like a concertina and stitched back in, via the anus -low risk but high recurrence)
		Haemorrhoids Tumour	Surgery if appropriate. Stoma as a last resort
Increased transit time with very loose stool	Infection Inflammatory bowel disease	*C. difficile* Ulcerative colitis Crohn's disease	Appropriate antibiotics Steroids and mesalazine
	Irritable bowel syndrome		Dietary advice, bulking laxative drugs as incontinence is more likely with liquid stool, loperamide
	Radiation proctitis		Sulfasalazine orally and as enemas
Neurological	Cerebral	PD Stroke	Sacral neuromodulation via an implanted device
	Spinal	Spinal cord injury	
	Peripheral nerve	Diabetic autonomic neuropathy	
Overflow	Secondary to faecal impaction		Laxatives and enemas; may need manual evacuation. Aim to avoid recurrence with diet, fluids, mobilisation, and regular laxatives
Poor mobility	Unable to reach the toilet, unable to reach in time	OA Stroke, PD	Reduce the distance to the toilet, use the commode Simplify clothing
Lack of awareness	Dementia Learning disabilities	See Chapter 8	Large signs over toilet doors Coloured toilet doors and seats

IBD, inflammatory bowel disease; OA, osteoarthritis; PD, Parkinson's disease.

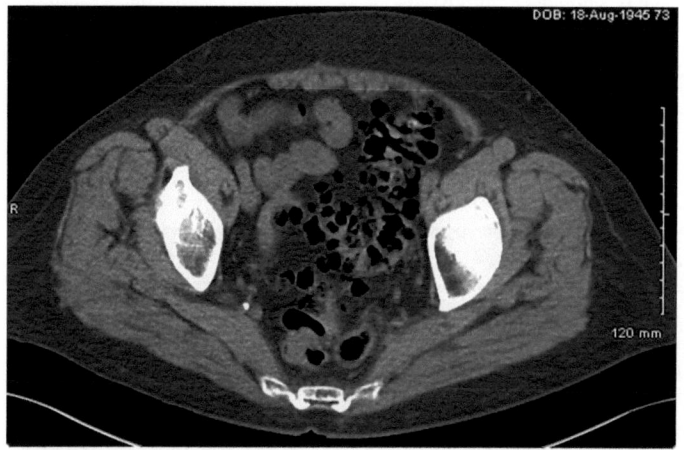

Figure 14.3 CT scan of a patient with pan-colonic diverticular disease showing multiple gas-filled diverticulae.

Investigation

- An erect CXR may show gas under the diaphragm if there has been a perforation.
- CT scanning of the abdomen may show colonic diverticula (Figure 14.3), pericolic fat stranding due to inflammation, bowel wall thickening, inflammatory masses, and abscesses.

Management

- Medical management in hospital includes:
  - Nil by mouth.
  - Wide-bore nasogastric tube.
  - Intravenous fluids (watch fluid balance and renal function carefully).
  - Antibiotics: often co-amoxiclav or cefuroxime plus metronidazole. Ciprofloxacin and metronidazole in penicillin allergy.
  - Good pain control, including opiates.
- Small abscesses can be drained percutaneously with CT guidance.
- Serious complications requiring surgical intervention are:
  - Peritonitis following perforation and faecal leakage.
  - Uncontrolled sepsis.
  - Fistula: e.g. bowel/bladder in men and bowel/vagina in women.
  - Obstruction.
  - Uncontrollable bleeding is due to small vessels stretched over a large diverticular mass.
  - Concern about a masked carcinoma.
- The most common surgical procedure is a Hartmann's procedure to remove the affected bowel and create an end-colostomy. The stoma can be reversed electively after a few months if the patient is well.
- The mortality of surgery in very frail older patients is high; explain this to the relatives to ensure expectation management.

Bowel ischaemia

Twenty per cent of cardiac output is used to supply the GI tract, so any significant drop is likely to affect the perfusion of the bowel and precipitate ischaemia.

At least two major mesenteric arteries must be compromised for bowel ischaemia to occur.

- Because of the poor anastomotic arrangement, the left side of the colon is the most vulnerable segment.
- Mesenteric angina: abdominal pain due to impaired bowel perfusion.
- Mechanism:
  - Arterial occlusion: 50% of cases.
  - Non-occlusive mechanisms (low flow): 20–30%.
  - Venous occlusion: 5–10%.

Factors associated with bowel ischaemia

- Embolisation, e.g. atrial fibrillation.
- Reduced cardiac output, e.g. hypotension and biventricular cardiac failure.
- Widespread atheroma.
- Drugs, e.g. oestrogens, antihypertensives, and psychotropic agents.
- Vasculitis, e.g. rheumatoid arthritis and polymyalgia rheumatica.
- Hypercoagulability.

Clinical course

Mild

- Post-prandial abdominal pain, diarrhoea, and weight loss.
- Mucosal swelling: the bowel wall may appear thickened on contrast CT scan.
- Recovery, plus or minus scarring (stricture).

Severe

- Sudden, severe pain but may be 'silent' with unexplained circulatory collapse.
- Movement of fluid into the bowel lumen, vomiting, diarrhoea, and shock.
- Rapid biochemical deterioration with hyperkalaemia and high lactate.
- Thickening of the bowel wall on contrast CT, sometimes with a target or halo appearance with IV contrast.
- Ischaemic bowel wall allows bacteria to cross from the lumen into the peritoneum, leading to peritonitis plus or minus septicaemia.
- Death is almost certain.

Management

Acute

- In mild disease, support fluids, broad-spectrum antibiotics, and heparin and treat the underlying cause to prevent a recurrence.
- In severe disease, consult colorectal surgeons to discuss resection; in most cases, supportive and palliative treatment is the mainstay.

Chronic

- Small, frequent meals; correct any nutritional deficiencies due to malabsorption.
- Consider warfarin/DOAC and treat any underlying arrhythmia.
- Peritonism makes laparotomy or palliative care mandatory.

Colorectal carcinoma

This is the most common malignancy of the GI tract and the second most common cause of death from cancer in the UK; it is rare in Africa and Asia. It is less aggressive than gastric or pancreatic adenocarcinoma; the 5-year survival of all newly diagnosed cases has improved to around 50%. Survival is stage-dependent, and screening has been introduced to improve early diagnosis. Eighty per cent of cases occur in people over the age of 60.

Clinical features

- Clinical presentation is often vague, but malaise, abdominal pain, change of bowel habit, rectal bleeding, tenesmus, or faecal incontinence, depending on the site of the lesion, are the usual pointers. Examination may reveal an abdominal or rectal mass or irregular hepatomegaly.
- Up to 30% of patients present with bowel obstruction; this confers a poorer prognosis as 40% have secondaries at presentation and <20% survive 5 years.
- Another acute presentation is with perforation (see Figure 14.4).

Investigation

Diagnosis is confirmed by rectal examination and sigmoidoscopy, followed by abdominal CT and/or colonoscopy for biopsy and molecular analysis and staging (see Figure 14.5).

Management

- The treatment plan will be discussed by a lower GI MDT. Fit older patients should be managed in the same way as their younger counterparts. The best option for cure of stage one and two disease is resection by a specialist colorectal surgeon in patients screened for frailty and optimised for surgery. Recovery is generally faster after laparoscopic surgery.
- Chemotherapy is increasingly offered to older patients for stage 3 patients with lymph node involvement. This is usually capecitabine with oxaliplatin (CAPOX) for 3 months.
- Patients with metastatic disease may be offered chemotherapy or targeted biologics. Monoclonal antibodies are promising; examples include pembrolizumab (for tumours with high microsatellite instability), cetuximab targeting epidermal growth factor receptors (EGFR), and bevacizumab targeting vascular endothelial growth factor (VEGF).
- Stoma specialist nurses have a key role in educating the patient and their family if a stoma is being considered. Some patients will accept a greater risk of local recurrence rather than having a stoma.

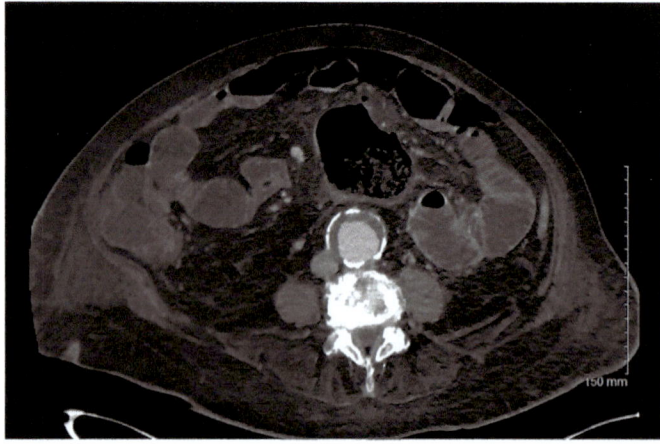

Figure 14.4 CT scan showing pneumoperitoneum due to perforation of sigmoid cancer. Note also the heavy aortic calcification, emphasising the comorbidity of older patients with colorectal cancer.

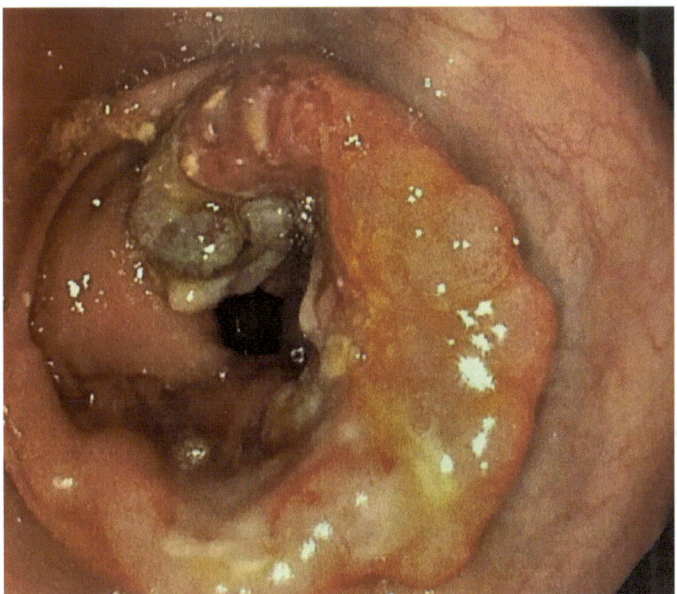

Figure 14.5 Colonoscopic view of adenocarcinoma in the colon. *Source*: Unknown Author/Wikimedia Commons/CC BY SA 3.0.

- Radiotherapy has a role in rectal cancers, as the rectum does not move like other parts of the gut, but older people may be more prone to complications, including VTE, hip and pelvic fractures, and the development of post-operative fistulae.
- Self-expanding intra-luminal stents offer some palliation for obstructive lesions.
- Patient education, support, and good palliative care when needed are essential.

Screening for bowel cancer

The UK uses the Faecal Immunochemical Test (FIT) to screen for bowel cancer in people aged 60–74 every 2 years. If the faecal Hb is greater than 10 mcg/g the patient is referred for colonoscopy.

Risk factors for carcinoma of the colon

- High red meat, processed meat, and animal fat intake.
- Low fibre intake from fruit and vegetables.
- Low physical activity.
- Obesity.
- High alcohol intake.
- Crohn's disease.
- Ulcerative colitis.
- Genetic tendency to form polyps (but the major genetic conditions, familial adenomatous polyposis and hereditary non-polyposis colon cancer, present when young).

Diseases affecting any part of the GI tract

GI bleeding

Older people are at increased risk of GI bleeds for several reasons. Many take antiplatelet therapy for cardiovascular and cerebrovascular disease. Some will be on a dual antiplatelet regimen and/or anticoagulants.

These patients should be co-prescribed a PPI and reviewed regularly to ensure that they are switched from dual to single platelet therapy as soon as clinically indicated.

In addition, most causes of GI bleeding become more common with increasing age, but 75% of cases are due to erosions or peptic ulceration.

- Hiatus hernia with oesophagitis.
- Varices.
- Mallory Weiss tear (after vomiting, but more common under 50).
- Gastritis and gastric erosions: older people taking NSAIDs have a sevenfold increased risk of bleeding compared with the same age group not taking such drugs.
- Gastric and duodenal ulcers.
- Carcinoma of the oesophagus and the stomach.
- Diverticular disease.
- Ischaemic bowel disease is sometimes difficult to differentiate from chronic inflammatory disease, e.g. Crohn's disease.
- Colonic polyps: 40% incidence in the over-65s in a post-mortem study.
- Colon cancer.
- Angiodysplasia.
- Haemorrhoids.

Acute upper GI bleed

This is particularly dangerous in older people, as the resulting hypotension may precipitate a stroke, MI, acute kidney injury or a fall causing a fracture. The mortality rate of acute GI bleeds in older people is 20%.

Symptoms include melaena with or without haematemesis or coffee ground vomit. Rectal blood from an upper GI lesion may be red rather than altered (melaena) if the bleeding is profuse. Other less localising symptoms include weakness, dizziness, increased confusion, and shortness of breath.

Management

- Assess haemodynamic status: remember that tachycardia will precede hypotension.
- In parallel, get more history from available sources and examine the abdomen and CVS.
- Get ITU support if help is needed to secure the patient's airway or if haemodynamically unstable.
- Risk stratification is done using scores such as the Glasgow-Blatchford Score (GBS).
- Insert two large bore cannulae.
- Replace volume with crystalloids.
- Measure baseline blood tests, including full blood count, prothrombin time, INR, and liver function tests; group and save.
- Recheck FBC within a few hours.
- Only transfuse if Hb drops to 70–90 g/L.
- If the patient is taking a DOAC, liaise with the haematology team for advice about local procedures for treatment with reversing agents.
- Endoscope within 24 hours if the patient is haemodynamically stable, as an emergency if not.
- Endoscopy not only shows the site of bleeding but also allows direct injection of a bleeding ulcer, which may help to stop bleeding. Gastric ulcers should be biopsied to look for malignancy.
- Give intravenous PPIs; there does not seem to be any advantage of a bolus versus infusion.

Acute lower GI bleed

- Massive lower GI bleeding is less common than from an upper GI source and is most often due to diverticular disease. Resuscitation follows similar lines.

- Acute, severe bowel ischaemia may present as rectal bleeding, and the ischaemia may be secondary to other pathology, e.g. a silent MI. A full assessment is therefore needed.
- Bleeding from the caecum in a patient with slow transit may present as melaena rather than red blood.

Chronic GI blood loss

Chronic GI bleeding is the most common cause of iron deficiency anaemia in older age in the UK (see Chapter 17). The bleeding site is often asymptomatic. Examination of both the upper and lower tract is needed in most cases. The discovery of a benign lesion should not prevent further exploration for more serious causes, provided the patient is sufficiently fit and willing to be investigated.

Investigation

Confirm the anaemia is due to iron deficiency (usually a microcytic anaemia with low serum iron; see Chapter 17).

- Consider whether GI bleeding is likely; faecal occult blood testing has been replaced by the FIT, as a negative test indicates that a significant colorectal pathology is less likely.
- Endoscopy of upper GI tract. Barium swallow is indicated for dysphagia.
- Flexible sigmoidoscopy followed by CT abdomen with oral and IV contrast to study the large bowel. Contrast CT of the abdomen is better tolerated than colonoscopy in frail older patients and gives extra information about the liver, pancreas, and lymph nodes. Barium enemas are rarely used.
- Colonoscopy, the gold standard, may require the patient to be hospitalised for bowel prep and, if poorly tolerated, the endoscopist may not reach the caecum. It is often used after CT to confirm an abnormality, biopsy or snare polyps, or to look for angiodysplasia.
- Radioisotope-labelled red cells during an episode may find the site of brisk intermittent bleeding of unknown cause.
- If no abnormality is found in the upper or lower bowel, capsule endoscopy is used to look for bleeding sites in the small bowel.

Treatment

- Specific treatment for the underlying causes.
- Iron supplements: oral ferrous sulphate if tolerated or intravenous iron.
- Transfuse only if haemoglobin is very low, e.g. less than 70 g/L or the patient has symptoms of heart failure or angina. (See chapter 17.)

The acute abdomen

This is a difficult diagnostic problem, but even more so in older age. The mortality rate in older patients may exceed 50%. There are four possible reasons for such depressing results:

1 Delay in presentation.
2 Atypical presentation, and the patient may downplay their symptoms.
3 The abdomen may appear benign on examination.
4 Increased frailty and comorbidities.

Perioperative care of older people undergoing surgery

The NCEPOD recommendations from 2010 are now embedded in the BGS guidelines:

- Review by senior surgeons/physicians with more input from geriatricians.
- Optimise assessment and management of all domains including medical, functional, psychological, and social.
- Better fluid balance, pain relief and nutrition to reduce complications such as AKI (Chapter 15) acute coronary syndromes, respiratory decompensation, and delirium.
- Review of all medications including venous thromboprophylaxis.
- Reduction of all risks for delirium.
- Optimise time to theatre; investigate and stabilise the patient but avoid delaying surgery in life-threatening conditions.
- Plan high-level post-operative care, e.g. high dependency or intensive care.
- Keep the patient and family well informed.
- Involve older patients in all research in this area, e.g. the National Emergency Laparotomy Audit (http://data.nela.org.uk/riskcalculator).

Common causes of acute abdomen in older people

- Ischaemic bowel, mortality rate can be as high as 50%.
- Ruptured abdominal aortic aneurysms.
- Bowel obstruction is commonly due to hernia, and adhesions (Figure 14.6), but also gallstone ileus and cancer in older people.
- Diverticulitis, occasionally leading to bowel perforation.
- Appendicitis.
- Peptic ulcer disease.
- Acute cholecystitis.
- Pancreatitis.
- Pyelonephritis.
- Abdominal pain can be due to non-abdominal pathology, e.g. acute MI, pneumonia, or an Addisonian crisis.

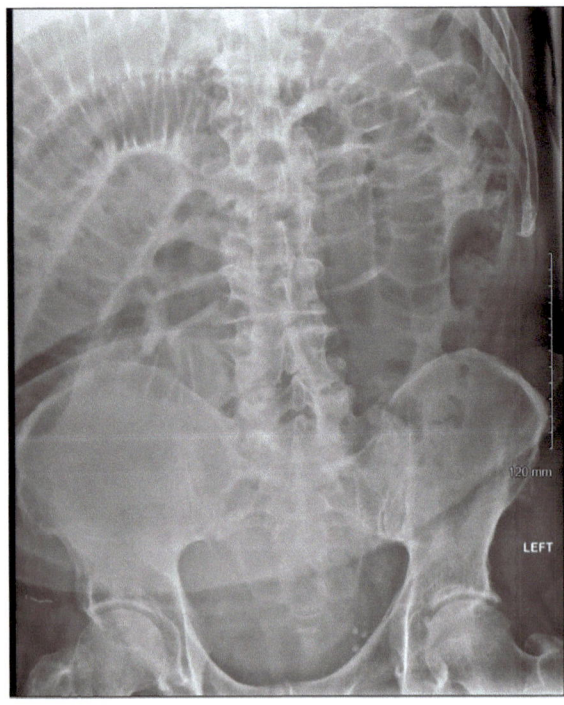

Figure 14.6 Abdominal radiograph showing small bowel obstruction due to adhesions. Note that the haustrations are visible across the whole bowel.

Useful pointers in the acute abdomen

- Abdominal scars from forgotten surgery.
- Check hernial orifices.
- Check lower limb pulses and use ultrasound to detect an aortic aneurysm.
- Check serum amylase: 50% of patients with acute pancreatitis are over 60.
- Do not forget ischaemic bowel.
- X-ray for fluid levels, free air in the peritoneal cavity, and distended bowel (e.g. coffee bean sign of sigmoid volvulus).
- Arrange an urgent CT scan.

Nutrition in older age

A range of physiological, psychosocial, and pathological factors affect nutritional status in later life.

The WHO defines clinically significant weight loss as a loss of >5% of usual body weight over 6–12 months.

- This is associated with increased morbidity and mortality.
- It affects 25% of over-65-year-olds living in the community and up to 60% of people in nursing homes.

Causes of unintentional weight loss

There is a tendency to lose weight in old age (in contrast to the weight gain common in middle age) but this is minor, around 0.1–0.2 kg/year, due to reduced body-water content, bone loss (osteoporosis), thinning of connective tissue, and the replacement of muscle with fat. Those who keep their lean body mass into old age have a better life expectancy than their shrinking peers. Significant weight loss is due to pathology.

- Oral and dental disease: review Table 14.1.
- Reduced olfactory, gustatory, and visual food perception reduces enjoyment of eating and, therefore, appetite.
- Reduced fluid intake is due to impaired thirst but also anxiety regarding toileting.
- GI disease, especially dysphagia, dyspepsia, and malabsorption.
- Cachexia syndromes: loss of muscle mass and other tissues due to the catabolism driven by tumour necrosis factor alpha (TNF-α) and interleukin 6 (IL-6) associated with chronic disorders, e.g. COPD, heart failure, and CKD.
- Other metabolic causes of weight loss include poorly controlled diabetes mellitus, thyrotoxicosis, and Addison's disease. Weight loss reflects the severity of the disease.
- Malignancy: GI malignancy accounts for 50% of cancers presenting with severe weight loss. The top 4 are gastric, colorectal, oesophageal, and pancreatic cancers.
- Psychiatric disease: the apathy of depression and self-neglect in some people living with dementia lead to weight loss. The paranoia of a psychosis may make food unacceptable. The hyperactivity of some demented and hypomanic patients may result in weight loss. Alcohol abuse should also be considered.
- Social isolation and loneliness, but also a change in environment, such as moving to a new care home or hospital admission.

- Reduced variety of food, including textures, e.g. older people being given a soft diet to reduce the risk of aspiration.
- Cost of living crisis.
- Loss of physical independence to shop, prepare food and feed oneself.
- Iatrogenic disease: impaired appetite may be due to unpalatable treatments, side effects, e.g. antibiotics (especially metronidazole and erythromycin), opiates, antidepressants, metformin, levodopa, or toxicity, e.g. digoxin. ACE inhibitors may cause a loss of taste or an unpleasant taste. Diarrhoea may be due to PPIs, cholinesterase inhibitors, misoprostol, or antibiotics. The burden of too many tablets may suppress appetite.
- Environment: Do not forget how unpleasant it is for patients in hospital to eat where they sleep, open their bowels, etc., and their proximity to others performing the same functions.

Diagnosis and management

- History: diet, appetite, taste, nausea, vomiting, dysphagia, abdominal pain, diarrhoea, change in bowel habit.
- Examination: cachexia, anaemia, dental health/fit of dentures, tongue, jaundice, lymphadenopathy, goitre, gross oedema, severe heart failure, obvious masses, organomegaly, and rectal examination.
- Assess mood and cognitive function.
- Baseline tests:
  - FBC: micro- or macrocytic anaemia.
  - LFTs: high ALP may be due to bone or liver metastases.
  - Remember that albumin is a poor marker of nutrition because it is a negative acute phase protein (i.e. levels drop in infection), moves to extravascular space during stress, is affected by fluid levels and liver function, and has a long half-life. However, a low albumin level is a predictor of increased morbidity and mortality.
  - TSH: suppressed in hyperthyroidism.
  - CRP and ESR: if normal, the cause is unlikely to be organic.
  - CXR: may show unexpected primary or secondary tumours.
  - Other tests, as indicated by the results of the above tests.
- Refer to the dietician team.
- Treat the underlying causes where possible.
- Explain to the patient and family when you recognise that this is an end-of-life event (see Chapter 22).

Assessment of nutritional status in old age

The Malnutrition Universal Screening Tool (MUST) is a straightforward scoring system that is validated for use in the community and in hospital. Factors indicating high risk are:

- Dietary history: reduced oral intake due to acute illness, score 1.
- Unintentional weight loss, score 1.
- BMI under >20 kg/m score 0, BMI 18.5-20kjg/m score 1, BMI < 18.5 kg/m score 2 (twice demi span may be substituted for height).

Total MUST score gives a risk for malnutrition:
0: low risk, 1: medium risk and 2 more: high risk.

Use the score to take appropriate action: refer to the dieticians, explore and treat the cause of the malnutrition, if possible.
Other red flags are:

- Reduced skinfold thickness.
- Reduced muscle power.
- Low blood levels of nutrients.
- Clinical evidence of nutritional disease.

A simple recipe for a good diet

- Eat wholemeal bread, not white bread.
- Have three portions of fresh vegetables daily.
- Eat two items of fresh fruit each day.
- Use 1/2 L (1 pint) of semi-skimmed milk daily for drinking and cooking.
- Have one small portion of meat or fish per day (preferably oily fish).
- Drink at least 2 litres of fluid a day.

Dietary deficiencies in older age

The most obvious are calories, protein, and fluid.

- **Vitamin B group:** refractory heart failure, macrocytic anaemia due to folate deficiency, peripheral neuropathy, dementia, vascular disease, and thromboembolism.
- **Vitamin C:** scurvy.
- **Vitamin D:** osteomalacia; supplementation recommended in all adults in the UK in winter.
- **Minerals:** iron, zinc, selenium are most readily obtained from animal protein and calcium from dairy foods. Those who follow a vegan or strict vegetarian diet or are eating very little are most at risk of deficiencies. Mineral deficiencies are often multiple. There are no common distinct deficiency syndromes, apart from iron deficiency anaemia. Zinc deficiency may be linked to macular degeneration.
- **Fibre:** diseases of 'Western civilisation'.

NB: The routine use of vitamins and mineral supplements has not been proven to benefit 'free range' older subjects. Even in vulnerable groups (people living in care homes or hospitals), there is no evidence for blanket supplementation, but if deficiencies are found, they should be corrected.

Management of subnutrition in the community

- Improve general health: treat underlying conditions.
- Encourage supervised meals, e.g. 'meals on wheels', luncheon clubs, meal preparation by home help, and microwave meals.
- Education of patients and carers.
- A balanced diet is the best source of nutrition, vitamins, and minerals. Supplements such as Fortisips and Forticreme should be used in addition to, not instead of, real food.

Management of subnutrition in institutions

According to Age UK, those admitted to hospital over the age of 80 are twice as likely to become malnourished as those under 50. The consequences are serious and lead to prolonged hospital stays due to:

- Poor healing and recovery.
- Increased risk of complications, e.g. infection, pressure ulcers, falling and depression.

    Attention must be paid to:

- Suitable foods, e.g. familiar, easy to swallow, enjoyable and energy-rich. Ask the patient or family what they like.
- Small, frequent meals and snacks.
- Protected mealtimes.
- Food and drink placed within reach.
- Provision of modified utensils.
- Help with feeding, when necessary, from food being cut up, to spoon feeding. A red tray system reminds staff who need extra help and encouragement.

How to encourage oral intake: food first

Avoid restrictive diets, e.g. for diabetes or to reduce aspiration risk	Often, energy poor Often not palatable
Offer the most calories at a time of day to suit the individual	Older people may eat the most calories at breakfast time. Consider hard-boiled eggs with toast or cereal bars
Finger food for people with dementia	People living with dementia often pace or are distracted at mealtimes, so put food in their hands and offer fruit with the skin still on
Small meals more often	A mid-morning snack and afternoon tea are useful
Offer foods of different tastes and textures	Add sweetcorn to sandwiches; try crunchy peanut butter on biscuits
Optimise oral health	Use dental fixatives, treat oral thrush, and consider artificial saliva
Add extra fat to normal food intake	E.g. cream to soup and porridge, butter to mashed potatoes, full-fat yoghurt
Use flavour enhancers	Herbs and spices, sugar and salt, unless specifically contraindicated
Food first: offer nutritious meals	Only offer supplements where intake is poor

---

- Eating in selected groups at a table increases both pleasure and intake.
- Enriched food, supplements, and artificial feeding (see Chapter 21).

Those most at risk in hospitals and care homes are people with end-stage disease or living with severe dementia. The best solution is provision of appetising, nutritious meals, but this takes weeks to make a difference, and improvement is unlikely towards the end of life.

Nasogastric feeding

Nasogastric (NG) tube feeding is used short-term in patients with functional bowels. A fine-bore feeding tube is inserted via the nose into the stomach for the delivery of nutrition and medications. Scenarios include acute dysphagia, which is expected to recover, or temporary poor oral intake due to an acute illness. Bridled loop NG tubes can be useful for patients with delirium or dementia who are likely to pull the tube out, but again, use should be short-term. Feeding into the lung is a 'never event' so it is essential to check the correct placement either with a gastric pH less than 5.5 or a CXR before starting the feed (see Figure 14.7).

Complications include aspiration, oesophagitis, stricture, GI bleeding, and very rarely perforation.

Percutaneous endoscopic gastrostomy tubes

If long-term treatment is contemplated, consider percutaneous endoscopic gastrostomy (PEG) feeding.

To place a PEG feeding tube, OGD is performed with a standard endoscope and gastric fluid is aspirated. The stomach is filled with air to approximate the stomach wall to the abdominal wall, and the endoscope light is used to shine through the anterior abdominal wall. A skin incision is made, and the feeding tube is introduced using the catheter-over-needle technique.

- In patients over 50, 18% die within 1 month of the procedure, 44% die within 6 months, 54% within 1 year, and 73% within 2 years.
- Only 9% of PEG-fed patients return to oral feeding, i.e. 90% have a PEG until death.
- Twelve per cent of patients are said to pull their own tubes out.

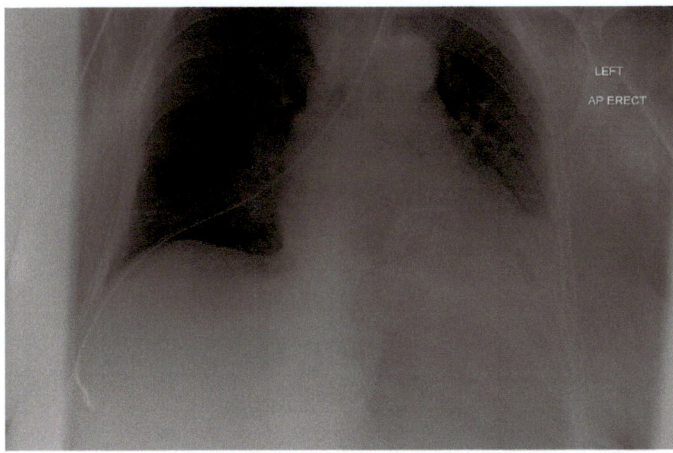

Figure 14.7 CXR shows a nasogastric tube inserted into the right main bronchus.

- Many hospitals have a multidisciplinary feeding team to discuss the appropriateness of each individual patient.
- In patients with dementia, there is no evidence that PEG feeding:
  ○ Reduces aspiration pneumonia.
  ○ Promotes pressure sore healing.
  ○ Improves functional status.
  ○ Provides comfort.
  ○ Prolongs life.
- For more discussion about the use of feeding tubes, see Chapters 9 and 21.

Total parenteral nutrition (TPN): is only indicated for older patients with non-functioning guts, e.g. high-output fistulas. It is given via a PICC line and should only be used for a specified time until a definitive procedure or decision is made. TPN is expensive but can improve nutritional status in as little as 7–10 days. Complications include line infections and fluid overload.

Refeeding syndrome: this occurs when a patient who has not been eating is started on nutritional support, most commonly NG feeding. This leads to dramatic shifts in electrolytes: hypophosphataemia, hypomagnesaemia, and hypokalaemia, thiamine deficiency, and fluid overload, which may lead to heart failure and arrhythmias. The key is to check levels daily and replace them as needed 30 min before feeding recommences.

Overnutrition

- Ageing is associated with the loss of up to 40% of fat-free mass in the form of skeletal muscle.
- Fat is distributed around organs, skeletal muscle, and the liver.
- The basal metabolic rate declines by 2–3% per decade after the age of 20.
- Physical activity also tends to reduce.
- The epidemic of morbid obesity in the Western world includes older people and is associated with higher rates of disability and morbidity.
- In the UK: 37% of men and 34% of women aged over 60 have a BMI ≥ 30 kg/m².
- The cost to the NHS of managing obesity is estimated to rise to £9.7 billion by 2050. This is because of the need for bariatric beds, pressure mattresses, clinic chairs, frames, commodes, etc.
- Whilst people with obesity remain well, they cope, but if they become sick and are admitted to hospital, they are at considerable risk of becoming immobile and needing significant support to regain mobility.
- The extra nutritional reserves they carry may be of benefit.

Carrying excess weight into old age can be detrimental to well-being through worsening of:

- Angina.
- Breathlessness.
- Glycaemic control and insulin resistance.
- Blood pressure.
- Arthritis in weight-bearing joints (hence pain and immobility).
- Depression and low self-esteem.
- Peri-operative complications.
- Rehabilitation outcomes.

However, multiple studies and meta-analyses suggest an 'obesity paradox' in that people over 65 years with a BMI of 28–31 kg/m² have the lowest overall mortality.

Management: weight-reducing diets, increased exercise where able. No quick fix is available, although drugs such as semaglutide and tirzepatide, glucagon-like peptide-1 receptor agonists, offer dramatic weight loss in younger adults, and trials are needed in older people.

📖 REFERENCES AND FURTHER READING

Bartlett D, O'Toole S (2019) Tooth wear and ageing. *Aust. Dent. J.* 64(S1):S59–S62. doi: 10.1111/adj.12681.

Christmas C, Rogus-Pulia N (2019) Swallowing disorders in the older population *J Am Geriatr. Soc.* 67:2643–2649. doi: 10.1111/jgs.16137.

Ko MS, Fung KZ, Shi Y, et al. (2016) Barrett's esophagus commonly diagnosed in elderly men with limited life expectancy. *J. Am. Geriatr. Soc.* 64:e109–e111. doi: 10.1111/jgs.14409.

NICE CKS (2023) *Dyspepsia – unidentified cause* https://cks.nice.org.uk/topics/dyspepsia-unidentified-cause

Tajiri K, Shimizu Y (2013) Liver physiology and liver diseases in the elderly. *World J. Gastroenterol.* 19:8459–8467. doi: 10.3748/wjg.v19.i46.8459.

Kim IH, Kisseleva T, Brenner DA (2015) Aging and liver disease. *Curr. Opin. Gastroenterol.* 31:184–91. doi: 10.1097/MOG.0000000000000176.

Köstenbauer JK, Gandy RC, Close J, et al. (2023) Factors affecting early cholecystectomy for acute cholecystitis in older people – a population-based study. *World J. Surg.* 47:1704–1710. doi: 10.1007/s00268-023-06968-9.

NICE CKS (2020) *Coeliac Disease.* https://cks.nice.org.uk/topics/coeliac-disease

Lancet Editorial (2019) *C. difficile* – rose by any other name. *Lancet Infect. Dis.* 19:449. doi: 10.1016/S1473-3099(19)30177-X.

Gov.UK (2023) *Data on C difficile infections* https://www.gov.uk/government/statistics/clostridium-difficile-infection-annual-data#full-publication-update-history

Fedor I, Zold E, Barta Z (2022) Microscopic colitis in older adults: impact, diagnosis, and management. *Ther. Adv. Chronic Dis.* 13:20406223221102821. doi: 10.1177/20406223221102821.

Ananthakrishnan AN, Shi HY, Tang W, et al. (2016) Systematic review and meta-analysis: phenotype and clinical outcomes of older-onset inflammatory bowel disease. *J. Crohns Colitis* 10:1224–1236. doi: 10.1093/ecco-jcc/jjw054.

NICE CKS (2023) Constipation in adults. https://cks.nice.org.uk/topics/constipation/management/adults

NICE CKS (2022) Faecal incontinence in adults. https://cks.nice.org.uk/topics/faecal-incontinence-in-adults

NICE CKS (2023) Diverticular disease. https://cks.nice.org.uk/topics/diverticular-disease

Monahan KJ, Davies MM, Abulafi M, et al. (2022) Faecal immunochemical testing (FIT) in patients with signs or symptoms of suspected colorectal cancer: a joint guideline from the Association of Coloproctology of Great Britain and Ireland and the British Society of Gastroenterology. *Gut* 71:1939–1962. https://gut.bmj.com/content/71/10/1939.

Millan M, Merino S, Caro A, et al. (2015) Treatment of colorectal cancer in the elderly. *World J. Gastrointest. Oncol.* 7:204–220. doi: 10.4251/wjgo.v7.i10.204.

Cancer Research UK: http://cancerhelp.cancerresearchuk.org For excellent statistics on cancers, patient information and up-to-date treatments see the relevant sections.

Alkhatib AA, Elkhatib FA, Alkhatib AA, et al. (2010) Acute upper gastrointestinal bleeding in elderly people: presentations, endoscopic findings, and outcomes. *J. Am. Geriatrics Soc.* 58:182–185. doi: 10.1111/j.1532-5415.2009.02633.x.

Chait MM (2010) Lower gastrointestinal bleeding in the elderly. *World J. Gastrointest. Endosc.* 2:147–154. doi: 10.4253/wjge.v2.i5.147.

NCEPOD (2010) *An Age Old Problem: A review of the care received by elderly patients undergoing surgery* www.ncepod.org.uk/2010report3/downloads/EESE_fullReport.pdf.

Desai J (2018) *BGS Guidelines for Peri-operative care of older people undergoing surgery.* www.bgs.org.uk/resources/peri-operative-care-for-older-patients-undergoing-surgery

Spangler R, Van Pham T, Khoujah D, et al. (2014) Abdominal emergencies in the geriatric patient. *Int. J. Emerg. Med.* 7:43. doi: 10.1186/s12245-014-0043-2.

McMinn J, Steel C, Bowman A (2011) Investigation and management of unintentional weight loss in older adults. *BMJ* 342:754–759. https://www.bmj.com/content/342/bmj.d1732.

NICE Nutrition support in adults (2012) www.nice.org.uk/guidance/qs24/chapter/quality-statement-1-screening-for-the-risk-of-malnutrition

Aubry E, Friedli N, Schuetz P, et al. (2018) Refeeding syndrome in the frail elderly population: prevention, diagnosis and management. *Clin. Exp. Gastroenterol.* 11:255–264. doi: 10.2147/CEG.S136429.

Samper-Ternent R, Al Snih S (2012) Obesity in older adults: epidemiology and implications for disability and disease. *Rev. Clin. Gerontol.* 22:10–34. doi: 10.1017/s0959259811000190.

McKee AM, Morley JE (2021) Obesity in the elderly. In Feingold KR, Anawalt B, Blackman MR, et al. editors. *Endotext [Internet].* South Dartmouth (MA). PMID: 30379513

INFORMATION FOR PATIENTS AND FAMILIES

AlzheimerUK: living with dentures: https://www.alzheimers.org.uk/get-support/daily-living/dentures-dementia

Coeliac UK: www.coeliac.org.uk/home

Patient information about C. difficile diarrhoea: https://patient.info/digestive-health/diarrhoea/clostridium-difficile-c-diff

St Marks guide to anal sphincter exercises: https://www.stmarkshospital.nhs.uk/wp-content/uploads/2014/05/Anal-sphincter-exercises-for-leakage.pdf

NHS 8 tips for healthy eating: https://www.nhs.uk/live-well/eat-well/how-to-eat-a-balanced-diet/eight-tips-for-healthy-eating

Association of British Dieticians, Foodfacts: Fibre: www.bda.uk.com/resource/fibre.html

All websites were acceswsed in September 2024.

15

Genitourinary medicine

Age-related changes

1 With increasing age, renal function is reduced to about 50% of the peak at 30 years old; glomerular filtration rate (GFR) declines by 6.3 mL/min/1.73 m^2 per decade.

2 Serum urea may remain in the normal range despite deteriorating renal function.

3 Creatinine reflects muscle bulk, so beware the frail elderly patient with a 'normal' level of creatinine.

4 The estimated glomerular filtration rate (eGFR) can be calculated using the creatinine, gender, and age. This only applies in steady states, not in an acute deterioration.

5 Both the ability to concentrate urine and the ability to process an extra water load quickly are impaired. This is one explanation for nocturia in old age. The maximum urine concentration falls from 1,300 to 850 mOsm/L.

6 There is loss of renal mass, affecting the cortex more than the medulla, in half of 'normal' elderly kidneys.

7 Reduced renal function is due to:
   (a) Loss and sclerosis of glomeruli, leading to fewer functioning nephrons,
   (b) Reduced renal blood flow, particularly to the cortex,
   (c) Diminished response to antidiuretic hormone (ADH).

8 These effects are exaggerated in hypertension, diabetes and after pyelonephritis.

9 The combination of ageing changes and systemic or renal disease may lead to a rapid, dramatic deterioration in renal function that does not resolve.

10 Atrophic changes occur in the urogenital tract of post-menopausal women as oestrogen levels fall, contributing to urinary incontinence (UI), dysuria, and discomfort.

11 In men, the size of the prostate increases, and cancerous foci become more common.

12 The incidence of an unstable bladder increases due to sudden, uncontrollable surges in bladder pressure secondary to contractions whilst filling (detrusor instability).

Acute kidney injury

Acute kidney injury (AKI) is defined as 'an abrupt (within hours) decrease in kidney function, which encompasses both injury (structural damage) and impairment (loss of function)'. It is a syndrome, and there is often a mixed aetiology (see Table 15.1). A period of renal hypoperfusion leads to ischaemia, an inflammatory response and acute tubular necrosis, although non-lethal cell injury is more common than frank necrosis.

In the acute situation, as recent renal function may not be known, the most useful criteria for recognition of AKI are a rise in serum creatinine of $\geq 26 \mu$mol/L within 48 hours or a fall in urine output in an adult to less than 0.5 mL/kg/hr for more than 6 hours. 'Injury' has replaced 'failure'

Table 15.1 Prerenal, renal, and post-renal causes of acute kidney injury common in older people.

Pre-renal	Renal	Post-renal	Inflammatory
Dehydration	Acute tubular necrosis due to ischaemia (usually a prerenal cause)	Ureteric stones	Allergic interstitial nephritis
Blood loss, e.g. GI bleed	Nephrotoxins, e.g. drugs, contrast agents	Prostatic hypertrophy	Drugs such as PPIs, NSAIDs, and antibiotics
Pump failure	Myoglobinuria secondary to rhabdomyolysis (after falling)	Prostate cancer	OTC medications, such as Chinese herbal medicine
Over-treatment of hypertension/CHF	Allergic interstitial nephritis	Gynaecological cancer	
Sepsis (vasodilation)	Systemic diseases – myeloma, gout, etc.	Bladder cancer	
Renovascular disease	Glomerulonephritides	Retroperitoneal fibrosis	

GI, gastrointestinal; PPIs, proton pump inhibitors; NSAIDs, nonsteroidal anti-inflammatory drugs; OTC, over the counter; CHF, chronic heart failure.

Geriatric Medicine and Elderly Care: Lecture Notes, Ninth Edition. Claire G. Nicholl, K. Jane Wilson, and Shaun D'Souza.
© 2025 John Wiley & Sons Ltd. Published 2025 by John Wiley & Sons Ltd.
Companion website: www.wiley.com/go/lecturenotesgeriatricmedicine9e

as even modest reductions in renal function are associated with worse outcomes. AKI warnings are now generated automatically from the biochemistry lab.

- AKI is common in older people on admission to hospital and is a frequent complication after admission.
- The ageing kidney does not have sufficient reserve to tolerate insults such as dehydration and sepsis, and pre-existing renal damage from cardiovascular disease, especially hypertension, diabetes and poor nutrition, increases the vulnerability of old kidneys.
- AKI is usually multifactorial, and iatrogenic factors such as drugs and inadequate fluid management often contribute.
- Twenty-nine per cent of the episodes of hospital-acquired AKI are in those aged 75–84 and 27% in those aged 85 and over.
- Older patients who develop hospital-acquired AKI have a high mortality rate, and those who survive may not recover baseline kidney function.
- Therefore, it is essential to check for reversible factors early in the admission.

History

- Consider all causes of volume depletion and hypotension: e.g. poor oral intake, vomiting, diarrhoea, GI bleed, sepsis, over-diuresis, ACS and antihypertensives. Acute-onset postural dizziness in the context of AKI suggests volume depletion.
- Ask about all drugs, including over the counter (OTC) herbal preparations, as some cause allergic interstitial nephritis. Check medications carefully, and ideally with a collateral source. The patient may not be taking their medication as prescribed – diuretics may be omitted if they have urinary incontinence.
- Ask about lower urinary tract symptoms (LUTS), pointing to a postrenal cause.
- Past medical history: prostate, bladder, ovarian, cervical, or uterine cancer.
- Review previous blood results to check baseline function. Does the patient have a known chronic kidney disease (CKD)?

Examination

- Assess fluid status (patients with oedema can still be intravascularly depleted). Check lying and standing blood pressure and heart rate. A postural drop and tachycardia indicate hypovolaemia.
- Fever, tachycardia, and low blood pressure suggest sepsis.
- Check the jugular venous pressure (JVP) carefully. Is this cardiorenal syndrome?
- Is the bladder palpable?
- Rectal examination; size and character of the prostate; constipation.
- Is there bruising/skin damage to suggest a long lie after a fall, leading to muscle damage and rhabdomyolysis?

Investigations

- Urgent electrolytes: hyperkalaemia is the most immediately life-threatening abnormality. Hypernatraemia is common in severe dehydration, with drowsiness leading to poor oral intake; the prognosis is extremely poor.
- Bicarbonate: low bicarbonate suggests metabolic acidosis.
- ECG to check for effects of hyperkalaemia (see Figure 15.1).
- FBC, CRP and ESR to check for sepsis or inflammation. A normocytic anaemia may suggest this is CKD.
- Glucose and HbA1c.
- Bone profile: high phosphate suggests CKD.
- ABG and lactate: is there acidosis?

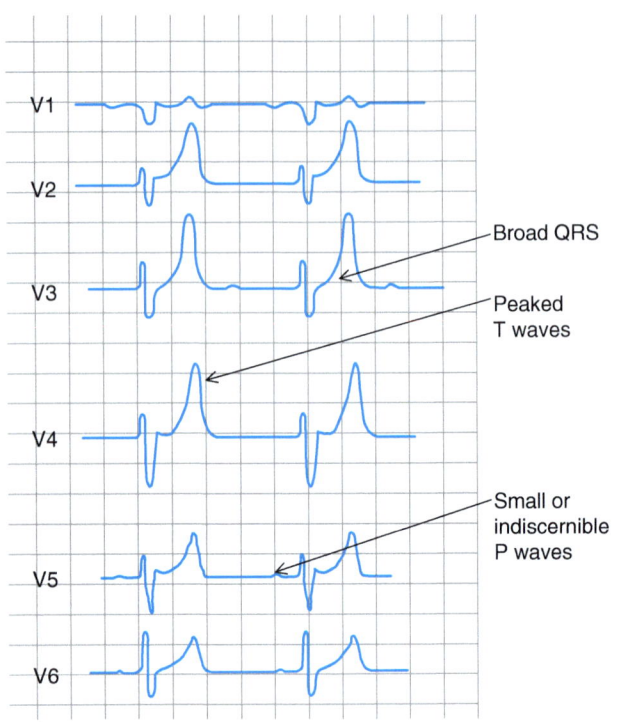

Broad QRS
Peaked T waves
Small or indiscernible P waves

Figure 15.1 ECG in hyperkalaemia. *Source*: Mikael Häggström/Wikimedia Commons/public domain.

- Blood cultures to find the source of sepsis.
- Tests for aetiology if glomerulonephritis is suspected.
- CXR: looking for cardiomegaly, pneumonia, pulmonary oedema, and infiltrates (vasculitis).
- Ultrasound: assess for bladder outflow obstruction (BOO), hydronephrosis and kidney size (bilateral small kidneys suggest CKD).
- Urinalysis: leucocytes and nitrites suggest infection; blood (non visible haematuria) and protein suggest renal disease.
- Midstream urine (MSU): microscopy for casts and culture.
- Further tests, guided by the initial results, might include creatine kinase, protein electrophoresis and Bence–Jones protein, uric acid, autoantibodies, and a CT scan.

Management

Treat hyperkalaemia urgently: intravenous calcium gluconate first (30 mL of 10% over 10 min; repeat after 5–10 min if ECG changes are still present) and then 50 mL of 50% dextrose with 10 units of Actrapid insulin over 20 min.

Monitor closely for subsequent hypoglycaemia, particularly in frail older patients with low body mass. Salbutamol nebulisation is often given as an adjunct to insulin-dextrose in severe cases. Consider Lokelma (sodium zirconium cyclosilicate), a non-absorbed cation-exchange compound, 10 mg tds for 72 hours.

- Fluid resuscitate: if in doubt as to whether the patient is dry, give 250 mL of 0.9% saline stat, review and repeat as needed.
- Catheter to relieve urinary obstruction and monitor urine output.
- Antibiotics for sepsis.
- Stop nephrotoxins, especially nonsteroidal anti-inflammatory drugs (NSAIDs) and diuretics, ACEi, ARBs and other antihypertensives if the patient is dry or hypotensive. Check ALL drugs on the chart in the BNF – do not rely on your memory.
- Reduce the dose of drugs metabolised by the kidneys, e.g. dalteparin and gentamicin.

- Daily weights help to guide fluid balance.
- Acute hydronephrosis: a nephrostomy tube is inserted under ultrasound guidance. If the hydronephrosis is secondary to a stone blocking the ureter, refer to urology for the insertion of a J–J stent. If the hydronephrosis is secondary to a tumour, it may be more appropriate to leave the nephrostomy in situ for symptomatic relief.
- Refer to nephrology for advice, including consideration of temporary haemofiltration in the intensive care unit for previously fit patients expected to survive the underlying cause. (This gives time to allow acute tubular necrosis to resolve.)

Managing complications

- Hyperkalaemia as discussed earlier.
- Acidosis: slow sodium bicarbonate infusion (seek specialist advice).
- Pulmonary oedema: give high-dose intravenous furosemide; consider IV GTN.
- Patients developing respiratory failure and encephalopathy have multi-organ failure, and the focus of care should be moved to symptom control.

Prevention of AKI

As ever, prevention is easier than cure.

- Maintain euvolaemia and correct hypovolaemia if detected.
- Look carefully for sepsis and treat it aggressively.
- There is still controversy about the dangers of iodine-based contrast media; current advice is to check eGFR if there is a history of CKD or diabetes and in those over 75. Discuss proposed imaging with radiology, and if considered essential, ensure good peri-procedure hydration with IV 0.9% sodium chloride.
- Recognise patients with CKD and manage them holistically.

Chronic kidney disease

CKD is defined as a reduction in kidney function or structural damage (or both) present for more than 3 months, with associated health implications. As explained earlier, interpret creatinine carefully because older people tend to have a lower muscle mass and therefore a lower creatinine level, whatever the renal function.

- CKD is diagnosed using eGFR, which is based on the MDRD (Modification of Diet in Renal Disease) calculation. MDRD GFR Equation (http://mdcalc.com)
- The Cockcroft–Gault equation includes weight and may be better for calculating doses of nephrotoxic drugs in older patients and patients at extremes of muscle mass. https://www.mdcalc.com/calc/43/creatinine-clearance-cockcroft-gault-equation

CKD is common: 70% of the over-70s have CKD 3 – this reflects vascular disease and renal ageing; these people are more likely to die from vascular disease than kidney failure. It has been suggested that a more appropriate GFR threshold for the diagnosis of CKD in those over 65 is <45 mL/min.

Common causes of CKD in older people

1 Diabetes mellitus.
2 Hypertension.
3 Obstructive uropathy.
4 Chronic pyelonephritis.
5 Cardiac insufficiency.
6 Nephrotoxic drugs.

Table 15.2 Stages of CKD.

Stage	Description	eGFR (mL/min/1.73 m²)
1	Normal or increased eGFR	≥ 90
2	Mildly decreased eGFR	60–89
3	Moderately decreased eGFR	30–59
4	Severely decreased eGFR	15–29
5	Kidney failure	< 15

7 Renovascular disease.
8 Myeloma.
9 Systemic vasculitis.

Symptoms

Table 15.2 shows the stages of CKD defined by eGFR. Symptoms appear usually only in CKD 4/5:

- Poor appetite.
- Nausea and vomiting.
- Tiredness.
- Breathlessness and peripheral oedema due to salt and water retention.
- Itching due to uraemia.
- Nocturia and polyuria due to being unable to concentrate urine.
- Restless legs.

Signs

The signs of possible causes may be present early in CKD, but the other findings are seen in end-stage kidney disease (ESKD).

- Fluid balance is variable: there may be hypovolaemia due to infection, dehydration, or fluid overload.
- Uraemic frost (anaemia plus uraemia).
- Bruising.
- Excoriation marks.
- Hypertension, or postural hypotension.
- Palpate for a palpable bladder or enlarged kidneys.
- Rectal examination for an enlarged prostate.
- Peripheral neuropathy.

Investigations

- As for AKI.
- Also, look for anaemia (decreased erythropoietin – epo – production from renal fibroblasts).
- Renal bone disease (increased PTH due to deficient 1α hydroxylation of vitamin D in proximal tubule mitochondria and phosphate retention).
- Sodium is sometimes low.
- Potassium may be raised and will need urgent management, as discussed earlier.
- Calcium may be low, normal, or high.
- Heavy proteinuria is suggestive of glomerular disease.
- Urine albumin-creatinine ratio (uACR): protein in the urine is a key marker of kidney damage. Most of the protein found in urine is albumin. A 'first catch' specimen should be tested – i.e. the first part of the urine stream from the first morning void.
  - Less than 3 mg/mmol (no proteinuria), no action is needed.
  - Between 3 and 70 mg/mmol, repeat the test within 3 months.
  - 70 mg/mmol or more, a repeat test is not needed as this indicates significant proteinuria.

- Repeat tests (typically 3 tests within 3 months) are required to confirm the presence of albuminuria. A patient is said to have albuminuria if 2 out of 3 tests are positive. CKD is present if the albuminuria persists for 3 months even if the eGFR is normal, and an abnormal uACR can be used to subdivide the stages of CKD.
- A biopsy is rarely helpful if both kidneys are small.

Management

The overall context, i.e. the patient's other comorbidities and cognition, must be considered, as well as their wishes.

The objectives are to:

1 Minimise progression.
2 Reduce complications.
3 Treat cardiovascular risk factors: if there are no contraindications, use aspirin and atorvastatin; target BP <140/80, if possible, without inducing symptomatic postural hypotension.
4 Control symptoms.
   - Encourage a healthy diet, such as the Mediterranean diet, to reduce BMI.
   - The best drugs to reduce blood pressure and proteinuria are ACEi and ARBs, but they reduce renal blood flow and may worsen renal function if the patient is hypovolaemic. Start with a small dose, and monitor!
   - Good diabetic control will support kidney function.
   - Sodium-glucose cotransporter-2 (SGLT2) inhibitors such as dapagliflozin and empagliflozin can also slow deterioration in kidney function, with or without proteinuria, but they should be avoided in people with T1DM as they can precipitate ketoacidosis.
   - Some trusts offer a renal MDT discussion for patients whose renal function has reduced to 15% to advise on the suitability of kidney replacement therapy (KRT), the management of anaemia and other complications.
   - Effective communication and education of the patient and their family are essential to improving concordance with fluid restriction, renal diet, blood sugar control and medications.

Complications

- Patients with severe fluid retention may need high-dose loop diuretics with the cautious addition of a thiazide, e.g. metolazone, watching the potassium.
- Review medications: avoid nephrotoxins, reduce doses and monitor levels where appropriate. See 'Drugs and the kidney' discussed later.
- Darbepoetin (recombinant human erythropoietin) injections/iron infusions for symptomatic anaemia.
- Hyperphosphataemia is due to reduced filtration of phosphate by the kidneys. It can be treated with phosphate binders. Calcium acetate is the first line, but if this is unsuitable, e.g. because of hypercalcaemia, sevelamer, a non-calcium-based phosphate binder should be offered.
- Chronic hyperkalaemia used to be managed with calcium resonium, but patiromer (Veltassa), a non-absorbed calcium-sorbitol cation exchange polymer, or sodium zirconium cyclosilicate (Lokelma), which exchanges potassium for hydrogen and sodium, are better tolerated and more effective. Both increase faecal potassium excretion by binding potassium in the lumen of the GI tract.
- The 'renal diet' (low sodium, potassium, and phosphate) is often unpalatable and is not necessary for end-of-life patients.
- Metabolic acidosis can be reduced with sodium bicarbonate tablets.
- Secondary hyperparathyroidism due to high phosphate levels affects calcium metabolism and leads to renal osteodystrophy. This can be treated with colecalciferol (D3).
- Palliative care when needed.

Kidney replacement therapy

Kidney replacement therapy (KRT) is started for patients with CKD 5 with complications such as fluid overload, symptomatic uraemia and electrolyte disturbances. In the UK in 2021, from registry data, 8,175 adult patients started KRT for ESKD at a median age of 63.7 years. About 25% were aged 65–74, 20% 75–84, and 3% ≥85 years. Most started with in-centre haemodialysis.

Studies on KRT in older people are observational and retrospective, and the outcomes depend on the age and frailty of patients taken on for dialysis. Life expectancy on dialysis is poor, and the improvement in quality of life is variable. For patients aged 75–84, 10% die within the first 90 days of starting dialysis and another 20% die in the following year (the top three causes being treatment withdrawal, infection, and cardiac disease). The alternative is conservative kidney management (CKM).

- KRT will not be recommended for patients with frailty, dementia, poor cardiac output, and multiple comorbidities, as it will not extend life expectancy and is unlikely to improve the quality of life.
- Selected patients with good self-care skills may manage continuous ambulatory peritoneal dialysis (CAPD) at home. This avoids the BP swings that occur with haemodialysis but has a significant risk of peritonitis.
- Withdrawal of dialysis when patients become frail or cachexic and the burden of dialysis is greater than the benefit usually gives a life expectancy of 3 weeks or less. The end of life can be managed at home or a hospice (see Chapter 22).

Intrinsic kidney disease

In older patients, specific kidney diseases are less common than pre- and post-renal causes of AKI, but glomerulonephritis is still an important cause of ESKD.

Nephrotic syndrome

In a series of patients aged over 50 (diabetics were excluded), the underlying cause, in order of incidence, was:

1 Membranous glomerulonephritis.
2 Proliferative glomerulonephritis.
3 Amyloid: usually secondary to a long-standing inflammatory disease, e.g. bronchiectasis or rheumatoid arthritis.
4 Minimal-change glomerulonephritis.

Diabetic nephropathy – common and increasing – has no distinctive features in old age.

Myeloma – more common in older people (see Chapter 17).

Renal stone disease – exclude excess vitamin D, gout, and hyperparathyroidism, all more common in older people.

Drugs and the kidney

In view of the changes to renal function that go with ageing and the increased risk of AKI and CKD, scrutinise every older patient's list of medications.

- Nephrotoxic drugs:
   - Antibiotics, e.g. gentamicin, vancomycin, and tetracycline.
   - Analgesics, e.g. NSAIDs and COX-2 inhibitors, disrupt the regulation of renal medullary blood flow and salt and water balance. This effect is exacerbated by diuretics and ACEi.

○ Disease-modifying anti-rheumatic drugs (DMARDs), e.g. penicillamine and gold.
- Too high a dosage of drugs with renal effects, i.e. diuretics, leading to dehydration, hypotension, and electrolyte imbalance, to the extent of causing marked renal failure. Remember to reduce/omit diuretics when patients are admitted with hypotension and dehydration, as in 'sick day rules'.
- Drug toxicity due to accumulation secondary to reduced renal excretion; the best example is digoxin.
- ACEi may precipitate renal failure in patients with silent renovascular disease.
- Long-term proton pump inhibitors (PPIs) are associated with an increased risk of CKD.
- Remember to check the BNF whenever prescribing for patients with AKI or CKD. It may be necessary to omit or reduce the dose of many medications, including metformin, allopurinol, dalteparin, ciprofloxacin, lithium, and digoxin.

Blood pressure and the kidney

- Renal diseases, such as chronic interstitial nephritis, may cause hypertension.
- Overtreatment of high blood pressure will impair renal function, but untreated hypertension may result in renal failure!
- About one-third of older patients with hypertension have impaired renal function.
- Hypotension, e.g. after haemorrhage, myocardial infarction, or pulmonary embolus, may result in renal shutdown and AKI, especially where renal function is already compromised by extreme old age or pathology.
- Renal artery stenosis (RAS) may first present as a marked deterioration in renal function after treatment with an ACEi. However, ACE inhibition is beneficial for other causes of CKD but should be started at a low dose. Renal function and electrolytes should be checked regularly.
- Bilateral RAS can also present with 'flash' pulmonary oedema, which is thought to be due to the combination of RAS and fluid overload plus diastolic ventricular dysfunction.

Urinary tract infection

Urinary tract infections (UTIs) are very common in older women: the incidence is 20% in women over the age of 85.

- In the UK (2022/23), there were 147,285 admissions with a primary diagnosis of UTI. Fifty-six per cent were people over 65 years old, and 12% were in the 80–84 age group.
- Female-to-male ratio: 2 : 1.
- *Escherichia coli* is the most common pathogen. Others include *Proteus mirabilis*, *Pseudomonas* and *Klebsiella*.
- Significant catheter-associated urinary tract infections (CAUTIs) account for around 10% of all hospital-acquired infections. Most trusts have protocols to reduce this. Only catheterise a patient when it is essential. Assiduous catheter care and removal as early as possible also reduce infection rates.
- Asymptomatic bacteriuria with no pyuria does not require treatment.
- Pyelonephritis is responsible for 20% of cases of renal failure, and therefore, needs to be completely treated.

Predisposing factors

- Poor fluid intake.
- Immobility.

- Decreased immune function.
- Loss of acidity of the female urethra, atrophic vaginitis, and urethritis – the genitourinary syndrome of menopause (GSM) – due to reduced oestrogen.
- Urinary stasis:
  ○ Incomplete voiding due to enlarged prostate, bladder diverticulae, weak bladder muscles.
  ○ Outflow obstruction of the urinary tract, including pressure from constipation.
- Constipation and poor perineal hygiene.
- Diabetes.
- Cognitive decline: ignoring the call to pass urine, leading to overflow incontinence; fiddling with a catheter.
- Urinary-tract stones.
- Urinary catheterisation.
- Medications: see Table 15.3.

Presentations

- Simple UTI: Increased frequency and dysuria are common, but there may be other vague symptoms such as nausea, vomiting and lethargy.
- Complicated UTI: a lower tract UTI but with features that make complications (treatment failure, persistent infection, or recurrent infection) more likely, e.g. an anatomical abnormality, an indwelling catheter, renal disease, or immunosuppression.
- Upper UTI or pyelonephritis: infection of one or both kidneys, usually caused by bacteria from the bladder – when the patient describes UTI symptoms plus fever, nausea/vomiting, or flank pain.
- CAUTI: asymptomatic bacteriuria is common and does not need to be treated. However, fever, pain, and raised inflammatory markers suggest developing sepsis – send cultures.
- New urinary incontinence: infected urine irritates the bladder mucosa.
- Increasing drowsiness due to worsening renal impairment.
- Other presentations in older people MAY be due to a UTI: delirium, falls, or malaise. It may be necessary to catheterise to obtain an uncontaminated urine specimen, or organisms may be isolated from a blood culture. NB: UTI is rarely the sole cause of the delirium!

Management

In men and women over 65 with clinical features of a UTI, NICE recommends sending an MSU, not doing dipstick testing, and having a lower

Table 15.3 Medications that increase the risk of UTIs.

Group	Mechanism	Examples
Anticholinergic drugs	Increased risk of urinary retention	Tolterodine, solifenacin, and TCA such as amitriptyline and antihistamines
PPIs	Reduce acidity of the GU tract, potentially promoting bacterial overgrowth	Omeprazole
Antibiotics – long-term	Disrupt the balance of commensal bacteria in the GU tract and select resistant organisms	Trimethoprim, cefalexin
Opioids	Constipation leading to outflow obstruction	Morphine, codeine

GU, genitourinary; TCA, tricyclic antidepressants.

threshold for starting empirical antibiotics – pending results – in men than women.

- Culture organisms from urine or blood.
- Appropriate antibiotics (see Table 15.4; but check trust guidelines because of local resistance patterns). NICE suggests first-line: either nitrofurantoin or trimethoprim; second-line: nitrofurantoin, if not already given, pivmecillinam or fosfomycin. A study linking primary care data to hospital records (over 300,000 UTIs in patients over 65) found that the 87% who received immediate antibiotics had fewer hospital admissions, positive blood cultures and lower mortality than those who had deferred or received no antibiotics. The paper and responses to it provoked discussion of methodological caveats, but they illustrate the difficulty for GPs in balancing antibiotic steward-ship with risk to individuals.
- Some older patients will need admission because of increased confusion/injury from falling/malaise.
- Patients with symptoms and signs of severe pyelonephritis should be admitted for IV antibiotics.
- A CAUTI will not be eliminated unless the catheter is changed. A prag-matic approach is to start antibiotics and change the catheter when the blood drug level would be high to reduce the colonisation of the new catheter.
- To reduce the risk of recurrence:
  - Maintain good fluid intake (greater than 1.5 L/day) – evidence base for effectiveness in care homes.
  - Reverse precipitating causes, if possible.
  - Trial of D-mannose (a health supplement, bought OTC), which may reduce the adhesion of bacteria to the urothelium and the fre-quency of UTIs.
  - Methenamine hippurate (1g bd) was non inferior to prophylactic antibiotics in reducing recurrence, had a reduced risk of developing multi-drug-resistant perineal bacteria and was cheaper (ALTAR study). It is hydrolysed to formaldehyde (bactericidal) in the acidic environment of the distal tubules of the kidney. NB: not relevant here, but do not use in pregnancy!

Obstructive uropathy

Some sources label obstructive 'uropathy' as conditions causing a block-age to the flow of urine and obstructive 'nephropathy' as the ensuing kidney disease, but they can be used synonymously. The blockage can be found anywhere along the urinary tract, from the renal pelvis to the urethral meatus. See Figure 15.2.

Bladder outflow obstruction

Bladder outflow obstruction (BOO) can be caused by problems in the bladder blocking the outflow tract or narrowing or compression of the urethra due to prostate pathology, stricture, advanced pelvic tumours or more rarely, a large cystocoele or inguinal hernia, muscle spasm or a foreign body. It can be iatrogenic following surgery for stress inconti-nence. It is more common in men because of prostate disease. If per-formed, urodynamic voiding studies show increased detrusor pressure and a reduced urine flow rate.

Benign prostatic hyperplasia

- By the age of 60, 50% of prostates have areas of hyperplasia of the glands and connective tissue. By 85 years, 90% of prostates are affected by BPH, i.e. this is part of normal ageing (sometimes, incorrectly, referred to as hypertrophy).
- Within the prostate, 5α reductase converts circulating testosterone to dihydrotestosterone (DHT), which acts locally to cause cellular proliferation.

Symptoms

LUTS are shown in Table 15.5. Post-micturition dribbling is also common.

- Fewer than half of all men with BPH develop symptoms.

Table 15.4 Overview of antibiotics for urinary tract infections (see local guidelines also).

Acute simple	Dose	Duration	Other considerations
Nitrofurantoin MR	100 mg bd	3 days for women 7 days for men 7 days if CAUTI	Avoid if CrCl >30
Trimethoprim	200 mg bd	3 days for women 7 days for men 7 days if CAUTI	Avoid if *E. coli* local resistance is high (30% in some areas) Avoid if patient has a blood dyscrasia
Fosfomycin	3 g sachet	Single dose	Can also be used as prophylaxis pre-transurethral surgery
Pivmecillinam	400 mg initially, then 200 mg tds	3 days for women or men (total of 10 tablets)	Remember, this is a penicillin
Upper tract/pyelonephritis: oral			
Cefalexin	500 mg bd to tds	7–10 days	Review culture results and change if necessary
Co-amoxiclav	625 mg tds	7–10 days	According to sensitivity
Ciprofloxacin	500 mg bd	7 days	Only if there is resistance to other antibiotics and the patient is warned about tendon rupture
Upper tract/pyelonephritis: IV			
Co-amoxiclav	1.2 g tds		Review cultures
Gentamicin	5–7 mg/kg once daily		Adjust daily doses according to serum gentamicin levels

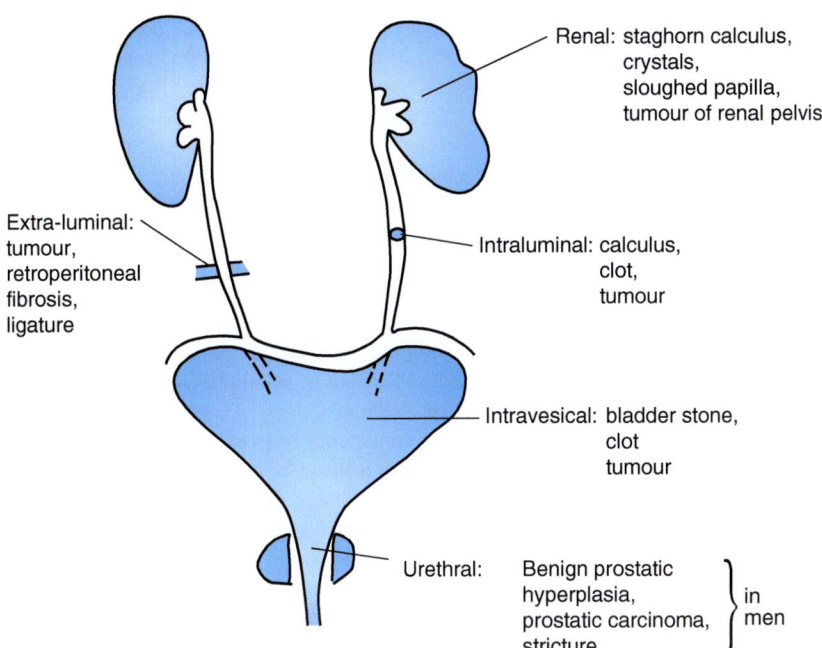

Renal: staghorn calculus,
crystals,
sloughed papilla,
tumour of renal pelvis

Extra-luminal:
tumour,
retroperitoneal
fibrosis,
ligature

Intraluminal: calculus,
clot,
tumour

Intravesical: bladder stone,
clot
tumour

Urethral: Benign prostatic
hyperplasia,
prostatic carcinoma,
stricture } in men

Figure 15.2 Causes of Obstructive Uropathy.

Table 15.5 Comparing storage and voiding symptoms.

LUTS	Storage symptoms Often, detrusor overactivity	Voiding symptoms Often, detrusor underactivity
	Urgency	Hesitancy
	Increased frequency: >8 times in 24 hours	Weak stream, splitting or spraying
	Nocturia	Straining
		Terminal dribble
		Sensation of incomplete emptying
	Urge incontinence	Retention and overflow incontinence

- Diagnosis: history, bladder diary, check for a distended bladder, rectal examination, measure post-void residual with a bladder scan, rectal ultrasound if there is doubt, urine dipstick, renal function.
- If suspicious nodules are detected on rectal examination, it may be appropriate to measure the prostate-specific antigen (PSA) after discussion about the implications. See cancer of the prostate, discussed later.

Management
Medical

A validated questionnaire (e.g. international prostate symptom score, or IPSS) can be used to monitor outcomes or guide referral.

- Lifestyle advice for all, especially those with symptoms of overactive bladder (see incontinence).
- Mild cases or patients who are at poor surgical risk can be effectively treated with selective alpha-adrenoceptor antagonists. There are alpha receptors in the smooth muscle, capsule of the bladder and bladder neck, and alpha-blockers relax the muscle. Tamsulosin has more α_1 specificity and causes less orthostatic hypotension than doxazosin or terazosin.

- 5α reductase inhibitors such as finasteride work by blocking the conversion of testosterone to DHT and inhibiting prostate growth. Warn the patient that it will take 6 months for the finasteride to reach optimum efficacy.
- The two classes of drug can be used together.
- An antimuscarinic, e.g. tolterodine, may improve associated overactive bladder symptoms.
- Botulinum A injections may be used for overactive bladder (OAB) syndrome with any of the other measures.

Surgical/interventional

- Transurethral prostatectomy (TURP) is the mainstay of treatment for severe symptoms, but complications include perioperative haemorrhage and absorption of irrigation fluids, urethral strictures, and incontinence. Repeat surgery is occasionally needed. If malignant cells are found in the chippings, the patient will be referred for MDT discussion.
- Minimally invasive procedures are being developed that can be performed as day cases under a local anaesthetic. Several modalities can be used to ablate prostate tissue and reduce outflow obstruction of the prostatic urethra. Common side effects are haematuria, infections, and urethral strictures. Rates of erectile dysfunction are variable. NICE has not updated guidelines recently, so the European ones are referenced. Be aware that when there are multiple options, usually there is no clear leader. There is limited data on long-term outcomes and the need for redo procedures. Examples include:
  - Transurethral incision of the prostate (TUIP) for small prostates in men unable to tolerate TURP.
  - Transurethral laser enucleation of the prostate, e.g. with a holmium laser (HoLEP), has a low recurrence risk and a low side effect profile.
  - Laser vaporisation (no histology).
  - UroLift: small clips in the prostate lift and hold the enlarged tissue away from the urethra.

Ongoing trials:
  - A temporary implantable nitinol device (iTIND) is a urethral stenting device.

- Water vapour thermal therapy (Rezum) uses water vapour injected via a catheter.
- Aquablation therapy uses robotic water jets.
- Prostate artery embolisation.

Prostate cancer

Prostate cancer is the most common cancer among men in the UK. Incidence rates are highest in men aged 75–79 years old. Prostate cancer can be indolent, i.e. 'many men die with it rather than from it'. However, invasive disease has a mean survival time of 4 years. The unpredictability of the clinical course makes management a challenge. The patient's preferences must be considered, and each patient must be offered an individualised treatment plan. Screening continues to be highly controversial because, despite much anecdotal evidence of improved outcomes in individuals, overall, treatment is thought to do as much harm as good.

Clinical features

- Often asymptomatic.
- There may be LUTS such as poor stream, post-micturition dribbling and nocturia, but usually only late in the disease. Erectile dysfunction is a rare symptom.
- Other symptoms may include haematuria, suprapubic pain, and rectal pain.
- If the cancer has spread, there may be bony pain, especially in the lower back, spinal cord compression, lower limb lymphoedema and cachexia.
- A rectal examination may be normal in early disease or may reveal a hard, craggy prostate.

Investigations

- The measurement of PSA is readily available but lacks sensitivity and specificity. The standard test measures the amount of free and bound PSA in the blood. Levels that usually lead to an investigation being carried out are age-related:
  - Between 60 and 69, >4.5 ng/mL.
  - Between 70 and 79, >6.5 ng/mL.
  - Above 79, use clinical judgement.
    An extremely high PSA suggests metastatic disease.
- Multiple prostatic biopsies were traditionally taken under transrectal ultrasound guidance (TRUS). Some centres now offer a local anaesthetic trans-perineal (LATP) prostate biopsy, which has a reduced risk of infection. Both methods of biopsy may be MRI-guided.
- Alternatively, if a TURP is done, the histology of the prostate chippings will be examined.
- The pathologist grades each sample of prostate cells to give a Grade Group from 1 (cells look similar to normal) to Grade Group 5 (very abnormal cells). This has replaced the Gleason score.
- Multiparametric MRI scans are useful in delineating local and widespread disease in patients who would be fit enough for radical treatments.
- Bone scintigraphy is a sensitive way of detecting bone metastases.

Assessment of the degree of spread

In localised disease, the tumour is completely inside the prostate gland (T1-2). Locally advanced disease includes a T3 tumour that has broken through the prostate capsule and may have spread to seminal vesicles and a T4 tumour that has spread to the bladder, rectum, or pelvic wall and there may be local LN involvement.

- If there is no evidence of distant spread (localised or locally advanced prostate cancer), the PSA level, tumour stage and Grade Group are considered, to classify the patient in a Cambridge Prognostic Group from 1 (low risk) to 5 (highest risk).
- Treatment is then planned by the MDT, considering the patient's general health, comorbidities, frailty, and wishes.
- If the Cambridge prognostic grouping is 1, 2 or 3, 'active surveillance' may be used with regular monitoring so that if the cancer starts to grow, management is changed to a strategy aiming at cure.
- This is different to 'watchful waiting' which is also used for localised prostate cancer, but for those who do not wish for or would not be fit enough to undertake curative treatment. There is monitoring, but this is less frequent and if the PSA rises or symptoms of spread develop, treatment starts aiming at palliation.
- Locally advanced prostate cancer may be treated with curative intent, but a period of control is more realistic for most older patients.
- If cancer has already spread to distant lymph nodes or other sites, typically the bones, this is metastatic and not curable, but it may respond well to a variety of treatments, several of which are appropriate for use in frail older people.

Management

A very wide range of treatment modalities is available, and centres may have different approaches. Patients and their families need written information about the range of options that would be suitable for the individual and their stage of disease.

Treatment aimed at cure

The main treatments aimed at a cure for localised cancer are radical prostatectomy and radical radiotherapy. They have very similar outcomes at 10 years: survival 98%, disease progression 8%, distant metastasis 3%, but different side effects.

- Radical prostatectomy is only indicated for men with cancer restricted to the prostate (some patients with locally advanced disease may be considered) with a life expectancy of over 10 years and no serious comorbidities. The procedure is usually laparoscopic and often robot-assisted. The prostate, seminal vesicles and local LN are removed. There are the usual risks of surgery. Long-term incontinence is a common side effect. The rates in the literature vary. Cancer Research UK states that 71% will have difficulty with bladder control at 6 months. This may improve with time and pelvic floor exercises but tends to worsen again with ageing. At 6 months, difficulty getting an erection affects 66% (treatment with phosphodiesterase type 5 inhibitors is often effective), and – the good news – problems with bowel control only occur in 1%.
- Radical radiotherapy is usually external radiotherapy, sometimes combined with internal radiotherapy – brachytherapy – in which radioactive seeds or a removable radioactive source are placed in the prostate tissue. Radiotherapy avoids the immediate risks of surgery but is still burdensome. After a planning visit, the therapy is usually given as an outpatient each weekday over 4–8 weeks so a great deal of time and money may be spent travelling and parking. After a couple of weeks of treatment, many people experience progressive tiredness, sore skin, and symptoms like cystitis due to bladder inflammation and diarrhoea due to radiation proctitis. These usually resolve over a few weeks after the treatment finishes. In comparison with surgery, at 6 months, incontinence is less of an issue at 38% (the same as those on active surveillance), erectile problems are intermediate at 48%, but problems with bowel control affect 5%. Other long-term side effects may develop, including lymphoedema, pelvic insufficiency fractures and rectal cancer.

Treatment aimed at control

The mainstay of treatment for prostate cancer that has spread or where the aim is control rather than cure is hormone therapy, more accurately androgen deprivation therapy (ADT), as prostate cancer is testosterone dependent (see Chapter 18).

Androgen deprivation therapy

- Bilateral subcapsular orchidectomy is simple, cheap, and effective and can be performed as a day case under local anaesthetic and testosterone falls rapidly. It is not often used because of the psychological impact. Prosthetic testes may be offered to preserve a normal appearance. The rapid fall in hormones which can be helpful if there is pain, means that early side effects particularly hot flashes can be marked.
- More commonly, drugs are used to reduce androgen stimulation of the tumour to levels found in castrated men. As well as drug-specific adverse effects, ADT treatments share a range of side effects:
  - Decreased libido and erectile dysfunction.
  - Hot flashes.
  - Gynecomastia.
  - Loss of muscle and an increase in body fat.
  - Osteoporosis: BMD should be monitored, and treatment started if needed.
  - An increased risk of developing T2DM.
  - A potential small increase in the risk of IHD.

ADTs may be used at various stages, including metastatic disease and in combination with other modalities. Response to treatment is usually monitored clinically and with serial PSA tests.

ADT medication

1 Luteinising hormone-releasing hormone agonists (LHRH agonists or LH blockers)
E.g. leuprorelin (Prostap) or goserelin acetate (Zoladex) sub cut every 4 weeks or 12 weeks. An initial tumour flare is prevented by giving an androgen receptor blocker for the first four weeks.
2 Gonadotrophin-releasing hormone antagonists or GnRH blockers
E.g. degarelix (Firmagon) sub cut every 4 weeks (less common).
3 Androgen receptor blockers
E.g. bicalutamide (Casodex) orally. These block androgen receptors on prostate cancer cells and increase testosterone, so they are usually used in combination with GnRH agonists. Gynaecomastia is common.
4 Androgen synthesis blockers
E.g. abiraterone orally. This blocks androgen production by prostate cancer cells, the testes, and adrenal glands. It must be given with prednisolone to reduce side effects.

At some stage, a prostate cancer, which has been well controlled on ADT, starts to 'escape' hormonal control, possibly due to clonal selection of hormone-independent malignant cells, and the PSA usually starts to rise. This may (unfeelingly) be referred to as 'castration-resistant prostate cancer'. The cancer is often metastatic at this stage.

Castration-resistant prostate cancer

Options at this stage include:

- A different ADT (often abiraterone with prednisolone or enzalutamide) or combination.
- Monotherapy with corticosteroids

Metastatic disease

- If there is macroscopic metastatic disease, chemotherapy with docetaxel and prednisolone may be offered (haematological side effects leading to anaemia and neutropenic infections are more frequent in older people).

- Palliative radiotherapy for bone pain due to symptomatic bone metastasis. A single treatment may suffice.
- Radioisotope therapy such as Radium-223 (which localises to bone metastases) for diffuse metastatic disease.
- A targeted drug, olaparib, with abiraterone and prednisolone, is NICE-approved for metastatic castration-resistant prostate cancer when chemotherapy is not clinically indicated.
- Lutetium-177-PSMA (tagged prostate-specific membrane antigen) is not NICE-approved (May 2024).

Symptomatic treatment

- Transurethral resection (TURP) may help relieve bladder-neck obstruction.
- IV zoledronate can be used to prevent or reduce pain from bone metastasis and reduce the risk of pathological fractures.
- Blood transfusions may improve the quality of life of patients with slowly progressive metastatic disease and severe anaemia.
- Usual approach to nausea.
- Referral for palliative care.

Haematuria

Haematuria (see Table 15.6) is a more common presentation now that many older patients are anticoagulated for atrial fibrillation. It is said to affect 2–30% of the adult population and is often divided into visible and non-visible haematuria. Visible haematuria always needs investigation. Nonvisible haematuria (NVH) suggested on the dipstick must be confirmed on microscopy (3 red blood cells per high-power field) before investigation. Microscopic haematuria may be idiopathic; people ≥60 years with unexplained NVH *and* either dysuria *or* a raised white cell count should be referred using a suspected bladder cancer pathway (NICE). In the US, the age alone would be sufficient for investigation.

Renal cell carcinoma

Renal cell carcinoma (RCC) is an adenocarcinoma and accounts for 85% of primary renal tumours. Most of the rest are urothelial tumours.

- The median age at diagnosis of RCC is 65–75 years.
- It is twice as common in men as in women.
- Risk factors include smoking, obesity (especially in women), and hypertension.
- Up to 30% of cases are asymptomatic and discovered incidentally on scans done for other reasons.
- RCC is associated with a high incidence of paraneoplastic syndromes secondary to the release of cytokines such as IL-6, erythropoietin and nitric oxide.

Symptoms

Haematuria (45%) only occurs once the tumour has invaded the collecting system.
Flank pain (40%).
Weight loss.

Signs

Flank mass: firm, not tender and moves with respiration.
Some patients present with pyrexia of unknown origin.
Symptoms from secondaries, e.g. lung, liver, or bone metastases.
Cachexia.

Table 15.6 Causes, investigations, and management of haematuria.

Cause	Investigations	Management
Bleeding diathesis	Abnormal clotting, low platelet count, abnormal platelet function	Review indications for anticoagulants, check liver function, and run a clotting screen
Glomerulonephritis	Urine microscopy is looking for casts. Autoimmune screen. Consider renal biopsy if appropriate	Nephrology referral
Urosepsis, pyelonephritis	MSU, blood cultures, and ultrasound	Antibiotics guided by MSU results treat predisposing factors
Renal cell carcinoma	Ultrasound or CT abdomen; urine cytology	Nephrectomy for early disease, embolisation for continuous haematuria
Ureteric stones/bladder stones	KUB, CT urogram, ultrasound	Extracorporeal shockwave lithotripsy, endoscopic removal, and preventative measures
Ureteric stricture	CT urogram, cystoscopy	May need stent insertion
Transitional cell carcinoma of the bladder	Cystoscopy	Transurethral resection of bladder tumour with regular review
BPH	Rectal examination, bladder ultrasound	Alpha-blockers, 5 alpha-reductase inhibitors, TURP
Carcinoma of the prostate	PSA, biopsy, MRI	Treat as appropriate
Urethra: e.g. trauma from a catheter, urethritis	Haematuria at the beginning of the stream	Fix the catheter appropriately
Contamination with vaginal blood	Obtain a clean catch specimen or use with a catheter if necessary	See vaginal bleeding
Immune complex disease, e.g. bacterial endocarditis	Blood cultures, echocardiography (see Chapter 12)	Treat the underlying condition

KUB, x-ray kidneys, ureter, and bladder.

Investigations

- U&E to check renal function.
- FBC may show anaemia of the chronic disease. More rarely, erythrocytosis occurs from excess erythropoietin. Neutrophilia and thrombocytosis are poor prognostic indicators.
- Bone function tests: calcium levels can be raised if the tumour produces elevated levels of parathyroid hormone-related protein or if there are lytic bone secondaries (high ALP).
- LFTs.
- LDH: a high level is associated with a poor prognosis.
- Urine cytology: is more useful for diagnosing urothelial tumours than RCC.
- Both ultrasound and CT scans can distinguish an RCC from simple cysts (see Figure 15.3) and visualise involvement of the renal vein and inferior vena cava.
- CT/MRI will show small tumours (cm) and contrast-enhanced CT/MRI of the chest, abdomen and pelvis are used for staging.
- Bone scintigraphy can be used to show bone secondaries.

Management

- All patients are discussed in the urology cancer MDT.
- For fit older people with non-metastatic disease, partial or radical nephrectomy may be curative.
- Some patients have very indolent disease and die with the RCC rather than from it.
- Patients with dementia, heart failure and kidney failure have the poorest outlook.
- RCC is generally resistant to chemotherapy.
- A variety of targeted and immunotherapy drugs are licensed for metastatic RCC, e.g. pembrolizumab plus axitinib. However, side effects may negate the limited benefits of treatment.

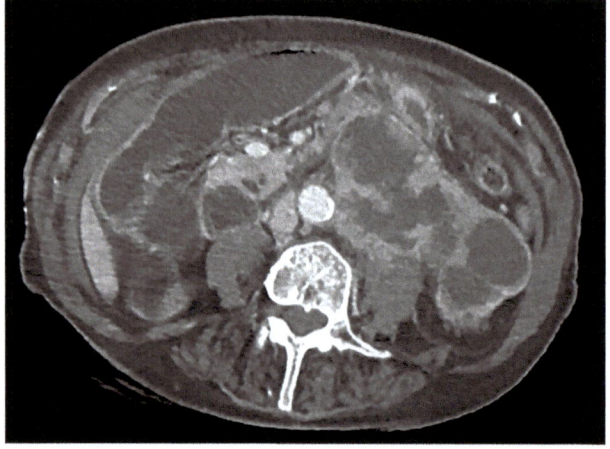

Figure 15.3 CT scan shows a large left-sided RCC with hydronephrosis. It is so large that it is compressing the duodenum, causing small bowel obstruction.

- Treatments for complications include radiotherapy for cord compression or bone metastases and renal artery embolisation, which can reduce severe haematuria.

Bladder cancer

Bladder cancer is the fourth most common cancer in men in the UK. The incidence of bladder cancer is highest in people aged 85–89 in the UK.

- Transitional cell carcinoma (TCC) accounts for 90%, squamous cell 5%, and adenocarcinoma only 2% of cases in the West.

- However, 75% of cases in the developing world are squamous cell carcinoma, thought to be due to infection with *Schistosoma haematobium*.
- TCC is four times more common in men than women. It may occur anywhere along the renal tract: the renal pelvis, ureter, bladder, or urethra.
- Fifty per cent of cases of bladder cancer are preventable. It is hoped that the incidence will fall as smoking becomes less common and fewer people are exposed to industrial chemicals such as beta-naphthylamine and benzidine.

Clinical features

- Painless, intermittent, visible haematuria. The amount may fluctuate.
- Sometimes patients report increased urinary frequency, urgency, or dysuria.
- Pain in the pelvis and weight loss are late features and suggest metastases.
- Often, nothing abnormal is found on examination.

Investigations

- Patients are usually sent to their local haematuria clinic on the 2-week wait path.
- Urine cytology has a low pick-up rate for low-grade carcinoma but has a 95% accuracy rate for high-grade disease.
- Flexible cystoscopy allows diagnosis and disease stratification; there is a wide range of disease burdens, from mild to advanced disease.
- Histology from more invasive procedures.

Management

- As always, patients are discussed in cancer MDTs, and patients should be involved in decision making. Cancer nurse specialists improve communication and continuity of care.
- 5-year survival rates are 80–90% if the tumour does not involve the bladder muscle.
- Most patients will benefit from a transurethral bladder tumour resection (TURBT), which can be done cystoscopically as a day case, under spinal or general anaesthesia. The histology indicates whether the tumour is restricted to the endothelium, has penetrated the connective tissue, or has invaded the muscle layer.
- As recurrence rates are up to 70%, patients need ongoing surveillance.
- Intravesical BCG (Bacillus Calmette–Guérin) is given weekly for 6 weeks followed by maintenance treatment as immunotherapy, to patients who have had a TURBT for superficial bladder cancer but are considered at high risk for recurrence. BCG-itis is a rare complication with miliary pulmonary and hepatic spread of the attenuated organism, requiring anti-TB chemotherapy.
- An alternative is a course of intravesical mitomycin C weekly for 6 weeks.
- Once the tumour has breached the muscle layer, cystectomy is the only cure, but this is very major surgery, and there are multiple side effects if the bladder is replaced by a pouch fashioned from a section of the bowel.
- Over 70-year-olds may be offered radiotherapy, but this causes proctitis in 10% of patients.
- Cisplatin-based chemotherapy is associated with multiple side effects in older people, including renal impairment, hearing impairment and peripheral neuropathy, and it is not usually recommended.
- Monoclonal antibody therapies such as pembrolizumab and enfortumab vedotin (an antibody-drug conjugate) are being used in trials in the UK for metastatic bladder cancer, but there is no consensus yet for their use in older patients.

Urinary incontinence

Urinary incontinence (UI) is defined as 'any involuntary urinary leakage'. Incontinence affects 50% of older people in hospitals and nursing homes and 40% of those living in the community. It is often concealed because of embarrassment. It is twice as common in women as in men because of the anatomy of the female urethra and low oestrogen levels which lead to reduced mucosal cohesion of the urethra, making it patulous. Many women have longstanding continence issues after childbirth, which worsen with ageing. Only 25% of affected women consult a doctor; it may be assumed that incontinence is normal with increasing age or that little can be done about it.

Overview of types

1. Stress UI: involuntary leakage on effort, sneezing or coughing.
2. Urgency UI: involuntary leakage associated with urgency.
3. OAB syndrome: urgency, usually accompanied by frequency and nocturia with or without incontinence (OAB-wet or OAB-dry) in the absence of urine infection or obvious disease.
4. Mixed: leakage with symptoms of stress *and* urgency.
5. Overflow UI: leakage from a full bladder.
6. Functional: inability to get to the toilet, e.g. arthritis, dementia (multifactorial).
7. Continuous: fistula (malignancy; in countries with poor obstetric care, obstructed labour can cause fistula, leading to constant bowel and bladder leakage).

Complications

UI markedly reduces health-related quality of life.

- Social
  - Embarrassment: – fear of losing bladder control or smelling urine.
  - Spiral of reluctance to go out, reduced fitness, isolation.
  - Carer stress: increased risk of moving to long-term care (second only to dementia).
- Psychological
  - Loss of self-confidence.
  - Sleep deprivation from nocturia.
  - Depression.
  - Fear of leaking may lead to the avoidance of sex.
- Physical
  - Skin irritation and maceration may lead to moisture lesions and ulceration (see Chapter 19).
  - Falls.
  - UTIs and the risk of hospitalisation.
  - Catheterisation and CAUTIs.
- Huge costs
  - The burden on older people and their carers is both practical (with the workload of extra washing) and financial (pads and new mattresses are expensive).
  - The estimated cost of UI to the NHS is £1.8 billion, with a further £270 million paid by affected individuals on pads, etc.

Treatable causes

The mnemonic 'diapers' is helpful in excluding easily reversible causes! See Table 15.7.

History

Bear in mind the reversible factors discussed above.

- Ask specific questions about the type of incontinence, i.e. urgency versus stress or mixed; see later.

Table 15.7 Treatable causes, examination, investigations, and management of UI in older people.

Cause	Examinations and investigations	Management
Delirium, dementia, and depression	Assess mental state and cognition. Exclude infection, constipation, and review medications	Treat the underlying cause, reorientate, toilet regularly; ensure toilets are well-signposted aconsider red toilet seats
Infection	MSU, CRP	Treat infection
Atrophic vulvovaginitis (GSM)	Pelvic examination	Topical oestrogen in females, e.g. Estriol 0.01% cream or gel twice weekly long-term
Pharmaceuticals: sedatives, caffeine, diuretics, doxazosin, antidepressants, and alcohol	Drug and alcohol history	Use alternatives if possible or try lower doses. Reduce caffeine and alcohol intake
Excess urine production	Serum glucose and calcium	Treat diabetes and hypercalcaemia
Restricted mobility	Joint and neurological examination	Physiotherapy, walking aids, commode, and adapted toilets
Stool impaction worsens overactive bladder syndrome	Rectal examination	Adequate fluid intake, regular laxatives, may need suppositories, or manual evacuation

- Red flag symptoms: chronic pain on passing urine (suggestive of interstitial cystitis), acute bladder pain (could be bladder stones), haematuria and frequent UTIs; need a specialist referral.
- Review medications: are there alternatives to diuretics that would not produce large volumes of urine? Alpha-blockers such as doxazosin cause incontinence by relaxing the bladder neck, so switch to a different antihypertensive if needed. Think laterally – can you treat the chronic cough causing the stress incontinence, e.g. by stopping the ACEi?
- Ask about prolapse, usually described as a sensation of 'something coming down' from the pelvis or a bulge, and whether it bothers the patient.
- Full medical and surgical history: especially obstetric, gynaecological, and urological.
- Social history: especially access to toilet(s) at home (downstairs/upstairs) and need for carer support.

Examination

- Examine the abdomen for a palpable bladder secondary to urinary retention. If the patient is obese, consider a bladder ultrasound or an 'in and out' catheter to exclude retention.
- DRE to assess prostate size in men, exclude faecal impaction and check the integrity of the anal sphincter in all patients.
- VE to exclude atrophic vaginitis and urethritis (GSM) and check for prolapse: a prolapse beyond the introitus pulls the bladder down, and intervention, e.g. a pessary, will be needed to improve symptoms. Asking the patient to perform a 'vaginal squeeze' will give a sign of whether they will understand pelvic floor exercises.

- Asking the patient to cough whilst standing with a full bladder is only useful if it is positive.
- General examination, including mobility, cognition, and neurology. If the patient can undress and get onto the couch independently, these are not major factors. Examine in more detail as needed:
  - Screen for cognition, especially where there is double incontinence.
  - Neurological examination to exclude spinal cord problems.

Investigations

- Bladder diary (see Figure 15.4).
- Urine dipstick.
- Further investigations such as urodynamics, cystometry and cystoscopy are not indicated prior to conservative management but are useful if surgery is planned or if there are concerns about an overactive bladder or bladder dysfunction.

Bladder diary

The patient should keep a bladder diary for at least 3 days. Suggest the patient buys a plastic measuring jug and a packet of wipes and carries these with the bladder chart in their bag. If housebound, use a 'cardboard hat' in the toilet. They should record:

- The volume and type of fluid drunk.
- The volume of urine passed.
- Whether they were continent or incontinent throughout the day and night.
- Any symptoms associated with leakage, such as sneezing, will help make the diagnosis.

Time	Type of fluid taken	Volume drunk (ml)	Volume of urine (ml)	How urgent: 0 = not urgent 3 = v urgent	Leakage with urgency	Leakage with activity	Number of pad changes
04:00			100	3	yes	no	
06:00			100	2	yes	no	
07:30	coffee	150					
10:00	coffee	150					
11:00			250	3	yes	no	
12:00	water	100					
13:00							

Figure 15.4 Example of a part of a bladder diary.

Normal values

- Fluid intake: 1.5–2 L; the type is recorded to check for caffeine and carbonation.
- Daytime voids: each 250–300 mL.
- Normal bladder capacity: up to 500 mL; an older woman with a low BMI might have a 300 mL bladder capacity.
- Daytime voids: 3–7.
- Nighttime voids: up to 3 per night.
- Urine output: 1–2.8 L in 24 hours.
- Polyuria >40 mL/kg body weight.
- Nocturnal polyuria is defined as >30% of total urine output being at night.

Management

General measures

These must be appropriate for the patient and their situation.

- Signposting the patient (and/ or carer) to education, advice, and self-help groups where appropriate.
- Fluid modification: avoid carbonated drinks (acidic), switch to decaffeinated hot drinks and reduce alcohol, as these irritate the bladder lining.
- Some older patients over-restrict fluid intake, and concentrated urine is an irritant to the bladder mucosa. Recommend drinking 1.5–2 L of fluid daily (avoiding the irritant drinks).
- Reduce weight by 5% to reduce the pressure of excess fat on the bladder and pelvic floor.
- Timed voiding or regular toileting.
- Treat constipation.
- Pelvic floor exercises: ideally, the first 6 weeks are supervised by a specialist physiotherapist. This is the most important intervention, as it can be much more effective than medication (see later).
- Radar key (access to disabled toilet facilities).
- Referral to continence advisor if there is no improvement with simple measures.
- OT input and provision of aids (commode, raised toilet seat, commode) if difficulty accessing the toilet is contributory.
- Clear signage and red toilet seats in hospitals and care homes.
- Laundry washing services are provided by some councils.
- Is attendance allowance warranted?

Types

Overactive bladder syndrome and urge incontinence

This is the frequent and urgent passing of small volumes of urine, sometimes with so little warning that the patient does not reach the toilet in time and has urge UI. This tends to be a larger volume than with stress UI. It is also associated with nocturia, which increases the risk of falling at night.

- It affects 10–16% of the general population and increases with age.
- It is due to detrusor instability and involuntary contractions of the detrusor muscle during the filling phase of the micturition cycle.
- Caffeinated, acidic and alcoholic drinks and comorbidities such as obesity, T2DM and UTI can worsen urgency.
- It can be associated with hyperreflexia in neurological conditions such as stroke, multiple sclerosis, and Parkinson's disease.

Medication

A Cochrane review confirms that antimuscarinic drugs reduce the number of urgency episodes per 24 hours.

- No anticholinergic drug is clearly superior to another. Tolterodine is often used first because of its familiarity.

- There is poor adherence to all these drugs. Most patients stop taking them within 3 months. They are not very effective, and common side effects include:
  - Dry mouth and eyes and constipation (though said to be less problematic with tolterodine.)
  - Other side effects include urinary retention, dizziness, and increased confusion.
- Many clinicians opt to use mirabegron, a beta-3 adrenoceptor agonist – that relaxes detrusor smooth muscle cells – for older women and certainly for those with cognitive impairment. It is more effective than a placebo, but long-term adherence is also poor. Blood pressure should be checked, as HT is a common side effect.

Procedures

- Botulism A: Botox can be injected into the detrusor muscle of the bladder to reduce bladder contractions, leading to reduced urgency and frequency lasting for several months before needing to be repeated. The risks include UTIs or urinary retention requiring temporary catheterisation.
- Surgical devices: the overactive bladder can be managed using sacral stimulation, where other treatments have failed. A lightweight (50 g) device, e.g. InterStim, is implanted above the buttock and stimulates the third sacral nerve. It has achieved 1-year success rates approaching 85% for controlling urgency, urge incontinence and nocturia.

Stress incontinence

This is the involuntary leaking of urine associated with increased intra-abdominal pressure, e.g. when sneezing, coughing, and exercising. In a study of 15,000 women, stress UI affected 10% of nulliparous women, 15% after C-section, and over 20% after vaginal delivery. Higher rates are seen in multiparous women and those who have had pelvic surgery. In men, the most common cause is sphincter damage after radical prostatectomy.

Conservative management

The patient should try all the strategies outlined above. Pelvic floor exercises can be very effective but only if they are carried out correctly, several times a day, and for weeks. There are lots of helpful YouTube clips for patients if access to a specialist PT is limited. Benefit is usually seen after 6 weeks but maximal improvement may take several months. Patients will need to continue maintenance exercises long-term, or the benefit is lost. Some patients benefit from biofeedback techniques so that they understand which muscles they should be contracting.

- Ring pessaries: useful for women with significant vaginal prolapse who are not fit for or do not wish to have surgery. They are circular or oval and made of silicone so that they are easily compressed to insert into the vagina. They can be used by sexually active women as they can be removed for cleaning and then reinserted.
- Shelf pessaries: made of more rigid plastic or silicone. They provide firmer support and are therefore used when ring pessaries keep falling out or the pelvic organ prolapse is more severe.
- Duloxetine: an SNRI that works at the level of the spinal cord, increasing urethral sphincter tone, is no longer recommended for older women.

Surgical procedures

- There has been a lot of controversy about the surgical management of stress UI because many women developed devastating chronic pain, haemorrhage, and immobility due to synthetic meshes. Currently, two minimally invasive procedures are available for older women who are still incontinent, despite the interventions covered earlier.
1 Periurethral bulking agents, such as collagen, improve continence. Collagen is injected into the urethral sphincter via a cystoscope

under local anaesthesia. The success rate varies between 48 and 75%, and the procedure needs to be repeated every 6–18 months.

2 Mid-urethral slings, such as tension-free vaginal tape (TVT), can be used to raise the middle part of the urethra and improve continence. This is done as a day case under local anaesthesia, so it is cheap, and recovery is fast. However, patients must be given time and clear information describing possible complications.

- Burch retropubic colposuspension is a traditional surgical technique where sutures are used to elevate the urethra and the bladder neck.

Mixed incontinence

This is a combination of the symptoms of stress and urge UI and is probably the most common presentation in older people. Most women benefit from starting conservative management, topical oestrogen, and a trial of an anticholinergic. If symptoms remain troublesome, a mid-urethral procedure may then be considered.

Overflow incontinence

Bladder outflow obstruction and detrusor underactivity can lead to urinary retention and overflow UI. This is most common in men with BPH but may also be secondary to prostatic carcinoma, constipation, or urethral stricture. It is also associated with neurological deficits, e.g. diabetes and MS. Exclude exacerbating constipation. If the cause is BPH, treatments include alpha-blockers such as tamsulosin, 5α reductase inhibitors such as finasteride or TURP. Urinary retention usually requires catheterisation to prevent obstructive nephropathy until the underlying cause is addressed.

Nocturia and nocturnal enuresis

These have a negative effect on quality of life: poor sleep patterns, disturbing their partner, and the risk of falling at night.

- There are usually multiple causes.
- Sensible lifestyle changes to start with are fluid restriction in the evenings and avoiding caffeine and fluid-containing foods such as fruit and rice later in the day.
- Nocturia due to BPH (with other obstructive symptoms) may respond to tamsulosin (caution – postural hypotension).
- Nocturia due to OAB syndrome (with urgency and urge incontinence) may respond to solifenacin or mirabegron.
- Patients with marked peripheral oedema are advised to lie on the bed for an hour in the afternoon to cause a diuresis prior to going to bed at night. Failing this, try a small dose of furosemide in the afternoon.
- If patients are on a calcium channel blocker, the associated leg oedema resolves overnight and results in a diuresis, so consider changing to another class of drug.
- Nocturnal polyuria is defined as producing greater than 1/3 of the 24-hour urine output at night; causes include diabetes insipidus and PD.
- Idiopathic nocturnal polyuria can be treated with low-dose desmopressin (25 mcg in women and 50 mcg in men) if there is no heart failure. Watch for hyponatraemia and weight gain due to fluid retention.

Containment strategies

Despite the measures described, input from the hospital or community continence team, and specialist referrals where appropriate, if incontinence is still an issue, the best containment strategy must be sought. Table 15.8 gives a comparison of the options. Further advice about different types of products is available online.

Urinary Catheters

Short-term catheters are usually made of latex because it is cheap, but it can cause local irritation and urethral trauma. Longer-term catheters are usually silicone. Most trusts use a care bundle approach to reduce the risk of infection. Bacteriuria is almost universal. The drainage system should be free-flowing and closed to reduce the introduction of infection. The catheter should be secured to the patient's thigh using a strap and connected to a leg bag attached to the patient's leg with a net support. At night, a larger bag is attached and should be hung from the bed so that the urine continues to drain by gravity.

Indications

- Acute urinary retention due to outflow obstruction or neurological causes.
- Chronic retention with hydronephrosis causing impaired renal function.
- Triple-lumen catheters are used for bladder irrigation post-surgery, haematuria, or clot retention.
- Intravesical treatment, e.g. for BCG (see bladder cancer discussion above).
- Preoperative abdominal or pelvic surgery.
- For monitoring urine output in acutely unwell patients.
- Keeping the skin dry allows macerated sacral pressure ulcers in an immobile, incontinent patient to heal.
- Patient choice for intractable incontinence, but risks must be explained.
- A catheter may make a protracted period of end-of-life care more comfortable.

Complications

- Chronic catheterisation leads to colonisation by bacteria such as *Proteus mirabilis*. This tends to make the urine alkaline, which leads to crystals forming that encrust and block the catheter. The patient can reduce the risk of this by drinking 1.5–2 L of fluid daily, including some citrated drinks to lower the pH. Encrustation and blockage of the catheter tip, especially in the presence of *P. mirabilis*, can lead to the formation of bladder stones.
- UTIs: catheters account for 86% of hospital-acquired UTIs. CAUTI should only be diagnosed when there are urinary symptoms and signs of sepsis. CAUTI is more common in women, patients who have had multiple catheterisations, when the catheter has been in situ for a long period and with poor hygiene. The risk is reduced by only putting in catheters when it is essential, optimal catheter care and taking out catheters as soon as possible. Giving prophylactic antibiotics on insertion, is not evidence-based is but often done pragmatically if a catheter is being replaced. The use of silver-alloy-coated catheters is no longer recommended.
- Trauma to the urethral epithelium during insertion and removal, especially if the catheter is pulled out with the balloon inflated by a confused patient.
- Chronic inflammation of the urethra can cause a urethral stricture, which might lead to obstructive uropathy.
- Urine bypassing catheter: try a catheter with a finer bore and an oral antispasmodic.
- The purple urine bag syndrome may occur in a catheterised patent with a UTI due to a variety if organisms, due to deamination of tryptophan and a series of reactions that produce blue and red compounds. Treat the infection and change the bag and catheter.
- Incontinence once the catheter has been removed: the risk can be reduced by using a valve that maintains bladder tone and gives the patient control over emptying the bladder.
- The use of a female (short) catheter in a man in error causes severe trauma if the balloon is inflated.

Table 15.8 Comparing advantages and disadvantages of containment strategies.

	Advantages	Disadvantages	Comments
Pad and pants	Convenient. Wide range of styles and sizes (see product advice website). Disposables cut down on laundry. A limited free supply may be available through the community continence service	Bulky pads may not be discrete. May be used in a care setting instead of regular toileting. May leak, so sheets and clothes still need washing. Cost, on average, £900 per year. Storage space. Environmentally unfriendly: 400 years to decompose.	Products that are more like normal underwear may be easier for patients with cognitive impairment. In developed countries, adult absorbent hygiene products already contribute more to waste than children's nappies – 4 to 10x by 2030!
Condom-type (conveen) catheters for men	Useful, especially at night. Not associated with UTIs.	Penis size may be too small to use. May fall off, causing leakage. Damage to the skin from the adhesive.	
Female urinals	May be useful if patient has control over urination but is functionally incontinent due to the inability to mobilise. Good for users who are not confused and may avoid long-term catheterisation	User must be able to lift her pelvis and hold onto the device at the same time	Need carers to bring and take away the urinal
Intermittent self-catheterisation (ICS)	No drainage system is needed. Useful for patients with MS	User needs good vision, dexterity, and cognition to perform the ICS and maintain hygiene	Contraindicated if the user is unable to retain urine in the bladder
Suprapubic catheter	Users can still have intercourse. No risk of trauma to the urethra. Reduced infection risk as it does not involve the genital tract and is away from the anus.	Urine may still leak from the urethra. Bladder spasm. Bladder stones	Main risks are at the time of insertion if the bladder is not distended: bowel perforation
Catheter with valve	User does not need a drainage system, and it promotes normal bladder tone and the urge to void	Not easy for users with poor dexterity or dementia with a lack of recognition of the urge to void	
Urethral catheter	Avoids incontinence. Maintains dignity. Keeps the skin dry	Risk of infection. Risk of blockage. Risk of trauma to the urethral lining	

Vaginal bleeding

Bleeding from the genital tract long after menopause must always be taken seriously because there are pre-malignant or malignant as well as benign causes. The patient may present with stained underwear or bed sheets.

If there is incontinence of urine, an anal lesion or pressure ulcer, the source of bleeding may be unclear.

- A physical examination should find the site.
- The heavier the bleeding, the more likely the cause is to be malignant.
- Ask especially about hormone therapy, either as a treatment for cancer or HRT.
- Ask about trauma (including abuse). Even very old women can be subject to this, either from sex or a foreign body in the vagina, such as a forgotten pessary.

Once you are sure that you are not dealing with haematuria or rectal bleeding, refer to gynaecology for further investigation.

Causes of post-menopausal bleeding

- Genitourinary syndrome of menopause (GSM) accounts for 60% of cases and responds to topical oestrogen cream.

- HRT: assess risk versus benefit for the individual.
- Ulceration from prolapse or foreign body, e.g. ring pessary.
- Endometrial hyperplasia, which may be premalignant.
- Benign tumours, such as cervical or endometrial polyps.
- Cancers of the endometrium (see Figure 15.5), cervix, vagina, and vulva.

Gynaecological malignancies

Cases are discussed in a gynae-oncology MDT.

Ovarian cancer

Around 7,500 women are diagnosed with ovarian cancer in the UK each year – the 6th most common cancer in women.

- Risk factors include age (highest risk at age 75–79), HRT, genetic predisposition (*BRCA* genes), obesity, endometriosis, diabetes, and asbestos exposure. Having had children, breastfeeding and having taken the oral contraceptive pill are protective.
- The early symptoms are vague and include early satiety, bloating, abdominal pain, needing to urinate more often, or changes in bowel habits.

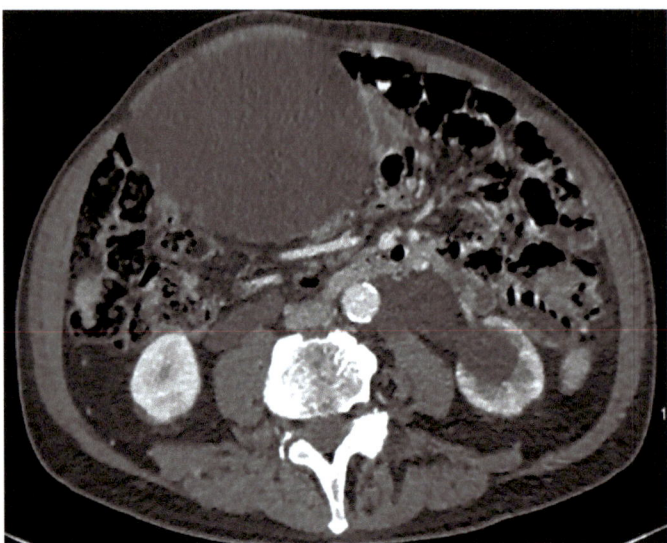

Figure 15.5 CT scan shows a large cystic endometrial cancer that is causing left-sided hydronephrosis (and a large femoral DVT, not visible in this cut).

- Patients with ascites or a pelvic or abdominal mass should be referred on a 2-week pathway.
- If the examination is normal, measure CA125 and if it is high (≥35 IU/mL), arrange an urgent ultrasound. If US suggests a mass, refer urgently, but if it is normal, review for other causes of a raised CA125, including heart failure.
- An image-guided biopsy will confirm the diagnosis.
- Because of its non-specific presentation, ovarian cancer is often diagnosed late. Debulking surgery and chemotherapy are common treatments if the patient is fit enough.

Endometrial cancer

Around 10,000 women are diagnosed with endometrial cancer in the UK each year – the 4th most common cancer in women.

- Risk factors include increasing age, obesity, diabetes mellitus, tamoxifen use, and unopposed oestrogen, e.g. oestrogen-only HRT.
- It is usually an adenocarcinoma, and because it typically presents with post-menopausal bleeding, patients often have early, surgically curable disease. After biopsy (via hysteroscopy) to confirm malignancy, if the patient is fit enough (frailty is more important than age), surgical staging (unusually) is used rather than extensive imaging.
- Standard treatment includes a total hysterectomy (usually laparoscopically), bilateral salpingo-oophorectomy and removal of lymph nodes.
- Locally advanced and advanced disease may be treated with radiotherapy, chemotherapy, and targeted therapies, but if the tumour is oestrogen or progesterone-positive, options include letrozole or megestrol.

Cervical cancer

Although it is thought of as a cancer of younger adults, because of the success of the cervical smear programme and now vaccination, half of all cervical cancer deaths in England are among women aged 65 years or older. It is almost always caused by the human papillomavirus. Treatment is surgery, if possible, but radiotherapy is another common choice for older people.

Vaginal prolapse

- Risk factors include trauma secondary to childbirth, striated muscle weakness and neuromuscular disease.
- Cystocoele: the bladder bulges through the anterior vaginal wall. This can be associated with stress incontinence, but a large cystocoele can impair bladder emptying.
- Rectocoele: bulging of the posterior vaginal wall by the rectum, which can impair defecation. Some women use a finger to push against the posterior vaginal wall to aid emptying.
- Conservative management consists of topical oestrogen, pelvic floor exercises and pessaries. Ring or shelf pessaries placed high within the vagina hold the uterus in place. They need to be changed 3–6 monthly and may cause vaginal discharge (especially if forgotten!).
- Surgery, e.g. anterior or posterior repair, for selected fit elderly women. Mesh is currently not being used on the NHS, and failure of the procedures or recurrence is common.

Disease of the vulva

Vulvar skin is sensitive to irritants, particularly in postmenopausal women, as ageing and oestrogen deficiency cause epithelial thinning. This results in an increased pH, which decreases the antimicrobial action of the skin. A decrease in lactobacilli and cell-mediated immunity further increased susceptibility to infection. Clothing and pantyliners can also cause abrasions, and a decrease in lipid production slows healing from injury.

- Because of its proximity to the anus, the vulva is prone to faecal contamination.
- If there is UI, the vulval skin can be permanently wet and macerated by ammonia.
- Scrupulous hygiene is of particular importance in older women, avoiding perfumed soap and wearing cotton underwear reduces the risk of many common conditions and vulval infections.

The most common symptoms are pruritus, discharge, and pain, or a lump may have been noted by the patient or their carer. Ask about co-morbidities including diabetes, atopy, and skin conditions including psoriasis and urinary and faecal incontinence. The most common cause of vulval itch and discharge in older women is candidiasis, which responds to topical 1% clotrimazole ointment or a single dose 500 mg pessary.

- For cases of itch with no discharge, rule out diabetes, jaundice, and uraemia.
- Allergic dermatitis responds well to topical steroids. Do not forget to avoid precipitants such as detergents or highly perfumed soaps.
- Lichen sclerosis is an autoimmune condition that affects older women. Initially, the vulval and perianal skin is red, but with time, the skin becomes paper thin and wrinkled, and white, shiny plaques may develop. A biopsy is needed to confirm the diagnosis, as it may be premalignant in 4% of cases. Treatment is with topical ultra-potent steroids such as clobetasol. Specialist management may be needed.
- Carcinoma of the vulva in older women is usually squamous cell. Early disease can be managed surgically with radiotherapy to the inguinal nodes. Invasive disease has an extremely poor prognosis.
- If the vulva looks beefy red, this may be Paget's disease; as in the breast, this is adenocarcinoma in situ.

Sex in later life

Many people continue to enjoy a sexual relationship until the end of life. A study in England in 2017 showed that 59% of men and 34% of women aged 70–79 years, and 31% of men and 14% of women aged 80 years or older, were sexually active. However, others stop having sex for a variety of reasons.

Age-related changes

1 Levels of oestrogen and testosterone fall and can cause decreased sexual drive.
2 Erectile dysfunction affects 15–25% of men by the age of 65. It is more common in men suffering from diabetes, hypertension, and renal disease, but stress, anxiety and depression play an important part. Drugs such as beta-blockers, alcohol, and luteinising hormone-releasing hormone (LHRH) agonists are also culprits. Premature ejaculation is less common.
3 Longer time for arousal.
4 Longer time to orgasm.
5 Reduced genital sensitivity.
6 Loss of lubrication in women.
7 Reduced satisfaction.

Chronic disease

- Reduced mobility, e.g. from arthritic hips, or a previous stroke.
- Anxiety about provoking myocardial or cerebrovascular events. However, the evidence suggests that sex with a familiar partner is unlikely to precipitate a fatal event.
- Low mood.
- Disinhibition in one partner secondary to dementia may be off-putting to the other partner.
- Moving to a residential home or into their children's home with reduced privacy.
- Loss of partner.

Societal attitudes

Ageism and stereotypes can negatively influence how society perceives sexuality among older people, including those who are LGBTQ+. This may cause older people to feel embarrassed about their sexual needs and therefore less likely to present with problems about their sexual health/wellbeing.

- Doctors need to be more willing to ask older people if they have concerns.
- Be aware that partners of people with neurological disorders, including PD and dementia, may also be experiencing problems – e.g. if the patient has hypersexuality – but be reluctant to seek help.

Advice for maintaining a healthy sexual life in later life

Recognise that sex does not have to be penetrative; other physical contact can also be pleasurable and satisfying.

- 'Use it or lose it'.
- Stop smoking.
- Avoid excess alcohol.
- Exercise to keep physically fit.
- Sex can reduce heart disease, blood pressure and stress.
- Consider intermittent self-catheterisation (ICS) or a suprapubic rather than urethral catheter for incontinence.
- Use lubricants and allow time for foreplay.
- Try various positions to find the most comfortable to allow for arthritic joints/weak limbs.
- Consider phosphodiesterase type 5 (PDE5) inhibitors, e.g. sildenafil or tadalafil, to achieve erection. (Use is contraindicated in patients taking nitrates or who have a history of recent MI or stroke.)
- Remember that sexually transmitted diseases are increasing in older people, so consider using a condom with a new partner.
- Feel able to seek help early for problems.

📖 REFERENCES AND FURTHER READING

Denic A, Glassock RJ, Rule AD (2016) Structural and functional changes with the aging kidney. *Adv. Chronic Kidney Dis.* 23:19–28. doi: 10.1053/j.ackd.2015.08.004.

Moore PK, Hsu RK, Liu KD (2018) Management of acute kidney injury: core curriculum. *Am. J. Kidney Dis.* 72:136–148. https://www.ajkd.org/article/S0272-6386(17)31141-1/fulltext.

UK Renal Registry (2023) *Acute kidney injury (AKI) in England – a report on the nationwide collection of AKI warning test scores from 2022.* https://www.ukkidney.org/sites/default/files/AKI_report_201223_FINAL.pdf

NICE Guideline 148 (updated 2023) Acute kidney injury: prevention, detection, and management. www.nice.org.uk/guidance/ng148

Kidney failure risk UK https://www.kidneyfailurerisk.co.uk/

Evans M, Morgan AR, Davies S, et al. (2022) The role of sodium-glucose co-transporter-2 inhibitors in frail older adults with or without type 2 diabetes mellitus. *Age Ageing*;51, afac201. doi: 10.1093/ageing/afac201.

NICE CKS (2024) *Chronic kidney disease.* https://cks.nice.org.uk/topics/chronic-kidney-disease

Alfano G, Perrone R, Fontana F, et al. (2022) Rethinking chronic kidney disease in the aging population. *Life (Basel)* 12:1724. doi: 10.3390/life12111724.

UK Kidney Association: *Renal Registry Data to 31/12/2021.* https://ukkidney.org/sites/renal.org/files/25th%20Annual%20Report%20Final%202.6.23.pdf

Kanbay M, Basile C, Battaglia, Y et al. on behalf of the EuDial Working Group of ERA (2024) Shared decision making in elderly patients with kidney failure. *Nephrol. Dialysis Transpl*; 39:742–751. https://academic.oup.com/ndt/article/39/5/742/7281724

NICE CKS (2023) *Urinary tract infection(lower) women (and equivalent for men).* https://cks.nice.org.uk/topics/urinary-tract-infection-lower-women

NICE CKS (2024) *Pyelonephritis.* https://cks.nice.org.uk/topics/pyelonephritis-acute

Gharbi M, Drysdale J H, Lishman H, et al. (2019) Antibiotic management of urinary tract infection in elderly patients in primary care and its association with bloodstream infections and all-cause mortality: population-based cohort study. *BMJ* 364:l525. doi: 10.1136/bmj.l525.

Wagenlehner F, Lorenz H, Ewald O, et al. (2022) Why d-mannose may be as efficient as antibiotics in the treatment of acute uncomplicated lower urinary tract infections – preliminary considerations and conclusions from a non-interventional study. *Antibiotics (Basel)* 11:314. doi: https://doi.org/10.3390/antibiotics11030314.

NICE CKS (2019) *LUTS in men.* https://cks.nice.org.uk/topics/luts-in-men

Cornu JN, Gacci M, Hashim H, et al. (2024) *EAU guidelines on non-neurogenic male lower urinary tract symptoms (LUTS).* https://d56bochluxqnz.cloudfront.net/documents/full-guideline/EAU-Guidelines-on-Non-Neurogenic-Male-LUTS-2024.pdf

Franco JVA, Tesolin P, Jung JH (2023) Update on the management of benign prostatic hyperplasia and the role of minimally invasive procedures. *Prostate Int.* 11:1–7. doi: 10.1016/j.prnil.2023.01.002.

Codelia-Anjum AJ, Berjaoui MB, Khondker A, et al. (2023) Procedural intervention for benign prostatic hyperplasia in men ≥ age 70 years – a review of published literature. *Clin. Interv. Aging* 18:1705–1717. doi: 10.2147/CIA.S414799.

Harding, C., Mossop, H., Homer, T., et al (2022). Alternative to prophylactic antibiotics for the treatment of recurrent urinary tract infections in women: multicentre, open label, randomised, non-inferiority trial (ALTAR). *BMJ, 2022,* 376. doi: 10.1136/bmj-2021-0068229

Cancer Research UK has detailed information about all genitourinary cancers including:

https://www.cancerresearchuk.org/about-cancer/prostate-cancer

https://www.cancerresearchuk.org/about-cancer/kidney-cancer

https://www.cancerresearchuk.org/about-cancer/bladder-cancer

https://www.cancerresearchuk.org/about-cancer/womb-cancer

https://www.cancerresearchuk.org/about-cancer/ovarian-cancer

NICE Guideline 131 (updated 2021) *Prostate cancer: diagnosis and management*: www.nice.org.uk/guidance/conditions-and-diseases/cancer/prostate-cancer

De Nunzio C, Lombardo R (2024) Best of 2023 in prostate cancer and prostatic diseases. *Prostate Cancer Prostatic Dis.* https://www.nature.com/articles/s41391-024-00790-7.

GP notebook (2021) *Haematuria.* https://gpnotebook.com/en-GB/pages/renal-medicine/haematuria

Pajunen H, Veitonmäki T, Huhtala H, et al. (2024) Prognostic factors of renal cell cancer in elderly patients: a population-based cohort study. Sci. Rep. 14:6295. https://www.nature.com/articles/s41598-024-56835-3.

NICE CKS (2024) *Incontinence – urinary, in women* https://cks.nice.org.uk/topics/incontinence-urinary-in-women

Harding CK, Lapitan MC, Arlandis S, et al. *EAU guidelines on management of non-neurogenic female lower urinary tract symptoms.* https://d56bochluxqnz.cloudfront.net/documents/full-guideline/EAU-Guidelines-on-Non-neurogenic-Female-LUTS-2024.pdf

Stoniute A, Madhuvrata P, Still M, et al. (2023) Oral anticholinergic drugs versus placebo or no treatment for managing overactive bladder syndrome in adults. *Cochrane Database Syst. Rev.* (5). Art. No.: CD003781. doi: 10.1002/14651858.CD003781.pub3.

Özcan C, Sancı A, Beyatlı M, et al. (2023) The efficiency and safety of mirabegron monotherapy for the treatment of urge incontinence in women aged >80 years. *Cureus* 15:e33685. doi: 10.7759/cureus.33685.

Brewster ET, Rounsefell B, Lin F, et al. (2022) Adult incontinence products are a larger and faster growing waste issue than disposable infant nappies (diapers) in Australia. *Waste Manag.* 152:30–37. doi: 10.1016/j.wasman.2022.07.038.

Chapple CR, Cruz F, Deffieux X, et al. (2017) Consensus Statement of the European Urology Association and the European Urogynaecological Association on the use of implanted materials for treating pelvic organ prolapse and stress urinary incontinence. *Eur. Urol.* 72:424–431. doi: 10.1016/j.eururo.2017.03.048.

NICE CKS (2021) *Symptoms suggestive of gynaecological cancers.* https://cks.nice.org.uk/topics/gynaecological-cancers-recognition-referral/diagnosis/symptoms-suggestive-of-gynaecological-cancers

Manda R, Tavakoli N, Stefanacci R, et al. (2021) Review: Management of vulvovaginal disorders in older women. *Ann. Longterm Care* 29:13–17. doi: 10.25270/altc.2020.4.00001.

Lee D, Nazroo J, O'Connor D, et al. (2016) Sexual health and wellbeing among older men and women in England: findings from the English Longitudinal Study of Ageing. *Arch. Sex Behav.* 45:133–144. https://eprints.whiterose.ac.uk/93296/1/ELSA-SRAQ_Pre-proofs.pdf.

Steckenrider J (2023) Sexual activity of older adults: let's talk about it. *Lancet Healthy Longev.* 4:E96–E97. doi: 10.1016/S2666-7568(23)00003-X.

 ## ADVICE FOR PATIENTS

Chronic kidney disease https://patient.info/kidney-urinary-tract/chronic-kidney-disease-leaflet

Prostate Cancer UK https://prostatecanceruk.org

AgeUK urinary incontinence www.ageuk.org.uk/information-advice/health-wellbeing/conditions-illnesses/urinary-incontinence

Disability Rights UK – how to order a radar key https://shop.disabilityrightsuk.org/products/radar-key

Squeezy App (pelvic floor exercises): this can be downloaded for a small fee, or patients can be invited to join Squeezy Connect, a free NHS version, by a participating clinic. https://squeezyapp.com

AgeUK Sex in Later Life: www.ageuk.org.uk/information-advice/health-wellbeing/relationships-family/sex-in-later-life/5-reasons-sexual-health

National Association for Continence: https://nafc.org

Continence Product Advisor (independent): https://www.continenceproductadvisor.org

All websites were accessed in April 2024.

16

Homeostasis and endocrinology

Ageing changes

There are changes in body composition, circulating hormones, neurotransmitters, and their receptors.

Body composition

1 ↓ lean body mass and body water and a relative increase in fat.
2 When marked this is known as sarcopaenia, which is a marker of physical frailty and has gained acceptance as a geriatric syndrome (see Chapter 4).

Hormone changes

Many hormones are affected by ageing but except for sex hormones the changes are not marked enough to warrant age-specific reference ranges. Even where plasma levels are similar there may be changes in circadian rhythm and feedback. Some of the changes have clinical consequences, e.g. impaired ability to concentrate urine resulting in nocturia, affect treatment (e.g. choice of first-line drugs for hypertension), and predispose to impaired homeostasis.

1 ↓ in both growth hormone (GH) and IGF-1, sometimes referred to as the somatopause. However, GH is not clinically useful as an anti-ageing therapy.
2 Oestrogen and progesterone in women ↓, follicle-stimulating hormone (FSH) and luteinising hormone (LH) ↑.
3 Testosterone in men ↓ (more gradual than the changes of menopause), FSH and LH ↑.
4 Insulin levels are often similar but less effective (due to insulin resistance): glucose tolerance diminishes.
5 Parathormone ↑.
6 Cortisol levels tend to be slightly ↑.
7 Antidiuretic hormone (ADH), also known as arginine vasopressin (AVP)↓ especially at night.
8 Atrial natriuretic peptide ↑.
9 Renin and aldosterone ↓.
10 Serum noradrenaline ↑ (but beta-receptors ↓) but adrenaline levels are ↓.

Adenomas are common in the anterior pituitary, thyroid, and adrenal glands and are usually of no clinical significance.

Fluid and electrolyte imbalance

Acutely unwell elderly patients are very often fluid-depleted or fluid-overloaded, and occasionally both.

Reasons for vulnerability to abnormalities of fluid balance

1 Reduced body water.
2 Inadequate intake due to:
   • Impaired thirst response.
   • Dementia or depression.
   • Immobility.
   • Reluctance through fear of being 'caught short'.
   • Swallowing difficulty.
   • Acute illness.
3 Increased loss:
   • Reduced concentrating ability by the kidney.
   • Diuretics.
   • Diabetes, diarrhoea, and vomiting.
   • Significant haemorrhage is more common.

Inadequate intake tends to result in shortage of water, initially affecting mainly the intracellular compartment and producing hypertonicity. This is correctly termed 'dehydration'. Symptoms include thirst (which may be blunted in older people), reduced urine output, confusion and drowsiness.

Increased loss results in loss of salt and water primarily causing a deficit in extracellular fluid or intravascular volume, and symptoms of volume depletion especially postural hypotension. Volume depletion may be isonatraemic, hyponatraemic or hypernatraemic depending on the composition of the fluid that is lost and the fluid it is replaced with (see the clear discussion by Asim). Salt and water loss are often replaced by water, tea, etc. Mixed salt and water depletion presents with confusion, weakness, reduced tissue turgor, tachycardia, and postural hypotension.

Hyponatraemia

This is the commonest electrolyte disturbance and is due to either too little sodium, too much water, or both. Do not treat the serum sodium level in isolation. If the result is very abnormal check whether it was taken from an arm attached to an intravenous infusion. Depending on the assay, high lipids, and high protein (e.g. myeloma) can give false results. The key is to make an accurate clinical assessment of the patient's fluid status. Decide whether the patient is volume depleted, euvolaemic, or fluid overloaded. The most accurate clinical finding in volume depletion is postural hypotension. Standard investigations in electrolyte disturbances include TSH and cortisol but abnormalities in these are rarely the cause in older people.

- If the patient is volume depleted, salt and water have been lost either through the kidneys (diuretics, especially thiazides, renal failure, osmotic diuresis), the gut (vomiting, diarrhoea, fistula, adenoma) or skin (burns).
- If the patient is oedematous, there is relative water excess due to fluid retention (in cardiac failure, liver failure or nephrotic syndrome) or excess water intake (i.e. occasionally overenthusiastic intravenous fluid supplementation after surgery).

Syndrome of inappropriate antidiuretic hormone secretion

If the urine is concentrated when it should not be (urinary sodium >30 mmol/L in the presence of hyponatraemia) and the plasma is dilute with a low plasma osmolality (<275 mmol/kg water), this is syndrome of inappropriate antidiuretic hormone secretion (SIADH).

- It is characterised by hypotonic hyponatraemia, concentrated urine, and a euvolaemic state.
- The impairment of free water excretion is caused by increased ADH release.
- It accounts for a third of all cases of hyponatremia.
- Accumulation of intracellular water in the brain causes confusion, headache, lethargy, coma, and seizures.

The level of sodium and the rate at which it falls are important: if it happens slowly brain cells have time to adapt to extracellular hypotonicity. Conversely, rapid correction may lead to the irreversible osmotic demyelination syndrome: paresis, dysphagia, dysarthria, diplopia, and loss of consciousness. In frail, older people aim to correct the sodium by not more than 8–10 mmol/L/24 hr.

The mechanism by which ADH affects water reabsorption in the renal collecting ducts is shown in Figure 16.1.

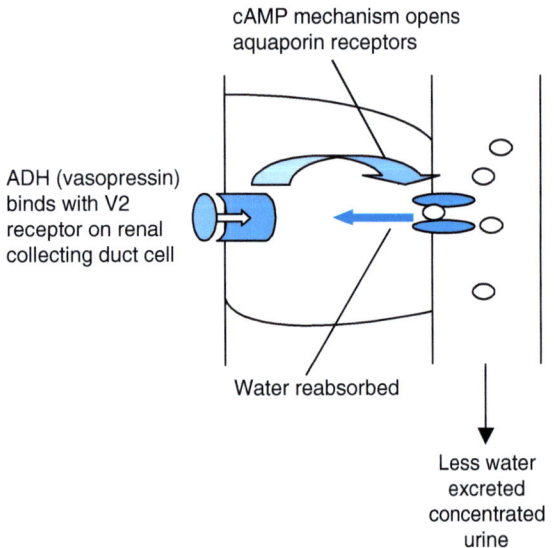

Figure 16.1 Mechanism of action of ADH at the collecting duct.

Causes

- Drugs, especially SSRIs, venlafaxine, opiates, antiepileptics, omeprazole.
- Malignancy, especially small-cell lung cancer.
- CNS disorders, e.g. subdural haematoma.
- Chest disease, e.g. pneumonia.
- Post-operative pain.

Treatment

Patients with severe hyponatraemia <120 mmol/L, those with rapid-onset hyponatraemia, and those with neurological impairment are at substantial risk of neurological consequences and should be considered for admission to a high dependency unit (HDU).

- Remove the underlying cause.
- Water restriction/intravenous infusion of normal or hypertonic saline as appropriate. Correct abnormalities slowly.
- Central venous access facilitates the assessment of fluid balance and frequent electrolyte testing.
- Drugs that promote free water excretion may be useful for chronic SIADH if long-term fluid restriction is poorly tolerated.
  - Demeclocycline (blocks the action of ADH on the tubule).
  - Vaptans, e.g. tolvaptan (an ADH-receptor antagonist). Rarely used acutely because of the risk of a too rapid correction. Risk of hepatotoxicity.

Hypernatraemia

This is usually due to water depletion in excess of sodium depletion and occurs when patients are unable to take in enough water to meet their needs.

- It is most common in older people with dementia and may be precipitated by water loss, e.g. in viral gastroenteritis, a heat wave or loop diuretics.
- It can also occur, usually in men, when obstructive uropathy is relieved.
- In people with diabetes mellitus exclude a hyperosmolar hyperglycaemic state (HHS).
- Central diabetes insipidus (DI) is due to ADH deficiency, e.g. after head trauma or nephrogenic DI; collecting duct insensitivity to ADH, e.g. due to lithium, present with polyuria and polydipsia; and are both rare in older people.

Seek endocrinology advice. Initial management for hypernatraemia is usually gradual rehydration with isotonic saline and oral fluids.

Oedema

Oedema is the presence of excess interstitial fluid in the tissues, which causes palpable swelling. Oedema develops when microvascular filtration exceeds lymph drainage for a sustained period. If oedema is present at knee level in a patient in a chair, check whether it extends up the back of the thigh; if it is present there too, lean the patient forward to check for a sacral pad. Bed-bound patients may have slim ankles but marked sacral oedema. Not all leg swelling is oedema, and not all oedema is due to heart failure (see Table 16.1).

Hypokalaemia

Low potassium is common in older patients, often due to diuretics or GI loss (remember the laxative abuser), exacerbated by inadequate dietary intake (especially fruit, vegetables, and meat). Primary aldosteronism is under-recognised. Sick older females may develop 'acute transient hypokalaemia', probably due to a shift into the cells, which usually

Table 16.1 Causes of leg swelling.

Raised venous pressure:
- Gravity (prolonged sitting).
- Cardiac failure.
- Pelvic mass.

The following causes are often unilateral:
- Venous insufficiency (side of hip surgery).
- DVT.
- Lack of muscle pump (side of hemiparesis).
- Chronic venous disease.

Note that in conditions that would cause bilateral oedema, an overactive muscle pump in one leg (e.g. tremor in PD) may result in the oedema appearing unilateral.

Fluid retention:
- Cardiac failure.
- Drugs (NSAIDs, steroids, calcium channel blockers, glitazones).
- Kidney failure.

Hypoalbuminaemia:
- Nutritional, hepatic disease or protein loss via kidney (dip-stick urine for protein).
- Leak from bowels or extensive skin loss.

Lymphatic obstruction:
- Usually malignancy or its treatment.
- Morbid obesity.

Inflammatory:
- Cellulitis – usually unilateral
- Ruptured popliteal (Baker's) cyst – usually unilateral.

self-corrects within a few days. Hypokalaemia exacerbates digoxin toxicity. Muscle weakness is typically seen if the potassium is <3.0 mmol/L. Check the ECG for U-waves. Replace potassium orally or by slow intravenous infusion in crystalloid if severe. If the response is poor, check for low magnesium (more likely on proton pump inhibitors), as correcting this helps.

Hyperkalaemia

This occurs in renal failure and rhabdomyolysis (which may follow a collapse and long lie). However, drugs are the common culprits. In old age, cardiac failure can often be managed with furosemide alone without needing the addition of potassium-retaining amiloride or spironolactone. A combination of an ACE inhibitor and spironolactone may be an evidence-based treatment for cardiac failure, but it will usually increase the risk of dangerous hyperkalaemia in older kidneys! For management, see Chapter 15.

Diabetes mellitus

Definition

Diabetes mellitus (DM) is a metabolic syndrome with heterogeneous aetiologies characterised by chronic hyperglycaemia and disturbances of carbohydrate, fat, and protein metabolism resulting from defects in insulin secretion, insulin action or both.

The WHO/NICE recommend an HbA1c cut point of ≥48 mmol/mol (6.5%) for the diagnosis of diabetes.

- **Advantages:** reflects average glucose over 8–12 weeks and avoids day-to-day variability; the test can be done at any time of day without fasting or a glucose load.
- **Disadvantages:** affected by anaemia, haemoglobinopathies, and red cell turnover (e.g. malaria and renal failure).

Other criteria include:

- Random plasma glucose of ≥11.1 mmol/L in a symptomatic patient or
- Fasting plasma glucose of ≥7.0 mmol/L

Epidemiology

The prevalence is higher in men and rises with age (see Figure 16.2). It is higher in people of South Asian, Chinese, African, and Afro-Caribbean heritage than White people in the UK. Since the 1990s, the number of people with diabetes has increased fourfold to around 5 million (4.3 million with a diagnosis and an estimated 850,000 who are yet to be identified). The increase is mainly due to population ageing and increasing obesity. Prevalence is also linked to social deprivation. 90% of adults with diabetes mellitus have the type 2 variant (T2DM). Half the diabetic population and a quarter of insulin users are older people. A 'ballpark' figure is that around 15% of people aged over 70 have known diabetes and 5% have undiagnosed diabetes. In care homes, around a quarter of residents have diabetes. The NHS spends at least £10 billion a year on diabetes (about 10% of its budget).

Prediabetes

The use of HbA1c in diagnosis has led to the identification of many people with prediabetes or non-diabetic hyperglycaemia (HbA1c 42–47 mmol/mol).

- Carries increased cardiovascular risk.
- Three out of four will go on to develop T2DM.

Lifestyle change, particularly moderate weight loss, has been shown to reduce or stop the progression of diabetes, and patients

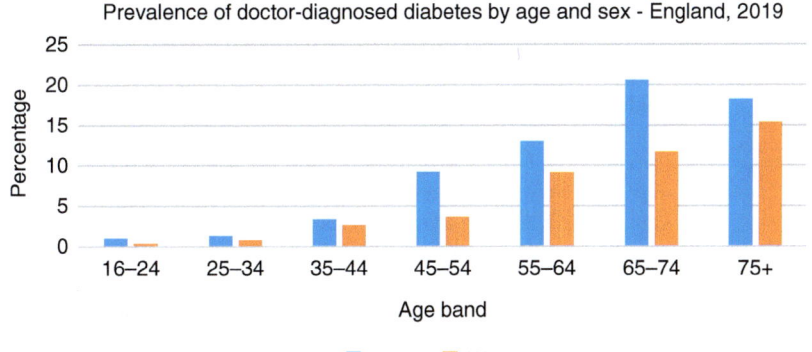

Prevalence of doctor-diagnosed diabetes by age and sex - England, 2019

Figure 16.2 shows the effect of age on the prevalence of diabetes in England.

should be offered a referral to the Diabetes Prevention Project. More work is needed on whether the cut points for diagnosis using HbA1c are equally applicable across the age range; older people typically have mildly raised fasting glucose levels but marked post-prandial hyperglycaemia.

Pathogenesis

The impairment of glucose tolerance in old age is mainly caused by reduced tissue sensitivity to insulin at the post-receptor level. There is also beta-cell dysfunction; the pancreas is less able to secrete insulin in response to a glucose load, and the rapid post-prandial spike of secretion is lost. The older diabetic usually has T2DM, although the number of type 1 graduates will increase steadily. Occasionally, type 1 diabetes occurs de novo in an older person.

Effects

Diabetics aged 65–75 have twice the cardiovascular and all-cause mortality of their non-diabetic peers, but thereafter mortality tends to revert towards normal for age. One-third has visual impairment, more often due to cataracts than to retinopathy, and the amputation rate is enormously increased. Cognitive and psychosocial function is often impaired. A common end-stage comprises poor cardiac function, renal failure, and marked oedema.

Management

This is becoming a lost skill for the average medical practitioner due to the advent of specialist nurse-led community teams who often supervise care. Diabetes management must be part of an integrated approach to cardiovascular risk and will depend on the circumstances of the patient; a frail nursing home resident requires different care than an otherwise fit and independent 75-year-old who should have access to the same resources as a younger person. Stopping smoking and treating high blood pressure and lipids continue to have high value in addition to good diabetic control.

The aims include:

- Enabling the patient to feel well.
- Avoidance of glycosuria was a traditional aim of diabetes management as osmotic diuresis gives rise to symptoms. The renal threshold increases with age, so tight control is not needed to achieve this. However, the mechanism of action of one of the groups of drugs used to manage diabetes, the sodium-glucose co-transporter 2 (SGLT2) inhibitors is to block glucose reabsorption in the proximal renal tubule resulting in glycosuria.
- Tight enough control to reduce complications in 'younger' older patients. Older people with diabetes should have an appropriate, individual HbA1c target. Good glycaemic control has a greater impact on microvascular than macrovascular complications. While the United Kingdom Prospective Diabetes Study (UKPDS) showed benefit in those <65 years old, there is limited evidence to confirm that tight diabetic control has the desired effect on cardiovascular risk and mortality in frail older patients.
- Hypoglycaemia (medication-related) is a more frequent occurrence in this population and can cause brain damage/injury/seizures/death. Therefore, this should be avoided, even if it leads to less-than-perfect glycaemic control.

The Action to Control Cardiovascular Risk in Diabetes (ACCORD) trial was terminated early due to increased mortality in the group with stricter glycaemic control. The Action in Diabetes and Vascular Disease: Preterax and DiamicroN Controlled Evaluation (ADVANCE) and the Veterans Affairs Diabetes Trial (VADT) did not show increased mortality

with tighter glycaemic control, but nor was there clear cardiovascular benefit, although nephropathy was reduced. Note that the mean age of participants in these studies ranged from 60 to 66 years.

General approach

The management of people with diabetes of all ages is multidisciplinary and, depending on severity, requires regular input and a comprehensive annual review, including weight, BP, foot check, injection site check if relevant, urine dip for microalbuminuria, blood tests for HbA1c, cholesterol, renal function, and retinal photography.

- Education: about diabetes and how lifestyle changes will help, and encouragement to join a programme such as DESMOND (Diabetes Education and Self-Management for Ongoing and Newly Diagnosed) and a local support group.
- Diet: weight reduction in the obese, reducing fat intake and ensuring that carbohydrates are of a high-fibre, unrefined, polysaccharide type. Because of the failure of the post-prandial insulin spike, the concept of the glycaemic index of food may be useful. Some carbohydrates are absorbed quickly, and blood glucose levels increase very rapidly ('high GI' foods), while others release glucose slowly and have little effect on blood glucose ('low GI' foods). Carbohydrates are ranked on a scale of 1–100, with glucose being used as the reference point of 100. GLP-1 analogues may be game-changing in future (see later).
- Exercise: highly beneficial (walking half an hour a day) or 'exercise snacking'. Any increase in physical activity is beneficial.
- Smoking: refer to the local quit service.
- Hypertension: treat vigorously if the patient can tolerate this. ACE inhibitors and ARBs have a particular role in reducing microscopic albuminuria. However, avoid causing postural hypotension.
- Hypercholesterolaemia: statins (at least up to 80 years).
- Foot care and regular chiropody: particularly important for older diabetics. Once foot complications occur, the patient's quality of life plunges, and the costs of care increase dramatically. An extended period in hospital usually culminates in an above-knee amputation.

Drug options for hyperglycaemia

If drugs are needed, many classes are available. Tablets can be given in various combinations (fixed-dose combinations are available) and used with injectable drugs. NICE produces flow charts to suggest the order in which the drugs should be used to achieve the individual's HbA1c target. If there are no contraindications or problems with tolerance, a typical order would be metformin, then add an SGLT2 inhibitor (good for the heart, BP and kidneys but caution with volume depletion/UTIs in older people). Then add one of a sulfonylurea, a dipeptidyl peptidase-4 (DPP-4) inhibitor, insulin or, if very obese, a glucagon-like peptide-1 (GLP-1) agonist. There is an increasing literature on deprescribing where older people are overtreated.

Oral drugs

- Metformin, a biguanide, decreases gluconeogenesis and increases the peripheral utilisation of glucose. It is traditionally first-line. Patients usually lose weight. Care must be taken if there is renal impairment (contraindicated if eGFR <30 ml/min). Increase the dose gradually to minimise GI side effects, and if these are unacceptable, try modified-release metformin. It is very unlikely to cause a hypoglycaemic event. Check the B_{12} level.
- Sulfonylureas augment insulin secretion from pancreatic beta cells by binding to sulfonylurea receptors. These drugs are highly likely to cause hypoglycaemia in older patients and so are avoided if possible.

If no other options are available, choose a sulfonylurea with a short half-life (glipizide), which reduces the risk of adverse effects.

- DPP-4 inhibitors, or 'gliptins', such as sitagliptin and vildagliptin, are orally active inhibitors of the enzyme that inactivates endogenous GLP-1. Physiologically, levels of GLP-1 rise in response to rising glucose after a meal and are responsible for the incretin effect, increasing pancreatic insulin secretion post-prandially. The therapeutic effects of DPP-4 inhibitors are therefore analogous to those of GLP-1 agonists/mimetics; they are less potent but weight-neutral and do not usually cause hypoglycaemia. They should be used cautiously in renal impairment.
- SGLT2 inhibitors or 'flozins' are secreted in the proximal tubules and resorb most of the glucose load undergoing filtration. They are associated with urinary tract infections and dehydration secondary to osmotic diuresis and are hence used with caution in older patients, but may be used first-line in younger patients with CKD. There is a risk of atypical ketoacidosis.
- GLP-1 agonists that can be given orally are becoming available (see later).

Rarely used

- Alpha-glucosidase inhibitor: acarbose, which delays starch absorption, is *often not well tolerated* because of flatulence but is safe and useful for those who can take it.
- Thiazolidinediones ('glitazones') activate the peroxisome-proliferator-activated receptor gamma (PPARγ) in the cell nucleus and increase glucose uptake and peripheral utilisation. They are *rarely used in older people* as they are contraindicated in heart failure. Unexpected osteoporotic fractures and cardiac side effects led to the withdrawal of rosiglitazone and a reduction in pioglitazone use.

Injectable drugs

- GLP-1 agonists
  GLP-1 agonists include exenatide, dulaglutide, and semaglutide. This class of injectable therapy for T2DM enhances post-prandial, glucose-dependent insulin secretion from the patient's beta cells. This has a physiological appeal; it makes hypoglycaemia less likely, and the drugs induce early satiety and thus weight loss. These are advantages over insulin in T2DM, which tends to cause weight gain and has the risk of hypoglycaemia. The early drugs in the class needed injecting once or twice a day. Several have been modified in various ways to increase their half-life and can be given weekly, e.g. once weekly exenatide, dulaglutide, and semaglutide. This would be a big advantage for older people who cannot manage daily insulin injections. Oral semaglutide is now available.
  - They are effective in reducing HbA1c and fasting glucose.
  - They reduce cardiovascular and cerebrovascular disease.
  - GI side effects are common, and more serious problems, including pancreatitis, have been reported.
  - The weight loss that can be achieved with semaglutide as Ozempic (and the larger dose in Wegovy – NICE-approved for weight loss in specialist obesity clinics) has been widely reported in social media.
  - Off-label and private prescribing has resulted in shortages for people with diabetes.
  - NICE guidance in 2024 still sets extremely tight limits on who should be offered GLP-1 agonists. Treatment is limited to people with T2DM attending hospital clinics with significant obesity and poor control, despite three drugs.
  - More data is needed, particularly on cardiovascular benefits and in older patients, but this group of drugs may be a game changer for weight loss in T2DM.
  - Tirzepatide, a novel dual GLP-1 and GIP (glucose-dependent insulinotropic polypeptide) agonist, appears even more potent at reducing HbA1c and weight.

- Insulin
  If control is poor (HbA1c ≥75 mmol/mol), it is a mistake to be too reluctant to start insulin, as this makes the person feel much better.
  - Combinations of insulin and tablets are increasingly used.
  - A single daily injection of insulin glargine or detemir can achieve adequate control with minimal risk of hypoglycaemia. This is useful if the patient cannot inject their own insulin and must rely on a visiting district nurse, as exact timing is not critical.
  - Even if good glycaemic control is not achieved, if the patient does not have the cognition, dexterity, or vision to give their own insulin, intensifying the regimen can be impractical.
  - A traditional twice-a-day mixed insulin regimen necessitates eating lunch at a fixed time and having an evening snack to avoid nocturnal hypoglycaemia and hence is useful for care home residents with regular mealtimes.
- Fit, active older people will manage a basal-bolus regimen just like younger people. Such patients should also be considered for newer technologies such as insulin pumps and continuous glucose monitoring (CGM), which can improve both diabetic control and quality of life in carefully selected patients.

Patients on any glucose-lowering drugs need further education to make sure they understand how and when to take the drug and how to recognise and manage hypoglycaemia. Glucose sweets should be carried for 'hypos' – blood sugar rises slowly after eating a Mars bar as the fat content delays gastric emptying! Check whether your patient drives and advise accordingly.

Hyperosmolar crisis (hyperosmolar hyperglycaemic state)

Diabetic crises and complications do not present any distinctive features in older people apart from the increased incidence of HHS.

- This typically occurs in patients with T2DM, which has often caused very few clinical problems.
- Infection is the most common trigger (look at the feet).
- It is a rare complication (1% of diabetic-related admissions) but has a mortality rate of up to 10%.
- An osmotic diuresis leads to insidiously progressive dehydration and hypotension, culminating in stupor or coma.
- There is still some endogenous insulin, so there is no switch to metabolic pathways that results in ketosis.
- Extreme hyperglycaemia, hypernatraemia, and uraemia are typical.
- Serum osmolality is often >320 mOsm/kg.

The aim in treating HHS is the steady correction of metabolic derangement. Remember that rehydration is more important than insulin.

- It is safest to give 0.9% (normal) saline, as this will be dilute in comparison with the plasma.
- Depending on the severity and the patient's cardiac status, give a litre over 1–2 hours initially.
- Continue with a litre over 2, 4, 6 hours, and so on, but the key is frequent monitoring.
- Aim for fluid input to exceed output by 3–6 L over the first 12 hr, ideally monitored by a central venous pressure (CVP) line and in an HDU.
- Ensure that there are no rapid changes in plasma sodium levels – aim not to reduce by more than 10 mmol/L/24 hr.

Hyperglycaemia often improves with rehydration alone, and insulin may not be required. The risk of venous thrombosis is high, so give prophylactic low molecular-weight heparin. Remember to consider precipitants, and antibiotics should be commenced if there is any hint of bacterial infection.

If it occurs, diabetic ketoacidosis is managed in the usual way.

Thyroid disease

Thyroid function tests

Normal thyroid function is usually preserved until at least 80 years of age, but in centenarians, TSH and free T3 levels may decline. In the seriously ill patient, the TSH, T3, and T4 levels may all be misleadingly low ('sick euthyroid syndrome'). Amiodarone and anticonvulsants often interfere with thyroid function tests (TFTs). Always check TFTs before starting amiodarone, and remember that this will interfere with radioiodine treatment. Both hypo- and hyperthyroidism are difficult to diagnose clinically in old age, and many geriatricians routinely check TSH in any significant illness.

Hyperthyroidism

Presentation is atypical – AF, heart failure, weight loss, proximal myopathy, functional decline. The thyroid may be nodular or impalpable – sometimes retrosternal.

- Treatment is carbimazole and a beta-blocker if the heart rate is high before definitive therapy with I^{131} (radioiodine).
- Carbimazole can be given at a dose aiming for a normal thyroid hormone level or at a dose sufficient to block all production with levothyroxine replacement (see BNF), updated 6-monthly.

Remember to give written advice about a sore throat on carbimazole (neutropaenia). The management of amiodarone-induced thyrotoxicosis is controversial. Some advocate ignoring a raised-free T_4 but treating the raised T_3 with carbimazole and steroids.

Hypothyroidism

Hypothyroidism affects 5% of people aged over 60, and it may be due to Hashimoto's disease, prior I^{131} treatment, surgery, idiopathic or, occasionally, secondary to pituitary failure. Clinical pointers include impaired cognition and slow-relaxing reflexes.

- Treatment is with levothyroxine 25 µg, with similar increments every 3–4 weeks until, on a daily dose of around 100 µg, the patient usually feels well and the TSH confirms euthyroidism.
- If a profoundly hypothyroid woman is admitted and 100 µg levothyroxine tablets are brought in with her, do not just write them on the chart – it is highly likely she has not been taking them. Get advice, and if in doubt build up from a low dose to avoid precipitating a cardiac event.

Adrenal disease

Cushing's syndrome

The commonest cause is iatrogenic: older people are often left on higher doses of steroids than they need, particularly for polymyalgia rheumatica, which usually burns itself out after a couple of years. Older people are particularly prone to fluid retention, heart failure, diabetes, proximal myopathy, skin thinning and bruising, and osteoporosis (always give bone protection), and high doses may lead to acute confusion ('steroid psychosis'). Around three-quarters of patients with endogenous corticosteroid excess have a pituitary tumour producing ACTH (Cushing's disease). Even less common are functional adrenal adeno-

mas, adrenal carcinoma, or ectopic ACTH secretion from bronchogenic or neuroendocrine tumours.

Addison's disease

Primary adrenal insufficiency may present acutely, usually when there is an acute, severe illness in a patient with iatrogenic adrenal suppression due to long-term steroid treatment. Chronic adrenal insufficiency is due to autoimmune destruction, metastases, or TB (the commonest cause worldwide) or infiltration, e.g. amyloid and haemochromatosis. You must consider the possibility if you are ever to make this diagnosis because the presentation is insidious even in middle age. Postural symptoms are common. If the patient is ill and suspicion is high, send a cortisol sample urgently and treat straight away with 100 mg hydrocortisone IV six hourly and fluids. Otherwise, do a short Synacthen test. Long-term treatment is hydrocortisone, ideally 10 mg in the morning, 5 mg at lunch, and 5 mg early in the evening, with 100 mcg fludrocortisone daily, then tailored to the individual.

Paraneoplastic syndromes

Paraneoplastic syndromes are a group of disorders that sometimes occur in malignancy and are not directly attributable to tumour invasion, tumour compression, or metastasis (see Table 16.2). They are due to tumour secretion of bioactive substances such as hormones, peptides including cytokines, exosomes (membrane-bound extracellular vesicles containing various compounds), or autoantibodies and cytotoxic T cells produced in response to the tumour and its products.

- With endocrine manifestations, the literature is inconsistent as to whether only ectopic hormone production is included or whether secretion (albeit unregulated) by a tumour in the tissue that usually produces that hormone is also included (strictly termed eutopic secretion).
- A wide range of organ systems can be affected, and symptoms can present before or after recognition of the underlying malignancy.

SIADH was first described as a paraneoplastic condition and is due to tumour cell production of ADH and atrial natriuretic peptide, which has natriuretic and antidiuretic properties. Hypercalcaemia occurs in up to 10% of all patients with advanced cancer and carries a poor prognosis. In paraneoplastic Cushing's syndrome, patients often present with symptoms before a cancer diagnosis is made. Unlike a pituitary source, paraneoplastic Cushing's syndrome does not respond to high-dose dexamethasone suppression. Drugs are used to inhibit steroid production; ketoconazole is first-line treatment. Tumour-associated hypoglycaemia is rare. The mediators are often not known, even in 'classical' syndromes.

Treatment is usually symptomatic and then that of the underlying malignancy, but the prognosis is often poor.

Autonomic nervous system

The autonomic nervous system (ANS) is the part of the nervous system most involved in homoeostatic mechanisms. There is age-related decline, but more obvious problems result from central or peripheral damage, e.g. diabetes, alcoholism, Parkinson's disease (multi-system atrophy is less common but more severe), uraemia, drug-induced neuropathies, amyloidosis, autoimmune disorders, and paraneoplastic syndromes. Common manifestations are orthostatic hypotension, erectile dysfunction, impaired bladder emptying, gastric paresis, diarrhoea, or constipation. A battery of tests for autonomic function may be used.

Table 16.2 Clinical presentations of paraneoplastic syndromes.

Organ system	Syndromes	Aetiology	Associations
Systemic	Cachexia, anorexia, fever	Complex, multifactorial, with a significant inflammatory component	Common, affecting >50% of people with malignancy. Particularly marked in lung, GI, and pancreatic cancers
Endocrine	Cushing's syndrome	Ectopic ACTH	Small cell lung cancer (SCLC), islet cell tumours, bronchial carcinoid
		Corticotrophin releasing hormone	
	SIADH	Ectopic ADH	SCLC, head, and neck cancer
		Ectopic atrial natriuretic peptide	
	Hypercalcaemia	Ectopic parathyroid hormone-related peptide (most common)	Squamous carcinomas, especially of the urinary tract and breast
		Lytic metastases are the second most common cause of malignant hypercalcaemia	Myeloma, renal carcinoma, lung cancer, thyroid cancer, melanoma
		Tumour secretion of vitamin D	Lymphomas and ovarian germ cell tumours
		Ectopic PTH is very rare	
	Hypoglycaemia	Big IGF-II	Sarcoma
		Insulin	Insulinoma or extrapancreatic secretion
	Carcinoid syndrome	Ectopic serotonin or bradykinin	Bronchial adenoma
			Gastric carcinoma
	Hyperaldosteronism	Ectopic aldosterone, e.g. from	Non-Hodgkin's lymphoma
			Adrenal adenoma
Haematological	Polycythaemia and thrombocytosis	Erythropoietin	Renal carcinoma, cerebellar haemangioma, uterine myoma, and hepatocellular carcinoma.
Renal	Nephrotic syndrome	Immune complex-mediated	Lung cancers, GI cancers
Rheumatological	Polyarthritis	?	Lung cancer, ovarian cancer
	Polymyalgia rheumatica	?	Myelodysplastic syndrome
	Hypertrophic osteoarthropathy	?	Lung cancer, especially adenocarcinoma
Dermatological	Acanthosis nigricans	?	Gastric adenocarcinoma
	Pemphigus	?	B-cell lymphomas
	Dermatomyositis	?	Breast, ovarian and lung cancers
Neurological			
CNS	Encephalitis	Anti-Hu, anti-Ma2 antibodies	Lung, especially SCLC, testicular, ovarian, and breast cancers
	Subacute cerebellar degeneration	?	SCLC
NMJ	Myasthenia gravis	Anti-acetylcholine receptor antibody	Thymoma
	Lambert-Eaton myasthenic syndrome	Anti-voltage-gated calcium channel antibody	SCLC, carcinoid
PNS	Autonomic neuropathy	?	SCLC
	Sensorimotor neuropathy	?	Lung cancer, myeloma. Lymphoma, breast

ACTH, adrenocorticotropic hormone; ADH, antidiuretic hormone; SIADH, syndrome of inappropriate ADH secretion; PTH, parathyroid hormone; big IGF-ii, pro-insulin-like growth factor-II

Accidental hypothermia

Clinical features

Hypothermia is defined as a core body temperature of <35° C. Above 32°C the features may be those of an underlying disease or functional decline. Lower temperatures may present with a loss of fine motor skills, slurred speech, and apathy. Below 27°C, 75% of the patients are coma-tose. Pancreatitis, hypoglycaemia, and ventricular arrhythmias are among the complications. The heart rate drops to 30–40 beats per minute at 27°C and continues to drop as the body temperature falls. J waves (not pathognomonic for hypothermia) may be seen on an ECG. Over 30°C, mortality is about 33%, but below 30°C it approaches 70%. Death certification records about 300 deaths from hypothermia annually in the UK, most of which are older people.

Although exposure on a picturesque mountain is what we may imagine, indoor accidental hypothermia is much more of a problem for the older people. Inadequately heated and insulated homes, rising energy bills, and social isolation (e.g. the housebound or after bereavement) are key risk factors. The most common presentation is following a fall, with a prolonged period on the floor, often only wearing nightwear.

Older people are more susceptible as they are less efficient at generating heat due to lower body mass, impaired mobility, a poor diet, and a reduced ability to shiver. They are also less able to vasoconstrict peripherally. The presence of co-morbidity such as stroke or CNS infection may affect central thermoregulation, and the 'hypo'-endocrinopathies may limit heat production. Excess alcohol intake can also predispose (peripheral dilatation, hypoglycaemia). The hypothermia associated with sepsis (so-called 'cold sepsis') is associated with worse outcomes. Opiates and benzodiazepines predispose to hypothermia, as can lithium toxicity.

Management

At a core temperature just below 35°C, it is reasonable to rewarm the patient at home and counsel to prevent recurrence, involving social services if there are concerns about self-neglect. More serious cases (30–34°C) have traditionally received gradual passive re-warming in hospital at 0.5–1.0°C per hour to avoid sudden, profound hypotension. Avoid instrumentation, which may precipitate serious arrhythmia. Below 30°C, some would argue that admission to the ITU is required. However, most older patients are managed on a ward with active rewarming using a 'Bair hugger' or forced-air warming system.

Other dangers of extreme weather

Although the number of deaths directly attributable to hypothermia in the UK is low, cold kills in other ways, and in an average year in England and Wales, there are 30,000 more winter deaths than non-winter deaths. Circulatory deaths are higher; platelets, haematocrit, blood viscosity, fibrinogen, cholesterol, and systolic BP all tend to rise on exposure to the cold. Respiratory illnesses are more common (typically influenza and, more recently, COVID-19) and slipping on icy pavements is a further hazard.

The incidence of strokes and the mortality rate also tend to rise among older people during heat waves (see Chapter 1).

📖 REFERENCES AND FURTHER READING

Asim, M., Alkadi, M. M., Asim, H. et al. (2019), Dehydration and volume depletion: How to handle the misconceptions. *World J Nephrol, 8*, 23–32. doi: 10.5527/wjn.v8.i1.23.

Biagetti B, Puig-Domingo M (2023) Age-related hormone changes and its impact on health status and lifespan. *Aging Dis.* 14(3):605–620. doi: 10.14336/AD.2022.1109.

NICE CKS *Hyponatraemia* https://cks.nice.org.uk/topics/hyponatraemia

BMJ Best Practice *SIADH* (2021) https://bestpractice.bmj.com/topics/en-gb/196

Hypernatraemia (2022) https://patient.info/doctor/hypernatraemia

Goyal A, Cusick S, Bhutta BS StatPearls (2023) *Peripheral Edema* https://www.ncbi.nlm.nih.gov/books/NBK554452

BMJ Best Practice *Hypokalaemia* (2022) https://bestpractice.bmj.com/topics/en-gb/59

BMJ Best Practice *Hyperkalaemia* (2022) https://bestpractice.bmj.com/topics/en-gb/60

NICE CKS *Type 2 Diabetes in an adult*, and linked pages (2024) https://cks.nice.org.uk/topics/diabetes-type-2/diagnosis/diagnosis-in-adults

Clement M Landmark trials in type 2 diabetes https://www.diabetescarecommunity.ca/living-well-with-diabetes-articles/diabetes-management-articles/landmark-trials-in-type-2-diabetes

Nauck MA, Quast DR, Wefers J, et al. (2021) GLP-1 receptor agonists in the treatment of type 2 diabetes – state-of-the-art. *Mol. Metab.* 46:101102. doi: 10.1016/j.molmet.2020.101102.

Yao H, Zhang A, Li D, et al. (2024) Comparative effectiveness of GLP-1 receptor agonists on glycaemic control, body weight, and lipid profile for type 2 diabetes: systematic review and network meta-analysis. *BMJ* 384:e076410. doi: 10.1136/bmj-2023-076410.

Shi Q, Nong K, Vandvik PO, et al. (2023) Benefits and harms of drug treatment for type 2 diabetes: systematic review and network meta-analysis of randomised controlled trials. *BMJ* 381:e074068. doi: 10.1136/bmj-2022-074068.

NICE CKS *Hypothyroidism* (2021) https://cks.nice.org.uk/topics/hypothyroidism

NICE CKS *Hyperthyroidism* (2021) https://cks.nice.org.uk/topics/hyperthyroidism

BMJ Best Practice *Cushing syndrome* (2023) https://bestpractice.bmj.com/topics/en-gb/205

BMJ Best Practice *Primary adrenal insufficiency* (2022) https://bestpractice.bmj.com/topics/en-gb/56

Medscape *Paraneoplastic syndromes* (2023) Santacroce L https://emedicine.medscape.com/article/280744-overview

BMJ Best Practice *Accidental Hypothermia* (2021) https://bestpractice.bmj.com/topics/en-gb/3000179

ONS (2023) W*inter mortality in England and Wales: 2021 to 2022 (provisional) and 2020 to 2021 (final)* www.ons.gov.uk/peoplepopulationandcommunity/birthsdeathsandmarriages/deaths/bulletins/excesswintermortalityinenglandandwales/2021to2022provisionaland2020to2021final

INFORMATION FOR PATIENTS AND FAMILIES

Diabetes UK provides a wide range of information for patients and professionals: www.diabetes.org.uk

All websites were accessed in September 2024.

17

Haematology

Age-related changes

Bone marrow

1 By the age of 65, bone marrow cellularity is reduced by 30%.
2 The rest of the bone marrow is replaced by adipocytes. This may be driven in part by changes in insulin-like growth factor (IGF) signalling and inflammatory cytokines secreted by the adipocytes, which might be a factor in the promotion of myelopoiesis.
3 Changes to the haematopoietic niche include a reduced number of osteoblasts, changes in the extracellular matrix, an increase in reactive oxidative stress causing errors in mitochondrial DNA leading to reduced mitochondrial function, and increased levels of cytokines such as CCL5 (chemokine ligand 5).
4 The fall in osteoblasts contributes to osteoporosis and reduced trabecular bone for haematopoiesis.
5 Haematopoietic stem cells (HSC) double in number but have impaired function. Although HSCs can produce all cell lines, single-cell transplant experiments have shown that there are myeloid-biased HSCs, lymphoid-biased HSCs, and balanced HSCs. The stem cells produce haematoprogenitor cells (HPCs) of the relevant lineage, common myeloid progenitors, and common lymphoid progenitors. With ageing, there is a skew towards the myeloid lineage and a reduction in lymphoid cells. This leads to increased inflammation/inflammageing, an increased risk of autoimmune diseases and myeloid cancers, and a reduced ability to fight infection.

Red cells

1 Haemoglobin levels fall with age; there is debate as to how much this represents normal ageing or the increased prevalence of pathology and chronic inflammation.
2 The WHO definition of anaemia is haemoglobin of less than 130 g/L in males or less than 120 g/L in females. The validity and relevance of this definition for older people are disputed. Some suggest that lower cut-offs should be used in old age (110 g/L in frail men and 100 g/L in frail women) to avoid over-investigation, which is burdensome, expensive, and often does not reveal a cause. However, using the usual adult normal range ensures that treatable causes of anaemia are not missed.
3 Others argue that there is no logic to having a lower figure in women after menopause, and this contributes to rates of anaemia being higher in men.

4 The mean cell volume (MCV) tends to be higher in older people because reticulocytes are released earlier into the peripheral circulation.
5 The red cell differential width tends to be higher because of increased anisocytosis.

White cells

1 Normal white cell counts are $4-11 \times 10^9$/L. The normal range is not altered for older people, but it is accepted that the usual white count is lower. However, there may still be a marked rise in total white cells in response to inflammation, trauma, and especially sepsis.
2 The number of circulating neutrophils is broadly stable in healthy ageing. However, neutrophils from aged individuals function less well with reduced chemotaxis, phagocytosis, and intracellular killing. Increased neutrophils are associated with frailty, and systemic inflammageing may result in neutrophils expressing an activated phenotype. In acute pathology (using a mouse model of stroke and comparing blood samples from young and old stroke patients), part of the worse outcome with age may be mediated by the prothrombotic signature of neutrophils produced by the aged bone marrow in response.
3 The lymph nodes and the lymphoid tissue of the GI tract and spleen are much reduced. The thymus is atrophied by middle age, but thymic remnants are thought to remain active into extreme old age.
4 Lymphocyte production is reduced in the marrow.
5 The number of naïve B and T cells that migrate from primary to secondary lymphoid organs is reduced and overall B and T cell numbers decline.
6 After production in the marrow, immature IgM+ B cells migrate to the spleen, where they differentiate into follicular or marginal zone B cells. Changes in B cells with ageing include altered DNA methylation, increased pro-inflammatory cytokine secretion, impaired class switching of antibodies, reduced antibody affinity, and increased autoantibody production.
7 CD8+ (cytotoxic T cells) are effector cells when initially activated, but a small proportion persist as CD8+ memory cells. These tend to accumulate with age, often due to persistent infections such as cytomegalovirus, and this leads to a skewed repertoire and may block space for naïve lymphocytes, impairing the response to new infections. CD4+ (helper T cells) differentiate into T_H1, T_H2, T_H17, and other cells that mediate cell-mediated immunity and T follicular helper cells $T_{FH}1$, 2, and 3, which provide classic helper functions to B cells to improve the humoral response. Once pathogens are eliminated, most CD4+ T cells undergo cell death, but around 5% persist as CD4+ memory cells. Treg

cells (regulatory T cells) are a specialised CD4+ subset for maintaining immune tolerance by suppressing an immune response. Natural killer T cells (NKT) decrease. Numerous changes have been described in ageing, and in such a complex interactive system, it is unclear which changes are primary. CD8+ numbers decline more than CD4+ cells. Changes include reduced T-cell receptor signalling and altered patterns of cytokine release. CD4+ cells tend to differentiate into T_H17 cells, which produce a massive proinflammatory cytokine response, which might contribute to inflammageing.

8　Impairment of phagocytosis by macrophages is also reported.

Plasma proteins

Conflicting reports on age changes relate to the difficulty in distinguishing changes due solely to age from those due to other factors, such as malnutrition or disease. The main points to emerge are:

1　Low levels of total protein and of the individual fractions are pathological.
2　Increased globulin fractions indicate disease; however, asymptomatic individuals with very high levels of gamma globulins may have monoclonal gammopathy of unknown significance (MGUS) rather than myeloma.
3　Abnormal immunoglobulins are increasingly common with age; they are present in about 3% of those aged >70 years and 20% aged over 90.
4　Autoantibodies are more prevalent with ageing, and the female preponderance is lost.

Anaemia

Anaemia is the most common blood abnormality. Estimates of the prevalence of anaemia in older people vary widely; prevalence increases with age and depends on the country, e.g. whether folate is supplemented and where the testing is done (a marker of health status).

Prevalence in the over-65s:

12% of those living in the community.
40% of older patients admitted to hospital.
47% of those living in nursing homes.

- Even mild anaemia is associated with frailty and a reduced quality of life.
- People with anaemia have a higher mortality rate, a greater risk of hospital admission, poorer mobility with a higher risk of falling, and reduced functional abilities.
- Anaemia worsens the symptoms of chronic conditions such as heart failure, angina, intermittent claudication, and cognitive impairment.
- In mild anaemia, clinical judgement is needed about how extensively to investigate.

Why anaemia develops

Anaemia is due to impaired red cell or haemoglobin production or red cell loss (see Figure 17.1).

History and examination

The symptoms of anaemia, such as tiredness, breathlessness, and general malaise, are too common and non-specific to add diagnostic value. Anaemia may exacerbate symptoms due to other pathologies. For example, a patient with a tendency to fall may fall more frequently if they develop anaemia.

Aspects of the history may suggest the cause:

- Speed of onset of symptoms,
- Previous surgery,
- Previous blood transfusions,
- History of chronic disease, e.g. heart failure, COPD, connective tissue disorders, CKD,
- Family history (pernicious anaemia and other autoimmune conditions),
- Medication and dietary change,
- Weight loss, GI symptoms and blood loss.

Physical examination may not be helpful, but look for pallor, jaundice, lymphadenopathy, abdominal organomegaly, rectal masses, neurological abnormalities, and chronic disease, which may direct you to the correct diagnosis.

Two important final points:

1　Remember that anaemia is an indication of disease and not a diagnosis.
2　There are more likely to be multiple causes in older patients.

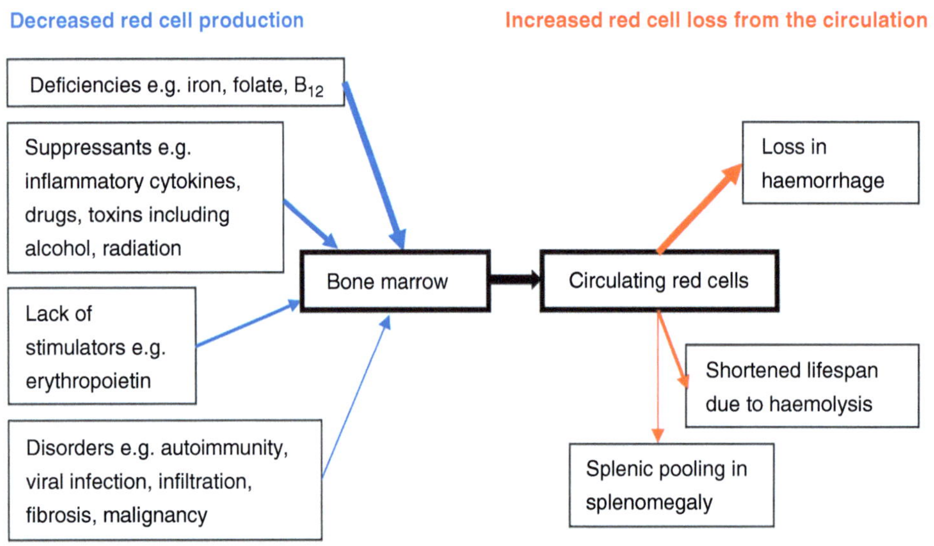

Figure 17.1 Mechanisms for acquired causes of anaemia.

Causes in older people

Note that these percentages are a guide to the order of magnitude, as figures depend on the population (Figure 17.2).

Investigations

A full blood count is needed to make the diagnosis, and the red cell size (mean corpuscular volume, MCV) and morphology often suggest the aetiology. Note the white count and platelets. Always request a peripheral blood film; it may lead you directly to the cause. White cell morphology will also be helpful, especially in myeloproliferative disorders.

Check the acute-phase response using the CRP. ESR reflects changes over days, whereas CRP changes over hours, and CRP is now the cheaper test. A retrospective study from the NHS clinical practice research database (137,009 patients, median age 55) found that overall CRP marginally outperformed ESR in the diagnosis of infection, and the tests were equivalent in cancer and autoimmune disease. ESR may be better if myeloma is suspected and may be better for monitoring giant cell arteritis. A protein-electrophoretic strip is needed to diagnose myeloma.

The MCV divides the anaemias into three groups, which leads to further logical investigation (see Figure 17.3).

Microcytic anaemias

Iron-deficiency anaemia

Iron-deficiency anaemia (IDA) is the most common cause of microcytic (low MCV) anaemia and affects 2–5% of the older population.

Summary of iron metabolism

Most diets contain about 10 g of iron. Meat-based food contains haem iron and plants contain non-haem iron. Haem iron can be absorbed with the protein. There are several steps for the absorption of mineral iron.

- In a low pH environment, a ferric reductase on the apical brush border of the duodenal enterocytes converts iron to ferrous iron ($Fe2+$), which is absorbed into the enterocytes via the divalent metal transporter 1 (DMT1).
- The iron may stay in the cell, be stored as ferritin (from which it may be released for use or excreted in the faeces when the cell dies), or be transported out of the enterocyte into the plasma by ferroportin, a basolateral transmembrane protein.
- If this occurs, it is reoxidised by hephaestin (named after Hephaestus, the Greek god of metal working) and bound to transferrin, which transports iron in the blood.

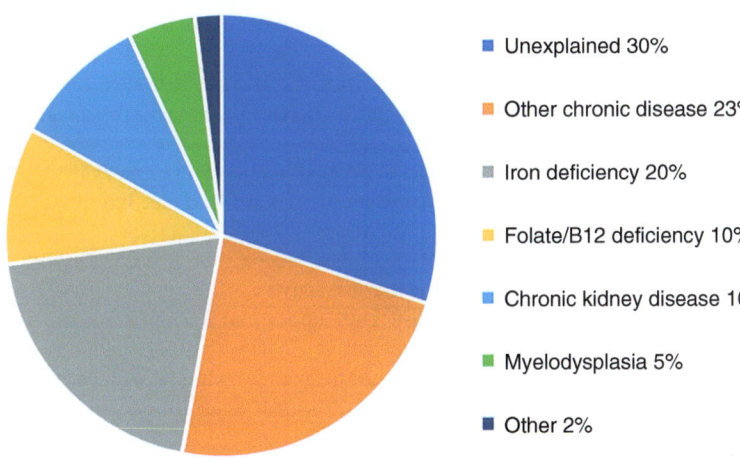

Figure 17.2 Frequency of underlying cause of anaemia in older people.

- Unexplained 30%
- Other chronic disease 23%
- Iron deficiency 20%
- Folate/B12 deficiency 10%
- Chronic kidney disease 10%
- Myelodysplasia 5%
- Other 2%

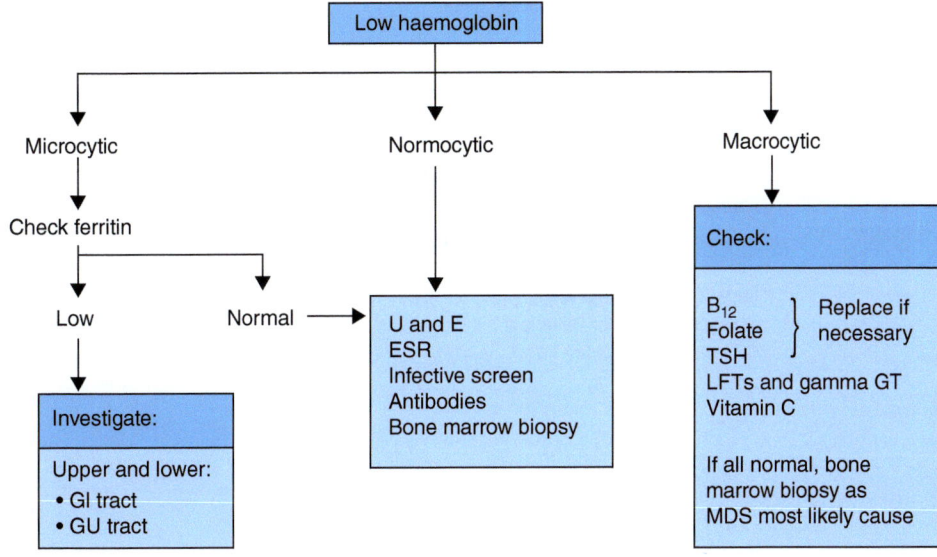

Figure 17.3 Investigation of anaemia depending on the MCV (MDS, myelodysplastic syndrome; GU, genitourinary tract).

Iron-bound transferrin enters red cells (and, to a lesser extent, hepatic and immune cells) by binding to transferrin receptors. The iron is released as ferric ions and can be incorporated into haemoglobin in erythroid precursors or stored. When red cells die after around 120 days, macrophages salvage the haemoglobin molecules, which are broken down, and the iron is transported back to the bone marrow in transferrin to produce new haemoglobin.

Most iron is stored as ferritin in macrophages and the liver. A smaller amount is sequestered as haemosiderin, but this does not release iron readily. Hepatocytes produce hepcidin, which is the major iron regulatory protein. It regulates the amount of iron absorbed by degrading ferroportin and the amount of iron released from iron-recycling macrophages. If iron levels are low, hepcidin synthesis is reduced, so iron absorption and release from macrophages are increased.

It is postulated that overexpression of hepcidin via IL-6 is one of the mechanisms causing the anaemia of chronic disease.

The aetiology of iron deficiency

1 Inadequate intake may be due to a restricted diet, e.g. strict veganism, an inability to shop or prepare meals because of a physical or mental disorder, or poverty.
2 Defective absorption may be a contributory (but rarely the sole) factor. Causes include chronic *H. pylori* infection, chronic peptic ulcer disease, achlorhydria secondary to chronic gastritis, previous gastrectomy, or small bowel disease. Remember drugs. Chronic proton pump inhibitor use may be under-recognised as a cause, as the IDA may be attributed to the indication for the PPI prescription! Oral calcium interferes with iron absorption. Look for clinical or biochemical evidence of malabsorption, such as steatorrhoea, osteomalacia, folate, and vitamin B deficiencies.
3 IDA is usually due to chronic blood loss, especially from the GI tract and, less often, from the genitourinary tract or elsewhere.

History

Symptoms may be non-specific.

- Ask about weight loss, problems swallowing, indigestion, change in bowel habit, black tarry stool, blood in the urine, haemoptysis, and postmenopausal bleeding. Do not forget to ask about alcohol intake.
- Restless legs syndrome is sometimes secondary to iron deficiency.
- Past medical history: peptic ulcer disease, gastrectomy, diverticular disease, bowel resection for carcinoma.
- Recent operations, hip fractures, trauma, etc.

- Document all drugs, including OTC medications, especially aspirin, ibuprofen, and Rennies.

Examination

See also Chapter 14 for the full gastrointestinal examination.

- General: pallor (difficult to discern in dark skin but may be evident in the conjunctiva) lymphadenopathy, or jaundice.
- Cardiac: tachycardia, hypotension, and murmurs if there is volume loss from bleeding.
- Mouth: stomatitis, telangiectasia around the mouth and palate.
- Hands: koilonychia (spoon-shaped nails associated with iron deficiency).
- Abdomen: epigastric tenderness, masses, scars from previous surgery, hepatomegaly, or splenomegaly.
- Rectum: check for masses and exclude melaena.

Investigations

- Peripheral blood film: the red cells are small, hypochromic and vary in size (anisocytosis) and shape (poikilocytosis). There may also be pencil cells and target cells.
- Red cell distribution width (RDW) may increase, reflecting greater variability in the size of the red cells. Remember that if there is also B_{12} or folate deficiency, the red cells may not be microcytic.
- A low serum ferritin level is good evidence of iron deficiency, as most of the body's iron is stored in this soluble form. However, it is an acute-phase protein and is likely to be high in inflammation, in which case the CRP will also be raised.
- Serum iron is a measure of ferric iron bound to serum transferrin. It is affected by multiple factors and is therefore a poor marker of iron deficiency.
- In iron deficiency, transferrin and total iron binding capacity (TIBC) are increased, but transferrin saturation is reduced (see Interpreting iron studies Table 17.1).
- A raised reticulocyte count implies bleeding or haemolysis with appropriate increased bone marrow activity.
- As 10–15% of patients have both upper and lower GI causes of anaemia, most patients need both an OGD with duodenal biopsies and, if colonoscopy is not appropriate, a CT abdomen with contrast (see Chapter 14).

Interpreting iron studies

Table 17.1 The interpretation of iron studies.

	Iron deficiency	Anaemia of chronic disease	Acute phase reaction	Iron overload
MCV	Reduced	May be normal	Normal	Normal
Ferritin 15–300 mcg/L (intracellular iron storage protein)	Low, but may be raised if there is infection/ inflammation	Raised	Raised	Markedly raised
Serum iron (ferric ions, Fe^{3+})	Low	Normal or low if iron is trapped in macrophages or there is a coexistent iron deficiency	Low	Raised
Transferrin	Raised	Low	Low	Normal or low
TIBC (available iron binding sites on transferrin)	Raised	Low		Low
Transferrin saturation (calculated by dividing serum iron by TIBC)	Low	Low	Low	Raised

Treatment

Oral iron

Mild iron deficiency can be treated with oral iron, such as ferrous sulphate.

- Oral iron should be continued for 3 months to replenish the iron stores.
- There is increasing evidence that oral iron is most effective if taken on alternate days. This is because oral iron downregulates the hepatocyte production of hepcidin and therefore reduces absorption.
- Oral iron can cause constipation or diarrhoea. Warn the patient that their stools will become black and gritty. Encourage the patient not to chew the tablets, or their teeth or dentures may become stained.
- If the response to oral iron treatment is not satisfactory (i.e. 20 g/L after 2 months), check that the patient is taking the tablets and that any bleeding has stopped. Also consider additional diagnoses that may explain the problem, such as co-existing anaemia of chronic disease. Consider giving ascorbic acid to increase absorption. Consider checking copper levels (see later).

Intravenous iron

The current formulations, e.g. Monofer, use iron with a carbohydrate shell, resulting in improved safety and fewer side effects than older preparations. Intravenous iron:

- Is indicated for patients with GI diseases that reduce absorption, including coeliac disease, gastric and duodenal disease, active colitis, plus CKD, and heart failure with a reduced ejection fraction.
- Is an option for Jehovah's Witnesses who are anaemic and decline blood transfusions.
- Can be given to improve haemoglobin preoperatively.
- Commonly causes mild side effects: nausea, headaches, and discomfort at the injection site.
- May result in arthralgia, myalgia, and fever around 1 week after the infusion.
- Rarely causes dangerous side effects but may cause anaphylaxis and hypophosphataemia. Importantly patients should be warned in writing of the risk of permanent staining of the skin if the cannula tissues.
- Should not be given when patients are septic (as during inflammation, hepcidin will be raised, reducing effective iron metabolism).
- Results in peak ferritin levels 2 weeks post-infusion, and which remain elevated for 5 weeks.

Blood transfusion

Although blood transfusion can be lifesaving, blood supplies are limited, and more importantly, transfusion is one of the riskiest interventions in routine medical use.

- Blood transfusion is essential after acute haemorrhage, such as a GI bleed, severe epistaxis, or major trauma. When there is volume loss, there is no need to give furosemide to prevent fluid overload.
- Injuries such as scalp lacerations, large haematomas and hip and pelvic fractures may cause substantial blood loss, which may not be obvious (especially in those taking a direct oral anticoagulant [DOAC] or warfarin).
- Transfuse if the patient is symptomatic or the Hb drops below 70 g/L; this more restrictive transfusion cut-off has helped to reduce transfusion reactions and the risk of infection.
- Patients with acute anaemia who are not shocked need full investigation, but emergency transfusions are not needed. Transfusions are given in the daytime, which is less disruptive and safer because the patients can be more easily monitored.
- Discuss the need for transfusion, the risks, and benefits and explain to the patient that after a transfusion they can no longer donate blood.

- Some people, including Jehovah's Witnesses will refuse blood transfusions.
- Patients with chronic anaemia may benefit from a transfusion. The usual cutoff is below 80 g/L, but the threshold may be higher if the patient has symptoms such as heart failure or angina. Usually, two units are sufficient; oral or IV furosemide is usually needed.
- Erythropoiesis-stimulating agents are used in CKD and with some chemotherapeutic regimens to avoid the need for transfusion.
- In conditions requiring regular transfusion, like some cases of myelodysplasia (MDS), transfusion is best carried out in an infusion centre.
- Regular blood donors can continue beyond the age of 70 if they remain well.

Thalassaemia trait

This will have been present since birth but is often asymptomatic and may have been overlooked or forgotten by an older patient. A mild microcytic anaemia is typical. Check haemoglobin electrophoresis if the patient has a relevant ethnic background.

Macrocytic anaemias

Macrocytic (high MCV) anaemias are much less common than anaemias due to iron deficiency or chronic disease. They are usually secondary to a deficiency of vitamin B_{12}, folic acid or, more rarely, thyroxine, or a high alcohol intake. In older people, myelodysplasia is also relatively common. Table 17.2 lists the causes of macrocytosis.

Mechanisms

There are three mechanisms that produce macrocytes:

1 Megaloblastosis: in B_{12} and folate deficiency, drug toxicity and myelodysplasia, DNA replication is affected. The bone marrow precursors are abnormal, the nucleus appears immature relative to the cytoplasm, and large nucleated RBCs may be seen. Megaloblastic changes affect all three haematopoietic cell lines. Neutrophils may be hypersegmented and anaemia, leukopenia, and thrombocytopenia all occur to varying extents.
2 In other macrocytic anaemias, the marrow is normoblastic. The cells are large because of the increased membrane surface area.
3 All conditions associated with reticulocytosis (e.g. haemolytic anaemia with a normal bone marrow) will cause a slight macrocytosis, as reticulocytes are about 20% larger than mature red cells.

Table 17.2 Causes of macrocytosis.

Folate deficiency

B_{12} deficiency

Alcohol excess

Hypothyroidism

Myelodysplastic syndromes

Liver disease

All causes of reticulocytosis

Drugs:

- Folic acid antagonists (e.g. methotrexate, phenytoin, metformin)
- Purine synthesis antagonists (e.g. 6-mercaptopurine, azathioprine, mycophenolate mofetil)
- Pyrimidine antagonists (e.g. cytosine arabinoside, zidovudine, leflunomide)

Spuriously raised MCV – cold agglutinins and paraproteins

Causes of macrocytosis

Vitamin B$_{12}$ deficiency

- B$_{12}$ deficiency affects 20% of those aged 85 and over. The frequency of the underlying causes varies in different populations.
- Pernicious anaemia (PA) is thought to be the cause of B$_{12}$ deficiency in 20% of older people in the UK.
- Gastric causes: total or partial gastrectomy.
- Intestinal causes: bacterial colonisation of intestinal strictures or diverticula and disorders of the terminal ileum, especially Crohn's disease.
- Food-bound cobalamin malabsorption is due to the inability to release cobalamin from food, usually due to chronic gastritis or chronic *H. pylori* infection.
- Drugs reducing B$_{12}$ absorption: chronic PPI use, metformin, and chronic alcoholism. Less likely to affect older people, nitrous oxide abuse impairs B$_{12}$ metabolism.
- A strict vegan diet.

B$_{12}$ stores in the liver last for up to 10 years, hence the lag between a pathology affecting B$_{12}$ absorption and clinical manifestations.

Pernicious anaemia

Pernicious anaemia (PA) is an autoimmune condition where there are antibodies to intrinsic factor or antibodies to gastric parietal cells so that they no longer produce intrinsic factor essential for absorbing B$_{12}$ from the diet. The incidence is said to be 1:10,000, with a female preponderance. Cancer of the stomach occurs in about 10% of cases, attributed to low stomach acid production. There may be a family history of other autoimmune conditions such as Hashimoto's thyroiditis, vitiligo, and Addison's disease.

Clinical features of B$_{12}$ deficiency

Symptoms and signs of anaemia include:

- A lemon tinge to the skin (jaundice secondary to mild haemolysis with pallor from the anaemia).
- Glossitis, anorexia, and weight loss.
- Hepatosplenomegaly and heart failure, in severe cases.
- Neurological signs are due to impaired myelin synthesis and patchy axonal loss, and there may be subacute combined (corticospinal and dorsal column) degeneration of the spinal cord and peripheral neuropathy. A T2 weighted MRI may demonstrate the lesions, especially in the dorsal cord (often thoracic). Signs may include a combination of UMN and LMN findings with reduced joint position sense, reduced vibration sense, peripheral neuropathy, spastic paraparesis, and ataxia. There may be cognitive impairment or, occasionally, severe delirium. These features may predate the haematological changes and worsen if folate is given when B$_{12}$ is low, so it is essential to load with hydroxocobalamin prior to giving folic acid when both are deficient.

Investigations

- The blood film contains large oval red cells and occasionally hypersegmented neutrophils. The reticulocyte count is reduced (they are abnormally fragile). Platelets may be low.
- The bone marrow is megaloblastic.
- Serum B$_{12}$ is low.
- Positive anti-intrinsic factor antibodies have high specificity for PA.
- The Schilling test is no longer available.
- If there is doubt about B$_{12}$ deficiency, serum total homocysteine levels can be measured. If there is B$_{12}$ deficiency, homocysteine cannot be converted to methionine, and therefore the levels are raised.

Treatment

- Hydroxocobalamin: 1 mg intramuscularly three times a week for 2 weeks, to replenish body stores, and thereafter, 1 mg every 3 months for life.

- This is essential when there are neurological deficits, pernicious anaemia, or other causes of malabsorption.
- There is often an associated iron deficiency, necessitating a course of oral iron.
- A blood transfusion is not indicated.
- Where the deficiency is not autoimmune, is dietary or is borderline, oral cyanocobalamin 50–150 mcg daily can be given. This preparation is not available on the NHS and must be bought over the counter. Oral cyanocobalamin is not indicated for patients with neurological deficits.

Folate deficiency

Folate deficiency is much more common than vitamin B$_{12}$ deficiency. Many countries have mandatory folic acid fortification programmes (US, Canada, Australia, Chile, and South Africa). In the UK, folate should be added to non-wholemeal flour (250 µg per 100 g of flour) by 2026. The measure is designed to reduce neural tube defects but will also reduce this common deficiency in older people. Folate deficiency is usually due to a poor diet or malabsorption, e.g. coeliac disease. Other factors are increased demand due to high cell turnover, e.g. lymphoma, infection and haemolysis. Anticonvulsant drugs and chronic alcoholism cause low levels by increasing the hepatic metabolism of folate. The body only stores sufficient folate for 6 months or so.

Clinical features

Symptoms and signs of anaemia include:

- Irritability, depression, confusion and occasionally dementia.
- Peripheral neuropathy and subacute combined degeneration of the cord (as with PA) occur in more severe cases.

Investigations

Red cell folate is low. Folic acid absorption tests are not used routinely. The peripheral blood and marrow picture is identical to that of vitamin B$_{12}$ deficiency.

Treatment

- Lifestyle advice: improve diet, reduce alcohol intake, and stop offending drugs when practicable.
- Oral folic acid 5 mg tablets are given daily for 4 months to replenish stores and then stopped; long-term use may mask a developing PA.
- Do not give folic acid until vitamin B$_{12}$ deficiency has been excluded to prevent the risk of precipitating subacute combined degeneration of the cord. If in doubt, give both vitamins concurrently; the patient may also need iron.
- Prophylactic use in malabsorption and patients with epilepsy taking anticonvulsants may be justified. Folate is routinely given to patients on methotrexate (methotrexate on Monday; folate on Friday is a useful memory aid).

Hypothyroidism

A macrocytic normoblastic anaemia can occur in over 50% of cases of myxoedema but is usually mild, never megaloblastic and responds slowly to levothyroxine replacement. It is thought to be caused by reduced renal erythropoietin production in response to the lower oxygen demand of a lower basal metabolic rate. Any co-existing iron deficiency will also require replacement. About 10% of patients also have autoimmune PA.

Vitamin C deficiency/scurvy

The macrocytic normoblastic anaemia of scurvy is commonly associated with other nutritional deficiencies. Ascorbic acid is necessary for the reduction of folate into its active metabolite. Clinical signs include bleeding gums (when the patient has teeth), vascular purpura secondary to fragile blood vessels, and occasionally blood loss can be severe. Vitamin C replacement, followed by a balanced diet, is curative.

Copper deficiency

Copper is essential for normal haematopoiesis. Copper deficiency is increasingly recognised. It may occur in dietary deficiency or due to zinc supplementation, enteropathies with malabsorption, after foregut surgery especially bariatric surgery and prolonged intravenous nutrition. Zinc, copper and, to some extent, iron compete for absorption. Copper deficiency can present as anaemia, which may be megaloblastic with myeloneuropathy, mimicking B_{12} deficiency. The serum copper level can be measured, and if it is low, oral supplementation is given.

Alcohol excess

This is a common cause of macrocytosis, but anaemia may be multifactorial (see later discussion).

Myelodysplasia

This typically shows a mild macrocytosis (see later discussion).

Haemolytic anaemias

Haemolysis is the premature destruction of red blood cells. When the bone marrow can no longer match the rate of haemolysis, the patient becomes anaemic. There is typically mild macrocytosis because of the reticulocytosis.

- Haemolytic anaemias are rare in older people and may be overlooked, especially as the blood film may not show any specific features.
- Autoimmune haemolytic anaemias (AIHA) are more common in older age as part of an autoimmune illness (e.g. SLE), due to antibody production secondary to infection (warm and cold antibodies following a viral infection) or drug-induced (e.g. cephalosporins, and methyl-dopa – which is still used in developing countries).
- Patients with hypersplenism may have a haemolytic element to their anaemia.
- Most patients with metal heart valves have minor haemolysis.
- Relevant investigations are those indicating increased red cell destruction, i.e. raised bilirubin level, lactate dehydrogenase and haptoglobin, raised reticulocyte count, and a positive direct antiglobulin test (Coombs' test) which detects red cells that are coated with antibodies or complement.
- Supportive management includes stopping culprit drugs, replacing folate and transfusions if severe.
- AIHA may respond to steroids, which reduce the production of autoantibodies by B cells.

Normocytic anaemias
Anaemia of chronic disease

This is now often called the anaemia of inflammation. It is usually a normochromic normocytic anaemia and does not respond to replacement of haematinics. It may be improved by treatment of the underlying condition.

- 75% of cases are associated with malignancy; the remaining cases are due to chronic infection or inflammation, such as rheumatoid arthritis, or chronic disease, such as congestive heart failure.
- Activation of the immune system by autoantigens, microbial molecules, or tumour antigens gives rise to the release of multiple inflammatory cytokines and free radicals that lead to an increase in hepcidin, which blocks gut iron absorption and iron release from reticuloendothelial cells. The production of red cells is impaired in this low iron environment, and is worsened by the inhibition of erythropoietin production. Red cell life span is also decreased.
- Ferritin is normal or high.
- There are increased levels of iron in the reticuloendothelial system.

- Anaemia of chronic disease can be differentiated from iron deficiency anaemia by measuring the number of transferrin receptors. They are upregulated in anaemia of chronic disease but normal in iron-deficiency anaemia. This assay is expensive and not yet widely used.

Mixed deficiency states

Patients who live on tea and toast may be deficient in folate, iron and vitamin C and can have normocytic anaemia.

Non-malignant disorders of the bone marrow

The peripheral red cells are usually normochromic and normocytic but may, on occasion, be macrocytic. There is usually a low reticulocyte count, so this does not give rise to macrocytosis. The underlying fault is pathology in the bone marrow, such as autoimmune disease, chronic viral infection, or infiltration. An aspirate or a trephine biopsy is needed for diagnosis.

Aplastic anaemia

Aplastic anaemia is a rare, potentially life-threatening failure of haemopoiesis characterised by pancytopenia and hypocellular bone marrow (without blasts or dysplasia), usually due to damage to stem cells. At least two of the following are needed for diagnosis:

1 Haemoglobin: <100 g/L,
2 Platelet count: <50 × 10⁹/L,
3 Neutrophil count: <1.5 × 10⁹/L.

Known causes of acquired aplastic anaemia are drugs (NSAIDs, antibiotics), toxins (benzene), and viral infections, but in up to 80% of cases, the trigger is not known. The pathogenesis is usually a CD4 T cell-mediated autoimmune attack on HSCs. It is most common at 10–25 and over 60 years.

Chemotherapy and radiotherapy may cause pancytopaenia, but this usually resolves after stopping treatment.

Management is supportive with blood and platelet transfusions and antibiotics for infection. More aggressive therapies include ciclosporin A, anti-thymocyte globulin, high-dose methylprednisolone, and stem cell transplantation, but these are rarely appropriate in older people where there is frailty or co-morbidity. The thrombopoietin mimetic eltrombopag has some efficacy but many limitations and multiple side effects.

Leucoerythroblastic anaemia

This is an anaemia with immature red and white cells in the peripheral blood. The marrow examination may reveal the malignant cells that have infiltrated and impaired function.

Mixed-picture anaemias

In clinical practice, many patients will be anaemic due to several causes, including deficiencies, blood loss, chronic inflammation, haemolysis, and marrow dysfunction. The MCV is variable depending on the dominant problem in an individual patient. The blood picture will only improve if the underlying conditions can be alleviated. The most common examples are discussed here.

Alcohol excess

This can cause or contribute to anaemia via several mechanisms:

- Bleeding from oesophagitis, gastric or duodenal ulceration, or varices.
- Anorexia.
- Dietary deficiency of folate.
- Direct effect of alcohol on the bowel, reducing absorption.

- Malabsorption from chronic pancreatitis.
- Suppressed marrow function.
- Hypersplenism from chronic liver disease with portal hypertension.

Chronic kidney disease

The anaemia in renal disease may be related to the underlying cause, e.g. myeloma or SLE or its treatment. In advanced kidney disease of any cause, erythropoietin production is reduced. Biologically fit older patients with chronic kidney disease and anaemia are offered subcutaneous recombinant erythropoietin or darbepoetin once any iron deficiency is corrected, usually with intravenous iron. Some common immunosuppressants cause macrocytosis.

Malignant disease

Usually there are several causes: anorexia, blood loss, anaemia of chronic disease, malabsorption, and/or haemolysis. Additionally, there may be marrow infiltration leading to the development of leucoerythroblastic anaemia.

Rheumatoid arthritis

In addition to 'anaemia of chronic disease', look for blood loss (NSAIDs), low folate due to poor nutrition and increased utilisation, B_{12} deficiency (autoimmune), and the effects of drugs such as methotrexate. Complications of rheumatoid disease (such as vasculitis or amyloidosis) increase the severity and complexity of the anaemia.

Haematological malignancies

The classification of haematological malignancies is increasingly complex, and diagnosis and active treatment require specialist haematology input. There are around 41,000 new cases per year in the UK. There is a tendency for older people to have more resistant cancer, more comorbidities, more functional and cognitive impairments, and they are still under-represented in trials. However, as Figure 17.4 shows, these are disorders of older people. As the diagnostic classification and understanding of molecular pathogenesis become more precise, targeted therapies may enable more older people to receive active treatment without overwhelming side effects.

To ensure consistency, all the figures for sex ratio, median age at diagnosis, and 5 year survival data are from the Haematological Malignancy Research Network (UK).

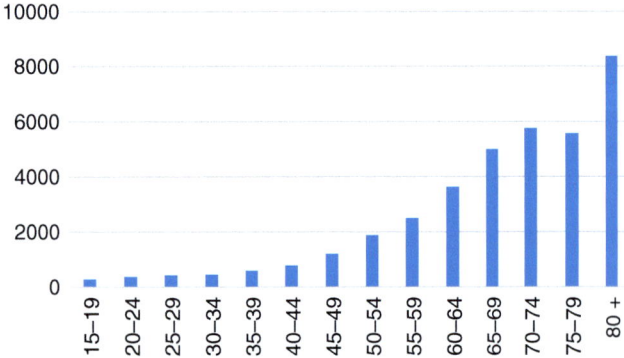

Figure 17.4 The estimated total annual cases of haematological malignancy in the UK by age band (HMRN data).

Myelodysplastic neoplasms

Skewing of the HSCs to myeloid progenitors with ageing leads to an increased risk of developing this heterogeneous group of clonal stem cell disorders. A mutant stem cell will multiply many times, suppressing the production of other cell lines. The stem cells retain the ability to differentiate into end-stage cells, but this happens in a disordered and ineffective manner. In the 2022 WHO classification, 'myelodysplastic syndromes' have been renamed 'myelodysplastic neoplasms' although the abbreviation remains MDS. The prognosis depends on the subtype but is worse than chronic leukaemias and many lymphomas. Any of the three cell lines can be affected. These clonal haematopoietic neoplasms are defined by cytopaenias and morphologic dysplasia.

- The incidence of MDS increases with age: M > F, median age at diagnosis: 76, 5-year survival: 26%.
- Most are spontaneous, but a few occur after chemotherapy or radiotherapy.
- Symptoms: 55% of patients will present with fatigue due to a refractory macrocytic anaemia (MCV >100), 20% present with excess bruising and bleeding gums due to thrombocytopenia, another 20% present with recurrent infections, and the rest will be asymptomatic.
- 25% are discovered incidentally on the blood film requested for another reason.
- On examination: pallor, bruising, signs of infection; only 10% have splenomegaly. Lymphadenopathy is rare.
- The blood film may show a single cytopaenia or, as the disease progresses, bicytopaenia, or pancytopaenia. There may also be giant platelets and juvenile neutrophils.
- The marrow is hypercellular due to stem-cell hyperplasia but has poor haemopoietic function.
- The clinical course is very variable. Some cases are indolent; others are aggressive with early transformation into acute myelocytic leukaemia (AML); or the patient may succumb to infection secondary to impaired white cell function.
- Most cases are managed with repeated blood transfusions (consider desferrioxamine to prevent iron overload).
- In view of toxicity, only fit older people with no serious comorbidities are considered for chemotherapy. Azacitidine, an epigenetic therapy that reduces DNA methylation, is relatively well tolerated, slows progression to AML in high-grade MDS, and is NICE-approved.

Myeloproliferative neoplasms

These heterogeneous malignant conditions are clonal HSC disorders, characterised by an overproduction of differentiated cells from the myeloid lineages in the bone marrow.

- The clinical features of the conditions overlap, but the predominant cells produced, and the speed of progression define the disease, and diagnosis is made based on the appearance of the blood film, bone marrow, and cytogenetics.
- Janus kinases (JAKs) are a family of cytoplasmic tyrosine kinases that link cytokine signalling from membrane receptors to signal transducers and activators of transcription. JAK2 transduces the signal from the erythropoietin, granulocyte-colony stimulating factor (G-CSF), and thrombopoietin receptors. Most patients with polycythaemia vera have the *JAK2V617F* mutation, which causes constitutive receptor activation. This *JAK2* mutation is also found in half of cases of essential thrombocythaemia, and myelofibrosis.
- Chronic myeloid leukaemia is classified in this group but is discussed with the other leukaemias. Mutations in the *CALR* (calreticulin) gene and *MPL* (named for myeloproliferative leukaemia, now identified as the thrombopoietin receptor gene) may be phenotypic drivers in *JAK2*-negative cases.

Polycythaemia vera

Initially, there is polycythaemia, a raised haematocrit and sometimes overproduction of white cells and platelets.

Median age at diagnosis: 70.7, M = F, 5-year survival 94%.

Over 10–15 years, myelofibrosis (around 10%) or AML (5%) may develop.

- Check oxygen saturation to exclude secondary polycythaemia; the erythropoietin level is usually low in polycythaemia vera (PV) and high in hypoxaemia.
- Symptoms due to hyperviscosity include headache, dizziness, vertigo, tinnitus, visual disturbance, angina, and claudication.
- May present with thrombosis or haemorrhage.
- Pruritus is secondary to the release of histamine, especially after a hot shower or bath.
- Gout results from increased cell turnover.
- On examination: facial plethora; splenomegaly; and less commonly, hepatomegaly (occurrence depends on disease stage).
- Treatment: venesection to reduce hyperviscosity, or hydroxycarbamide, which is well tolerated, and aspirin.

Essential thrombocythaemia

Essential thrombocythaemia (EV) results in uncontrolled production of platelets and episodes of thrombosis and haemorrhage. The long-term risk of myelofibrosis and leukaemia is lower than with PV. Hydroxycarbamide and aspirin are used.

Median age at diagnosis is 71.7, F > M, and 5-year survival is 88%.

Primary myelofibrosis

Neoplastic transformation of an early HSC stimulates angiogenesis in the marrow and polyclonal proliferation of fibroblasts, causing bone marrow fibrosis. This results in anaemia, high or low white cells and platelet counts, and extramedullary haematopoiesis. Splenomegaly is very common, which may be massive ; causing the patient to complain of abdominal or shoulder tip pain. Hepatomegaly is common, and portal hypertension may develop. Other symptoms include weight loss, fatigue secondary to anaemia, and frequent infections secondary to white cell dysfunction. Primary myelofibrosis (PMF) may progress to marrow failure. Management in older people is symptomatic.

Median age at diagnosis is 73.4, M > F, and 5-year survival is 57%.

Overlap syndromes, which share features of myelodysplastic and myeloproliferative neoplasia, are increasingly recognised.

Leukaemias

Leukaemias are a group of cancers of the white blood cells and their precursors that arise in the bone marrow and the abnormal cells are found in the blood. There are four broad categories: myeloid or lymphocytic, and acute, or chronic.

AML (acute myeloid leukaemia, all types): median age at diagnosis 73, M > F, 5-year survival 13%.

ALL (acute lymphoblastic leukaemia): M ≥ F, when diagnosed at 40+, 5-year survival 27%.

CML (chronic myeloid leukaemia): median age at diagnosis 59, M ≥ F, 5-year survival 82%.

CLL (chronic lymphocytic leukaemia): median age at diagnosis 72, M > F, 5-year survival 83%.

Until recently, the high toxicity of conventional chemotherapy for acute leukaemias meant that the best choice for older people was usually supportive and then palliative management. As molecular mechanisms are becoming better understood, targeted and biological therapies are showing benefits with fewer side effects, and more trials are including older people.

Acute myeloid leukaemia

Acute myeloid leukaemia (AML) may develop in patients with PV, ET or PMF, aplastic anaemia, and myelodysplastic syndrome, or it may develop directly. It is more common in the Western world and in men, as the most common risk factor is the transformation of MDS.

- The development of the haemopoietic precursors is arrested at an immature stage. In AML, the bone marrow contains at least 20% blasts.
- Normal maturation of all cell lines is affected, leading to anaemia, thrombocytopenia, and neutropenia.
- The patient may present with symptoms and signs of anaemia, bleeding, or sepsis.
- AML is aggressive, and most older patients are best managed with good supportive care, including blood and platelet transfusions and antibiotics, as necessary.
- Robust, older patients with high performance scores may be treated intensively, but non-intensive treatment may still be the best choice. Options include azacitidine, low-dose cytarabine, and venetoclax, a drug that targets overexpression of BCL2 (B cell lymphoma) proteins in AML cells, making them more sensitive to either of the other drugs. Hydroxycarbamide may be used if the white count becomes high.

Acute lymphoblastic leukaemia

Acute lymphoblastic leukaemia (ALL) is thought of as a disease of childhood, but it has a bimodal age distribution, and the highest incidence in adults is in those over 75 years old.

- There are B-cell and, more rarely, T-cell types.
- Prognosis is usually extremely poor.
- The Philadelphia chromosome (see later) occurs in about 25% of adult cases.
- Where indicated, treatment of ALL combines prolonged chemotherapy (remission induction, consolidation, and maintenance) and supportive measures. Standard chemotherapy, e.g. high-dose cytarabine, methotrexate, vincristine, cyclophosphamide, doxorubicin, and a steroid, is far too toxic for older people. Some success is seen with lower-dose regimens without doxorubicin and biologicals such as blinatumomab, which targets different antigens on B and T cells. Blinatumomab attaches to T cells and malignant B cells, enabling T cells to find and destroy the cancer cells. During this process, T cells are activated, creating more killer T cells.

Chronic myeloid leukaemia

Chronic myeloid leukaemia (CML) is less common than CLL. It is of interest because it is the best understood genetically. Reciprocal translocation of genes between the long arms of chromosome 9 and chromosome 22 creates the Philadelphia chromosome (the truncated chromosome 22 fused with a short segment of 9 results in the *BCR-ABL1* fusion oncogene). This results in a constitutively activated tyrosine kinase, which triggers uncontrolled cell division.

Clinical features

- Weight loss, anorexia, and night sweats due to hypermetabolism.
- Tiredness and frequent infections are due to bone marrow failure.
- Early satiety and left upper quadrant pain from splenomegaly, which may be massive
- More rarely, leucostasis causes priapism, visual impairment, and hyperuricaemia.

Investigations

The peripheral blood film demonstrates:

- Leucocytosis, 50–200 × 10⁹/L, with the full spectrum of myeloid cells.
- Normochromic normocytic anaemia.
- Platelet count is often elevated but may be normal or low.
- Raised uric acid due to high cell turnover.
- Bone marrow is hypercellular with granulocytes.
- Philadelphia chromosome may be detected in the peripheral blood or bone marrow.

Treatment

Usually, the disease remains in the chronic phase for 3–5 years. If it is not treated, it will progress to the acute blast phase. When the disease enters its acute phase, deterioration may be rapid, with median survival being 3–6 months. Philadelphia-positive CML can be treated in the chronic phase with oral imatinib, which is a BCR-ABL kinase inhibitor that is usually well tolerated.

Chronic lymphatic leukaemia

Chronic lymphatic leukaemia (CLL) is caused by the clonal expansion of immature B cells, which resemble normal lymphocytes but are functionally incompetent. They also have an abnormally long survival rate because of suppression of apoptosis.

The aetiology is unknown, but there is a genetic element; it arises at a younger age in successive generations of affected families. Small lymphocytic lymphoma (SLL), which is a type of non-Hodgkin's lymphoma, is essentially the same disease as CLL and is treated in the same way; the difference is that CLL arises in the marrow and SLL in the lymph nodes or spleen.

- Around 3,800 new cases of CLL occur a year.
- 30% of cases are detected incidentally on a blood film, e.g. pre-operative assessment.
- It does not require treatment if it is asymptomatic.
- May convert to an acute disorder.

Clinical features

- May be asymptomatic for years; an incidental diagnosis is stressful to the patient and their relatives.
- Fatigue, night sweats, loss of appetite.
- Lymphadenopathy is most common in the neck, and axillae, but can be widespread (Figure 17.5).
- Anaemia.
- Splenomegaly in 40%.
- Hepatomegaly in 15%.
- Purpura and bruising are secondary to the low platelet count.
- May present with pruritus.
- Infections; occasionally presents with florid herpes zoster.

Investigations

The blood film contains multiple small lymphocytes, as high as 300 × 10⁹ lymphocytes/L, with occasional smudge cells (lymphocyte remnants due to fragility of the cells, also called smear cells).

There may be normocytic normochromic anaemia or AIHA.

Bone marrow aspirate shows replacement of the normal marrow with lymphocytes.

Treatment

Older people often have a benign form of the disease, which requires no treatment, and survive for up to 10 years.

The mainstay of treatment for those with more aggressive disease is steroids plus alkylating agents such as chlorambucil.

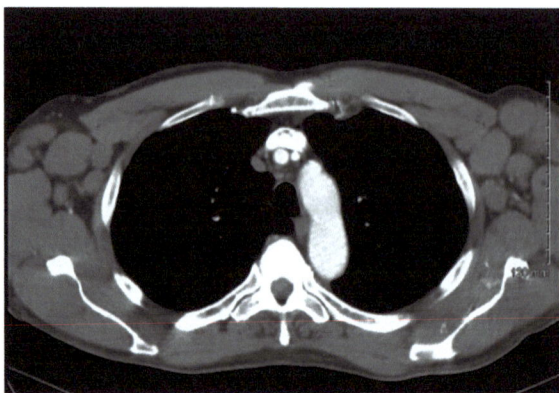

Bilateral enlarged axillary lymph nodes

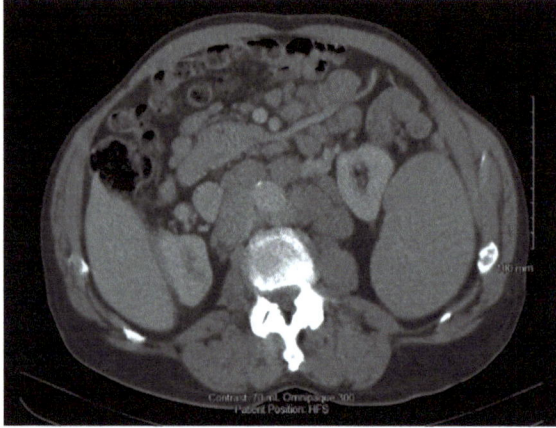

Retroperitoneal, para-aortic, and mesenteric lymph node enlargement, and splenomegaly

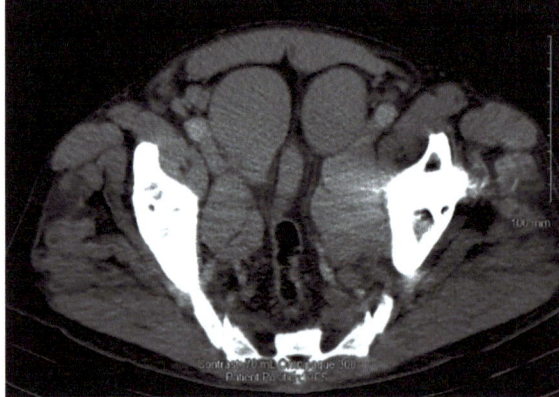

Bilateral iliac lymph node enlargement

Figure 17.5 CT scans with contrast in a 79-year-old male with CLL (with thanks to James Tanner, Radiology, CUH).

The monoclonal antibody rituximab is also useful; it targets CD20 on B cells. Survival in these cases is usually 3–5 years. Ibrutinib is sometimes used for CLL that has relapsed.

Myeloma syndromes

Multiple myeloma

Myeloma is a clonal plasma cell proliferative disorder characterised by the production of large amounts of immunoglobulins/parts of immunoglobulins that form the monoclonal paraprotein 'M band'. There are about 6,000 new cases a year in the UK. It is more common in black populations and at older ages. The median age at diagnosis is 72 years,

M > F, 5-year survival 50%. The aetiology is unknown, but possibilities include toxins and the human herpes virus HH8. There may be a genetic component, as it can occur in family clusters.

Clinical features

Common

- Malaise secondary to a normocytic anaemia due to three mechanisms:
  1 Shift from myeloid to lymphoid progenitors,
  2 Overproduction of plasma cells in the bone marrow, suppressing other cell production,
  3 Failing kidneys produce less erythropoietin (EPO).
- Bone pain in vertebrae or ribs and pathological fractures occur in 70% of cases in some series. Enhanced osteoclastic activity and suppressed osteoblast activity lead to lytic bone lesions, fractures, and hypercalcaemia.
- Recurrent infections secondary to immunoparesis and neutropaenia.
- Renal failure is due to deposition of immune complexes in the glomeruli and tubules, and sometimes the development of amyloid. Renal function can also deteriorate secondary to hyperuricaemia and nephrocalcinosis due to hypercalcaemia.
- Bleeding is secondary to impaired platelet function.

Less common

- Confusion secondary to hypercalcaemia.
- Rarely, hyperviscosity syndromes,
- Amyloidosis: normally the kidneys filter light chains. However, in myeloma, excessive numbers of light chains are produced and become misfolded and aggregate into amyloid fibrils which block the glomeruli leading to proteinuria and amyloid kidney.
- Cord compression.

Investigations

- FBC demonstrates a normochromic normocytic anaemia.
- The red cells form rouleaux.
- There is thrombocytopenia.
- Markedly raised ESR, greater than 100.
- Increased plasma viscosity.
- Hypercalcaemia.
- Increased creatinine in 50% of cases.
- Serum protein electrophoresis detects an abnormal M (monoclonal) band, usually IgG. IgA is the next most common, with IgM, IgD, and IgE types all rare.
- In an IgG myeloma, IgM and IgA levels tend to be low (suppressed).
- Usually more light chains than heavy chains are produced; in 20% of cases, only light chains are produced (kappa or lambda) so a serum-free light chain (sFLC) assay is needed for diagnosis. Light chain myeloma is associated with more kidney damage as light chains tend to block the renal tubules.
- Free light chains in the urine are known as Bence–Jones protein (BJP); the sFLC assay is more sensitive, so if this is available, there is no need for BJP.
- BM biopsy: in myeloma, the bone marrow contains more than 10% plasma cells.
- A CT skeletal survey is used to look for lytic bone lesions. These are caused by overexpression of the receptor activator of nuclear factor kappa-B ligand (RANKL), leading to increased osteoclast activity.

Treatment

This depends on how the patient presents.

- Careful fluid balance for renal failure, and dialysis in selected cases.
- Fluids and bisphosphonates such as intravenous zoledronate or pamidronate for hypercalcaemia. Some studies show that patients treated with bisphosphonates do better long-term.
- Radiotherapy for bone pain due to lytic lesions and cord compression (must be done as an emergency to prevent irreversible neurological damage).
- Analgesia including opioids are often needed.
- Treat infections, usually bacterial respiratory infections.
- VTE prophylaxis.
- Myeloma treatment has been changing rapidly, and this is an active area for clinical trials that now include older, frailer patients. Non-frail older patients who are unsuitable for stem cell transplantation (there is a cut off of 65 years old currently) can now receive DRD: daratumumab (Darzalex), lenalidomide (Revlimid), and dexamethasone. Daratumumab is a synthetic antibody that binds to a protein on the surface of myeloma cells called CD38. When daratumumab attaches to CD38, it makes the myeloma cell more visible to the immune system. Lenalidomide binds to an E3 ubiquitin ligase complex and modulates its substrate specificity, resulting in the proteasomal degradation of specific disease-related proteins.
- Bortezomib, a proteasome inhibitor, is another recent option, especially for patients with rapidly deteriorating renal function; however peripheral neuropathy is often dose-limiting.

Smouldering myeloma

This is defined as a raised M band ≥30 g/L. The bone marrow contains 10–60% clonal plasma cells, **but** there is no evidence of end organ damage. There is a 10% chance per year over the first 5 years of progression to myeloma, which then slows.

Monoclonal gammopathy of unknown significance

A monoclonal band is present but <30 g/L, the bone marrow contains less than 10% clonal plasma cells, and there is no end organ damage. There is a much lower risk of progression to myeloma compared with smouldering myeloma: 1% per year for the first 5 years.

MGUS → smouldering myeloma → multiple myeloma, but not all cases progress.

Lymphomas

Lymphomas are group of cancers of the white blood cells that arise in the lymphatic system. There are around 16,000 new cases of lymphoma each year.

There are two main types of lymphoma:

1 Hodgkin's lymphoma (HL): usually a disease of adolescents and people in their 20–30s, but there is a second peak in 80-year-olds. Reed–Sternberg cells are pathognomonic of HL; they are multinucleated giant cells found in the peripheral blood. The clinical features include lymphadenopathy, which is typically localised. It may be accompanied by constitutional 'B symptoms' such as fever, drenching night sweats and weight loss. Survival in classic HL is markedly worse with increasing age; 5-year survival is 54% if the diagnosis is made at 70–79 years. The effect of age is much greater than the effect of disease stage.

2 Non-Hodgkin's lymphoma (NHL): This is not an entity but a diverse group, with over 60 subtypes making up nearly 90% of new lymphomas in a year. About 90% of NHL cases arise in B cells, 9% in T cells, and 1% in natural killer (NK) cells. The incidence increases with age from around 50 years, peaking at 80 years. Any lymphoid tissue may

be affected (up to 20% of cases arise in the GI tract, bone, liver, or CNS). Symptoms include general malaise, pyrexia of unknown origin, night sweats, pruritus, and weight loss. Hepatosplenomegaly is more common in NHL. Compression of neighbouring structures may also lead to symptoms, e.g. superior vena caval obstruction. Cerebral lymphoma presents with subacute progression of confusion or other neurological symptoms such as dizziness. It is more common in immunosuppressed patients. The two most common subtypes account for around half of cases.

i Diffuse large B-cell lymphoma: M > F, median age at diagnosis: 71, 5-year survival 61%. Accounts for 13% of all haematological malignancies.

ii Follicular lymphoma: M = F, median age at diagnosis 67, often indolent, 5 year survival 84%. A chromosome 14/18 translocation results in the deregulation of the *BCL2* protooncogene.

Walderströms macroglobulinaemia

Although it is rare, there is an indolent subtype of NHL, lymphoplasmacytic lymphoma (LPL), due to malignant expansion of B cells and plasma cells in the bone marrow. Waldenström's macroglobulinaemia is a subtype of LPL. Over 90% have a mutation in the *MYD88* gene that turns on pathways that sustain the growth and survival of WM cells. The cancer cells produce large amounts of IgM antibody M protein. The deposition of M protein leads to hyperviscosity, lymphadenopathy and neuropathies.

Investigations

- Blood film: lymphocytic leucocytosis, normochromic normocytic anaemia, plus thrombocytopenia.
  ESR: often raised.
  CRP: often extremely high with no evidence of infection.
- LDH: high as increased cell turnover releases more lactate dehydrogenase (LDH).
- CT or MRI abdomen, pelvis, and chest: shows the presence and distribution of lymphadenopathy.
- PET-CT: has the advantage of detecting metabolically active lymph nodes which are more likely to give positive histology.
- Excision lymph node biopsy: for classification of the subtype, immunophenotyping, cytogenetic analysis, and DNA sequencing.
- Bone marrow biopsy: only needed in advanced disease.

Treatment

Depending on histology and staging as well as the performance status and frailty of the patient, the agents used most frequently are cyclophosphamide and chlorambucil, often given with steroids. This is obviously a problem when patients have comorbidities including diabetes, osteoporosis, heart failure, etc. Thus, each patient must be assessed individually to determine whether they would benefit from chemotherapy.

Disorders of coagulation

Clotting disorders

Deep vein thrombosis (DVT) is the most common clotting problem in geriatric practice.

Age alone is a risk factor, but most patients also have other precipitants, such as immobility, trauma (accidental and surgical), underlying malignancy, inflammatory disorders, and dehydration.

Other conditions in which the blood has increased viscosity, e.g. myeloma, polycythaemia, hyperosmolar non-ketotic diabetic coma, and hypothermia, also increase the risk of venous thrombosis.

- All older people in hospital are at increased risk of venous thromboembolism and should be offered prophylactic low-molecular weight heparin unless there is a contraindication. Thromboembolic deterrent stockings (TEDS) are useful in reducing post-phlebitic syndrome. See Chapter 9 for more information about venous thromboembolism.

Bleeding disorders

The most common cause of prolonged bleeding is medical treatment or overtreatment with anticoagulants. There are now more indications for older people to be anticoagulated, including atrial fibrillation, ventricular thrombus, prosthetic heart valves, treatment of DVT/PE, post surgery prophylaxis and cancer associated thrombosis.

- Older people taking warfarin are at greater risk of complications because of changing pharmacodynamics and interactions with antibiotics such as ciprofloxacin. High INRs not complicated by haemorrhage or shock can be managed by withholding warfarin and monitoring, or giving a small dose of vitamin K orally (assuming the warfarin is to be continued). If there is severe haemorrhage with hypovolaemic shock or bleeding into a confined space, then the warfarin should be reversed with IV vitamin K and IV reconstituted dried prothrombin complex, e.g. Beriplex.
- Direct oral anticoagulants (DOACs) have made anticoagulation easier and removed the need for monitoring. However, even with DOACs, there is a risk of bleeding; patients who fall frequently often have repeat CT head scans to rule out intracerebral bleeds. If necessary, dabigatran can be reversed by idarucizumab (a monoclonal antibody fragment that binds to dabigatran). Apixaban and rivaroxaban can be reversed by andexanet alfa (a recombinant form of factor Xa protein).
- Other older patients at risk are those with reduced platelet function on dual antiplatelet therapy or thrombocytopenia. This may be due to their underlying pathology, as in aplastic anaemia or autoimmune idiopathic thrombocytopenia, or resulting from aggressive chemotherapeutic regimes for myeloproliferative and other neoplastic diseases. The risk of serious haemorrhage, e.g. stroke, is much higher in older people.
- The increasing use of thrombolysis (see Chapters 9 and 12) is another example of older patients experiencing both greater benefits and greater risks. Careful selection is needed to avoid the increased risk of bleeding, especially into the brain.
- Older people with renal impairment are at increased risk of bleeding due to functional platelet disorders.

Disseminated intravascular coagulation

Older people are more susceptible to disseminated intravascular coagulation (DIC) because of the proinflammatory state associated with ageing.

- In DIC, thrombosis and haemorrhage co-exist. The initial thrombotic element is usually silent, but the consumption of coagulation factors in the process leads to uncontrolled bleeding. Likely precipitants in older age are sepsis, disseminated malignant disease, trauma, and fulminant liver failure.
- More recently, severe COVID-19 has caused coagulopathies through the activation and consumption of clotting factors.
- Only sepsis is likely to respond to active treatment. Supportive treatments are blood transfusions for bleeding, Beriplex and fresh platelet transfusions.

- In general, 50% of patients die, and this percentage is even higher in the very frail population.

Iron overload disorders

These are often diagnosed late, as the symptoms come on insidiously due to the slow accumulation of non-transferrin-bound iron in the liver, joints, pancreas, thyroid and other endocrine organs, bone, and heart. Symptoms include fatigue, darkening of the skin, joint pain, fractures (due to osteoporosis) and if there is cardiac involvement, palpitations, shortness of breath, and oedema.

Ask about:

- Family history of haemochromatosis.
- Recurrent blood transfusions.
- Excess alcohol intake.

On examination: bronze discolouration of the skin, raised JVP, displaced apex beat, hepatomegaly, jaundice, ascites.

Investigations: markedly raised ferritin, i.e. over 1,000 mcg/L; elevated transferrin saturation > 50%; LFTs often raised; raised HbA1c; and high TSH.

Once evidence of iron overload is established, MRI modalities such as T2* can be used to document the iron level in key organs.

Causes

- Hereditary haemochromatosis: the most common genetic variant in the UK is *HFE* C282Y (H for high and Fe for iron). This variant occurs in around 10% of people with European ancestry. This is recessive, so two copies of the variant are needed. However, for poorly understood reasons, even with two copies, most people do not develop iron overload. In general, males who develop iron overload tend to do so at a younger age than females because of the effect of menstruation.
- Chronic liver disease: alcoholic liver disease, metabolic dysfunction-associated steatotic liver disease and hepatitis C (due to low levels of hepcidin).
- Recurrent blood transfusions for sickle cell disease, thalassaemia, and MDS.

Treatment

The mainstay is venesection, initially weekly until ferritin is down to 20–30 mcg/L and then as needed. Once the ferritin is within the normal range, the blood can be donated.

If venous access is difficult, an oral iron binder such as desferrioxamine may be used.

Lifestyle changes: reduce alcohol intake, avoid iron and vitamin C supplements, but there is no evidence that reducing meat in the diet makes a difference.

📖 REFERENCES AND FURTHER READING

Hoffbrand V, Steensma DP (2019). Hoffbrand's haematology, essentials 8th edn. Wiley-Blackwell, Oxford. https://download.e-bookshelf.de/download/0013/2652/68/L-G-0013265268-0037033783.pdf

Phillips R, Wood H, Weaving G et al. (2021). Changes in full blood count parameters with age and sex: results of a survey of almost 900,000 patient samples from primary care. BJH, doi: 10.1111/bjh.17290.

Kovtonyuk LV, Fritsch K, Feng X, et al. (2016). Inflamm-aging of hematopoiesis, hematopoietic stem cells, and the bone marrow microenvironment. *Frontiers in Immunology* 14(7): 502, doi: 10.3389/fimmu.2016.00502

Stauder R, Vakent P, Theurl I (2018) Anemia at older age: etiologies, clinical implications, and management. *Blood* 131: 505–514, doi: 10.1182/blood-2017-07-746446

Gado K, Khodier, VA et al. (2022). Anemia of geriatric patients. *Physiology International* 109:2, 119–1345, doi: 10.1556/2060.2022.00218.

Watson J, Jones HE, Banks J et al. (2019) Use of multiple inflammatory marker tests in primary care: using clinical practice research datalink to evaluate accuracy. *British Journal of General Practice* 69:e462–e469, doi: 10.3399/bjgp19X704309.

Guralnik J, Ershler W, Artz A et al. (2022) Unexplained anemia of aging: Etiology, health consequences, and diagnostic criteria. *Journal of the American Geriatrics Society* 70:891–899, doi: 10.1111/jgs.17565

Moretti D, Goede JS, Zeder C et al. (2015). Oral iron supplements increase hepcidin and decrease iron absorption from daily or twice-daily doses in iron-depleted young women. *Blood* 126:1981–1989, ISSN 0006-4971, doi: 10.1182/blood-2015-05-642223.

Rund, D. (2021). Intravenous iron: do we adequately understand the short- and long-term risks in clinical practice?. *British Journal of Haematology* 193:466–480, doi: 10.1111/bjh.17202.

NICE Guidelines on Blood Transfusion (2015) www.nice.org.uk/guidance/ng24

Joint UK Blood Transfusion and Tissue Transplantation Services Professional Advisory committee: Jehovah's Witnesses and blood transfusion (transfusionguidelines.org)

NICE *Guidelines for B12 and folate deficiency*: https://cks.nice.org.uk/topics/anaemia-b12-folate-deficiency

Maquet J, Lafaurie M, Sommet A et al. (2020) Autoimmune Hemolytic Anemia: a disease of the elderly and the very elderly with increased mortality and increased rates of hospitalization for thrombosis and infection. *Blood* 136(Supplement 1), ISSN 0006-4971, doi: 10.1182/blood-2020-137545.

Weiss G, Ganz T, Goodnough LT (2019). Anemia of inflammation. *Blood* 133:40–50. https://ashpublications.org/blood/article/133/1/40/6617/Anemia-of-inflammation.

BMJ Best Practice (2022) *Aplastic anaemia in adults* https://bestpractice.bmj.com/topics/en-gb/96

Ponikowski P, Voors AA, Anker SD et al. (2016). ESC guidelines for the diagnosis and treatment of acute and chronic heart failure. *European Heart Journal* 37:2129–2200. (section 11.12 – treatment with IV iron). https://academic.oup.com/eurheartj/article/37/27/2129/1748921#109987048.

Khoury JD, Solary E, Abla O et al. (2022). The 5th edition of the World Health Organization classification of haematolymphoid tumours: myeloid and histiocytic/dendritic neoplasms. *Leukemia* 36:1703–1719, doi: 10.1038/s41375-022-01613-1

Pizzi M, Croci GA, Ruggeri M et al. (2021). The classification of myeloproliferative neoplasms: rationale, historical background and future perspectives with focus on unclassifiable Ccses. *Cancers (Basel)* 13(22):5666, doi: 10.3390/cancers13225666

Haematological Malignancy Research Network (UK data) https://hmrn.org

Panitsas F, Kothari J, Vallance G et al. (2018). Treat or palliate: outcomes of very elderly myeloma patients. *Haematologica* 103(1):e32–e34, doi: https://doi.org/10.3324/haematol.2017.173617

Myeloma UK *Myeloma and MGUS A Guide for GPs* (2021) www.myeloma.org.uk/wp-content/uploads/2023/04/Myeloma-UK-Myeloma-and-MGUS-A-Guide-for-GPs.pdf

Côté J, Kotb R, Bergström DJ et al. (2023). First line treatment of newly diagnosed transplant ineligible multiple myeloma: recommendations from the Canadian myeloma research group consensus guideline consortium. *Clinical Lymphoma Myeloma and Leukemia* 23:340–354, doi: 10.1016/j.clml.2023.01.016

Jamil A, Mukkamalla SKR *Lymphoma* Statpearls https://www.ncbi.nlm.nih.gov/books/NBK560826

White K, Faruqi U, Cohen AT (2022) New agents for DOAC reversal: a practical management review. *British Journal of Cardiology* 29:26–30d, doi: 10.5837/bjc.2022.001.

Geyer-Roberts E, Akhand T, Blanco A et al. (2022). Disseminated intravascular coagulation in varying age groups based on clinical conditions. *Cureus* 14(4):e24362, doi: 10.7759/cureus.24362

INFORMATION FOR PATIENTS AND FAMILIES

NHS Blood and Transplant website: https://www.nhs.uk/conditions/blood-transfusion

British Dietetics Association website: Iron Food Fact Sheet: https://www.bda.uk.com/resource/iron-rich-foods-iron-deficiency.html

Haemochromatosis UK: www.haemochromatosis.org.uk

Blood Cancer UK: https://bloodcancer.org.uk

Cancer Research UK: https://www.cancerresearchuk.org/about-cancer/blood-cancers

Leukaemia https://www.cancerresearchuk.org/about-cancer/leukaemia

Myeloma https://www.cancerresearchuk.org/about-cancer/myeloma/treatment

Myelofibrosis https://www.cancerresearchuk.org/about-cancer/myelofibrosis

Lymphoma https://www.cancerresearchuk.org/about-cancer/lymphoma

All websites were accessed in September 2024.

18

Oncogeriatrics

This is a new chapter, reflecting the change over the last 5 years in oncology, with older people being considered for more active management. The British Geriatrics Society now has a special interest group in oncology. We have included an initial section on the basic principles of drug treatment for cancer. This has grown very rapidly; the terminology is complex, and even recent graduates struggle to have an overview. A stream of new options is being approved for clinical use, and they are easier to grasp if you can fit them into a framework.

Treatments for cancer

Chemotherapy

Chemotherapy is the use of drugs to stop or slow the growth of cancer cells. Chemotherapy cannot distinguish between cancer cells and normal cells, but it works because cancer cells grow and divide more quickly than normal cells. Toxicity results from the effects on normal cells. Most chemotherapy interferes with DNA, RNA, or protein synthesis or stops them from working properly. The cell may die because of direct toxicity, or apoptosis may be triggered.

Drugs with different mechanisms of action are usually used in combination to improve efficacy, reduce toxicity, and prevent the development of resistance. The drugs are not targeted at an individual's cancer, but different drugs are used for cancers from various organs, depending on the histology.

Chemotherapy can be used in several ways:

- **Neoadjuvant:** before the primary treatment.
- **Adjuvant:** with the initial therapy.
- **Combined:** with other modalities, such as radiation.
- **Palliative:** in metastatic cancer, to extend life expectancy or improve quality of life.

Classification by mechanisms of action

Drugs used in chemotherapy are classified in various ways; this is a simplified classification based on the main mode of action. Some of the drugs have other uses, e.g. in immunosuppression and some were derived from antibiotics.

1 **Alkylating agents:** reactive alkyl groups cross-link DNA strands and inhibit replication and transcription. Act on multiple stages of the cell cycle.
   - Nitrogen mustards, e.g. chlorambucil, cyclophosphamide, and melphalan.
   - Nitrosoureas (which can cross the blood–brain barrier), e.g. lomustine.
   - Platinum analogues, e.g. cisplatin.

2 **Antimetabolites:** interfere with DNA and RNA synthesis by acting as false metabolites or blocking key enzymes. S phase specific. (Purine/pyrimidine base + sugar is a nucleoside, + phosphate is a nucleotide.)
   - Purine (adenine and guanine) analogues, e.g. 6-mercaptopurine.
   - Pyrimidine (cytosine, thymine, and uracil) analogues, e.g. gemcitabine, fluorouracil, and capecitabine (5-FU prodrug).
   - Folate antagonists: inhibit dihydrofolate reductase, impairing nucleotide formation, e.g. methotrexate.

3 **Topoisomerase inhibitors:** act on these nuclear enzymes, which are essential in DNA replication, transcription, chromosome segregation, and recombination. All cells have two major topoisomerases: type I, which makes transient single-stranded cuts in DNA, and type II, which cuts and passes double-stranded DNA. These cuts allow the DNA to be unwound or untangled. The inhibitors block the cutting or inhibit the repair. Topo I inhibition leads to S1 phase arrest and cell death. Topo II inhibition arrests cells in the G2 pre-mitosis phase.
   - Topoisomerase I inhibitors, e.g. irinotecan.
   - Topoisomerase II inhibitors, e.g. doxorubicin, etoposide.

4 **Anti-microtubule agents:** act directly on the cytoskeleton by interfering with microtubule function, disrupting the mitotic spindle, and inhibiting mitosis at the metaphase/anaphase junction. Taxanes bind preferentially to beta-subunits of tubulin, stimulating microtubule polymerisation and the formation of stable microbundles. Vinca alkaloids bind to alpha- and beta-subunits of tubulin in the S phase of the cycle, inhibiting the polymerisation of tubulin, which leads to the disruption of the microtubule assembly during mitosis.
   - Taxanes, e.g. paclitaxel, docetaxel.
   - Vinca alkaloids, e.g. vinblastine, vincristine.

5 **Oxidative damage:** G2 arrest in the cell cycle results from damage to DNA.
   - Glycopeptide antibiotics, e.g. bleomycin.

Common side effects

The side effect profile depends on the drug, but many side effects are common because of toxicity to tissues with high cell turnover, e.g. skin, GI tract, and blood.

- Asthenia.
- Nausea and vomiting.
- Diarrhoea.
- Fever or chills.
- Hair loss.
- Anaemia, neutropaenia, and thrombocytopaenia.
- Stomatitis.
- Peripheral neuropathy.
- Brain fog.

Neutropaenic sepsis is a common cause of admission. Some drugs have major long-term toxicity, such as cardiac damage with anthracyclines and lung fibrosis with bleomycin. Each side effect is graded from 0 to 4.

Geriatric Medicine and Elderly Care: Lecture Notes, Ninth Edition. Claire G. Nicholl, K. Jane Wilson, and Shaun D'Souza.
© 2025 John Wiley & Sons Ltd. Published 2025 by John Wiley & Sons Ltd.
Companion website: www.wiley.com/go/lecturenotesgeriatricmedicine9e

Targeted therapy

Targeted therapy targets the specific changes in cancer cells that help them grow, divide, and spread. Hormone therapy was the first targeted therapy to be used – the improvement following orchiectomy for advanced prostate cancer in 1941 demonstrated proof of principle, and anti-androgen drugs followed. At presentation, prostate cancer of any stage is hormone-responsive, so the individual's cancer cells are not tested for receptors. However, in breast cancer (BC), each patient's cancer cells must be analysed for hormone receptors, as the pattern is variable. Tamoxifen for oestrogen-positive (ER+ve) breast cancer was introduced in 1972 in the UK.

Hormonal treatment is discussed here, but the label 'targeted therapy' is usually reserved for two newer families of therapies that target specific changes in an individual's cancer cells: monoclonal antibodies (first approved was rituximab for lymphoma in 1997) and small-molecule inhibitors (first approved was imatinib for CML in 2001).

Monoclonal antibodies are used when receptor targets are overexpressed on the outside of cancer cells. Small molecular inhibitors are used to target processes within the cell. Some can be targeted by both methods. For example, there are two classes of anti-EGFR/ HER (epidermal growth factor receptor/ human epidermal growth factor receptor) drugs: monoclonal antibodies against the extracellular domain and small-molecule inhibitors, which can bind to the intracellular catalytic site.

Hormones

Use is limited to cancers that are hormone-sensitive, which include:

- **Breast cancer:** can be oestrogen- or progesterone-receptor-positive or both. Aromatase inhibitors are used post-menopausally to block oestrogen production from androgens, e.g. letrozole. Tamoxifen blocks oestrogen receptors and can be used pre- and post-menopausally for ER+ve BC.
- **Prostate cancer:** is androgen-dependent. Gonadotropin-releasing hormone (GnRH) produced by the hypothalamus stimulates the pituitary to produce luteinising hormone (LH) **and** follicle-stimulating hormone (FSH). However, GnRH is also known simply as LHRH. LH causes the Leydig cells of the testis to produce testosterone, whereas FSH acts on the Sertoli cells to stimulate spermatogenesis. There are several ways of reducing testosterone production or its effects:
  - LHRH blockers (e.g. degarelix).
  - LHRH agonists, also referred to in patient literature as LH blockers (e.g. goserelin).
  - Androgen receptor blockers (e.g. enzalutamide).
  - Androgen synthesis inhibitors inhibit CYP17 and also prevent adrenal synthesis (e.g. abiraterone).
  The use of LHRH agonists is counterintuitive, but after causing a temporary increase in LH and testosterone (the so-called 'testosterone flare'), high sustained LHRH downregulates its receptors in the pituitary, causing LH release and hence testosterone production to be markedly reduced. The effect of the flare is prevented with an androgen receptor blocker. LHRH antagonists do not cause a testosterone flare.
- **Uterine cancer:** progesterone may be used in advanced uterine cancer.

Monoclonal antibodies

Monoclonal antibodies (mAbs) are used in several ways to treat cancer:

1 Attach to cell surface receptors such as epidermal growth factor receptor (EGRF) to block interaction with signalling molecules or their receptors (e.g. cetuximab for RAS wild-type metastatic colorectal cancer).

2 Block signals that enable cancers to develop a blood supply. Some cancer cells produce vascular endothelial growth factor (VEGF), which attaches to receptors on capillaries, promoting growth; antiangiogenic mAbs block this.

3 Activate the body's natural immune response.
   i Promotion of antibody-dependent cell-mediated cytotoxicity.
   ii Activate complement-dependent cytotoxicity.
   iii BiTEs, or bispecific T cell engagers, are antibodies with two specificities that bring T cells and cancer cells together to improve cancer cell elimination.
   iv Checkpoint inhibitors.
      Normal T cells have multiple 'checkpoint' proteins on them to switch them on and off as needed. Some cancer cells express high levels of proteins, which switch off T cells and stop them from attacking the cancer cells. There are checkpoint blockers that block the inhibitory receptors or their ligands to turn the T cells back on again, including:
      - CTLA-4 (cytotoxic T lymphocyte-associated protein 4), e.g. ipilimumab for melanoma.
      - PD-1 (programmed cell death protein 1) on the T cell, e.g. pembrolizumab for Hodgkin lymphoma.
      - PD-L1 (programmed cell death ligand 1) on the cancer cell, e.g. atezolizumab for some lung cancers (see Figure 18.1).

4 Deliver radioactive molecules or toxins to the inside of the cells through attachment to cellular receptors (conjugated mAbs). Monoclonal antibodies are too big to get across the blood–brain barrier, but a conjugated mAb could be used with a technique to open the blood–brain barrier around a brain tumour, e.g. using focused ultrasound.

The naming of monoclonal antibodies

Understanding this may help you remember individual monoclonals.

Monoclonals in current use have the stem-mab, like a family name.

The substem identifies how the antibodies were generated, with the three most common sources being:

1 **Chimeric human-mouse:** xi.
2 **Humanised mouse:** zu.
3 **Fully human:** mu.

An additional substem describes the target, e.g. tu for tumour, ci for circulation and li for immune system.

The prefix is like a given name – chosen by the drug company to identify their product. Thus:

- Rituximab (ri-tu-xi-mab) is a chimeric monoclonal directed against a tumour antigen.
- Bevacizumab (beva-ci-zu-mab) is a humanised mouse monoclonal directed against a circulatory antigen.

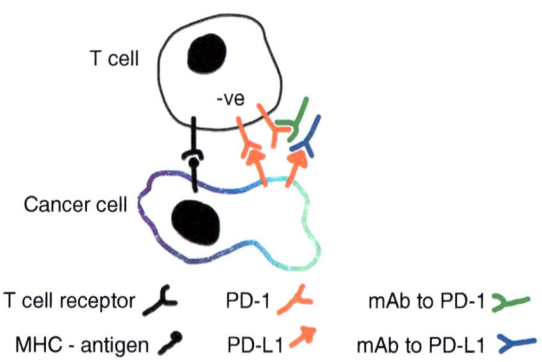

Figure 18.1 Diagram shows how monoclonal antibodies can block the binding of PD-1 to its ligand, removing the inhibitory effect on the T cell.

- Ipilimumab (ipi-li-mu-mab) is a fully human monoclonal directed against an immune system target.

Over 800 mAb names have been selected, so in 2021, the WHO introduced a new system that is simpler but less obvious as it gets rid of the -mab stem. There will be four stems:

Group 1: tug for **u**nmodified immuno**g**lobulins.
Group 2: bart for anti**b**ody **art**ificial (monospecific full-length immunoglobulins with any genetically engineered modification).
Group 3: mig for **m**ulti-**i**mmuno**g**lobulins (immunoglobulins of any format with more than one specificity).
Group 4: ment for frag**ment** (all monospecific fragments that do not contain an Fc domain).

The stems will be preceded by an infix that indicates the target class, as prior to 2021, but with a bigger range of immune targets, and the prefix will still be the given name. At present, mAbs with new names are still in clinical trials.

Small molecule inhibitors

Small-molecule inhibitors (-ibs) target specific proteins that are deregulated due to mutations, translocations, or overexpression in oncogenic pathways.

- They are usually taken orally, and as they are small, get into cells and may get into the CNS.
- Many target kinases in cell surface receptors, downstream in intracellular signalling cascades, and in the cytoplasm. Many kinases are protooncogenes and become oncogenes when mutated so that the cell keeps dividing. Kinase inhibitors can be selective or multikinase inhibitors.

Targets
These include:

1 **Tyrosine kinase inhibition:** -sub stem '-tin-ib'. Imatinib, the first in class to be approved, is an ABL kinase inhibitor, blocking the aberrant kinase produced by the fused Philadelphia chromosome in CML. EGFR (also known as HER1) consists of four receptor tyrosine kinases, and inhibitors are used in HER+ve breast cancer (e.g. neratinib), where HER2 is overexpressed, and in non-small cell lung cancer (NSCLC) with *EGFR* mutations (e.g. gefitinib). Anaplastic lymphoma kinase (ALK) fusion proteins are part of the insulin receptor family and drive aberrant proliferation and cell survival through the PI3K/AKT/mTOR (phosphatidylinositol-3-kinase/AKT/mammalian target of rapamycin), MAPK (mitogen-activated protein kinase) and JAK/STAT (Janus kinase-signal transducer and activator of transcription) pathways. Inhibitors (e.g. lorlatinib) are used for ALK-positive NSCLC with brain metastases.
2 **Cyclin-dependent kinase (CDK) inhibition:** '-cicl-ib'. The cell cycle is essential for cell proliferation. CDKs are cell cycle activators. Normal cells contain many inhibitors or cell cycle checkpoints. Increased activation and decreased inhibition are seen in several cancers, so inhibitors are used (e.g. palbociclib for HER-ve advanced breast cancer).
3 **Proteasome inhibition:** '-zom-ib' proteosomes function as a protein recycling centre, so inhibiting the system causes a buildup of unwanted proteins, causing cell death (e.g. bortezomib for myeloma).
4 **PARP (poly [ADP-ribose] polymerase) inhibition:** '-par-ib' Cells have two normal mechanisms to repair DNA. One is controlled by DNA repair genes such as *BRCA-1* and *BRCA-2*. In some breast and other cancers, these genes are mutated, so the cell cannot use this pathway. PARP inhibitors block the remaining DNA repair pathway, resulting in multiple double-strand breaks and increasing apoptosis of the cancer cells (e.g. olaparib).
5 **Angiogenesis inhibition:** '-an-ib' (e.g. tivozanib for advanced renal cell cancer).
6 **BRAF inhibition:** '-fenibs' The *BRAF* gene encodes a serine-threonine protein kinase called B-raf, which affects how cells divide and grow. *BRAF* gene mutations occur in several cancers, most commonly melanoma. If the *BRAF* gene is faulty, it affects mitogen-activated protein kinase (MEK). MEK is also involved in cell division and can make cancer cells keep dividing out of control (e.g. dabrafenib, a BRAF inhibitor, with trametinib, a MEK inhibitor for advanced melanoma).
7 **P13K inhibition:** '-lisibs' (R-idelalisib for relapsed CLL)

Small-molecule inhibitors have their own range of side effects, which can be severe. Drug resistance tends to develop as the cellular metabolism adapts. They may be used in combination with other treatments, including chemotherapy, but trials are always needed.

Immunotherapy

Immunotherapy is a broad term for anticancer treatments that enhance the immune response and include some of the treatments already discussed.

T-cell transfer therapy

There are two main types: tumour-infiltrating lymphocyte therapy and CAR T-cell therapy. Both involve collecting the patient's immune cells, growing them up in vitro, and transfusing them back after depleting the patient's own B cells. Lymphocytes are extracted from the tumour or blood and may be tested to find those with the best anti-tumour activity. In CAR T, the T cells are engineered to produce CAR, a chimeric antigen receptor, which will allow the T cells to attach to the cancer cells. Currently, treatment is expensive, availability in the UK is extremely limited and side effects can be very severe, including infection (as B cells are also killed), encephalopathy, cytokine release syndrome and tumour lysis syndrome. However, it highlights how understanding pathogenetic pathways will lead to individualised treatment.

Vaccines

BCG acts as a non-specific immune stimulant in bladder cancer. Specific vaccines are being developed; they direct the immune system to target the cancer rather than targeting the cancer directly. A vaccine is approved in the US for advanced prostate cancer. The patient's peripheral blood mononuclear cells are cultured with recombinant prostatic acid phosphatase-macrophage colony-stimulating factor. The resulting activated antigen-presenting cells are infused back into the patient.

Oncolytic viruses

Oncolytic viruses are a form of immunotherapy that uses viruses to infect and destroy cancer cells.

Monoclonal antibodies

Described earlier under targeted therapy.

Surgery

The aim of cancer surgery is to remove the cancer with an adequate margin of normal tissue whilst causing minimal morbidity. Many solid tumours require the removal of draining lymph nodes for staging or to achieve local control. The use of sentinel node biopsies in some cancers, e.g. breast cancer, reduces lymphatic damage and hence lymphoedema. Older people are more likely to be diagnosed with cancer following an emergency surgical presentation such as bowel obstruction or a perforation when outcomes are worse (see Chapter 6).

Radiotherapy

Radiotherapy uses high-energy ionising radiation to damage the DNA of the cancer cells and destroy them, but some normal tissue is damaged too. It can be used with the intent to cure, but it is more often used to reduce the chance of recurrence and for symptom relief. It can be administered externally, usually by a linear accelerator (Linac), or internally. Radiation oncology teams include clinical oncologists, therapeutic radiographers, medical physicists and medical engineers, nurses, and the wider MDT. The team plans the treatment for the individual patient, including the dose and number of fractions. The location is marked using tattoos, and masks and moulds may be used to keep the patient still. Fractionation increases the number of visits and duration of the therapy but reduces late side effects by giving normal tissues time to recover. The number of visits needed may be particularly burdensome for older people if they no longer drive and must rely on transport.

External radiotherapy

3D conformal radiotherapy (3DCRT) is designed by a computer programme with the information from the patient's CT, MRI and sometimes PET scan to follow the shape of the tumour (sometimes with the draining lymph bed) as closely as possible. Image-guided radiotherapy (IGRT) uses a check scan once the patient is positioned for the radiotherapy. Intensity-modulated radiotherapy (IMRT) allows different doses of radiation to be given across the field to minimise the damage to critical normal tissues near the tumour. Stereotactic radiotherapy is even more precise and may be delivered by a CyberKnife, which has a rotating arm to deliver radiation from different angles.

Internal radiotherapy

Brachytherapy

Radioactive implants are placed in the tumour, either to give high-dose radiotherapy when the source is positioned via applicator tubes and then removed or low-dose radioactive 'seeds' which are left in situ. This is an option for prostate cancer.

Radioisotopes

The commonest treatment is radioactive iodine (iodine 131 for thyroid cancer). This is not suitable for people with dementia who need care, as the patient needs isolation for 3 days because of their radioactivity.

Common side effects

These depend on the site and are dose-dependent. Fatigue and skin changes like moderate sunburn are common and develop a couple of weeks into the course. Irradiating mucus membranes cause ulcers and, in the gut, diarrhoea. Initial swelling may be critical in some situations, e.g. SVC obstruction and spinal cord compression; high-dose steroids are given. Late effects are often due to fibrosis, and second malignancies may occur years later.

Cancer in old age

Incidence

There are around 376,000 new cases of cancer each year in the UK. The four most common types of cancer, as in Europe as a whole, are female breast, bowel, prostate, and lung, and these make up over half of new cases each year.

Cancer is primarily a disease of older people. The peak rate of cancer cases in the UK occurs at 85–89 years (see Figure 18.2). There is some evidence that the fall after the age of 90 is due to a decrease in the likelihood of cancer in extreme old age, but part of the drop may reflect a lack of investigation. A third of new cases occur in people aged 75 or over, and this will increase as the population ages.

Older people have more cancer for several reasons:

- The incidence increases with age, at least to the age of 90. This is partly due to biological reasons including increasing genomic instability and epigenetic changes, longer exposure to risk factors, a proinflammatory environment, and weakening immune surveillance.

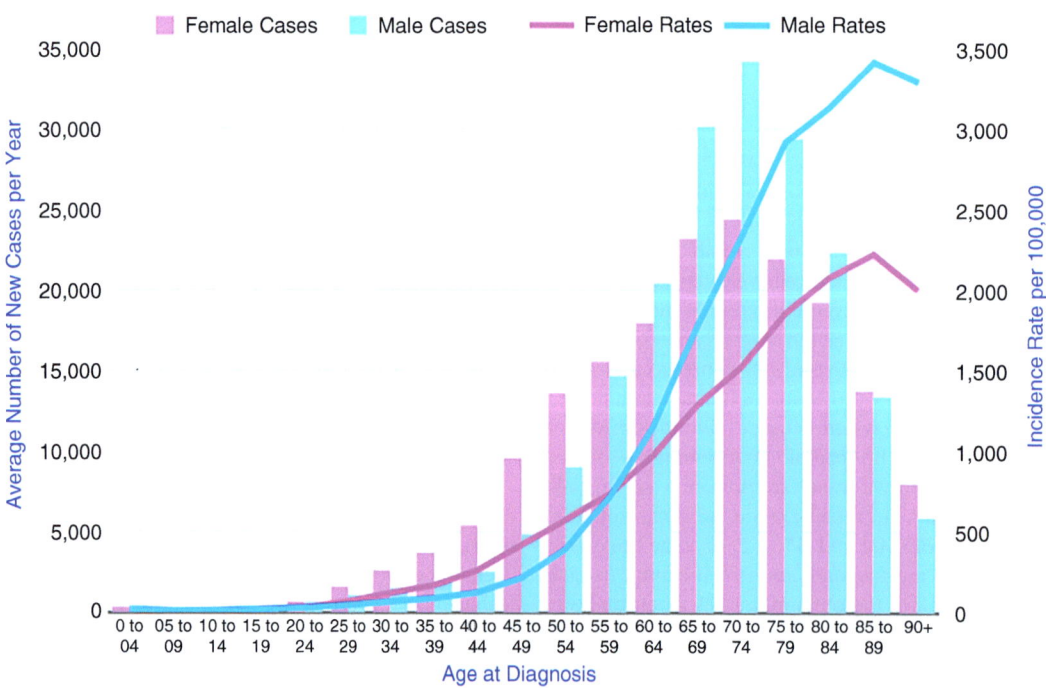

Figure 18.2 Incidence of all cancers (excluding non-melanoma skin cancer) Cancer Research UK data 2016–2018.

- Treatment of some cancers in middle age has improved so that although the cancer may not have been cured, it become a chronic disease – e.g. breast cancer.
- Second malignancies may occur after the treatment of a first malignancy.
- Cancer tends to present later in older people.
  - Routine screening programmes do not extend into old age.
    - **Breast:** women are not automatically invited for a mammogram after 70 but have the right to be screened every 3 years if they wish by contacting their local breast screening unit directly.
    - **Bowel:** people are not sent Faecal Immunochemical Testing (FIT) kits after 74, but people can contact the free bowel screening helpline for a kit every 2 years.
    - **Lung:** targeted screening with a low-dose CT scan for ex- and current smokers up to the age of 74 was recommended in 2022 but is yet to be implemented nationally.
  - Older people tend to have more comorbidities and symptoms, so the significance of new symptoms may not be appreciated.
  - It is now less common to see a GP face-to-face so opportunities for opportunistic diagnosis have been lost.
  - Doctors may be reluctant to investigate.
  - Waiting lists for investigations and treatment if cancer is found are long, particularly since the COVID-19 pandemic.

Diagnosis

Many older people with suspected cancer will be referred directly to an organ specialist team, e.g. gastroenterology (in principle, to be seen within 2 weeks). Others, often with less specific symptoms or incidental findings like a breast lump, are seen by geriatricians as outpatients or following emergency admission. Patients with a breast lump are then sent straight to the breast clinic. Otherwise, the geriatrician will usually make the diagnosis with input from an organ specialist if needed, e.g. for a colonoscopy, arrange basic staging and then refer on to oncology.

People in their 80s and 90s can still be very shocked at receiving a diagnosis of cancer, and the usual guidance about breaking bad news, arranging symptomatic relief and ongoing support applies.

Cancer of unknown primary

Sometimes the first presentation of cancer is with metastases, typically in the lungs, liver, bones, lymph nodes, or skin. Blood tests for tumour markers, biopsy and scans may reveal a primary, but in 2% cases, the primary cannot be identified; this is more common in older people – 60% of these occur in the over-75s. This makes specific treatment more problematic and adds to the feeling of uncertainty for the patient.

The oncology MDT team

There is an oncology multi-disciplinary team for cancers of different sites. This may be organised in your trust for common cancers or regionally. It includes surgeons and clinical oncologists specialising in radiotherapy and chemotherapy. With their therapy and technical colleagues, they will decide on the treatment plan. Specialist nurses provide much of the communication and support for patients. All patients, even those who clearly need palliative care, are referred to the team to improve the recording of cancer statistics. Give the team an accurate and detailed picture of an older person's overall clinical condition, particularly if they are active, not frail and want active management, or have distressing symptoms that could be alleviated, even if the plan will be palliative.

Over and undertreatment

Many cancer treatments are very burdensome for patients of all ages and impose considerable physiological as well as psychological stress. Older people must not be denied treatment with curative intent because of their age alone. However, geriatricians may have seen the oncology team gathered around a side room, discussing the encouraging shrinkage of the lymph nodes on the latest scan, when a glance at the owner of the lymph nodes suggests that, unfortunately, this is no longer relevant. The patient's view about the treatment they would want is central, but full information about the options must be given. There is a balance to be struck; decisions are hampered by the lack of inclusion of older patients in oncology trials. Undertreatment is more common.

The global challenge

The complexity of the diagnosis and management of cancer, with its reliance on high-tech imaging, accurate pathology, and good supportive care, makes it particularly challenging in less economically developed countries. Apart from in Africa, populations are ageing rapidly, so many more people need treatment.

Survival

Cancer survival is improving (albeit with marked variations between countries, with the UK being a poor performer), but this is mainly for patients younger than 75 rather than older patients. However, the Australian data shows that survival gains can be made in older people, even from a good baseline (see Table 18.1).

Treatments offered to older people

Older people are offered less treatment. The National Audit of Breast Cancer in Older Patients (NABCOP) has been pivotal in documenting the effect of age in England and Wales. As well as showing considerable geographic variation, older women present later and are less likely to have surgery, radiotherapy, or chemotherapy (see Table 18.2).

Radiotherapy for older people

Radiotherapy is underused in older people. A study of patients with bone metastases ($n = 558$) showed no difference in response rates for up to 3 months after treatment completion. In a large study of palliative radiotherapy for metastatic lung, breast, prostate, or colorectal cancer

Table 18.1 Age-standardised 5-year net survival for colon cancer according to period of diagnosis (Arnold et al.).

	Australia	UK
Under 75		
1995–1999	62%	51%
2000–2004	66%	55%
2005–2009	70%	60%
2020–2014	73%	64%
75 and older		
1995–1999	53%	38%
2000–2004	57%	42%
2005–2009	61%	45%
2020–2014	65%	46%

Table 18.2 Aspects of treatment for breast cancer according to age in England and Wales (NABCOP).

For women diagnosed between 2014 and 2019	Age band		
	50–69	70–79	80+
Metastases at presentation	3%	6%	8%
Surgery for early invasive BC (EIBC)	97%	91%	55%
Radiotherapy after breast-conserving surgery	60%	50%	27%
Chemotherapy for ER-negative, HER2-negative, and node-positive EIBC	74%	47%	5%

NABCOP, National Audit of Breast Cancer in Older Patients; BC, breast cancer; EIBC, early invasive breast cancer

(n = 63,221), 42% of the patients aged 66–69 received palliative radiotherapy. Multivariate analysis found that in comparison with this group, there was a steady reduction in the use of radiotherapy that was based on age alone (see Figure 18.3).

Guidelines for treating older people

NICE and international guidelines all state that treatment decisions should be based on clinical need and patient fitness, not age.

Performance scores

Oncologists have long used performance scores as a guide to the overall health of their patients prior to treatment. Two commonly used scores are shown in Table 18.3.

These scores and their changes with treatment do predict outcomes, but scoring has high inter-observer variability. Also, poor scores can be due to chronic conditions, e.g. PD or the acute effects of cancer, and good scores may miss conditions that are markers of frailty, such as the tendency to fall and mild cognitive impairment.

Assessment of frailty

Over the past 5 years, there has been considerable interest in the use of frailty to aid decision making for cancer treatment (see Figure 18.4).

There is now considerable data to suggest that the assessment of frailty gives better information than a traditional performance score.

Table 18.3 Common performance scores used in oncology.

ECOG (Eastern Cooperative Oncology Group) score		Karnofsky scale	
0	Normal activity	100	Normal; no evidence of disease
		90	Able to perform normal activities with only minor symptoms
1	Symptomatic and ambulatory; cares for self	80	Normal activity with effort; some symptoms
		70	Able to care for self but unable to do normal activities
2	Ambulatory: >50% of the time; occasional assistance	60	Requires occasional assistance; cares for most needs
		50	Requires considerable assistance
3	Ambulatory: <50% of the time nursing care needed	40	Disabled; requires special assistance
		30	Severely disabled
4	Bedridden or chairbound	20	Very sick; requires active supportive treatment
		10	Moribund

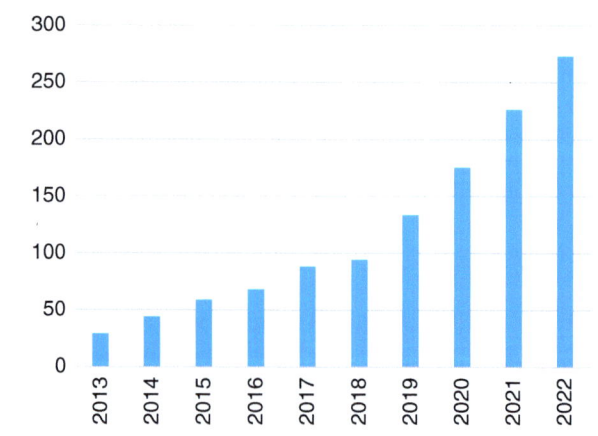

Figure 18.4 Publications in PubMed for the search query 'frailty, cancer and treatment' by year since 2013.

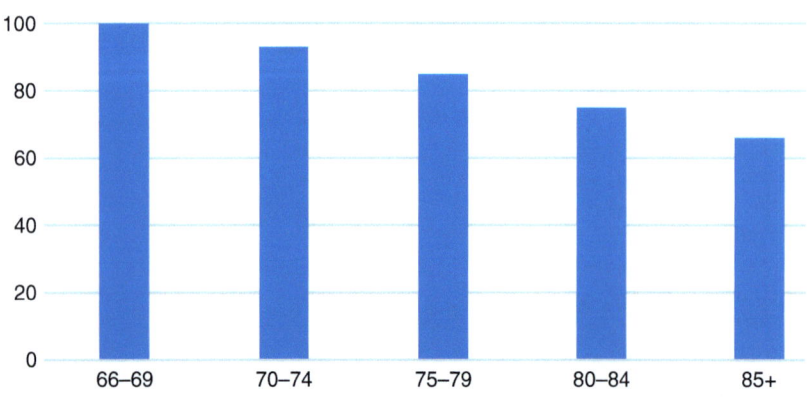

Figure 18.3 Percentage of patients receiving palliative radiotherapy relative to those aged 66–69 years (Wong).

To quote from the 2022 NABCOP report: 'In the same way that we would not treat breast cancer (BC) without knowing the ER and HER2 status, we should not treat BC in those aged 70+ years without a formal assessment of frailty'. This is still rarely done but needs to become routine practice.

From 2014 to 2019, women aged 80+ who were fit or had mild–moderate frailty were a little more likely to get surgery, with an increase from 62% to 69% (remember, the average life expectancy at 80 is over 9 years).

Where there is outcome data, the relative survival of fit older women receiving surgery was comparable to that of younger women, and overnight hospital admission within 30 days of adjuvant chemotherapy was not related to age but was related to frailty at all ages.

Full comprehensive geriatric assessment may be the gold standard (leading to a new sub-speciality of geriatric oncology) with evidence of benefit from assessment and intervention in an RCT that reduces serious chemotherapy-related toxicity (Li et al.), but this will not be widely available. A simple frailty score such as the Rockwood clinical frailty score (CFS) may be a practical option, but prospective studies are needed.

Trials in older people

As well as assessing frailty, another approach is to consider lower-dose chemotherapy in older patients, and data is beginning to appear. A multi-centre open-label randomised trial in frail older people with advanced gastro-oesophageal cancer found that reduced-intensity chemotherapy improved patients' experience without compromising anticancer control.

 ## REFERENCES AND FURTHER READING

Cancer Research UK *Chemotherapy* https://www.cancerresearchuk.org/about-cancer/treatment/chemotherapy

Amjad MT, Chidharla A, Kasi A (2023) *Cancer Chemotherapy* StatPearls https://www.ncbi.nlm.nih.gov/books/NBK564367

Choi E, Buie J, Camacho J, et al. (2022) Evolution of androgen deprivation therapy (ADT) and its new emerging modalities in prostate Cancer: an update for practicing urologists, clinicians and medical providers. *Res. Rep. Urol.* 14:87–108. doi: 10.2147/RRU.S303215.

Zahavi D, Weiner L (2020) Monoclonal antibodies in cancer therapy. *Antibodies (Basel)* 20(9):34. doi: 10.3390/antib9030034.

Eltarhoni K, Kamel F, Ihebunezie K, et al. (2022) Therapeutic antibodies in cancer treatment in the UK. *Int. J. Mol. Sci.* 23:14589. doi: 10.3390/ijms232314589.

Lythgoe MP (2022) No new 'mabs' in medicine – new nomenclature for monoclonal antibodies. *Br. J. Pharmacol.* 179:5338–5339. https://doi.org/10.1111/bph.15953

Liu G-H, Chen T, Zhang X, et al. (2022) Small molecule inhibitors targeting the cancers. *MedComm* 3:e181. doi: 10.1002/mco2.181.

Cancer Research UK *Immunotherapy* https://www.cancerresearchuk.org/about-cancer/treatment/immunotherapy

Shiravand Y, Khodadadi F, Kashani SMA, et al. (2022) Immune checkpoint inhibitors in cancer therapy. *Curr. Oncol.* 29:3044–3060. doi: 10.3390/curroncol29050247.

Cancer Research UK *Radiotherapy* https://about-cancer.cancerresearchuk.org/about-cancer/treatment/radiotherapy

Cree A, O'Donovan A, O'Hanlon, S (2019) New horizons in radiotherapy for older people. *Age and Ageing* 48 (I5):605–612. doi: 10.1093/ageing/afz089.

Cancer Research UK *Cancer incidence by age* https://www.cancerresearchuk.org/health-professional/cancer-statistics/incidence/age#heading-Zero

Arnold M, Rutherford MJ, Bardot A, et al. (2019) Progress in cancer survival, mortality, and incidence in seven high-income countries 1995-2014 (ICBP SURVMARK-2): a population-based study. *Lancet Oncol.* 20:1493–1505. doi: 10.1016/S1470-2045(19)30456-5.

National Audit of Breast Cancer in Older Patients (NABCOP). *Annual Report* (2022). https://www.nabcop.org.uk/reports/nabcop-2022-annual-report

Campos S, Presutti, R, Zhang L, et al. (2010) Elderly patients with painful bone metastases should be offered palliative radiotherapy. *Int. J. Radiat. Oncol.* 76:1500–1506. https://www.sciencedirect.com/science/article/abs/pii/S0360301609004386.

Whalen G. Principles of Surgical Oncology. In: Pieters RS, Liebmann J, eds. Cancer Concepts: A Guidebook for the Non-Oncologist. Worcester, MA: University of Massachusetts Medical School; 2016. doi: 10.7191/cancer_concepts.1022

Wong J, Xu B, Yeung HD, et al. (2014) Age disparity in palliative radiation therapy among patients with advanced cancer. *Int. J. Radiat. Oncol.* 90:224–230. doi: 10.1016/j.ijrobp.2014.03.050.

Gomes F, Lewis A, Morris R, et al. (2020) The care of older cancer patients in the United Kingdom. *Ecancermedicalscience* 14: 1101 https://ecancer.org/en/journal/article/1101-the-care-of-older-cancer-patients-in-the-united-kingdom.

Seghers PAL, Alibhai SMH, Battisti NML, et al. (2023) Geriatric assessment for older people with cancer: policy recommendations. *Glob. Health Res. Policy* 8:37. doi: 10.1186/s41256-023-00323-0.

Hall PS, Swinson D, Cairns DA, et al. (2021) Efficacy of reduced-intensity chemotherapy with oxaliplatin and capecitabine on quality of life and cancer control among older and frail patients with advanced gastro-oesophageal cancer: the GO2 Phase 3 Randomized Clinical Trial. *JAMA Oncol.* 7:869–877. doi: 10.1001/jamaoncol.2021.0848.

Li D, Sun CL, Kim H, et al. (2021) Geriatric assessment-driven intervention (GAIN) on chemotherapy-related toxic effects in older adults with cancer: a randomized clinical trial. *JAMA Oncol.* 7:e214158. doi: 10.1001/jamaoncol.2021.4158.

INFORMATION FOR PATIENTS (AND NON-SPECIALIST DOCTORS)

Cancer Research UK: excellent, up-to-date, and detailed information, including detailed statistics about individual cancers. https://www.cancerresearchuk.org

All websites were accessed in October 2023.

19

Dermatology

Age-related skin changes

Ageing of the skin is usually a combination of intrinsic chronological ageing and premature ageing due to sun exposure.

Intrinsic factors

Skin changes due to ageing are most obvious in areas of the body not usually exposed to the sun, such as the lower abdomen and buttocks. Atrophy of the epidermis due to a reduced number of cells makes the skin look more translucent.

1 The dermis has fewer mast cells and fibroblasts, and elastin in the elastic fibres degrades, so the skin loses its elasticity.
2 Ageing fibroblasts produce less extracellular matrix, leading to fibrosis.
3 Reduced epidermal turnover and repair of damage to the skin lead to poor wound healing (up to four times slower than in younger people).
4 Skin becomes drier due to the reduction in sebum secretion, which is more marked in women.
5 Reduced sweating, due to both reduced numbers and function of sweat glands, impairs the body's ability to cool down.
6 Reduced subcutaneous fat impairs the ability of the body to maintain its temperature and makes the skin more vulnerable to damage from shearing (see discussion about the development of pressure ulcers) or direct trauma from falling.
7 Increased capillary fragility leads to bruising under the skin, also known as senile purpura.
8 Reduction in the production of vitamin D3 from 7-dehydrocholesterol.
9 The reduced number of melanocytes reduces protection from UV rays.
10 Age-related proliferation of capillaries causes pink cherry angiomas (also known as Campbell de Morgan spots) on the arms and trunk. The prevalence said to be 75% in over 70-year-olds.
11 Proliferation of immature keratinocytes leads to seborrheic keratoses – well-demarcated, waxy-feeling, pigmented (yellow, brown, or black) macules found on the trunk, under the breasts, over the spine or in the scalp.

Extrinsic factors

Photo-ageing: inflammageing due to the sun's ultraviolet rays is most visible on the face, ears, bald scalp, forearms and back of the hands.

- Changes include increased pigmentation/patchy depigmentation, e.g. 'liver' spots or lentigines (named for their colour, not their aetiology) on the back of the hands, elastosis (thick, furrowed skin), telangiectasia, and precancerous lesions such as actinic keratosis.
- Actinic (or solar) keratosis starts as a small, rough area of skin but may develop into a larger (3–10 mm) hyperkeratotic plaque. It is more common in men. Treatment options include emollients, factor 30 sunscreen, topical 5-fluorouracil, photodynamic therapy, and surgical excision. If left untreated, it may develop into a squamous carcinoma.

Some studies suggest that both intrinsic skin ageing and photo-ageing can be improved with topical retinol.

Cigarette smoking produces more facial lines and atrophy because of increased collagen and elastin breakdown plus increased free radicals, slowing cellular repair.

Air pollution containing hydrocarbons causes pigment spots.

Direct heat produces erythema ab igne: a localised, red/brown network pattern of skin damage due to atrophy of the epidermis, telangiectasia, and hemosiderin deposition. It is often seen on the shins of older people who sit in front of a fire, or on the abdomen from a hot water bottle/heat pad applied to soothe chronic pain (or on the thighs from extended use of laptops).

Poor nutrition and hydration exacerbate all skin injuries, including pressure ulcers and burns.

Topical treatments: over-drying from soaps, etc. Use aqueous cream as a soap substitute. Skin thinning can result from chronic topical steroid use.

Vascular damage

Leg ulcers are a common, serious, and expensive condition in geriatric practice, with a prevalence of 1–2% in over 65-year-olds. Most are due to venous insufficiency, arterial disease, diabetes, or a mixture. The aim is to treat the underlying cause and promote healing of the ulcer itself by keeping it clean, warm, and hydrated to promote capillary growth. Experienced nurses with input from a tissue viability team will select an appropriate dressing from the many options – trial data is very limited despite the millions of pounds spent on dressings.

Chronic venous disease is due to raised venous pressure secondary to varicose veins, previous pregnancy, previous deep vein thrombosis, or after lower limb surgery or trauma (see Table 19.1).

- Exacerbated by immobility (standing or sitting), weight gain, and smoking.
- Early signs include capillary flare and varicose veins, which may be painful.
- Over time, chronic venous hypertension leads to further dilatation of the veins, which may leak red cells. This causes localised

Geriatric Medicine and Elderly Care: Lecture Notes, Ninth Edition. Claire G. Nicholl, K. Jane Wilson, and Shaun D'Souza.
© 2025 John Wiley & Sons Ltd. Published 2025 by John Wiley & Sons Ltd.
Companion website: www.wiley.com/go/lecturenotesgeriatricmedicine9e

Table 19.1 Differences between arterial and venous leg ulcers.

	Arterial	Venous
History of onset	Usually recent	Often months/years
Pain	Present	Often absent
Site	Over toe joints, under heels, over malleoli, and on anterior shins	Gaiter area of the leg
Appearance	Small, clean, punched out	Large, weepy, infected, surrounding hyperpigmentation or eczema
Pulses	Absent or bruits in proximal vessels (not invariable in diabetes)	Present unless obscured by oedema or mixed picture
Proportion	15%	70%

inflammation, so fibroblasts are stimulated to produce collagen, thus creating a vicious cycle of increasing inflammation and localised tissue breakdown. The breakdown product of the red cells (haemosiderin) causes brown pigmentation. Capillary leakage leads to oedema. Ongoing fibrosis causes lipodermatosclerosis, the 'inverted champagne bottle' appearance of the lower legs. Chronic inflammation leads to poor wound healing, leading to venous ulceration.

- Venous ulcers usually occur in the distal third of the lower leg, in the medial gaiter area, and tend to be superficial and non-painful except when they are dressed.
- Prevention: if the ankle brachial pressure index (ABPI) is greater than 0.8, use graduated compression stockings. Advise the patient to elevate their legs (suggest greater than hip height for 30 min three to four times per day), increase mobility to engage calf muscle pumps, reduce obesity, and encourage good nutrition.
- Refer for a Doppler venous ultrasound to assess reflux in the veins. Reflux in the small saphenous vein plus reflux in the deeper veins may be associated with a greater risk of the progression of chronic venous disease. These patients should be offered more aggressive treatment, such as foam sclerotherapy.
- The mainstay of treatment is compression bandaging (two to four layers), a skilled clinic procedure as the grading needs to have the greatest compression at the ankle, tapering to below the knee. The bandages and dressing are usually changed one to three times a week.
- Treatment includes oral antibiotics to cover infection common pathogens: *Staphylococcus aureus*, *Pseudomonas aeruginosa*, beta-haemolytic streptococcus, and occasionally MRSA.
- Extensive venous ulcers occasionally require surgical debridement, i.e. the excision of dead tissue to promote wound granulation, and may need skin grafting.
- Once the ulcer is healed, care and compression stockings are needed to prevent recurrence.

Arterial ulcers develop because of poor blood supply from the peripheral arterial system (see Table 19.1).

- Address vascular risk factors: smoking, high cholesterol, hypertension, and diabetes before ulceration occurs, if possible.
- Arterial ulcers are painful, often have sharp edges, and are found on the malleoli.
- The legs are pale and cool, and capillary refill time is prolonged.
- Pulses are difficult to palpate, check ABPI and arrange arterial duplex studies.

- Refer for revascularisation, usually angioplasty for a localised lesion or reconstructive surgery for more extensive disease. Once the blood supply has been improved, skin grafting may be needed.
- Infection can cause rapid deterioration, and admission may be needed for IV antibiotics to reduce the likelihood of wet gangrene and amputation.

Diabetic ulcers are usually associated with peripheral neuropathy and peripheral arterial disease.

- Prevent with well-fitting, supportive shoes, good diabetic control, treating tinea pedis with terbinafine, checking sensation, and restoring blood flow if necessary.
- Older people with diabetes may need help with daily inspections of their feet and shoes.
- Regular review by podiatrists is essential to reduce the risk of harm from sharp or long toenails.
- Maintaining good foot health reduces the risk of amputation.
- If ulcers develop, the patient should attend a specialist diabetic foot clinic. Treatment is debridement, antibiotics, and sometimes off-loading in a plaster boot.

Vasculitic ulcers are less common. Ulcers are often multiple, necrotic, and deep, and there may be evidence of vasculitic lesions elsewhere, e.g. nailfold infarcts. Suspect if the inflammatory markers are high or if the patient has a known vasculitis. Confirm with a skin biopsy.

Malignant ulcers: suspicion may be raised by a non-healing ulcer; occasionally, biopsies of chronic leg ulcers show squamous cell carcinoma.

Pressure injury

Pressure injury occurs when an area of skin and the tissues below are damaged by being placed under pressure sufficient to impair its blood supply. This is usually over a bony prominence: ischial tuberosities (30%), sacrum (30%), and heels (13%). Shear (within lax tissues) and friction (between the skin and the sheet) may contribute. Pressure injuries can be significant before the skin breaks, resulting in an ulcer. Pressure ulcers are a common cause of potentially avoidable harm to older people in the community (poor equipment, long waits for an ambulance after a fall) and in the hospital.

Pressure ulcer statistics

A range of figures, some of which use very old data, are quoted for the incidence, prevalence, and cost of pressure ulcers. In the UK, over 200,000 adult patients had a pressure ulcer in 2017/2018 an increase of a third in 5 years (data from >560 GP practices). A cross-sectional survey (2021) in 36 hospitals in England found a prevalence of 9% in 10,000 patients, 55% of whom were aged 70+. According to NHS Improvement (2018), treating pressure damage costs the NHS more than £3.8 million *every day*. In June 2022, 2.6% of patients developed a pressure ulcer following hip fracture (in the England National Hip Fracture Database, see Chapter 10).

Risk factors

1 Patient

Factors include: serious illness (especially with hypotension), impaired sensation (especially spinal injury), any cause of impaired mobility so patients cannot reposition themselves, significant cognitive impairment, bony deformity, poor circulation, obesity, sarcopaenia, malnutrition, poor skin, urinary and faecal incontinence, previous or current ulcer. In the context of terminal illness, the focus should be on comfort rather than healing.

2 Environment
- Accidental, e.g. a long lie on the floor.
- Inappropriate equipment, e.g. bed, chair, wheelchair, bed rails without pressure relief.
- Injurious devices, e.g. poorly fitting plaster casts, rigid neck collars, urinary catheters, nasal cannulae, and oxygen tubing (can cause painful ulcers in the nose and behind the ears).

3 Insufficient nursing time
Lack of turning, poor manual handling, e.g. friction from sheets, left-on bedpan, poor hygiene.

Consequences

Pressure ulcers cause considerable morbidity, increase mortality fivefold, and the cost of treatment and litigation is huge.

Pressure ulcers are:

- painful and perpetuate the cycle of reduced mobility.
- associated with longer hospital stay: 4–10 days on average (data from 2003 and 2011)!
- a potential source for systemic infection and osteomyelitis.

The aetiology is often mixed: ageing physiology + illness + environment. Prevention is much better than cure.

Assessment and management of skin health

The **ASSKING** model is a helpful strategy for assessing and managing skin health (see Figure 19.1).

A. Assess the risk for all older people on admission to hospital or a care home and those at home with a sudden decrease in mobility. Most settings use a risk tool, e.g. the Waterlow score, and any ulcers are documented on body maps and with photos.

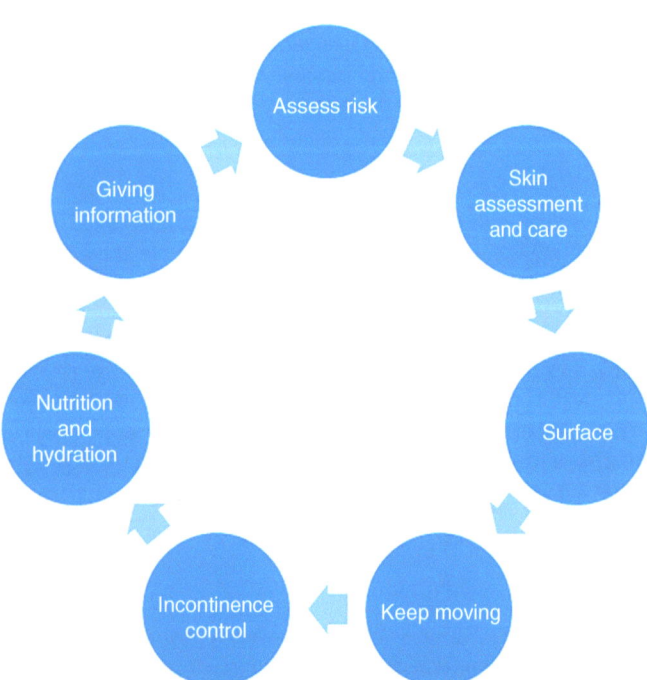

Figure 19.1 The ASSKING model (NHS England).

S. Skin assessment and care: review skin health over pressure areas, check for colour changes, heat, and non-blanching erythema, and apply barrier creams to the skin over bony prominences.

S. Surface: High-specification foam mattresses are standard in NHS hospitals. Consider the need for additional protection such as inflatable boots/overlays, and air mattresses (see Figure 19.2).

K. Keep moving: encourage patients to change position at least 4 hourly, turn those that cannot move themselves.

I. Incontinence management: keep vulnerable skin clean and dry.

N. Nutrition and hydration: encourage a good diet and plenty of fluids.

G. Giving information to other staff, the patient and family to maximise opportunities for prevention. If an ulcer is developing, explain why and what is being done.

Staging of pressure ulcers

Stage I: non-blanchable (extra care is needed to assess dark skin); may be warm, oedematous, or indurated.

Stage II: partial-thickness, presents as an abrasion or blister.

Stage III: full-thickness skin loss and damage to subcutaneous tissue down to the underlying fascia.

Stage IV: full-thickness tissue loss with exposed bone, tendon, or muscle.

A suspected deep tissue injury (SDTI) is an area of soft tissue damage due to pressure or shear at the bone-muscle interface that has not yet ulcerated. It usually appears as a dark bruise and may evolve rapidly into a deep ulcer, despite optimal treatment, as the underlying damage has already happened.

Unstageable: full-thickness tissue loss in which the depth of the ulcer is completely obscured by slough (will be III or IV if the slough is removed, but a dry adherent eschar over a heel should not be removed).

Management

This is multidisciplinary.

- Ward nurses/district or community nurses take the lead, and ongoing skin and pressure area care is essential.
- Specialist: The tissue viability nurse (TVN) will advise on difficult cases.
- Ward doctor: analgesia, coordination, communication with family.
- Microbiology: swab wounds for guidance about antibiotic use IF there is systemic infection. The course will be extended if there is associated osteomyelitis.
- Additional help from the diabetes team, radiology (imaging such as MRI to investigate underlying osteomyelitis), or surgical team (for debridement or skin grafting) may be needed.

Dressings for ulcers

There is a huge range of dressings available. Some are very expensive. Most studies comparing their efficacy involve small numbers, and there is little hard evidence. Your hospital will use a range of dressings, and the senior nursing staff on the ward usually decide which to use. Basic principles are shown in Figure 19.3.

Special circumstances

- Debridement may be needed for the removal of non-viable tissue.
  - Autolytic: occlusive dressing.

(a) waterproof profiling mattress

(b) 'air bed' with alternating pressure relieving mattress system

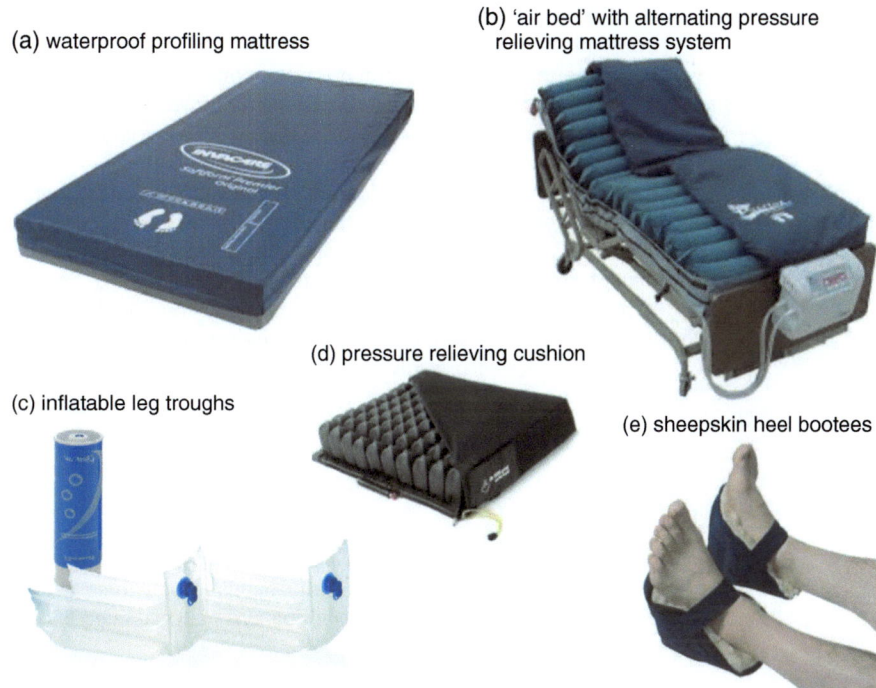

(d) pressure relieving cushion

(c) inflatable leg troughs

(e) sheepskin heel bootees

Figure 19.2 Common pressure-relieving equipment. *Source*: 19.2a: Invacare Corporation and 19.2b: Tech Ventures LLC.

Mepore film – an example of self-adhesive transparent dressings

DuoDerm – an example of hydrocolloid dressings

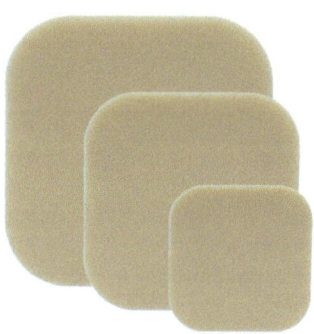

Kalostat – an example of an alginate dressing

Intrasitegel – an example of hydrogel to be applied to an irregular sloughy wound

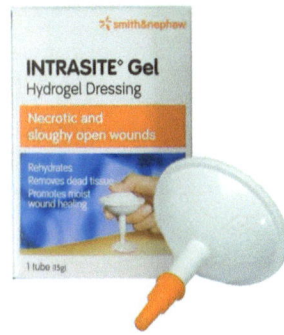

Figure 19.3 Dressings for ulcers.

- ○ Enzymatic: e.g. inject collagenase, less popular.
- ○ Sharp: surgical, most rapid, painless in necrotic tissue, sterile environment is not needed.
- ○ Larval (maggot) therapy: if debridement is needed but there is vascular insufficiency (Figure 19.4).
- Negative pressure or vacuum-assisted wound closure (VAC): used for a large cavity, e.g. after debridement of a sacral wound (Figure 19.5).

Moisture-associated skin damage

Moisture-associated skin damage (MASD) is often midline damage to the skin due to moisture from urine or stool but may be due to other sources of moisture, such as stomas.

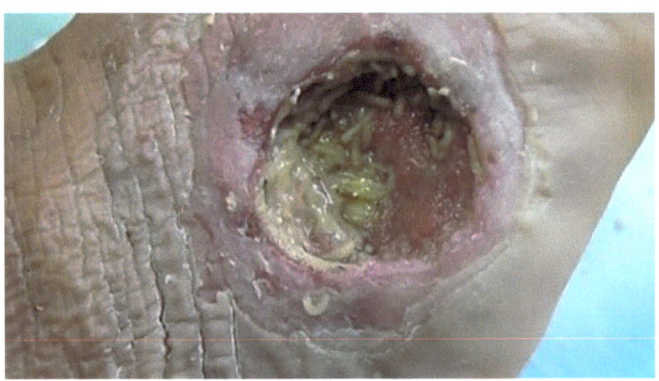

Figure 19.4 Larval therapy (free-range) for a malleolar ulcer in a diabetic foot. *Source*: Aleksey Nosenko/Wikimedia Commons/CC BY 3.0.

- MASD should be documented and reported in addition to pressure ulcers.
- Prevent by careful cleaning and drying the skin, and use of a barrier cream such as zinc oxide.

Cellulitis

Cellulitis is an acute bacterial infection of the dermis and subcutaneous tissue, most commonly affecting the lower limbs (accounting for 60%), upper limbs, and face.

- The incidence is 0.2 to 25 per 1,000 person years, depending on the population.
- Once it has occurred, the risk of recurrence is around 14%, and the more episodes, the greater the risk of further recurrence.
- Symptoms include acute onset of pain, swelling, and redness of the affected area.
- On examination, the skin is erythematous, hot, swollen and sometimes blisters. Check for lymphangitis, i.e. redness over the lymphatics demonstrating that the infection is in the lymphatics, and lymph node involvement. Look for a break in the skin that allowed bacteria to enter, e.g. trauma, especially pretibial lacerations, which heal slowly, insect/dog bites, ulcers, or tinea pedis causing maceration in the toe webs.
- Cellulitis can complicate chronic conditions such as lymphoedema, leg oedema, venous insufficiency, and obesity. People with diabetes, a neuropathy, immunocompromise, and IV drug users are at higher risk.
- Note bilateral red legs are not usually due to cellulitis; this is more commonly venous eczema or lipodermatosclerosis. It is important to differentiate to prevent unnecessary repeated courses of antibiotics and hospital admissions.
- The most common pathogens are *Streptococcus pyogenes* and *Staphylococcus aureus*. *Strep. pneumoniae* and *Haemophilus influenzae* are more likely in traumatic wounds, burns, infection associated with diabetes, immunocompromise, or cancer.
- Initial treatment in the community is usually oral flucloxacillin 500 mg to 1 g four times daily for 5–7 days (clarithromycin if penicillin-allergic). If the infection is close to the eyes or nose, use co-amoxiclav 500/125 mg three times daily for 7 days.
- Indications for admission for intravenous antibiotics include failure to respond to oral antibiotics, rapid spreading, increasing pain or swelling of joints, suggesting a deeper infection and systemic symptoms.
- It may be necessary to exclude a coexisting DVT.
- Rapidly spreading infection with crepitus and severe tenderness of the skin should raise the suspicion of necrotising fasciitis, which should be referred urgently to plastic surgery for consideration of aggressive debridement.

Burns

Older people may be at increased risk of burns because of syncope (e.g. due to standing in a hot kitchen), arthritic hands causing them to drop pans/cups of hot liquid, peripheral neuropathy or reduced safety awareness due to delirium or dementia.

Classification

Burns are classified according to the depth of tissues affected:

1 First degree: damage to the superficial epidermis, which will be red and painful.
2 Second degree: damage to the epidermis and upper layer of the dermis causing redness, mottling, weeping, and blistering.
   (a) Partial thickness: superficial dermal – blistered and painful.
   (b) Partial thickness: deep dermal – typically white, but there may be non-blanching erythema; reduced sensation but painful to deep pressure. Scarring occurs on healing.
3 Third degree: full thickness of the epidermis and dermis, sometimes down to the subcutaneous tissue. The skin may look white, brown, charred red, blackened, and be painless or develop a constant dull ache. Most require skin grafting.
4 Fourth degree: damage extends into underlying fat or muscle.
5 Fifth degree: down to muscle and bone.
6 (Sixth degree: involving bone, usually identified post-mortem.)

Management

In a serious burn, get the patient away from the heat source and use the ABCDE approach.

- If possible, submerge the affected area in cool water for 20 min.
- Cover loosely with cling film.
- Do not attempt to remove anything stuck to the burn.

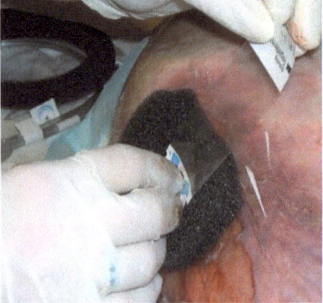

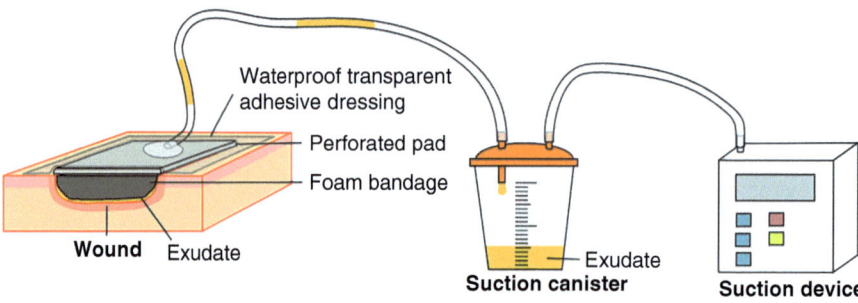

Waterproof transparent adhesive dressing

Perforated pad

Foam bandage

Wound Exudate

Exudate

Suction canister

Suction device

Figure 19.5 Application of a KCl wound vac dressing to a large sacral wound and a diagram to show the negative pressure wound therapy system. *Source*: Noles 1984 / Wikimedia Commons / Public domain. A loose necktie/https://en.m.wikipedia.org/wiki/File:NPWT_diagram.svg.

- All electrical and chemical burns, any burn bigger than 1% of the patient's total surface area (larger than their hand), burns to the face, neck, hands and feet, and all full-thickness burns need treatment in the emergency department.
- Complications, including infection, will also need specialist review.
- Ensure the patient has had full tetanus immunisation, especially if the wound is contaminated.
- NB healing burns are susceptible to UV damage, so advise patients to stay out of strong sunlight.

Pruritus (itch)

This is common in older people, who are predisposed to dry skin because of ageing changes as discussed above. Pruritus is important because it can:

- Significantly reduce quality of life;
- Prevent patients and their partners/carers from sleeping;
- Cause depression and agitation;
- Be frustratingly intractable, especially if applying creams is difficult because of arthritis or compliance is limited because of dementia.

The itch–scratch cycle occurs because scratching causes inflammation of the skin, which releases mediators including histamine, serotonin, prostaglandins, and cytokines, which trigger unmyelinated C nerve fibres that fire off to the thalamus via the spinothalamic tract. Motor fibres from the cortex lead to more scratching, and the cycle continues. Eventually the skin is damaged, and its barrier function is breeched, allowing superadded infection to occur. See Table 19.2 for more specific causes of itch and an outline of treatment.

An approach to management

- Take a good history to make a diagnosis where possible.
  - A new onset itch might suggest a reaction to a new drug or infestation.
  - Heat often worsens itch.
- Careful examination to exclude infestation/infection or other cause, as shown in Table 19.2.
- Routine blood tests to exclude a metabolic or systemic cause: FBC, ferritin, urea, bilirubin, alkaline phosphatase, and TSH.
- Encourage the patient to drink plenty (at least eight glasses) of water per day.
- Avoid hot baths.
- Avoid soap (because of its drying effect); use aqueous cream as a soap substitute.
- Pat the skin dry and avoid rubbing.
- Moisturise within 5 min of leaving the bath, preferably with a ceramide lipid-based emollient that traps the absorbed water and reduces evaporation.
- Educate the patient to avoid scratching: trim fingernails!
- Use steroid creams or ointments for short periods only for true inflammatory eczema.
- Consider antihistamines at night for sedative effects.
- Cooling preparations, e.g. menthol cream, may help by masking the itch.

Other important skin conditions in geriatric medicine

1 **Shingles** presents with crops of vesicles which then scab, in a dermatomal distribution. The subsequent post herpetic pain, debility, and risk of chicken pox to others present the most serious aspects of this condition.

2 **Intertrigo** is a moist rash that is often secondarily infected with fungi, e.g. Candida. It is especially common in obese individuals where there is skin-to-skin contact under pendulous breasts, abdominal aprons and between the buttocks. Better personal hygiene and treatment with antifungal (e.g. clotrimazole) preparations are required.

3 **Drug reactions** can present as any lesion, from eruptions to purpura. Pathological thinning of the skin secondary to chronic steroid use is another common example.

4 **Rosacea** typically occurs in older women with fair skin and is characterised by erythema, telangiectasia, and pustules on the nose, cheeks, and forehead. Occasionally, men develop a severe form with hypertrophy of the sebaceous glands and skin of the nose, producing a disfiguring rhinophyma. It seems to be triggered by stress, high temperatures, hot drinks, and alcohol. Treatment includes oral tetracyclines, topical metronidazole, or topical permethrin. Laser therapy can reduce the appearance of telangiectasia and rhinophyma.

5 **Bullous pemphigoid** is the most common autoimmune blistering condition and usually occurs in patients aged 60 to 80+ years. It presents with itching and blisters. The blisters may be large and tense because the immunological lesion is subepidermal, targeting the basement membrane. IgG autoantibodies are directed to hemidesmosomal bullous pemphigoid antigens. Mouth ulceration occurs in around a third of patients and is minor. The skin changes may be localised, and in practice, the blisters often burst.

Bullous pemphigoid can be triggered by drugs including furosemide, penicillins, gliptins (e.g. sitagliptin), and cancer treatments including PD-1 inhibitor immunotherapies and checkpoint inhibitors. Patients are typically younger, and if the culprit drug is stopped, resolution can be rapid. There is an association with neurological conditions such as stroke, dementia, and Parkinson's disease. The mechanism is unclear.

Treatment is with oral steroids, at a high dose initially until the lesions are under control, and then a lower maintenance dose. It usually remits spontaneously (after months or years), but while it is active, good management is needed to avoid sepsis.

6 **Pemphigus vulgaris**, another blistering autoimmune disorder, is much rarer (affects 3 in 100,000) and more serious. Remember, pemphigu**S** is **S**erious and **S**uperficial. IgG autoantibodies bind to desmoglein 3 molecules on the surface of keratinocytes, causing loss of cell-to-cell adhesion, leading to severe, extensive superficial blistering and erosions of the skin. The blisters are so superficial that they burst very quickly and may not be seen. In 50% of cases, there are also antibodies to desmoglein 1. The lesions tend to start in the mouth and spread to other areas of the skin. It is a life-threatening condition because of the high risk of secondary bacterial infection and the extreme loss of protein.

The mainstay of treatment is high-dose steroids. Other options for immunosuppression include azathioprine, mycophenolate, cyclophosphamide, and rituximab.

Malignant diseases of the skin

Fair-skinned (Fitzpatrick type 1 and 11) people exposed to the sun are at the highest risk. There is an increasing incidence of skin cancer because of increased longevity and the opportunity for sun exposure. Until the 1980s, most sun creams had an SPF of 2–6!

Basal cell carcinoma

Basal cell carcinoma (BCC) is the most common skin malignancy (accounts for 80%), and usually occurs in sun-damaged skin. It arises as a pearly papule, usually on the upper face (70%), ears or scalp. It slowly, but inexorably, enlarges. Metastatic spread is extremely rare.

Table 19.2 Causes, clinical features, and treatments of itch in older people.

Cause	Clinical features	Examples	Treatment
Xerosis	Abnormal maturation of keratocytes causes dryness and roughness of the skin with a fine scale.	Very common with no underlying pathology, PVD, and neurological disease.	Avoid soap and use emollients.
Eczema	Erythema, classically over flexure surfaces. Exacerbated in winter, dry conditions, or exposure to allergens. Venous	Atopic Seborrhoeic Contact Venous	Emollients, short course topical steroid cream Nizoral shampoo. Remove/avoid allergens See Chapter 12
Psoriasis	Erythematous plaques with silver scale, commonly over extensor surfaces Tear-drop lesions on the trunk Lesions on the palms and soles	Exacerbated by stress, alcohol, and beta blockers Guttate psoriasis triggered by streptococcal infections Pustular psoriasis	Topical calcipotriol and steroids PUVA treatment
Lichen simplex chronicus	Localised raised plaques caused by habitual scratching.		Consider covering with an occlusive non-adherent dressing to break the cycle
Drugs	Ask about new medications	Opiates Phenothiazines Aspirin Quinine	Stop suspected medications whenever possible
Urticaria	Raised weals due to type 1 hypersensitivity reaction to, e.g. drugs, food, cold, sunlight	Sensitivity to, e.g. penicillin, nuts	Avoid precipitants and short course of steroids
Lichen planus	Pruritic, purple, polygonal, papules on flexures of the wrist, but can affect other areas, including the buccal and genital mucosa	May be triggered by exposure to gold or mercury in dental fillings, hepatitis C	Topical steroids are systemic in severe reactions.
Dermatitis Herpetiformis	Very itchy vesicles on extensor sites, buttocks, back and scalp	Gluten enteropathy, but may be subclinical	Avoid gluten in diet
Pityriasis rosacea	Itching red rash on trunk in 'Christmas tree' distribution		Usually self-limiting. If necessary, try sedating antihistamine
Bullous pemphigoid	Irritating deep blisters	See text	Oral steroids
Infestation	Straight or 's' shaped burrows in finger webs and wrists. Check other members of the household/care home. Likely to produce a generalised allergic rash due to scratching.	Scabies	Shower/bathe in antibacterial soap. Topical permethrin solution. Wash clothes and bed clothes. Treat contacts
Infection	Dermatophytes	Candida in intertriginous areas Tinea corporis Tinea cruris	Topical antifungals such as clotrimazole or terbinafine
Neoplasia	Fever, weight loss, and itch	Mycosis fungoides Lymphoma	Treat as appropriate
Metabolic	Hypothyroid facies Uraemic frost Jaundice Iron deficiency	Hypothyroidism End-stage renal disease Liver disease IDA	Levothyroxine See Chapter 15 Ursodeoxycholic acid Look for and treat causes.

IDA, iron deficiency anaemia; PUVA, psoralen and ultraviolet A light therapy; PVD, peripheral vascular disease.

Subtypes:

- Nodular: most common: look for a rolled edge, telangiectasia, and often a central ulcerated area.
- Superficial: slow-growing erythematous lesion on a sun-exposed area.
- Morphoeic BCC: looks like a white scar that slowly enlarges and can be infiltrative or spread perineurally.

- Pigmented BCC: brown/black pearly nodule that can be difficult to distinguish from a malignant melanoma.

Diagnosis can be made clinically by dermoscopic examination or biopsy if the lesion is large.

A BCC is easily removed in the early stages by curettage. It is preferable to remove BCCs when they are small to preserve nearby organs such as the eyes, ears, and nose. If the BCC is close to the eye, it is better to surgically excise the lesion to determine the margin of the tumour. Larger lesions may require radiotherapy. If they are ignored, they can cause significant local destruction, hence the common name 'rodent ulcer'.

Bowen's disease: intra-epidermal epithelioma

These lesions appear as single, scaly, erythematous plaques, usually in sun-exposed areas. They are squamous-cell carcinomas (SCCs) that have not invaded beyond the epidermis. They are treated with cryotherapy, surgical excision, or radiotherapy.

Actinic keratosis

Lesions commonly occurring on the face or balding scalp secondary to sun damage: red, scaly macules due to accumulation of abnormal keratinocytes.

- Only 3% progress to squamous cell carcinomas, but can be difficult to distinguish from an SCC, so a shave or punch biopsy is needed.
- Uncommon in people with olive or dark skin.
- Multiple lesions are a red flag for significant sun exposure.

Cutaneous squamous-cell carcinoma

Cutaneous squamous-cell carcinoma (cSCC) is less common than BCC. It presents as a reddened, indurated ulcer, nodule, or plaque. cSCC often arises in already sun-damaged skin, e.g. in a solar keratosis or a patch of Bowen's disease, but also in other situations where the skin has been damaged, such as chronic venous ulcers of the lower leg or a longstanding cutaneous horn. The patient may report pain, bleeding, or rapid growth. It may metastasise to lymph nodes. Once the diagnosis is confirmed by biopsy, it should be excised or treated with radiotherapy.

Mohs' micrographic surgery

This is used for aggressive BCCs and cSCCs. The tumour and a 1–2 mm layer of normal tissue is excised. This sample is frozen and reviewed under a microscope. If there is tumour present, a further excision is made, and the procedure is repeated until the skin margins are cancer-free. This balances minimal skin loss with the greatest chance of complete resection, but is a lengthy procedure.

Malignant melanoma

In the UK, 25% of new cases of malignant melanoma are diagnosed in people over 75.

- These are expanding pigmented lesions, again usually, but not always, arising in sun-exposed skin.
- Lesions require early, wide excision because of the high risk of metastases. Refer under a 2-week wait to dermatology.
- Survival depends on the stage, and rates have improved overall but are worse in the over-80s. There may be a role for immune checkpoint inhibitors, but currently too few over 75 year olds have been included in clinical trials to demonstrate efficacy and side effects in older people.

- Support for veterans developing skin cancers after sun exposure whilst working in the Armed Forces may be available at: https://www.gov.uk/guidance/armed-forces-compensation-scheme-afcs

Hair and nails

Age-related changes

1 Hair: the ageing of hair follicles reduces the amount of melanin produced so that the hair loses its colour. Scalp hair loses colour earlier than body hair. A single hair has a lifespan of 2–7 years. With age, hair becomes thinner and more brittle. Male pattern baldness is obviously more common, but baldness may also occur in women at an advanced age. Body hair is lost in the same order as its acquisition. Facial hair increases in women.
2 Nails tend to grow more slowly, may turn yellow, and become thicker and more brittle.

Pathological changes

- Retention of hair colour was said to indicate hypothyroidism, but this is anecdotal. However, dry, brittle hair is a sign of hypothyroidism.
- Exaggerated hair loss may indicate hypopituitarism, Addison's disease, or be a consequence of cytotoxic therapy.
- Toenails may be neglected because of difficulty cutting them due to visual impairment, arthritis, or stroke disease and fungal infection is common. Without podiatry, which became very difficult to access during the COVID-19 pandemic, a ram's horn nail – onychogryphosis – may develop.
- Brittle and deformed nails may indicate systemic disease, e.g. deficiencies such as calcium or iron.
- Clubbing, pitting, and white bands may suggest systemic disease.
- Discomfort due to toenail deformity and neglect can seriously impair mobility.
- Extra care is needed with nail maintenance in patients with peripheral vascular disease and neuropathy, especially diabetics.

📖 REFERENCES AND FURTHER READING

Linos E, Chren M, Covinsky K (2018) Geriatric dermatology – a framework for caring for older patients with skin disease. *JAMA Dermatol.* 154:757–758. doi: 10.1001/jamadermatol.2018.0286

Labropoulos N (2019) How does chronic venous disease progress from the first symptoms to the advanced stages? A review. *Adv. Ther.* 36(Suppl 1):13–19. doi: 10.1007/s12325-019-0885-3.

NICE CKS (2023) *Leg ulcer – venous* https://cks.nice.org.uk/topics/leg-ulcer-venous

Guest J, Fuller G, Vowden P (2020) Cohort study evaluating the burden of wounds to the UK's National Health Service in 2017/2018: update from 2012/2013. *BMJ Open* 10:e045253. doi: 10.1136/bmjopen-2020-045253.

Parfitt G, Fletcher J, Stephenson, et al (2021) National audit of pressure ulcer prevalence in England: a cross sectional study. *Wounds UK* 17:45–55. https:wounds-uk.com/journal-articles/national-audit-pressure-ulcer-prevalence-england-cross-sectional-study/.

NICE Clinical Guideline [CG179] (2014, updated 2019) *Pressure ulcers: prevention and management* www.nice.org.uk/guidance/cg179/chapter/1-Recommendations#prevention-adults

NHS Improvement (2018) *Pressure Ulcers: revised definition and measurement* https://www.england.nhs.uk/wp-content/uploads/2021/09/NSTPP-summary-recommendations.pdf.

Young C (2021) Using the 'aSSKINg' model in pressure ulcer prevention and care planning. *Nursing Standard* 36:61–66. doi: 10.7748/ns.2021.e11674.

Patel M, Lee SI, Levell NJ, et al. (2020) An interview study to determine the experiences of cellulitis diagnosis amongst health care professionals in the UK. *BMJ Open* 10:e034692. doi: 10.1136/bmjopen-2019-034692.

NICE CKS (2023) *Burns and scalds* https://cks.nice.org.uk/topics/burns-scalds

Garcovich S, Colloca G, Sollena P, et al. (2017) Skin cancer epidemics in the elderly as an emerging issue in geriatric oncology. *Aging and Disease* 8:643–661. doi: 10.14336/AD.2017.0503.

INFORMATION FOR PATIENTS

Diabetes UK *How to look after your feet*: www.diabetes.org.uk/guide-to-diabetes/complications/feet/taking-care-of-your-feet

British Association of Dermatology patient leaflet on *Mohs micrographic surgery*: www.bad.org.uk/pils/mohs-micrographic-surgery

All websites were accessed in September 2024.

20

Eyes and ENT

The Eyes

Age-related changes

1 The eyes appear sunken due to the loss of periorbital fat.
2 Eyelid changes are mainly due to reduced connective tissue elasticity and weak eye muscles, and can be corrected surgically if they are severe.
   - Ectropion (out-turned eyelid) is common and contributes to epiphora (watery eye) as the laxity of the eyelid displaces the lacrimal punctum, so tears drain less effectively. This can co-exist with dry eyes.
   - Entropion (in-turned eyelid) is less common but important as the lashes can irritate the cornea.
   - Mild ptosis (drooping of the upper eyelid) with some hooding is often seen, but check pupils and eye movements to exclude pathology (unilateral – Horner's and 3rd nerve palsy, bilateral – myasthenia or myopathy).
3 The conjunctiva thins and yellows (cosmetic), but conjunctival vessels are more fragile, leading to a greater risk of conjunctival haemorrhages.
4 Reduced tear production leads to dry eyes. All three components of the tear film are affected: the reduced number of Meibomian glands reduces the lipid layer; fewer lacrimal glands lead to a reduction in the aqueous layer; and the reduced function of conjunctival goblet cells reduces the mucin layer. Hence, many older people need hydrating eye drops.
5 The cornea becomes less sensitive, so foreign bodies or ulceration may be overlooked.
6 Arcus senilis, the pale ring at the edge of the cornea caused by the deposition of calcium and cholesterol esters, is common but not clinically significant, in contrast with arcus juvenilis in young adults, which suggests hypercholesterolaemia.
7 Yellowing of the sclera occurs due to dehydration and deposition of lipids.
8 Muscles in the iris atrophy, so the pupil becomes smaller (miosis); less light reaches the retina, reducing vision in low light, especially at night (nyctalopia).
9 The lens yellows and becomes less elastic, reducing blue/green discrimination and causing presbyopia – Greek for 'old eyes', the gradual loss of ability to focus on near objects that is almost universal from around 40 years. Some degree of clouding of the lens – cataract formation – is almost inevitable with advanced old age.
10 The vitreous network of collagen and hyaluronic acid degenerates, causing the appearance of floaters. Shrinkage and liquefaction may pull the vitreous away from the retina, increasing the risk of retinal detachment. Patients reporting the sudden onset of 'a curtain coming down' or sudden increase in floaters need urgent ophthalmological review.
11 The retina thins, and dark adaptation is further slowed by the reduced regeneration rate of rhodopsin by the rods.
12 Transmission in the optic nerve and tracts slows, so visual-evoked responses are longer, but this is not clinically significant.
13 Older people have more difficulty picking out figures from complex backgrounds (central processing).

Examination of the retina

Pupils are small in older people, so it is usually necessary to dilate them to examine the fundi. Tropicamide 0.5% drops are usually used. This is a short-acting parasympathetic antagonist. Reversal with pilocarpine is rarely needed and can be painful. The risk of acute-closed-angle glaucoma is minimal but beware of the small eyeball with a shallow anterior chamber. If in doubt, dilate only one pupil with phenylephrine 10%, reverse with thymoxamine 0.5%, and leave the other eye for a subsequent occasion.

Loss of vision

Prevalence

In the UK, two million people have visual impairment, and the prevalence rises markedly with age. About 20% of over 75-year-olds are affected, rising to 50% of over 90-year-olds. There are many causes (see Figure 20.1) but in older adults, most new cases are due to macular degeneration, glaucoma, diabetes, cataracts and lack of correct prescription spectacles. Some ethnic groups have an increased prevalence of eye disease: people with Black African and Caribbean heritage are more at risk of glaucoma, and South Asian people are more at risk of diabetic eye disease.

Globally, at least 2.2 billion people have vision impairment that would have been preventable, or treatable in at least one billion. In sub-Saharan Africa, it is estimated that over 85% of people with presbyopia do not have any appropriate glasses. The main causes of blindness in older people globally are the same as in high-income countries but a wider range of issues are seen, such as severe pterygium and corneal opacification from various causes, including injury, and sequalae from childhood, such as vitamin A deficiency and infections like trachoma and measles.

Geriatric Medicine and Elderly Care: Lecture Notes, Ninth Edition. Claire G. Nicholl, K. Jane Wilson, and Shaun D'Souza.
© 2025 John Wiley & Sons Ltd. Published 2025 by John Wiley & Sons Ltd.
Companion website: www.wiley.com/go/lecturenotesgeriatricmedicine9e

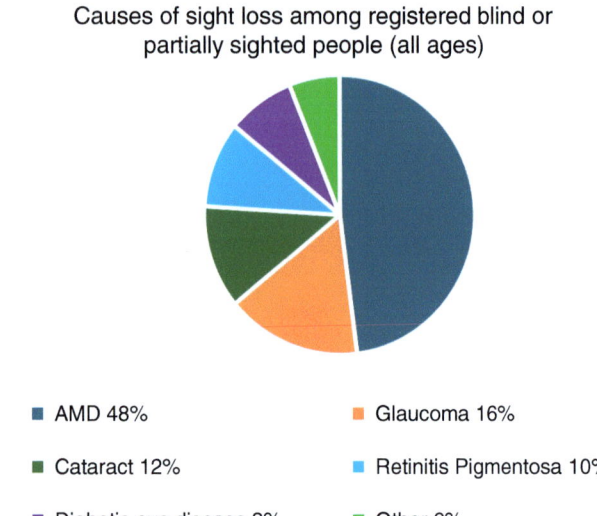

Causes of sight loss among registered blind or partially sighted people (all ages)

- ■ AMD 48%
- ■ Glaucoma 16%
- ■ Cataract 12%
- ■ Retinitis Pigmentosa 10%
- ■ Diabetic eye disease 8%
- ■ Other 6%

Figure 20.1 Main causes of blindness in people in the UK (by percentage). RNIB. AMD, age-related macular degeneration.

Consequences

Poor vision has many consequences for physical and mental health, and social functioning. It has been linked to loneliness, social isolation, anxiety, fear, depression, and thoughts of suicide. People with visual impairment sometimes have visual hallucinations (Charles Bonnet syndrome), which vary from flashes and lines to complex images. These have no significance, but sufferers may fear they are developing dementia and need reassurance.

Visual loss is a risk factor for reduced mobility and falls (see Chapter 11). It has a marked effect on quality of life causing many practical difficulties and independence is reduced:

- Cooking: buying and preparing food, using appliances, pouring liquids.
- Mobility: loss of driving, going out alone, crossing roads, using public transport.
- Communication: phone, writing, using a computer, recognising friends.
- Reading and hobbies: letters, TV listings, sewing, and crafting.
- Medication: taking tablets, self-injecting, measuring blood sugar.
- Roles: are lost, e.g. the ability to care for grandchildren.

Visual loss often interacts adversely with other common pathologies in older age, e.g. hearing loss, dementia, and osteoporosis. People with visual impairment are at increased risk of developing delirium if admitted to hospital. They may miss visual cues or misinterpret what they see, e.g. a jacket draped over a chair looks like a headless person and is terrifying. The risk of delirium is even higher if the person is also deaf.

Unsurprisingly, visual impairment is associated with an increase in all-cause mortality.

Overview of causes of visual impairment

Have a logical approach, and then learn what is common.

- Consider problems in the eye (working back from cornea to retina), its blood supply, and central connections.
- Also, consider whether it is an eye disease or a systemic disorder with eye involvement.

Causes of visual impairment

A practical clinical classification is to consider the speed of onset and whether the eye looks normal or is swollen and inflamed.

Gradual loss

- Age-related macular degeneration: central vision is lost but peripheral vision is maintained.
- Cataracts.
- Glaucoma: central vision is maintained until late in the disease.
- Retinopathy (diabetes mellitus).
- Uncorrected refractive problems.
- Iatrogenic disease.

Sudden loss in a quiet (normal looking) eye

- Central retinal artery occlusion – secondary to embolus from carotids or heart valve.
- Central retinal vein occlusion – more common in hypertension or hyperviscosity syndromes.
- Retinal detachment – sudden increase in floaters, flashes, and a dark 'curtain' over the vision.
- Vitreous haemorrhage – more common in diabetics.
- Ischaemic optic atrophy – secondary to giant-cell arteritis or atherosclerosis.
- Stroke (effects depend on the site of damage – see Chapter 9).

Sudden loss in a red, painful eye

- Acute-angle-closure glaucoma
  Note: if one eye is affected, the other is at risk.

General management of visual loss

This depends on the condition and is specialist-led, but general management is (of course) multidisciplinary.

1 Be suspicious and look for this.
   Patients may not notice gradual impairment, particularly if the problem is loss of visual fields, and patients with dementia may not report problems with acuity. The author will always remember the aptly named Mrs Dark, who had moderate dementia and was being 'encouraged' to move into care because of frequent falls. A brief examination showed dense bilateral cataracts, and surgery enabled her to stay at home with her husband.
2 Refer
   People aged 60+ (any age with diabetes or over 40 with a family history of glaucoma) can self-refer to a high-street optometrist for a free eye examination, but may be unaware of this as younger people have to pay. There may be a home-visiting service. Acute problems should be referred directly to ophthalmology.
   - Diagnosis: may be treatable.
   - Access to low-vision services: assessment and loan of magnifiers, telescopic aids, etc.
   - Registration as visually impaired: if desired.
3 Education: information about conditions, aids, and appliances – see Figure 20.2.
4 Therapy services: OT and PT may improve independence.
5 Social services: signposting for advice about benefits and care assessment.
   A caution about rehousing – an older person with sight loss may remain safer and more independent in familiar surroundings than in a 'more suitable' new flat.
6 Check whether your patient drives.

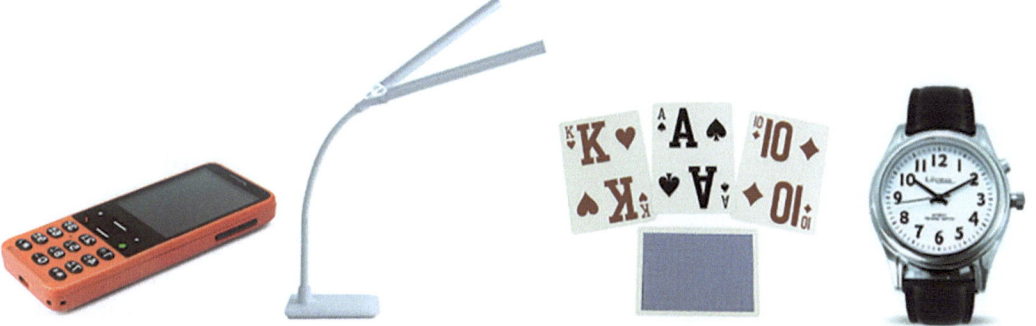

Figure 20.2 Widely available aids for people with impaired vision.

Simple measures to assist patients with visual impairment

1 Check visual acuity – provision or change of lenses may help. Lenses should have a reflective coating to reduce glare.
2 Keep patients and spectacles together, especially in hospitals.
3 Keep the spectacles clean.
4 Insist on task-appropriate lighting – good light is the best visual aid. Shield the bulb from the eye line. Most people will benefit from a bright light to read, but others must avoid glare. Avoid a bright sitting room and dim hallways or toilets.
5 Be aware of the benefits of increased contrast, e.g. edges of stairs, doorframes, and toilet doors in the hospital ward, as well as recommending this at home.
6 Make sure that ward and hospital information is in a suitable, large font, and well set out.
7 Encourage the patient to be registered as visually impaired.
8 Be aware of the range of low-visual aids that enable people to remain independent at home and know how to refer to the local service. Examples include phones with large buttons, talking clocks, magnifying glasses for reading; an integrated marker helps patients with AMD keep their place when reading (see Figure 20.2).
9 Check whether appropriate people have applied for Attendance Allowance.
10 Promote contact with a support charity, e.g. the Royal National Institute for Blind People, the Macular Society, or Glaucoma UK.
11 Maintain maximum hearing ability.
12 Encourage subscriptions to talking newspapers, talking-book libraries, audiobooks online, etc.
13 Look for and offer treatment for depression.

Legal aspects in the UK

Vision required for driving a car

The rules for driving are complex – see the DVLA website.

Vision (with glasses if needed) must be at least Snellen 6/12 (i.e. able to read a normal registration plate from 20 m), and visual fields must be within acceptable limits.

Criteria for being registered as sight impaired

If registration is desired, optometrists must refer to an ophthalmologist who will assess the visual acuity and visual fields and provide certification if the criteria are met:

Severely sight impaired/blind:
Acuity of less than 3/60 with a full field.
Acuity between 3/60 and 6/60 with a severe reduction of fields, such as tunnel vision.
Acuity of 6/60 or above but with a very reduced field of vision, especially if a lot of sight is missing in the lower part of the field.

Sight impaired/partially sighted:
Acuity of 3/60 to 6/60 with a full field.
Acuity of up to 6/24 with a moderate reduction of fields or central blurriness.
Visual acuity of up to 6/18 if a large part of the field or extensive peripheral vision is missing.

Not all people with visual impairment are registered, but this should be encouraged.

The advantages of registration include:

- Half-price TV licence.
- Help with the council tax bill.
- Leisure discounts.
- Travel concessions.
- Blue badge parking permit for the person's driver.
- Blind person's allowance – an extra tax-free allowance of £3,070 (2024–2025), regardless of age or income.
- Strengthens the case for eligibility for Attendance Allowance (e.g. if help is needed to choose clothes. read and reply to mail, walk around safely, and take part in social activities).

Common causes of visual loss

Age-related macular degeneration

Age-related macular degeneration (AMD) affects people aged 50 and over and becomes more common with advancing age. It is the most common cause of visual impairment in the developed world. It affects 600,000 people in the UK currently and is predicted to double by 2050 as the population ages.

- Usually bilateral, but may affect one eye earlier or more than the other.
- As the macula is damaged, central vision is affected most, with peripheral vision being preserved. Loss of central vision means loss of face recognition and difficulty reading, but peripheral vision enables the person to walk around independently.

Risk factors for AMD

- Older age.
- Female preponderance.
- Positive family history.
- Smoking (inhibits complement factor H).
- Hypertension.

- Having white ancestry, especially with light-coloured eyes.
- High-fat diet.
- Obesity.
- Diet low in omega 3 and 6, vitamins, carotenoids, and minerals.

AMD can be divided into two broad types: dry and wet (see Table 20.1). Any stage of dry AMD can develop into wet AMD.

Dry macular degeneration

- Dry (non-exudative) AMD tends to develop slowly over months or years but is not always progressive.
- Drusen (German for pebbles) are yellow extracellular deposits of lipid and protein that develop below the retinal pigment epithelium (RPE), which sits on Bruch's membrane. A few small drusen are not significant, but a large number of larger drusen is an early sign of dry AMD.
- The pathogenesis is not understood but includes activation of the complement cascade and inflammation, with changes in membrane permeability limiting nutrient delivery to and waste removal from the retina. It is not known why some eyes progress to advanced dry AMD, whereas in others wet AMD develops.
- Areas of degeneration of the RPE cells and the overlying retinal photoreceptors (which depend on the RPE for trophic support) develop and coalesce to form patchy areas called geographic atrophy. Drusen and geographic atrophy are visible on fundoscopy.
- There is no treatment for AMD, but patients should be encouraged to stop smoking, and there is some evidence suggesting that antioxidant supplements may be protective.
- People with dry AMD should be asked to monitor their vision (e.g. by sticking a paper with grid lines on the fridge), as if there is sudden loss of acuity or straight lines appear to become wavy, they may be developing the wet form, which needs urgent assessment for treatment.
- Advanced degeneration can result in a complete central defect (scotoma).

Wet macular degeneration

- Wet (exudative) AMD is more rapidly progressive and causes more visual impairment.
- Starts as dry AMD; 10–15% of patients progress to the wet type.
- Wet AMD is characterised by choroidal neovascularisation. Low levels of oxygen are detected and stimulate the release of vascular endothelial growth factor (VEGF). This in turn stimulates the production of new vessels growing into the choroid, which are fragile and 'leaky'. Exudation of fluid, proteins, and lipids or bleeding and then scarring further damage the macula.
- Anti-VEGF treatments include ranibizumab (Lucentis), bevacizumab (Avastin – off-label use), and aflibercept (Eylea). These are administered by intravitreal injection, given monthly for 3 months, and then at varying intervals, depending on response. Treatment and follow-up may need to be continued for up to and beyond 2 years to preserve vision. Newer drugs may enable a longer interval between injections.
- For treatment to be given, the patient must fulfil the NICE criteria:
  - Best corrected vision: between 6/12 and 6/96.
  - No permanent structural damage to the central fovea.
  - Lesion less than 12-disc areas in greatest linear dimension.
  - Evidence of disease progression, i.e. vessel growth or loss of visual acuity.
  - Reasonable response to treatment.
- Side effects of treatment include conjunctival haemorrhage, eye pain, vitreous floaters, vitreous haemorrhage, retinal detachment, and increased intraocular pressure.
- In trials, anti-VEGF therapies prevented deterioration in vision in most patients, and in 40% of cases, vision improved. In clinical practice, the common treatments appear similar and overall stabilise vision for 2 years, followed by some deterioration.
- Photodynamic therapy: intravenous verteporfin, a light-sensitive drug, followed by a cold laser to seal new vessels, is second-line treatment.
- The understanding of the genetics of AMD continues to advance. Genome wide association studies (GWAS) have identified over 30 genes with variants associated with an increased risk of AMD. A number of these are involved in the complement system, including complement factor H (*CFH*), which limits activation of the alternative pathway; complement component 3 (*C3*); and serpin peptidase inhibitor (*SERPING1*), a C1 inhibitor. This supports the role of complement activation and inflammation in the pathogenesis.

Cataracts

Cataracts have been recognised since antiquity and are so called because vision is blurred as if seen from behind a waterfall. Surgical treatment dates back to India around 600 BCE, when a needle was used to push the opaque lens aside! Cataracts are very common; in the UK, 30% of people aged 65 or older have a cataract affecting the vision in one or both eyes, easily detected and corrected, resulting in a marked enhancement of quality of life. However, worldwide, 12 million people are blind due to cataracts.

- Early symptoms include increased glare from sunshine or headlights when driving in the dark and difficulty reading small print despite reading glasses.
- There is a gradual, painless loss of visual clarity and sharpness, then acuity.
- People may report halos around lights, monocular double vision, or polyopia (multiple images), and reduced colour vision, especially of blue.

Types

1 Central: early visual loss.
2 Peripheral: late visual loss but vision impaired by the scattering of bright light.

Pathogenesis is multifactorial.

Table 20.1 Differences between dry and wet AMD.

	Dry AMD	Wet AMD
Frequency	85–90% of all AMD	10–15%
Symptoms	Asymptomatic until late stage.	Sudden loss of central vision over days to weeks.
	May notice a loss of central acuity.	
	Peripheral vision preserved.	Metamorphopsia (shape distortion)
	Sudden deterioration of vision suggests progression to wet AMD.	
Appearance	Focal hypo- or hyperpigmentation, numerous large, confluent, or soft drusen, geographic atrophy	Abnormal blood vessels seen under the retina may leak and scar
Progression	May be static for long periods.	Evolves from dry AMD
		May deteriorate rapidly, and loss of acuity is severe
Management	Stop smoking	Rapid assessment
	Diet	Intravitreal anti-VEGF drugs
	Antioxidant supplements?	Photodynamic therapy
	Support	Support

Risk factors for cataracts

- Ageing.
- Ethnicity: higher in people of Asian background.
- Female gender.
- Family history.
- Diabetes mellitus.
- Hypertension.
- Past eye injury.
- Iatrogenic, e.g. steroids.
- Smoking.
- Poor nutrition.
- Environmental – excessive sunshine (ultraviolet light) – the reason for increased incidence in the tropics.

Examination

- Look for loss of the red reflex in dense cataracts (see Figure 20.3).
- Check visual acuity.
- Fundoscopy (you are unlikely to get a clear view, but attempt this before referring).

Surgery

Treatment is the removal of the cloudy lens. According to NICE guidelines, timing should depend on the needs of the individual, but many areas have acuity criteria for referral to ophthalmology. Contraindications are:

- Early stages.
- Where vision is compromised by other ocular co-morbidities such as severe macular degeneration or retinopathy.
- Severe dementia.

This is usually a day-case procedure under local anaesthesia. The patient needs to be able to lie flat for 20 min and keep still. The procedure is around 15 min from end to end. The pupil is maximally dilated and anaesthetised, and iodine drops are used to prevent infection. The eye is clamped open. The patient sees a bright light, not the approaching scalpel! A small incision is made in the anterior chamber of the eye. A phaco probe is inserted. Phacoemulsification is the process of fragmenting the opacified lens with ultrasound. This debris is washed out, leaving the lens capsule intact. An artificial lens is inserted into the capsule.

The power of the new lens is selected to optimise vision. The patient usually opts for normal distance vision and after surgery will need glasses for close work.

Post-operative care

After surgery, drops are used to reduce the risk of infection and inflammation. A combination preparation is convenient, e.g. Tobradex, (tobramycin and dexamethasone), four times a day for 2 weeks and then twice a day for 2 weeks. If the patient will not manage this, a plan is needed. If the patient struggles to self-administer drops, there are a variety of dispensers (see Figure 20.4).

Complications of treatment

1. Dilatation of the pupil may precipitate glaucoma.
2. Lens implant: possible failure and risk of infection. The risk of endophthalmitis is reduced by using povidone–iodine drops just prior to the incision and antibiotic eye drops post-op.
3. Posterior capsular opacification: may occur several months after the cataract extraction and is treated by yttrium aluminium garnet (YAG) laser capsulotomy.

Glaucoma

Glaucoma is a group of eye diseases that cause progressive optic neuropathy, in which intraocular pressure (IOP) is a key modifiable factor. Glaucoma is usually associated with a raised IOP and is characterised by:

- Visual field defects.
- Changes to the optic nerve head such as pathological cupping (the cup takes up more of the disc) or, as a late sign, pallor of the optic disc - optic atrophy due to loss of retinal ganglion cell axons,

Visual loss due to glaucoma is irreversible, so detection and prevention of deterioration are the key priorities. Glaucoma is the cause of the visual loss in 16% of those registered blind or partially sighted in the UK. After the COVID-19 pandemic, there was a significant backlog in diagnosis and therefore treatment.

Classification

In adults, there are two main types, classified according to the angle between the iris and the cornea.

1. Primary open-angle glaucoma (POAG): a chronic painless disorder that gradually impairs vision.
2. Primary angle-closure glaucoma (PACG): this is also most commonly chronic and painless, as the angle opens and closes, but the presentation may be acute, a painful, sight-threatening medical emergency, or sub-acute.

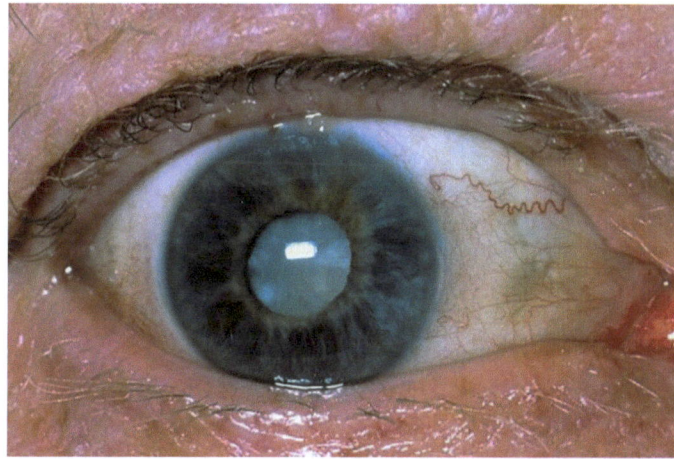

Figure 20.3 Cataract in right eye with loss of red reflex: National Health Service/https://www.nhs.uk/conditions/cataracts/Public domain.

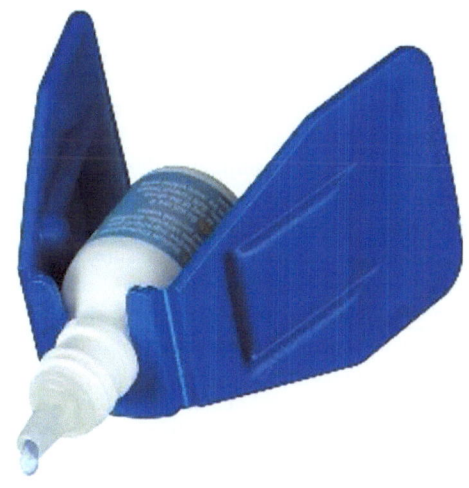

Figure 20.4 One type of aid for using eye drops – The AutoSqueeze™.

Table 20.2 Differences between acute and chronic glaucoma.

	Acute – angle-closure	Chronic – open-angle or less commonly, angle-closure
Symptoms	Sudden pain in the eye, blurred vision, reduced acuity, vomiting, and prostration	Insidious peripheral field loss leads to tunnel vision; family history is common (relatives get free eye tests)
Signs	Eye tense and red, irregular fixed pupil, cornea and conjunctiva congested	Raised pressure on tonometry; scotomas on field testing; cupped disc
Pathology	Sudden impairment of anterior chamber drainage – may be precipitated by dim light, anticholinergics and mydriatics	Gradual increase in intraocular pressure – idiopathic deterioration in the trabecular mesh or due to the narrow angle
Treatment	A medical emergency. Constrict the pupil, lower intraocular pressure with acetazolamide and drops, and use topical steroids to reduce inflammation. Antiemetics and analgesia. A definitive procedure, e.g. laser iridotomy to both eyes.	Laser trabeculoplasty (for POAG) in the affected eye Laser iridotomy (for PACG) in both eyes Eye drops as needed.

POAG, primary open angle glaucoma; PACG, primary angle closure glaucoma.

The difference between acute and chronic glaucoma is summarised in Table 20.2.

There are also secondary causes of both open-angle and angle-closure glaucoma after conditions such as uveitis, vitreous haemorrhage and eye trauma or surgery.

Pathogenesis

Intraocular pressure (IOP) is maintained by the balance of production and drainage of aqueous humour.

- Aqueous produced by the ciliary body flows out through the pupil into the anterior chamber and is absorbed through the trabecular mesh into Schlemm's canal and into the venous system or the minor uveosclero outflow pathway.
- Pressures between 11 and 21 mmHg are considered normal. Pressures above this are called ocular hypertension.
- Depending on factors in an individual, at an IOP greater than 21 mmHg, nerve damage starts to develop, and the person is said to have glaucoma.
- Occasionally, damage occurs at 'normal' pressures, presumably because the optic head is susceptible.
- In open-angle glaucoma, the absorption of the aqueous is impaired.
- In angle-closure glaucoma, the flow of aqueous is intermittently or completely obstructed. One eye may be more affected than its pair.
- High IOP damages the optic nerve head with subsequent loss of retinal ganglion cells, causing variable peripheral visual field loss, most commonly arcuate defects in the nasal fields.
- The defects are often asymmetrical, so the patient does not appreciate the loss when using both eyes.
- Another reason for the late presentation is that the macula is spared until there is very advanced field loss with tunnel vision.
- If the macula is affected, complete blindness results, in contrast with AMD, where some navigational vision remains.
- AMD and glaucoma may coexist, with a poor prognosis for vision.

Primary openangle glaucoma

POAG is silent and progressive. It is usually detected by opticians during routine eye tests; referral to ophthalmology is advised when the IOP is 24 mmHg or more, with some evidence of retinal damage. The aetiology is unclear but may include age-related changes to the trabecular mesh and Schlemm's canal.

- Risk factors include increasing age, family history, being of African or Caribbean descent, and myopia; possibly T2DM and HT, but these patients get more eye tests.
- Treatment (both for POAG and ocular hypertension thought likely to progress to POAG) is aimed at reducing IOP; best practice is to offer 360° selective laser trabeculoplasty (SLT).
  - A low-energy laser is used to improve the drainage of aqueous fluid through the trabecular mesh.
  - SLT is cost-effective, reduces the need for multiple eye drops for life, and can be repeated.
  - The procedure may cause some discomfort, transient blurred vision, and hyperaemia.
- If SLT is unsuitable or additional treatment is needed, eye drops are used.
  - Topical prostaglandin analogues, e.g. latanoprost/travoprost, increase aqueous outflow at the uveoscleral junction.
  - Beta blockers, e.g. betaxolol drops, reduce the production of aqueous by the ciliary body.
  - Alpha agonists, e.g. brimonidine drops, reduce the production of aqueous.
  - Carbonic anhydrase inhibitors, e.g. brinzolamide drops, reduce the production of aqueous but are less effective, so they are used as adjuncts.
  - The patient must be shown how to use eye drops correctly and educated to continue medication.
  - If drops cause an allergy, preservative-free preparations are available.
- If there is no improvement, surgical trabeculectomy is used to improve aqueous flow.

Primary angle closure glaucoma

PACG is much less common than POAG, but it accounts for half of global glaucoma-related blindness. The presentation may be acute, subacute (intermittent) or chronic.

- The aetiology is due to the anatomy of the eye, with a shallow anterior chamber. When the iris dilates, aqueous cannot pass between the lens and the iris and out through the pupil into the anterior chamber (pupillary block). This can be intermittent. If the block persists, pressure from the continued secretion of aqueous fluid pushes the peripheral iris forward and closes the angle, resulting in a rapid (hours) and severe (>40 mmHg) rise in IOP.
- Risk factors include increasing age (the lens gets fatter) so PACG is most common in the sixth and seventh decades, female sex as the anterior chamber is more shallow, family history, being of Asian or Chinese descent, and long-sight.
- Acute angle-closure causes blurred or reduced vision in a very painful red eye, often with headache, nausea, and vomiting.
  - The patient may also describe halos around lights secondary to corneal oedema.
  - There may be a precipitating event causing pupillary dilatation, such as exposure to dim light or anticholinergic medication.
  - The eye is tender with a mid-dilated, irregular, and non-reactive pupil.
  - Visual acuity is reduced.
  - The intraocular pressure will be very high.
  - Slit lamp examination may show corneal oedema.
  - Arrange emergency admission and start oral acetazolamide to reduce aqueous production, plus topical treatment - pilocarpine

(which constricts the pupil and helps open the drainage angle), beta blockers, and steroids (to reduce inflammation). Analgesia and an antiemetic will reduce distress.

  - ○ IV acetazolamide may be used, and drops may be continued while arranging definitive management.
  - ○ Interventions include laser iridotomy (in the outpatient department), phacoemulsification for coexisting cataracts, iridoplasty or iridectomy.
  - ○ A procedure is usually performed on both eyes to prevent an attack on the unaffected eye.
- Subacute presentation is similar but less severe, and symptoms often resolve spontaneously on lying down (the pupil block resolves), so it may not be recognised.
- Chronic PACG presents like chronic POAG. The pupil block is intermittent. Synechiae (adhesions) may form between the iris and the trabecular meshwork, further limiting aqueous outflow.
- There is a significant risk of acute closure as well as the progression of visual loss in both subacute and chronic PACG, so a bilateral procedure is done to relieve pupil block, and drops are used as for POAG (with the addition of pilocarpine).

Giant-cell arteritis

See also Chapter 10.

Giant cell arteritis (GCA) is a chronic systemic vasculitis that can threaten vision. It is characterised by granulomatous inflammation of the walls of large and medium-sized arteries.

- Rare before 50; the highest incidence is in women aged 70–79.
- Risk factors include Northern European extraction and smoking.

It most commonly affects the extracranial branches of the carotid artery.

It can also affect the ophthalmic artery, the first branch of the internal carotid artery, branches of which include the posterior ciliary arteries, which supply the choroid and optic nerve, and the central retinal artery. Symptoms may include:

- A new headache usually localised to the temporal region, which may be tender; scalp tenderness when combing the hair; jaw ache secondary to ischaemia of the masseter muscles; or occipital headache secondary to occipital artery claudication.
- Systemic illness with low-grade fever, fatigue, anorexia, and weight loss.
- Overlap with symptoms of polymyalgia rheumatica (PMR): proximal muscle pain and early morning stiffness in 40–50%. (GCA should be actively excluded in people presenting with features of PMR).
- Visual disturbances include loss of vision, change in colour vision, photopsia – the perception of flickering lights or flashes, and diplopia. Visual loss may occur in up to 30% and may be transient (a cause of amaurosis fugax) or permanent. The most feared sequel of GCA is permanent visual loss secondary to arteritic anterior ischaemic optic neuropathy (AAION) due to occlusion of the posterior ciliary arteries. Permanent loss often follows a transient episode, and if loss occurs in one eye the other eye is at risk. Involvement of the central retinal artery may result in a central retinal artery occlusion. Diplopia results from ischaemia to the eye muscles.

Signs may include:

- Tender, thickened temporal arteries.
- Abnormalities on fundoscopy including a pale swollen disc with occasional splinter retinal haemorrhages and cotton wool spots.
- Signs of arteritis elsewhere.

The diagnosis is supported by:

- Raised ESR and CRP.
- Normocytic normochromic anaemia, thrombocythaemia, mildly raised alkaline phosphatase, and reduced albumin.
- Vascular ultrasonography: this may show the halo sign due to wall thickening.

Confirmation is by:

- Temporal artery biopsy. This should not delay treatment but should be done as soon as possible and within 2 weeks of starting treatment. The classical histological appearance is a panarteritis consisting of lymphocytes and macrophages with or without granuloma formation, intimal thickening, and fragmentation of the internal elastic lamina.

Management

With eye involvement, refer urgently to ophthalmology and rheumatology.

Treatment is high-dose oral steroids (80–100 mg prednisolone per day) or IV methylprednisolone without delay. 75 mg aspirin may reduce ischaemic events, and tocilizumab (anti IL-6) may be used. For details of monitoring, steroid weaning according to the clinical picture, ESR and CRP, and steroid sparing agents, see Chapter 10. The disease often lasts for up to 2 years. Don't forget gut and bone protection

Dry eyes

Dry eyes affect 5–30% of older people.

- More common in women and usually idiopathic, although it can be part of a connective disorder such as Sjogren's syndrome.
- Due to ageing changes as described earlier: reduced lacrimal glands, conjunctival glands, and eyelid changes.
- Symptoms include intermittent itching and a gritty feeling.
- Exacerbated by polypharmacy: anticholinergics, e.g. antihistamines, PD medications, antipsychotics, and tricyclic antidepressants, plus topical treatments for glaucoma.
- Benzalkonium is a preservative often added to eye drops and can itself cause irritation.
- Can lead to blurred vision, although it does not affect visual acuity.
- Treatment is with artificial tears. Hyaluronate drops are more effective than hypromellose.

Painful eyes

1 Angle closure glaucoma (acute) as above.
2 Infection:
  (a) Conjunctivitis: erythema of the conjunctiva with visible fine blood vessels. Often self-limiting, secondary to contact allergy or ocular manifestation of a viral infection such as a cold. Purulent discharge suggests bacterial infection, e.g. with *Staphylococcus aureus* or *Haemophilus*. Treat with chloramphenicol eye drops.
  (b) Blepharitis: red, itchy, inflamed eyelids, sometimes with crusting of the eyelashes in the mornings. The patient may complain of gritty eyes. May be due to irritation from cosmetics or infection, often viral. Prevent with good eyelid hygiene, e.g. washing with diluted baby shampoo. Golden crusting may suggest infection with *S. aureus*. If infected, treat with chloramphenicol ointment.

(c) Uveitis: inflammation of the uveal tract (iris, ciliary body, and choroid), the middle part of the eye. Can be due to infection, but also systemic inflammatory diseases and drugs. Best managed by ophthalmology.
(d) Herpes zoster ophthalmicus: suspect when there is a classical shingles rash on one side of the forehead, around the eyelids and conjunctiva. A lesion on the side of the nose (Hutchinson's sign) shows that the nasociliary branch of the trigeminal nerve is affected, flagging an increased risk of eye involvement. The patient may develop conjunctivitis, episcleritis, keratitis, or iritis and needs an urgent ophthalmology review and consideration of IV aciclovir.

3 Trauma, e.g. corneal abrasion or a foreign body.

Ear, Nose, and Throat

Ears

Age-related changes

1 Wax becomes more viscous and needs removal in one-quarter of older people.
2 Age-related hearing loss (presbycusis) is insidious, symmetrical, and progressive. It tends to affect higher pitched sounds the most. Consonants, e.g. s, f, h, and th, and word endings are missed, impairing word discrimination in speech. High-frequency sounds are lost because the outer hair cells of the organ of Corti (located in the basal cochlear) are more vulnerable to free radical damage.
3 The brain is slower at processing auditory information.
4 'Recruitment' may lead to people with hearing impairments saying, 'no need to shout'. Soft sounds, e.g. <50 dB, may be inaudible, but slightly louder sounds, e.g. >80 dB, are uncomfortable or distorted. This occurs as more neurones are switched on or 'recruited' to try to compensate for the loss of hair cells.
5 Around 70% of people over 70 have hearing loss and should be considered for a hearing aid.
6 Impaired hearing leads to impaired health.
7 The WHO predicts that by 2030, age-related hearing loss will be in the top 10 health burdens (more common than cataracts and diabetes) in the UK and other economically developed countries.
8 Progressive loss of hair cells in the semi-circular canals impairs balance.
9 Degeneration of otoliths in the saccule makes benign paroxysmal positional vertigo (BPPV) more common.
10 A reduction in the number of vestibular nerve cells contributes to an increased risk of dizziness with age.

Loss of hearing

Prevalence

Around 12 million people in the UK have hearing loss greater than 25 dB. The loss is severe or profound at around 900,000. The number of people affected will increase as there is a strong relationship with age.

- 40% of over-50s.
- 70% of people over 70.

Most older people have mild to moderate hearing loss (see Table 20.3).

Consequences

- Social isolation and withdrawal from friends and family, especially at large gatherings.

Table 20.3 Degree of hearing impairment in people aged over 70 years (range in dB with the quietest sound heard).

Loss	Population	Loss in dB	Impact
No significant loss	30%	0–24	
Mild	27%	25–39	Difficulty following conversations in a noisy room
Moderate	36%	40–69	Difficulty following a one-to-one speech
Severe	6%	70–94	May have to lip-read/sign even with hearing aids
Profound	1%	>94	Likely to rely on lip-reading/signing

- Depression and anxiety.
- Increased risk of accidents because of reduced awareness of auditory warnings.
- Associated tinnitus.
- Associated dizziness and unsteadiness increase the risk of falls.
- Increased risk of developing delirium when admitted to hospital due to increased disorientation, missing cues, hot drinks and meals, and misinterpreting the environment.
- Hearing loss is associated with dementia, and the benefits of hearing aids have been shown in the UK Biobank population. People with hearing loss without hearing aids had an increased risk of *developing* all-cause dementia (HR 1.42 [95% CI 1.29–1.56]); no increased risk was found in people with hearing loss with hearing aids (1.04 [0.98–1.10]). This is an important study, as people with dementia may not get or manage hearing aids, which is a confounding factor in studies showing that people with dementia and deafness do not wear aids.

Causes of hearing impairment

Sensorineural deafness

This is the inability to transduce sound information into usable neural signals. It is most commonly due to damage to the cochlear hair cells, but it also includes damage to the auditory nerve (peripheral sensorineural loss). Deafness due to damage in central auditory pathways from the cochlear (spiral) nuclei to the auditory cortex (the superior temporal gyrus) is central hearing loss. Most auditory information goes to the opposite cortex, but some is relayed ipsilaterally for binaural processing, and there are descending feedback circuits. Because of the bilateral connections, deafness is a very rare result of a brain stem or cortical stroke. However, central deafness may be a bigger component of the hearing difficulties in old age than previously realised.

- Presbycusis: age-related hearing impairment, usually bilateral. Risk factors: genetic predisposition, low socioeconomic status, noise exposure, smoking, hypertension, diabetes, and vascular disease.
- Noise-induced: occupational or environmental causes include construction work, heavy industries, shooting and loud music in rock/orchestral musicians and their audiences. Ear protectors are essential.
- Ototoxic drugs, e.g. gentamicin, high-dose furosemide and chemotherapy, especially platinum drugs.
- Nerve compression, e.g. vestibular schwannoma/acoustic neuroma (unilateral) and Paget's disease of the bone (usually bilateral). Schwannomas are benign and very slowly progressive tumours; the dilemma is choosing when to operate, as surgery always causes hearing loss.

- Meniere's disease (idiopathic endolymphatic hydrops), the classic triad of vertigo, tinnitus and hearing impairment, is rare but can be debilitating.
- Blunt head trauma without a temporal bone fracture may cause labyrinthine concussion with hearing loss and vertigo.
- Cerebrovascular disease: the main arterial supply, the labyrinthine artery (also known as the internal auditory artery), comes off the basilar artery, or sometimes the anterior inferior cerebellar artery, and divides into the anterior vestibular and common cochlear arteries. Complete occlusion of the labyrinthine artery leads to sudden deafness and vertigo, so ipsilateral deafness can occur in posterior circulation strokes. However, the vertigo tends to dominate the clinical picture.
- 'Graduates' with early onset deafness: familial, congenital, e.g. maternal rubella, childhood illness.

Conductive deafness

This is due to disorders of the external and middle ears, reducing the transmission of sound from the environment to the inner ear. Causes include:

- Impacted wax (cerumen).
- Otosclerosis (usually fixation of the stapes) is often familial and usually presents at 30–50 years of age.
- Post-infective, e.g. chronic suppurative otitis media.
- Ruptured ear drum secondary to a blow to the head.
- Cholesteatoma.
- Paget's disease of the bone, as discussed earlier.

Schwannomas and serious conductive forms of deafness in older people are treated surgically; although cochlear implants are useful in profound presbycusis, they are currently deemed too expensive for this indication in the NHS.

In the history, ask about: speed of onset, duration, and progression; whether it affects one or both ears; other ear symptoms – pain and discharge – and associated symptoms – vertigo and tinnitus.

Management of hearing impairment

- Check for wax. If present, administer softening drops, e.g. sodium bicarbonate or olive oil, and then refer for micro-suction if necessary. This service is increasingly unavailable in primary care and may need to be paid for.
- If deafness persists after wax removal, refer to audiometry.
- If the audiogram shows markedly asymmetrical loss, refer to the routine ENT clinic. An MRI of the internal auditory meatus is used to look for a schwannoma.
- Ask if the patient thinks they are deaf. If they do not, they are unlikely to use a hearing aid.
- If appropriate, refer to the local hearing aid service (often on the high street, as hospital audiology provision has been reduced).
- Educate the patient and their family about assistive technology.
  ○ Environmental aids, e.g. flashing telephones and doorbells, vibrating-pillow alarm clocks and smoke alarms (see Figure 20.5).
  ○ Advise about the use of the 'T' switch, used in conjunction with induction loop systems to amplify television, phones, at cinemas, etc.
  ○ Educate the patient/family about national charities and local support groups.

Digital hearing aids

- These are now standard NHS provision.
- Sound is digitally processed, so the quality is better than older analogue aids.

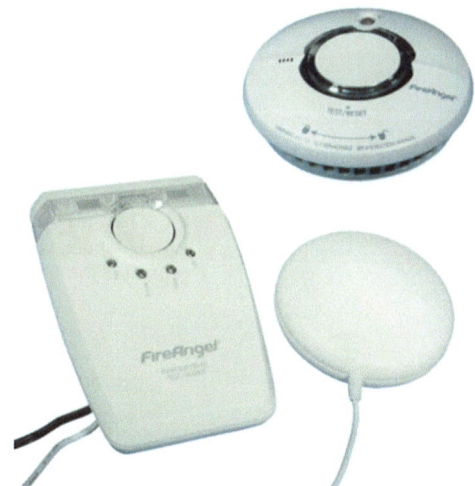

Cushion; large button amplified telephone

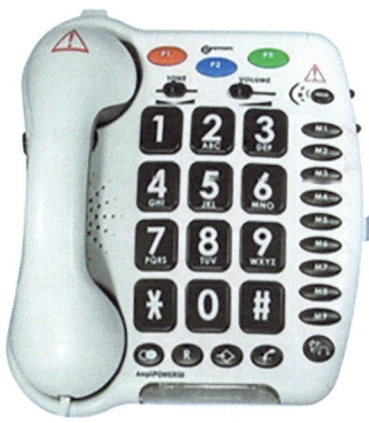

Figure 20.5 Smoke detector with wireless connection to strobe light and vibrating pad to put under a pillow or cushion.

- A soft dome is used rather than a mould, so individual fitting is not needed for mild to moderate loss.
- Feedback is the whistling that occurs when sound waves escape the ear canal, hit the hearing aid microphone, and are amplified again. Feedback is reduced as aids are programmed to filter it out, but they may still whistle, especially if wax is building up.
- Volume control is automatic.
- The aid is programmed for the individual's pattern of frequency loss, amplifying these frequencies more.
- More sophisticated aids have directional microphones, which help in environments such as restaurants.
- They may have several programmes, e.g. to compensate for background noise, concerts, or meetings. Top-of-the-range models switch programmes automatically, but this is reflected in increased cost.
- Technology is improving all the time. Standard NHS aids (2024) have Bluetooth connectivity for use with mobile phones, tablets and televisions.
- Batteries are free for NHS users. Some aids are rechargeable.

Getting the most from hearing aids

- Warn the patient that even the best hearing aids can only amplify sound and cannot restore normal hearing. Otherwise, people are so put off by the general increase in noise that they do not persevere.

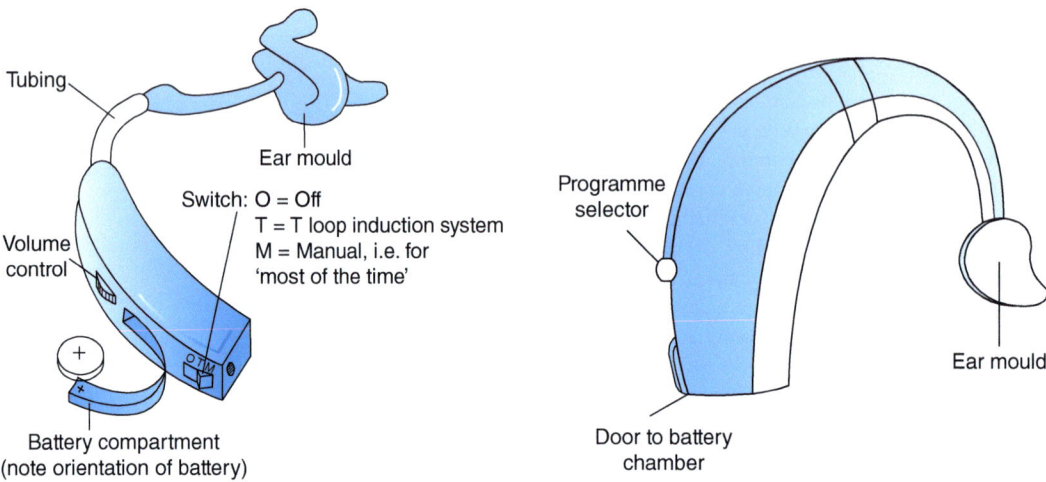

Figure 20.6 Behind-the-ear analogue (right) and digital hearing (left) hearing aids.

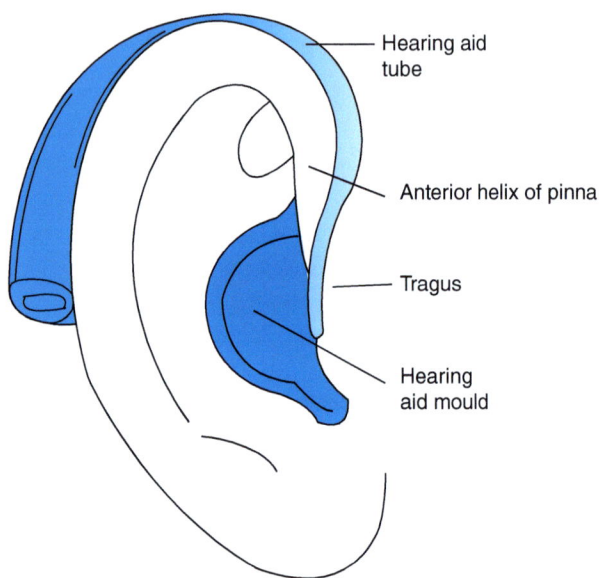

Figure 20.7 Correct insertion of a behind-the-ear hearing aid. Watch the video of how to insert a hearing aid from Northampton General Hospital: https://www.youtube.com/watch?v=CymbnS0thgw

- People do better the more they practise with the aid early on (brain plasticity). Around 40% of hearing aids are not used, so there is interest in auditory training (phone apps and computer software) to improve use, hearing outcomes and satisfaction.
- Bilateral aids are prescribed even if the loss is unilateral.
- If feedback is troublesome, check for wax in the ear and tubing and make sure that the volume is not too high. The dome needs replacing every 3–6 months, as it becomes rigid. If whistling persists, contact the provider.
- Teach maintenance of the aid, i.e. cleaning of the tubing and battery replacement (see Figure 20.6).
- Follow-up to encourage use of the aid is essential; volunteers can help.
- Behind-the-ear aids are still the most frequently available via the NHS. See Figure 20.7 for correct insertion.

- In-the-ear aids have the advantage of being discrete, but they are easily plugged with wax, are awkward if manual dexterity is reduced, and are easily lost, especially in hospitals. They are unsuitable for patients with severe otitis externa (inflammation of the pinna and ear canal).
- Body-worn hearing aids are the most powerful and are used by people with profound hearing loss.
- People who can afford it and want to avoid waiting lists can go directly to a private hearing aid provider (who may also do NHS work). Costs range from £500 a pair to over £3500 for high-end aids. Follow-up will be with the provider.

How to communicate with people who have hearing impairment

- Do not shout, as this just increases the distortion of your voice (recruitment) and lips (making it more difficult for lip-readers).
- Speak clearly and slowly, but not in an exaggerated way.
- Face the patient and make sure your face is well lit to assist lip-reading.
- Do not obscure your mouth.
- Ask the patient if they can hear you, lower the pitch of your voice, or try rephrasing your question.
- Check that any hearing aid is correctly inserted and that the battery is functioning.
- All clinical areas should have a simple portable microphone and headphones, or 'communicator'.
- If all else fails, write down your questions/answers.

Face masks and hearing impairments

During the COVID pandemic, mask-wearing caused additional communication problems, particularly in areas with high background noise like the ED and busy ward bays. Masks block low-amplitude high-frequency sounds, reducing the clarity of speech for patients and staff with hearing impairments Masks with clear plastic windows facilitate lip reading but block out more sound. Other solutions that may help include whiteboards, a personal amplifier, and online consultations.

Tinnitus

Tinnitus is the sensation of sound in the ears that does not come from an external source.

- Noises in the ears may be continuous or intermittent. Often described as rushing, buzzing or roaring. If sentences are heard, a psychiatric cause should be suspected.
- Most commonly associated with presbycusis; one theory is that the noise is generated by the brain to replace the sound that is 'missing'.
- Can be noise-induced.
- Over seven million adults in the UK have tinnitus.
- Affects over 20% of those aged over 65.
  - Severe symptoms in 5%.
  - Incapacitating in 0.5%.
- Pulsatile tinnitus: the noise beats in time with the pulse suggesting a vascular lesion such as an arteriovenous malformation or a glomus tumour.
- Discontinue implicated drugs: aspirin, NSAIDs, loop diuretics, aminoglycosides.
- Refer intrusive tinnitus (sleep disturbance) and unilateral tinnitus (to exclude a schwannoma) to ENT.
- Treatment:
  - Research suggests that patients respond better to being advised that tinnitus is often self-limiting than to negative suggestions such as 'nothing can be done'.
  - Hearing aids are helpful if the tinnitus is associated with hearing loss.
  - Advise the patient to minimise stress and tiredness, which tend to aggravate the symptoms.
  - Sometimes a noise generator (tinnitus masker), which produces 'white noise', is helpful.
  - Fill quietness with music or predictable noises, such as a fan, just above the volume of the tinnitus.
  - If the tinnitus causes depression, antidepressants may be helpful.
  - There is evidence that cognitive behavioural therapy improves quality of life for people with tinnitus, including those with depression.
  - Encourage contact with self-help organisations, e.g. British Tinnitus Association.

Vertigo (dizziness)

See chapter 11.

Other common ear problems in older people

Otitis externa, inflammation of the skin of the ear canal, causes itch. Discomfort and discharge are common. Hearing may be impaired by debris in the canal. Keep it clean and dry. Aural toilet may be needed. Treat with combination steroid and antibiotic (e.g. neomycin) drops.

Herpes zoster affecting the facial nerve (Ramsay Hunt syndrome) may present with severe pain, vesicles on the external ear canal and posterior pinna, facial paralysis, loss of taste on the anterior two-thirds of the tongue, and decreased lacrimation on the involved side. Remember, this lower motor neurone lesion will affect the forehead on the same side as the facial droop.

The nose

Age-related changes

1 Appearance: the skin thins, and the sebaceous glands are more active, causing the tip to sag.
2 A reduced sense of smell is attributed not only to fewer olfactory nerve receptors but also to age-related inflammation in the nasal passages. The olfactory cortex may also be affected (anosmia may precede Parkinson's disease).
3 Degeneration of the septal cartilage may change the shape of the nasal cavity, reducing airflow and causing the sensation of nasal congestion.
4 The thinning of the nasal epithelium, combined with a tendency to dehydration, can cause thickening of the mucus. There is a tendency to slower mucociliary clearance, which may lead to an increased incidence of postnasal drip, coughing and sneezing but also contribute to allergic rhinitis.
5 Reduced nasal blood flow can lead to lower temperatures and humidity in the nasal passages, leading to dryness and crusting.

Common conditions

Rhinitis

Inflammation of the nasal mucosa: associated with congestion or rhinorrhoea, itching, postnasal drip and sneezing, crusting, cough, olfactory loss, and nasal dryness. The symptoms can impair sleep, and the oedema can predispose to sinusitis by reducing drainage.

Allergic

This is IgE mediated and triggered by dust, pollen, or moulds. Antihistamine nose drops (azelastine) are first line, followed by cromoglicate or steroid sprays.

Non-allergic

- Viral infection: colds
- Autonomic (vasomotor) rhinitis: response to a physical trigger, including a change in temperature or humidity, or a chemical irritant such as the smell of food or perfume. Often copious clear rhinorrhoea. Saline sprays may help, but steroid sprays are usually given.
- Medication-induced: a wide range of drugs can cause rhinitis, mainly by changing the balance of vasoconstriction and dilatation or through inflammatory mediators.
  - One of the commonest is rebound after stopping decongestant nose drops, e.g. pseudoephedrine and xylometazoline (alpha-agonists). The mechanism is unclear – possibly tachyphylaxis.
  - Alpha-1 blockers, e.g. doxazosin and calcium channel blockers, e.g. amlodipine (vasodilation).
  - Some people develop a triad of asthma, eosinophilic rhinosinusitis and nasal polyps after ingestion of aspirin or a COX-1 inhibitor NSAIDs (leukotriene and prostaglandin release). ACE inhibitors, e.g. lisinopril (bradykinin, substance P, and histamine release).

Epistaxis

Most nose bleeds are from the anterior part of the nose. Posterior bleeds are more serious and more likely to require hospital treatment.

They are more common in older people because of:

- Frequent use of blood thinners, including aspirin, clopidogrel, DOACs, and warfarin.
- Co-existing nasal pathologies, including allergic rhinitis.
- Co-morbidities, including hypertension and heart failure.

Management: resuscitate if there is massive blood loss. Initial tamponade: ask the patient to hold their nose firmly below the bony bridge for at least 10 min, sitting forward to avoid swallowing the blood.

If there is ongoing bleeding, refer to the ENT team to perform cautery on any visible bleeding points or nasal packing.

Nasal polyps

These are shiny growths of inflammatory tissue that form in the nasal passage and cause congestion, postnasal drip, cough, reduced taste and smell, and headaches. In older people, treatment is usually oral or intra-nasal steroids.

Catarrh

This is build-up of mucus in the nose, sinuses, or throat and can be associated with an URTI or an allergic response. It can be more troublesome for older people as the mucus may be thicker and mucociliary clearance is less efficient, as is cough.

Management: avoid allergens where possible, non-drowsy oral or topical antihistamines, and topical steroids.

The Throat

Age-related changes

1 Laryngeal cartilage calcifies, and cricoarytenoid joints involved in opening and closing the vocal folds become stiffer.
2 Calcification and ossification of the cartilage and laryngeal muscles lead to weakness.
3 Vocal folds atrophy and become bowed.
4 After the menopause, the number of mucus glands is reduced making the mucus drier and more difficult to clear, which can lower the pitch of the voice. In men, the vocal speaking pitch may rise.
5 In addition, there is a component of reduced pulmonary function, including increased rigidity of the rib cage, leading to reduced air flow over the vocal cords.

All these changes lead to impaired voice production and quality. Speaking becomes tiring. The voice is breathier, and higher notes may cut out whilst singing.

Tips to maintain a healthy larynx in older age

- Stop smoking.
- Reduce alcohol intake.
- Drink 8 glasses of water per day.
- Regular exercise.
- Healthy diet.
- Check hearing (to avoid shouting).
- Use it or lose it.
- Singing is good!

MDT approach to improving the voice

Voice clinics with specialist ENT surgeons and speech and language therapists provide an MDT approach. SLTs may prescribe a course of vocal exercises, and vocal cords can be injected with filler if necessary.

Pathology causing changes to the voice

- Laryngitis.
- Vocal cord nodules.
- Allergies.
- Smoking.
- Irritants.
- Foreign body.
- Acid reflux.
- Long-term inhaled steroids.
- Laryngeal cancer.
- Thyroid disease.
- Recurrent laryngeal nerve palsy.
- Neurological conditions: PD, stroke, multiple sclerosis.
- Spasmodic dysphonia.
- Blunt trauma, e.g. due to a blow, endotracheal tube, or bronchoscopy.

Oropharyngeal dysphagia

Changes in the tissues of the throat may lead to leakage of food or fluids into the trachea on swallowing (aspiration). This is another common problem for older people – see Chapter 14.

📖 REFERENCES AND FURTHER READING

EYES

The College of Optometrists. A useful website about assessing vision in older people: DOCET; The Ageing Eye: Adapting the Routine-Community Practice: https://docet.info/course/view.php?id=140

GBD 2019 Blindness and Vision Impairment Collaborators (2021) Causes of blindness and vision impairment in 2020 and trends over 30 years, and prevalence of avoidable blindness in relation to VISION 2020: the Right to Sight: an analysis for the Global Burden of Disease Study. *Lancet Global Health* 9:e144–e160. doi: 10.1016/S2214-109X(20)30489-7.

World Health Organization *World report on vision.* Geneva: (2019) Licence: CC BY-NC-SA 3.0 IGO. https://www.who.int/publications/i/item/9789241516570

Ehrlich J, Ramke J, McCleod D, et al. (2021) Association between vision impairment and mortality: a systematic review and meta-analysis. *Lancet Global Health* 9:E418–E430. doi: 10.1016/S2214-109X(20)30549-0.

GOV.UK *Visual disorders: assessing fitness to drive* (2021) https://www.gov.uk/guidance/visual-disorders-assessing-fitness-to-drive#minimum-eyesight-standards--all-drivers

RNIB *The criteria for certification* www.rnib.org.uk/your-eyes/navigating-sight-loss/registering-as-sight-impaired/the-criteria-for-certification

NICE guideline [NG82] (2018) Age-related macular degeneration www.nice.org.uk/guidance/ng82

Hammadi S, Tzoumas N, Ferrara M, et al. (2023) A key consideration with complement-based therapies for age-related macular degeneration. *J. Clin. Med.* 12:2870. doi: 10.3390/jcm12082870.

Guymer R, Campbell T (2023) Age-related macular degeneration. *Lancet* 401:1459–1472. doi: 10.1016/S0140-6736(22)02609-5.

Corazza P, D'Alterio, FM, Kabbani J, et al. (2021) Long-term outcomes of intravitreal anti-VEGF therapies in patients affected by neovascular age-related macular degeneration: a real-life study. *BMC Ophthalmol.;* 21, 300. doi: 10.1186/s12886-021-02055-6.

Tajran J, Mohamed M, He Y, et al. (2023) *Photodynamic therapy* https://eyewiki.aao.org/Photodynamic_Therapy_(PDT)

NICE guideline [NG77] (2017) *Cataracts in adults: management* www.nice.org.uk/guidance/ng77

NICE Glaucoma [NG81] (2022) *Glaucoma: diagnosis and management* www.nice.org.uk/guidance/ng81

Dave S, Meyer J (2022) *Closed angle glaucoma* StatPearls https://www.ncbi.nlm.nih.gov/books/NBK559098

Mukhtyar C (2021) *Giant cell arteritis* BMJ Best Practice http://bestpractice.bmj.com/topics/en-gb/3000249

Sharma A, Hindman H (2014) A predisposition to dry eyes. *J. Ophthalmol.* doi: 10.1155/2014/781683MSD manual.

Eye disorders https://www.msdmanuals.com/en-gb/professional/eye-disorders

INFORMATION FOR PATIENTS AND RELATIVES

The Royal National Institute for Blind People: www.rnib.org
Macular society: www.macularsociety.org
Glaucoma UK: https://glaucoma.uk

EARS

RNID *Facts and Figures, Prevalence on hearing loss and tinnitus* (2018) https://rnid.org.uk/about-us/research-and-policy/facts-and-figures

WHO: *World report on hearing* (2021) World Health Organization, Geneva http://www.who.int/publications/i/item/9789240020481

Jayakody D, Friedland P, Martins R, et al (2018) Impact of aging on the auditory system and related cognitive functions: a narrative review. *Front. Neurosci.* 12. doi: 10.3389/fnins.2018.00125.

Lawrence BJ, Jayakody DMP, Bennett RJ, et al. (2020) Hearing loss and depression in older adults: a systematic review and meta-analysis. *Gerontologist* 60:e137–e154.

Pittman C, Ward B, Nieman C (2021) A review of adult-onset hearing loss: a primer for neurologists. Curr. *Treat. Options Neurol.* 23:20. doi: 10.1007/s11940-021-00674-4.

NICE CKS *Hearing loss in adults* (2019) https://cks.nice.org.uk/topics/hearing-loss-in-adults

Jiang F, Mishra S, Shrestha N (2023) Association between hearing aid use and all-cause and cause-specific dementia: an analysis of the UK biobank cohort. *Lancet Public Health* 8:e329–338. doi: 10.1016/S2468-2667(23)00048-8.

Chodosh J, Weinstein B, Blustein J (2020) Face masks can be devastating for people with hearing loss. *BMJ* 370:m2683. doi: 10.1136/bmj.m2683.

INFORMATION FOR PATIENTS AND RELATIVES

The Royal National Institute for Deaf People: www.rnid.org
YouTube video from the University of Nottingham with excellent communication tactics: https://www.youtube.com/watch?v=gssPxFtB0e8
www.actiononhearingloss.org.uk
www.deafcouncil.org.uk/CAMTAD.htm
www.yourlocalcinema.com – gives information about whether a loop system or subtitles are available.
The British Tinnitus Association: www.tinnitus.org.uk

NOSE

Pinto J, Jeswani S (2010) Rhinitis in the geriatric population. *Allergy Asthma Clin. Immunol.* 6:10. doi: 10.1186/1710-1492-6-10.

THROAT

Crawley B, Dehom S, Thiel C, et al. (2018) Assessment of clinical and social characteristics that distinguish presbylaryngis from pathologic presbyphonia in elderly individuals. *JAMA Otolaryngol. Head Neck Surg.* 144:566–571. doi: 10.1001/jamaoto.2018.0409.

ENT Health – patient advice: http://www.enthealth.org/throat

All websites were accessed in September 2024.

21

Legal and ethical aspects

Introduction

Most older patients pose no more ethical or legal problems than other adults. However, in a few cases, particularly where there is mental as well as physical frailty, problems are numerous. The COVID-19 pandemic raised ethical issues with accusations of 'ageism'. Ethical problems are often resistant to dogmatic resolution. Remember the four basic moral commitments (Beauchamp and Childress, see Page, 2012):

1 Respect for autonomy (confidentiality, informed consent).
2 Beneficence.
3 Non-maleficence.
4 Justice:
   - Fair distribution of scarce resources (distributive justice – relevant to ageism).
   - Respect for people's rights (rights-based justice).
   - Respect for morally acceptable laws (legal justice).

For any ethical issue, a framework can help you consider the issues. One example is:
   The Ethics Grid (Seedhouse, see Shale, 2020):

1 Describe the details of the case.
2 List management options and consider the practicalities for each, including:
   - Any disputed facts or evidence.
   - The degree of certainty around the facts.
   - Likely effectiveness of the action.
   - The risk.
   - Resources available.
   - Wishes of others.
   - Codes of practice.
   - The law.
3 Look at the consequences to find the most beneficial outcome for:
   - Yourself.
   - A particular group.
   - The individual.
   - Society.
4 Remember duties:
   - Tell the truth.
   - Keep promises.
   - Do most good.
   - Do the least harm.
5 Remember the core ethical concepts:
   - Respect/create autonomy.
   - Serve needs first.
   - Respect people equally.

Confidentiality

Older people have the same rights as everyone else to confidentiality. This sometimes surprises relatives! If older people are dependent on others, the family will need to be kept informed, but do discuss this with the patient first. If the person cannot consent, you will need to do this in their best interests.

Consent

Consent must be sought for all medical interventions, although this will often be a very informal process and sometimes only implied. Without it, the health care professional has committed the crime of *battery*. Written forms are used for surgical procedures and research involving drug trials or other interventions, although oral consent is equally valid in law. Consent must be *informed,* which means that the doctor must provide the necessary information, and ambiguities can arise concerning how much information was given and whether it was easy to understand. Consent must also be voluntary, i.e. no pressure must be exerted on the patient.

Age discrimination

Ageism is much debated and is said to remain widespread throughout the NHS. In a book on geriatric medicine, the easy option would be to make a sweeping condemnation of it as an evil like racial or gender discrimination. It became a hot topic during the COVID pandemic, when there was pressure to discharge people from hospitals to ensure that beds were available for the expected influx of people with COVID. There were suggestions that older people, particularly those with frailty, should not be admitted to hospitals, and if they were, there was reluctance to admit them to ICU beds. Age discrimination is often based on three rational but misconceived beliefs:

- Older people do not benefit from high-tech interventions as much as younger people. There is usually data that indicate just how beneficial each intervention is for older subjects. Fitness/frailty is usually more predictive than chronological age.
- The potential quantity and quality of life are too low to justify the procedure under consideration. Life expectancies for otherwise well older people are surprisingly high, and quality of life can only be assessed by that person and is consistently underestimated by doctors and others.

Geriatric Medicine and Elderly Care: Lecture Notes, Ninth Edition. Claire G. Nicholl, K. Jane Wilson, and Shaun D'Souza.
© 2025 John Wiley & Sons Ltd. Published 2025 by John Wiley & Sons Ltd.
Companion website: www.wiley.com/go/lecturenotesgeriatricmedicine9e

- To make such interventions available to older patients is to deny them to younger ones. It is not the role of physicians to compare how deserving their patients are, but unfortunately, decisions must be made. Because of the shortage of ICU beds, admission may mean that someone else must be moved out. Politicians should accept responsibility for rationing when resources are inadequate. If asked, older people are often very altruistic about resource allocation, but this may change as the baby boomer generation reaches old age.

Decisions on prioritising patients must be based on the patient's capacity to benefit, not on grounds of age.

Driving in later life

Younger drivers have more accidents than older ones! Overall, in 2021, around a fifth of all killed or seriously injured (KSI) casualties from collisions involving cars were in collisions that involved a young car driver. Older people tend to have low mileage, so the actual risk is even lower. However, UK *law* obliges drivers to surrender their driving licence at the age of 70. A new 3-year licence is issued, which can be renewed every 3 years on completion of a declaration of good health. The Driver and Vehicle Licensing Agency (DVLA) accepts that functional ability is more important than age but recognises that comorbidities, frailty, and cognitive decline may all impair driving ability. The data provide a case for a formal check at the age of 85.

Certain conditions, many common in old age, make the individual unfit to drive. The doctor must explain this to the patient and document it. Anyone with a medical condition 'likely' (a 20% likelihood of an event in 1 year for a car driver) to cause a sudden disabling event at the wheel, or who is unable to control their vehicle for any reason, must not drive. Successful treatment may allow driving to be resumed after a specified period.

These conditions include those causing:

- Transient loss of consciousness (TLoC), e.g. epilepsy, symptomatic cardiac arrhythmia, cough syncope, poorly controlled diabetes.

- Symptoms that would distract from driving, e.g. severe vertigo, angina at rest, severe heart failure.
- A high risk of sudden death, e.g. abdominal aortic aneurysm (AAA) >6.5 cm.
- Uncorrectable visual impairment, particularly significant field defects.
- Progressive neurological impairment, e.g. dementia and PD – driving is usually possible in the early stages but, at some point, becomes too risky.

Many disease episodes and procedures have defined driving bans:

- **Uncomplicated acute coronary syndrome (ACS) with no revascularisation:** 4 weeks
- **Post-CABG:** 4 weeks
- **Post-pacemaker:** 1 week

The rules are nuanced; check the DVLA website for details and the duration of any bar:

- **Single transient ischaemic attack (TIA):** must not drive for 1 month but need not notify DVLA.
- **Multiple TIAs over a short period of time:** must not drive and MUST notify DVLA; can resume driving at 3 months if no further episodes.

Advice for older drivers includes:

- Avoid distractions such as chatty passengers.
- If a long journey is unavoidable, take adequate breaks.
- If the route is unfamiliar, make advance preparations and allow plenty of time.
- Avoid rush hour and night driving.

Two ethical dilemmas are common:

1 A patient with a disorder listed by the DVLA refuses to stop driving.
2 A patient with a progressive disorder, e.g. dementia, insists that they are fine to drive when others disagree.

When advising someone to stop driving, it may help to frame the discussion in terms of: 'the other drivers on the road, so much more traffic, drivers are less courteous these days, if someone else did something

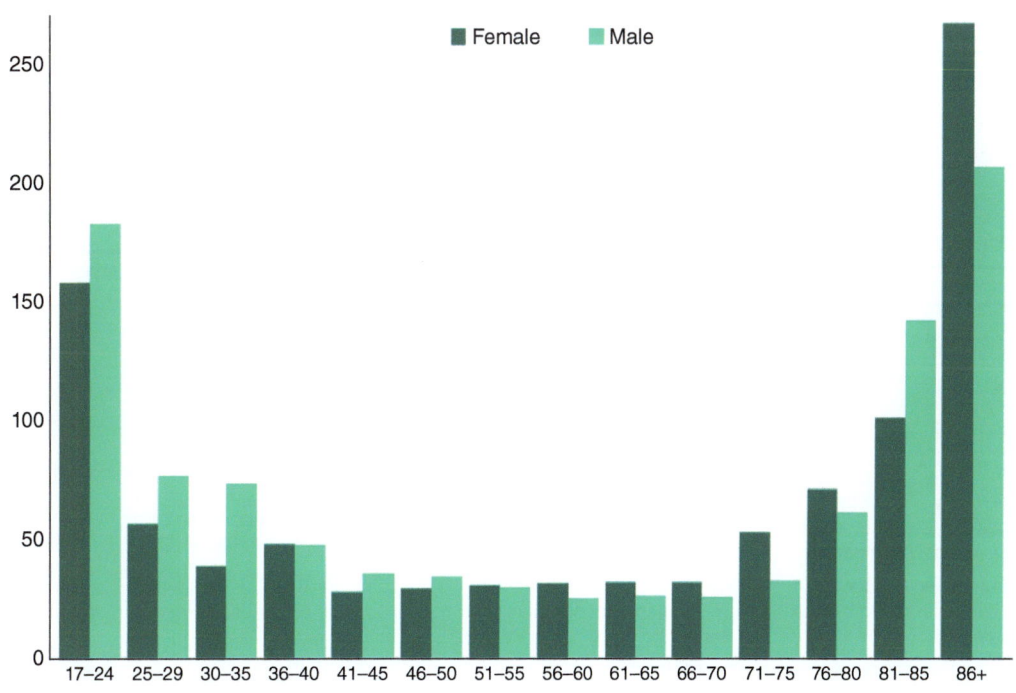

KSI car driver casualties per billion miles driven, by age and sex, Great Britain: 2021 UK Government Younger Driver Factsheet, 2021

silly it might take longer for you to weigh up the options' etc. If you fail to persuade them to give up driving, a family member may be prepared to try, particularly if they have experienced a terrifying ride as a passenger.

- Suggest seeking the opinion of a professional driving instructor or a session at a driving mobility centre, (staffed by therapists, fee for assessment, but enabling where appropriate).
- If a patient continues to drive after advice to stop, the doctor's duty to public safety overrides the usual duty of confidentiality, and the doctor must inform the DVLA (tell the patient also).

Notifiable diseases

Remember, there is a statutory duty to inform the local health protection team. COVID is the most common of the long list of infections, which also includes TB and food poisoning.

The Human Rights Act

The Human Rights Act 1998 has been in force across the UK since 2000. The Act incorporates rights set out in the European Convention on Human Rights into domestic law. It applies to all public bodies, including the NHS and social services. The articles that are most relevant to health care are:

Article 2: Right to life and positive duty on public authorities to protect life.
Article 3: Prohibition of inhumane and degrading treatment.
Article 8: Right to respect for private and family life.
Article 10: Freedom of expression and right to information.
Article 14: Right not to be discriminated against.

The Mental Health Act

The Mental Health Act (MHA) 1983, revised in 2015, is the main piece of legislation guiding the compulsory inpatient admission and treatment of mental health problems in England and Wales (see Table 21.1). If the person is detained under the MHA, this takes precedence over the Mental Capacity Act (see later).

Most people in psychiatric hospitals are informal patients who have agreed to admission; 25% are compulsorily detained or 'sectioned' under the Act.

The Mental Capacity Act

The Mental Capacity Act (MCA) 2005 came into force in 2007. It is a statutory framework to:

- Empower and protect people who may lack the mental capacity to make their own decisions.
- Enable people to plan for a time when they may lack capacity.

If you have a patient who lacks capacity, the MCA will affect how you consult family and friends, and the patient may need an advocate, particularly where:

- They are to be discharged from the hospital to different accommodations.
- Decisions are to be made about 'serious medical treatment', defined as providing, withdrawing, or withholding treatment where:
  ○ There is a fine balance between benefits/burdens and risks, e.g. deciding whether to amputate a gangrenous foot in a patient who has just had a stroke.

Table 21.1 Sections under the Mental Health Act.

Section	Use	Applicant	Signatory	Duration
Section 2	Admission for assessment	AMHP, or very rarely, the nearest relative	Two doctors: a Section 12 approved doctor and, usually, the patient's GP	28 days
Section 3	Admission for treatment	AMHP, or very rarely, the nearest relative	As above	Up to 6 months, unless the consultant discharges the patient, renewable
Section 4	Emergency admission	As above, but must have seen the patient in the last 24 hr	Any doctor	72 hr Used rarely
Section 5	Holding power	A doctor can detain a patient needing treatment (including for a physical illness). A psychiatric nurse can detain an informal patient for 6 hr until the clinician in charge arrives	The hospital manager is informed by the doctor that an application for compulsory admission 'ought to be made'	72 hr
Section 7	Guardianship. Used rarely, a guardian is appointed to direct the affairs of an incapacitous person	As above	Two registered practitioners. The guardian is LA Social Services or their appointee	Up to 6 months, renewable
Section 135	Warrant to search for and remove a person to a place of safety	A magistrate issues a warrant on sufficient grounds of mental illness and being unable to care for themselves	Doctor, an AMHP, accompanied by a police officer can enter any premises where the person is believed to be	36-hr maximum

AMHP, Approved Mental Health Professional; Section 12 approved doctor, usually a psychiatrist - both have specific training in the MHA. LA, local authority.

- ○ The choice of treatments is finely balanced, e.g. type of chemotherapy in advanced breast cancer.
- ○ What is proposed would have serious consequences for the patient.
- They are to be included in drug trials.

Five principles underpinned by the MCA

1 There is a presumption of capacity, unless demonstrated otherwise.
2 Individuals should be supported in making their own decisions.
3 People retain the right to make an eccentric or unwise decision.
4 Others must act in the best interests of the patient.
5 If an intervention is needed, it should be the least restrictive.

Assessment of capacity

This is only considered if the patient has an 'impairment of brain function'. For older people, this is usually dementia or a stroke. Capacity is decision- and time-specific, i.e. a person may be able to decide what to eat and to make a will but may not be able to decide about returning home. However, the situation may be different the next day.

To have capacity, the person must be able to:

- *Understand* information relevant to the decision (consequences of deciding one way or another or failing to make the decision).
- *Retain* that information for long enough to decide (even though they may then forget a decision has been made).
- *Use* that information as part of the process of making the decision.
- *Communicate* the decision (by any method, including sign language, or squeezing the hand).

Advance decisions

The MCA puts the status of advance decisions on a statutory footing. A person:

- Can specify what treatment they would NOT want and under what circumstances.
- Cannot demand treatment.

The advance decision must have been made when the person had the capacity to be valid. It only applies to the circumstances described; e.g. 'I do not want resuscitation if I cannot speak after a stroke' will not influence treatment after a heart attack. To refuse life-sustaining treatment, the advance decision must be in writing, signed, witnessed, and specify 'even if life is at risk'. See Chapter 22 for more information.

Lasting Power of Attorney (England)

This is how a person with capacity can choose who will look after their affairs in the future if capacity is lost.

- The donor confers authority on the *attorney* (a person of their choice, usually a relative or friend) to make decisions about all or any of:
  - ○ The donor's health and personal welfare.
  - ○ The donor's property and affairs.
- The Lasting Power of Attorney (LPA) must be registered by the Office of the Public Guardian, which manages administration for the Court of Protection (see later).
- If your patient lacks capacity and has a health LPA, you must discuss their treatment with the attorney.

A person with financial means who does not have the capacity to take out an LPA should be referred to the Court of Protection. An application may be made by a relative, a solicitor or a doctor. A medical certificate is required, and the court will usually appoint an interested relative or other suitable person as a *deputy* to function as the patient's agent but not to dispose of assets. If the only income is benefits, an individual can apply to the Department of Work and Pensions to act as an *appointee*

to deploy them for the person's benefit. Scottish law differs in detail (see references), but the principles are similar.

The Court of Protection

This specialist court makes decisions on financial or welfare matters for people who lack capacity. It:

- Declares whether a person has capacity if there is a dispute.
- Makes decisions about health care/treatment.
- Makes decisions about property/financial affairs.
- Appoints deputies to have ongoing authority.
- Makes decisions in relation to LPAs.
- Makes decisions about deprivation of liberty.

The court can issue a declaration that the proposed treatment would be lawful. In considering the patient's best interests, the court will be guided by the *Bolam test,* which asks whether the treatment would be supported by a responsible body of medical opinion. An approach to the court is best made through the trust's legal services or, in an emergency, through the duty manager. If it is uncertain whether a refusal to be treated reflects depression, seek a psychiatric opinion. Capacitous people are allowed to make unusual decisions ('Ms. B' vs. NHS 2002), and their wishes should be respected. The public guardian and their office run the affairs of the court. It is a criminal offence to mistreat a person who lacks capacity.

Independent mental capacity advocates

Most people who lack capacity have support from family or friends (or an attorney or deputy). If there is no such person (or they are 'not practicable or appropriate' to consult) and a decision is needed about serious (not emergency) medical treatment or a change of accommodation (as mentioned above), there is a duty to instruct an independent mental capacity advocate (IMCA).

IMCAs need to be able to access and copy health/social care records. VoiceAbility, a charity, is one of the UK's largest providers of advocacy services.

The duties of an IMCA

- Support the person who lacks capacity and represent their views and interests to the decision maker.
- Obtain and evaluate information.
- Ascertain the person's wishes, feelings, beliefs, and values.
- Ascertain alternative courses of action.
- Obtain a further medical opinion if necessary.
- Challenge a decision, if necessary, in the patient's interests.

Testamentary capacity

Testamentary capacity means mental competence in the single connection of drawing up (or revoking) a will. To be capable of this act, a person needs to:

- Understand the nature of such an act.
- Have a reasonable grasp of the extent of their assets, so an assessing doctor must have some idea of the patient's circumstances.
- Be aware of which persons have a claim on their property.
- Be free of delusions that might distort their judgement.

Deprivation of Liberty Safeguards

The Deprivation of Liberty Safeguards (DoLS), an amendment to the MCA, have been used in England and Wales since 2009. The safeguards provide legal protection for vulnerable adults (mainly with learning disabilities and dementia) who are not detained under the MHA but are in a hospital or a care home. These adults lack the capacity to consent to care or treatment, and their freedom is restricted to keep them safe – they are not allowed to leave and are constantly supervised. Care should be the least restrictive possible and contact with family or friends should be encouraged. If hospitals and care homes (referred to as the managing authority) are depriving people of their liberty, this needs to be authorised by a supervisory body, usually the local authority (LA).

Liberty Protection Safeguards

It was planned to replace DoLS with Liberty Protection Safeguards (LPS), which should be simpler to use, but this has been postponed, and may not happen. Three assessments would be needed for LPS:

1 Capacity assessment.
2 Medical assessment (to confirm a qualifying mental disorder – usually dementia for older people).
3 A necessary and proportionate assessment to check the balance between any restriction and the harm it is designed to prevent.

LAs *and* NHS trusts *and* Integrated care boards (ICBs) would be 'Responsible Bodies'.

A family member or appropriate person must be consulted.

The legislation was intended to apply to people living at home as well as those in hospitals or care homes.

The Care Act

The Care Act 2014 replaced the National Assistance Act 1948, and 'Section 47', which enabled a LA to remove a person in need of care from their home, was repealed. The Care Act aims to help improve people's independence and lists the duties of social services. It sets out a single route for establishing an entitlement to care and support for all adults who need care. This includes an assessment of needs, a decision about whether the needs are eligible, and a financial assessment where necessary.

Safeguarding

Adult safeguarding duties apply to any adult who:

- Has care and support needs.
- Is experiencing or is at risk of abuse or neglect.
- Is unable to protect themselves because of their care and support needs.

There are differences between the safeguarding frameworks in the four UK nations. In England, safeguarding adults is a statutory duty for councils with adult social services responsibilities (CASSRs) under the Care Act. The six principles are:

1 **Empowerment:** supporting people to make their own decisions.
2 **Prevention:** it is better to act before harm occurs.
3 **Proportionality:** the least intrusive response to the risk.
4 **Protection:** support and representation for those in greatest need.
5 **Partnership:** services working within their communities.
6 **Accountability**.

After an initial confidential discussion, if there are grounds for suspicion, the matter must be pursued through interdisciplinary channels. There will be a safeguarding lead for vulnerable adults in your trust who will liaise with the team in social services.

A competent older person has the right to choose to remain in a setting where there is a risk of or actual abuse, if they wish to do so. For many older victims, abuse may have become normalised and accepted, which can create barriers to getting help. They may be reluctant to admit what is going on; they may be dependent on their abuser for support or company; or they may have a caring role for their abuser which they are reluctant to leave. Support must be offered to make the situation as safe as possible. Vulnerable people without capacity must be protected.

Elder abuse

The abuse of older people, often referred to as 'elder abuse', is a global public health problem.

Elder abuse is a single or repeated act, or lack of appropriate action, occurring within any relationship where there is an expectation of trust, that causes harm or distress to an older person. It overlaps with domestic abuse, and several types of abuse may coexist. Abuse can happen anywhere, from the person's home, even when they live alone, to day facilities, care homes, and hospitals (institutional abuse). The perpetrator may be a stranger but is usually known to the victim.

A review of 52 studies in 28 countries from diverse regions estimated that over the preceding year, 1 in 6 people aged 60 years and older were subjected to some form of abuse (Yon et al. 2017). Two-thirds of staff working in institutions reported perpetrating abuse in the past year (Yon et al. 2018).

Hourglass, the UK charity previously known as Action on Elder Abuse, produces clear information and has a 24/7 phone helpline. Hourglass estimates that around one million people over 65 are victims of abuse each year in the UK. Old age abuse is hard to detect and takes many forms.

Types of elder abuse

- **Psychological or emotional (the most common):** threats of harm, verbal abuse, shouting, swearing, blaming, humiliating, isolating, and coercive control.
- **Physical:** rough handling, pushing, punching, slapping, burning, restraining, overdosing, or withholding medication.
- **Financial:** 'asset-stripping', theft, refusal to pay for personal items or appropriate care.
- **Neglect:** withholding food, drink, warmth, and access to support and medical care.
- **Sexual:** any non-consensual sexual activity; this can be particularly difficult in a spousal relationship where one partner has dementia.
- **Cultural:** forcing a vegetarian to eat meat, not helping a Muslim patient to wash before prayer.

Risk factors for Elder Abuse

Victim

- Heavy dependency (such as needing help with personal care, transferring on and off toilet/bed) and communication difficulties.
- Dementia.
- Behavioural problems and aggression.

Shared

- Poor housing.
- Poor long-term relationship.

Carer

- Excessive alcohol consumption.
- Changed lifestyle due to a caring role.
- Divided loyalties, e.g. elderly parent and child.
- Health problems, including psychiatric.
- Role reversal, ageing child, and aged parent.
- Isolation, real or perceived.

Detection of abuse

Although the diagnosis is difficult to substantiate, there are warning signs:

- Recurrent falls and accidents, unexplained fractures.
- Multiple bruising, especially clear thumbprint bruises to arms or bruises or burns to unusual areas such as flexure surfaces.
- Injury similar in shape to an object.
- The patient tries to hide a part of the body from examination.
- Patient is withdrawn, frightened (especially of the carer), anxious, and makes an effort to please.
- Sudden changes in the patient's character.
- Difficulty gaining access to the patient.
- Isolation of the patient in one room of the home or care setting.
- Carer complaining of 'nerves' or of being under stress.
- Refusal by the patient and/or carer to accept necessary support services.

Restraint of confused patients

In caring for people, it is sometimes necessary to carry out actions that limit their freedom of movement. If a person has the capacity, measures to make them safer are discussed with them. However, if a person is confused (usually, in an older person, because of delirium, dementia or a combination), restraint may be required. Restraint is used in hospitals, care homes and at home. If any restraint is used, the method, the reasons, the discussions with those close to the patient, and the arrangements for review should be documented. The least restrictive option should be chosen, and DoLS documentation may be needed. The need for restraint is reduced by diligent care and an enabling environment. However, a risk-averse culture, poor staffing, and a rising tide of complaints and litigation increase the use of restraint, e.g. the prevention of falls by any means, may be a higher priority for managers than respect for dignity and autonomy.

Emergency sedation of the acutely confused patient

In a hospital, the trust security team will come to a ward if an extremely agitated patient is endangering themselves, other patients, or the staff. It is permissible under common law to hold the patient down to administer an injection as a last resort and for their own protection if other physicians would regard it as appropriate and if reasonable people would want the treatment themselves to enable investigation and treatment of the underlying cause. The procedure is distressing to everyone and can usually be avoided (see also Chapter 8).

Chemical restraint

More controversial is the longer-term administration of drugs, often antipsychotics or benzodiazepines, to calm behaviour and make the patient easier to manage. A key question is whether the medication is for the benefit of the patient or the staff. Covert medication should only be used if it is essential, discussed with the family, and must be properly documented.

Physical restraint

This includes the use of extra bandaging, mittens, or boxing gloves to make it harder for the patient to remove IV lines and catheters. Trunk or limb belts are not used on UK wards but are more common in other settings (ICU) and countries.

Bedrails may seem like a sensible precaution to reduce falls out of bed, but confused patients often find a way over them and then fall from a greater height or risk entrapment injury. Nursing a patient on a very low bed or a mattress on the floor may be preferable, but this is also a form of physical restraint and bad for the nurses' backs. Tilting chairs are rarely used except if a competent patient who likes to sit out would otherwise slide off the seat, but restraint may be less obvious if a patient is 'wedged' in a normal chair by their bed table or in a wheelchair with a fixed table.

Environmental restraint

This includes one-to-one supervision (which can be of great benefit if the carer is skilled and develops rapport with the patient), the use of a side room, which makes noisy behaviour easier to tolerate but is isolating, and electronic devices. A common method to reduce the risk of falls is a buzzer attached to a pad on which the patient sits; it sounds when the patient stands. This works best if the area is well-staffed and the patient is dealt with straight away – they may want to use the toilet or stretch their legs; otherwise, it may just agitate the patient, their neighbours, and any doctors trying to do a ward round. Mobile patients can be fitted with an electronic tag that triggers an alarm if the patient leaves the hospital ward. Other methods include doors that, although not locked, are difficult to open, e.g. with two different handles that must be used simultaneously. In a person's home, rooms or stairs may be barricaded, the gas supply to the cooker may be disconnected, with hot meals delivered instead, and various forms of electronic monitoring may be used. Full discussion within the MDT, and with the family and good documentation are essential.

Ethical issues relating to life-supporting interventions

Treatment and care towards the end of life

The GMC provides detailed guidance on decision making for doctors in the UK treating patients approaching the end of their lives, including patients whose death is imminent and those with:

(a) Advanced, progressive, and incurable conditions.
(b) General frailty and co-existing conditions who are expected to die within 12 months.
(c) A risk of dying if there is a sudden acute crisis in an existing condition.
(d) Life-threatening acute conditions caused by sudden catastrophic events.

The most difficult decisions often relate to whether or not to start a treatment or withdraw a treatment that might prolong the patient's life. The benefits, burdens, and risks of treatment for a frail older person may be difficult to gauge.

General ethical and legal principles apply. There is a presumption in favour of prolonging life, but there is no absolute obligation to do this. The doctor and wider health care team should discuss the clinical options. If the patient has capacity, the options and their consequences should be explained. With the patient's permission, it is best to involve those close to them. If the person lacks capacity, check whether there is a relevant advance decision. If not, the doctor must consult with any legal proxy and others close to the patient to find out what the patient themselves would have wanted. Patients or those close to them have no legal right to demand clinically inappropriate treatment. If there are different views within the team or family, seek a formal second opinion. Resource constraints are a real factor, and the GMC acknowledges that there may be competing duties towards the wider population, e.g. over the availability of ICU beds.

Clinically assisted nutrition and hydration

Nasogastric (NG) or percutaneous gastrostomy (PEG) feeding and intravenous or subcutaneous fluids are medical treatments (GMC and British Medical Association [BMA]). Because of the complexity of decision making in this area, some trusts have a multidisciplinary 'feeding issues team' to discuss the risks and benefits of assisted nutrition for individual patients.

- If a patient lacks capacity and cannot eat or drink enough to meet their needs, the doctor must assess whether providing clinically assisted nutrition or hydration would be of overall benefit.
- As with other treatments, the patient's wishes are the key issue. If the patient has a registered health and welfare LPA, the attorney is the lawful decision maker. Discuss what the patient would have wanted if known or their best interests with input from the attorney if appointed, family, friends, or an IMCA. If, after discussion, the doctor and healthcare team still consider that the treatment would not be of benefit, there is no obligation to provide it. However, as well as a full explanation, a second opinion should be offered.
- Even food and drink by mouth (basic care rather than treatment) may lead to choking and aspiration.
- NG tubes look unsightly to the family, are often pulled out by patients (even when bridled), and are associated with reflux and aspiration. Placing a PEG tube in a frail patient has risks, including death. Skin infections, tube blockage, and aspiration occur, and patients may also pull these out.
- Stroke, terminal cancer, and advanced dementia are common situations where feeding and hydration issues arise. In stroke, except where the prognosis looks hopeless, it should initially be assumed that recovery is possible, so hydration and nutrition are generally provided. Many cancer patients can express their wishes, and in the later stages, the clear trajectory of the illness may make the timing of decisions easier.

Patients with advanced dementia are perhaps the most difficult. Oropharyngeal dysphagia and aspiration are common. Eating and drinking, even in small amounts, may be a last remaining pleasure. The drive to eat and drink is basic. Keeping a patient 'nil by mouth' and tube-feeding them when they cannot understand why they are not offered food or drink may be both unkind and futile, as tube-feeding does not prevent aspiration. Speech and language therapists and dieticians can provide useful input. Generally, the best approach is to offer 'comfort feeding' with the safest texture of food (usually puree), when the patient is alert and well positioned, pausing if aspiration is suspected. This is time-consuming and requires skill. Traditionally, fluids have been thickened, but thickened fluids worsen quality of life, are often refused, lead to dehydration and good evidence that they reduce aspiration is lacking. It may be best to offer plain cold water, and foods like jelly and ice cream contribute to fluid intake. However, giving what the patient wants, slowly and carefully is pragmatic. If the patient does not take enough, it is unlikely they are experiencing hunger or thirst.

The loss of the desire to eat and drink is a normal part of the dying process. It can be distressing to watch a visibly dehydrated terminal patient. However, it may be considered that 'the ethical situation is not that the patient is failing to drink and therefore will die, but that the patient is dying and therefore does not wish to drink'. Good mouth care is essential. In England, Wales and Northern Ireland, the withdrawal or withholding of clinically assisted nutrition and hydration from a patient in a persistent vegetative state needs a court review, but this is rarely encountered in old age.

(See Chapter 8 for evidence that tube feeding in advanced dementia is not beneficial.)

Cardiopulmonary resuscitation

Every clinical setting you work in will have a policy on CPR and how decisions are documented. Find out what it is before your first 'crash call'.

CPR is an emotionally charged topic. This has been amplified by media attention, which has led to the widespread misconception that a 'do not attempt cardiopulmonary resuscitation' (DNACPR) decision is the major determinant of life or death during an admission. There is pressure on staff to introduce this topic at their first encounter with the patient. It is important, but it only applies to cardiorespiratory arrest.

There is robust outcome data from the annual audit of CPR attempts in UK acute hospitals. The COVID pandemic affected figures in 2020–2021:

- Between 2014 and 2019, the number of in-hospital cardiac arrests attended by resuscitation teams fell despite an increase in admissions, so either fewer patients had a cardiac arrest or the identification of people who might benefit from CPR improved.
- About half of attempts at resuscitation are successful; survival to hospital discharge has increased steadily to 20–25%.
- Outcomes after attempted resuscitation are best in otherwise fit patients on coronary care. Survival to discharge after an arrest on a ward in acute hospitals is 14%.
- Outcomes are worse with increasing age. In acute hospitals, 15% patients aged 75–84, and 11% patients aged 85+ were discharged alive in comparison with 18% aged 65–74. The very elderly patients will have been identified by their teams as having the possibility of a successful resuscitation, so this is NOT the same as the outcome in a typical 85-year old.
- Frailty may be a better predictor than age. Sample sizes are smaller in studies, but Ibitoye found that no frail patients (CFS > 4) survived to discharge, in contrast with 26% of the non-frail. Other studies do not show such a clear effect, but all publications and meta-analyses have shown that frailty is associated with worse outcomes after resuscitation (Hamlyn et al., 2022).

A DNACPR decision should be taken by the most senior doctor available, ideally after discussion with the patient, the team and, with the permission of the competent patient and the family, regularly reviewed and recorded in the notes, together with the reason.

A DNACPR order is appropriate:

- Where CPR is not in accordance with the sustained wishes of the patient.
- Where the patient has a poor quality of life that they do not wish to be prolonged.
- Where successful CPR would be followed by a quantity and quality of life that would be unacceptable to the patient.

Where CPR is unlikely to be successful, there is still an expectation that this will be discussed with a competent patient, although the discussion should not be forced on them if they do not want it. If the patient does not wish to discuss it, seek permission to talk to those close to them. If you make a DNACPR decision for a patient who lacks capacity, you must consult with any legal proxy, or others close to the patient at the earliest practicable opportunity. This should include a careful explanation that the intention is to spare the patient treatment that will be of no benefit.

If a competent patient insists on receiving CPR that the team deems futile, there is no legal obligation to provide it. However, it is sensible to offer a second opinion. Another option, although this is contentious, is to offer limited CPR intervention.

A DNACPR decision is NOT a proxy for other decisions and does not imply 'not for treatment'. The patient must continue to receive appropriate management. An increasing number of areas in England and Scotland use the ReSPECT process (Recommended Summary Plan for Emergency Care and Treatment) to document decisions about a wider range of treatments towards the end of life. The Resuscitation Council UK website has the latest version of the form and a clear explanation (see Chapter 22).

If a patient who has a DNACPR order has an incidental problem, e.g. they choke on a food bolus, this should be treated. A DNACPR order may be revoked or suspended if circumstances change, e.g. for a planned surgical procedure.

If your patient is discharged to another setting, ensure that any decision about CPR is communicated and that proper documentation accompanies the patient.

Admission to the intensive care unit

The usual reason for emergency medical ICU admission is for ventilation or for life-threatening respiratory failure due to airway obstruction, pneumonia, neurological disorders, or drug overdose. The dilemma is to avoid deaths from a reversible cause (asthma, Guillain–Barré syndrome) but to avoid prolonging life (usually prolonging death) when the prognosis is hopeless (end-stage emphysema, motor neurone disease, advanced dementia with aspiration pneumonia).

If your patient is deteriorating and ICU admission might be an option, get an opinion before the patient has a respiratory arrest on the ward. Many trusts have an ICU outreach service. Ask them to assess the patient and explain this to the relatives. This assessment from another team often reassures the family that everything sensible has been done. Always listen to the family if they are concerned that their relative's condition is deteriorating; patients and families have a right to request a second opinion (Martha's Rule). Other considerations are similar to those governing CPR: the patient's and relatives' wishes and the previous quality of life. The trajectory of many chronic conditions that will result in respiratory failure, e.g. COPD, is predictable, so advance planning is best. Age per se is not a bar to ventilation.

Euthanasia

Euthanasia, the active and intentional termination of a person's life, remains illegal in the UK. Support for assisted dying is around 80% amongst the British public, but doctors have been reluctant to support this. In 2019 the RCP changed its position on this from opposition to one of neutrality, as did the BMA in 2021. Further debate is ongoing in the UK Parliament in 2024.

- **Voluntary euthanasia:** the deliberate and intentional hastening of death at the request of a seriously ill patient. This is legal in Belgium, Luxembourg, the Netherlands, and Spain in Europe, as well as in Columbia, Canada, New Zealand, and six states of Australia.
- **Physician-assisted suicide:** the patient takes a lethal cocktail that has been prescribed or provided by the physician at the patient's request. Assisted suicide is legal in Switzerland, and several US states have followed the example of Oregon and Washington.

It is acceptable morally and legally to administer increasing doses of sedative and analgesic drugs that may, incidentally, shorten life (which they seldom do) if the doctor's intention is to provide effective pain relief – the so-called 'double effect'. When you are prescribing drugs such as morphine for end-of-life care, make it clear in your notes that the aim is pain relief.

To withhold potentially life-prolonging treatment is sometimes called *passive euthanasia,* and some ethicists regard it as morally indistinguishable from active euthanasia. But, as we have seen, no doctor is obliged to initiate or continue treatment that they consider futile.

While suicide or travelling abroad to receive assisted suicide is not illegal, facilitating suicide is a criminal offence. To date, neither a doctor providing a report, nor any accompanying person has been prosecuted for helping a patient to travel abroad to end their life, but this remains contentious.

Death certification and the role of the coroner

UK death certification and the coronial system were reformed following the Shipman scandal. The UK health service has commissioned NHS trusts to implement learning from deaths policies, including the formation of medical examiner's offices, with the intention of collaborating with local authority coroner's offices. The purpose of these reforms is to facilitate *independent* scrutiny of causes of death and, hence, provide reassurance to the public. Rules for verifying and certifying death also changed during the COVID pandemic; most of those provisions have been repealed, but some persist.

After a person dies, the first step is 'confirmation of death' (if seen by a doctor), but other designated professionals may do this: 'verification of death' (if seen by a nurse) or 'recognition of life extinct' (if seen by a paramedic). This is the recorded time of death, although the family may be aware that the person took their last breath earlier. Registered nurses and paramedics with appropriate training can verify expected adult deaths at home, including care homes and nurses usually verify deaths in nursing homes, hospitals, and hospices. There must be a DNACPR decision or signs of irreversible death (e.g. rigor mortis) or CPR must be attempted.

A medical certificate of cause of death (MCCD) enables the deceased's family to register the death. It provides a permanent legal record of the death. A doctor who attended during the patient's lifetime (usually in hospital during their last illness) has a legal responsibility to complete a MCCD. The new MCCD was launched in September 2024. It is now signed by the Medical Examiner **and** a member of the clinical team (see Figure 21.1). There is no longer a separate cremation form, and the MCCD includes details of ethnicity and removal of implantable medical devices.

Medical examiners

After some delay, this role became a statutory requirement in September 2024 for hospital trusts and primary care in England and Wales. Medical examiners are senior medical doctors with additional training who are contracted for a number of sessions a week to examine all deaths in the trust. They perform 'proportionate reviews' of medical records and discuss the case with the clinical team.

They seek to answer three questions:

1 What caused the death?
2 Does the coroner need to be notified?
3 Was the care before death appropriate?

The purpose is to:

- Provide *independent* scrutiny of all deaths. Medical examiners can therefore not review cases that they have been directly involved with.
- To ensure referrals to the coroner are appropriate.

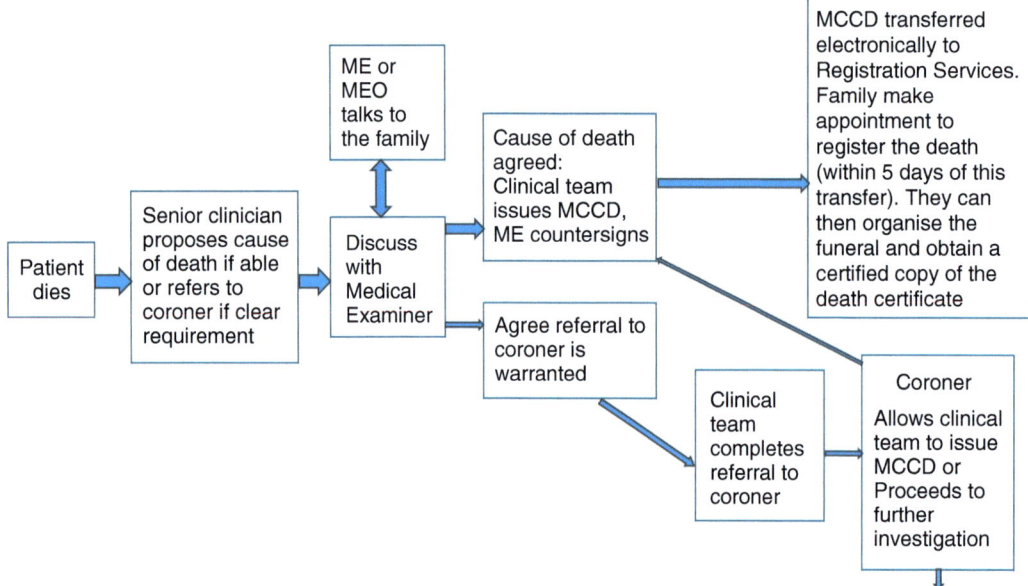

Figure 21.1 System for death certification. MCCD, medical certificate of cause of death. ME, medical examiner; MEO, ME's office.

- Allow relatives with questions to approach a doctor who was not involved in the deceased's care.
- Improve the quality of death certification and, hence, mortality data.

In a trust, there will be several medical examiners with office support from the bereavement office and in an area several GPs will have this role. There is a National Medical Examiner, whose office provides regular update bulletins, and whose responsibility it is to govern the service at a national level.

The coroner

A coroner (procurator fiscal in Scotland) is an independent judicial office-holder appointed by a LA to investigate certain deaths in their area. They are now usually lawyers with no formal medical training. Coroners investigate deaths that were violent or unnatural, where the cause of death is unknown, or if a death occurred in detention. Their staff – coroner's officers – are usually civilian police. Coroners either decide that a death certificate can be issued, arrange a post-mortem, or open an inquest. There are no special rules for the deaths of older people, but as most people die in old age and falls are a common reason for admission, there is often more contact between medicine for older people and the coroner's office. If a patient falls on your ward and breaks a hip or sustains a subdural, keep exemplary notes, as if they die, there will usually be a coroner's inquest.

All deaths, whether in a hospital or the community, will be reviewed by a medical examiner who will usually advise if a referral to the coroner is needed. If there is doubt or disagreement, a referral to the coroner is required. The following deaths should be reported:
Deaths due to:

- Poisoning, toxic substances, medical or recreational drugs (including *acute, but not chronic,* alcohol poisoning).
- Violence, trauma, or injury, e.g. RTA and *falls*.
- Self-harm.
- Neglect, including self-neglect (but self-neglect due to the natural progression of an illness such as dementia does not require notification unless there was neglect by others).

- A person undergoing any elective medical or surgical procedure or treatment. Deaths following surgery are likely to be referred; death after surgery for a fractured neck or femur almost always occurs, as there is usually a preceding fall.
- An occupational disease, e.g. asbestosis.
- An unknown cause.
- Any cause in any type of state detention (a DoLS order alone is not included).

Medical devices to remove prior to cremation

This list is growing, in addition to pacemakers and defibrillators (which must be inactivated before removal), remember implantable loop recorders, radioactive implants for prostate brachytherapy and Fixion intramedullary nails – the saline-filled chamber forms steam and can explode.

 REFERENCES AND FURTHER READING

Page K (2012) The four principles: can they be measured and do they predict ethical decision making? *BMC Med Ethics* 13: 10, doi: 10.1186/1472-6939-13-10.

Shale S (2020) *Ethics in NHS integrated care systems.* https://www.clearer-thinking.co.uk/ethics-in-nhs-integrated-care-systems/

DVLA *Assessing fitness to drive: a guide for medical professionals* (updated 2022). http://www.gov.uk/government/publications/assessing-fitness-to-drive-a-guide-for-medical-professionals

UK Government Department of Transport National statistics. *Reported road casualties in Great Britain: younger driver factsheet,* 2021 Published November 2022. https://www.gov.uk/government/statistics/reported-road-casualties-great-britain-older-and-younger-driver-factsheets-2021/reported-road-casualties-in-great-britain-younger-driver-factsheet-2021

Yon Y, Mikton KR, Gassoumis ZD, et al. (2017) Elder abuse prevalence in community settings: a systematic review and meta-analysis. Lancet Global Health 5(2):e147–e156. https://www.ncbi.nlm.nih.gov/pubmed/28104184.

Yon Y, Ramiro-Gonzalez M, Mikton C, et al. (2018) The prevalence of elder abuse in institutional settings: a systematic review and meta-analysis. Eur. J. Public Health. https://www.ncbi.nlm.nih.gov/pubmed/29878101.

Siegrist-Dreier S, Barbezat I, Thomann S, et al. (2022) Restraining patients in acute care hospitals – a qualitative study on the experiences of healthcare staff. *Nursing Open* 9:1311–1321. doi: 10.1002/nop2.1175.

CQC *Covert administration of medicines* (2022) www.cqc.org.uk/guidance-providers/adult-social-care/covert-administration-medicines

National Cardiac Arrest Audit: Public report 2022-23. https://www.icnarc.org/wp-content/uploads/2024/05/NCAA-Summary-Statistics-2022-23.pdf.pdf

Ibitoye SE, Rawlinson S, Andrew Cavanagh A, et al. (2021) Frailty status predicts futility of cardiopulmonary resuscitation in older adults. *Age Ageing* 50:147–152. doi: 10.1093/ageing/afaa104.

Hamlyn J, Lowry C, Jackson TA, et al. (2022) Outcomes in adults living with frailty receiving cardiopulmonary resuscitation: a systematic review and meta-analysis. Resuscitation Plus 11:100266. doi: 10.1016/j.resplu.2022.100266.

GMC Ethical Guidance. This has links to all the relevant GMC guidance. http://www.gmc-uk.org/ethical-guidance

BMA Ethics website. This is open to non-members and has links to a range of topics covering the issues discussed above and more, including the Ethics toolkit for medical students, Clinically assisted nutrition and hydration, Mental Capacity Act Toolkit, DoLS, Adult safeguarding, Domestic abuse, Physician assisted dying, and Decisions relating to CPR. https://www.bma.org.uk/advice-and-support/ethics

AgeUK *Worried about someone's driving?* https://www.ageuk.org.uk/information-advice/travel-hobbies/driving/worried-about-someones-driving/

Driving mobility www.drivingmobility.org.uk

Mind Mental Health Act. This is easier to read than the government guidance. https://www.mind.org.uk/information-support/legal-rights/mental-health-act-1983/about-the-mha-1983/

VoiceAbility. www.voiceability.org

NHS England *Liberty Protection Safeguards.* https://www.e-lfh.org.uk/programmes/liberty-protection-safeguards

SCIE *Care Act Assessment and eligibility* (2022). www.scie.org.uk/care-act-2014/assessment-and-eligibility

Hourglass, the UK's only charity focused on the abuse and neglect of older people. https://wearehourglass.org

RCP *Supporting people who have eating and drinking difficulties* (2021). www.rcplondon.ac.uk/projects/outputs/supporting-people-who-have-eating-and-drinking-difficulties

O'Keeffe ST, Lazenby-Paterson T, Collins L et al. (2023) Thickened fluids and risk of dehydration. *J Am Med Dir Assoc* 24: 2018–2019. doi: 10.1016/j.jamda.2023.08.017

Gov.UK Guidance for medical practitioners completing medical certificates of cause of death in England and Wales (Dec 2024) https://www.gov.uk/government/publications/medical-certificate-of-cause-of-death-mccd-guidance-for-medical-practitioners/guidance-for-medical-practitioners-completing-medical-certificates-of-cause-of-death-in-england-and-wales

Ministry of Justice *Guidance for registered medical practitioners on the Notification of Deaths Regulations* (2022). https://assets.publishing.service.gov.uk/government/uploads/system/uploads/attachment_data/file/1062499/registered-medical-practitioners-notification-deaths-regulations-25-march-2022.pdf

NHS England *The national medical examiner system.* https://www.england.nhs.uk/establishing-medical-examiner-system-nhs

All websites were accessed in September 2024.

22

Palliative care

What is palliative care?

Palliative care embraces the interdisciplinary, holistic assessment and management of people who have a life-limiting illness. Palliative care also embraces the families and friends of those who are dying. End-of-life care is the final phase of palliative care, but the definition used by the NHS is vague, described as support for people who are in the last few hours, days, months or even a year or more of their lives. This is partly because the trajectory of dying differs depending on the illness (see Figure 22.1).

The Lancet Commission on the Value of Death (2022) suggests that in high income countries, we have lost a balanced relationship with death as dying has moved from the context of family, community, and culture to sit within the health care system. Health care has a role, but interventions at the end of life are often excessive, may increase suffering, exclude contributions from family and friends, and consume resources inappropriately.

A useful resource, Dying Matters, Hospice UK's campaign, encourages people to have conversations about death and dying. It is intuitive that older people with multiple co-morbidities are more likely to die, but we often shy away from this idea; even health care staff may see death as a failure of treatment. 'With the End in Mind' by Dr Kathryn Mannix, a palliative care specialist, is recommended reading.

Five priorities for the care of the dying person

In the UK, the Leadership Alliance for the Care of Dying People, a coalition of 21 national organisations, published One Chance to Get It Right (2014). This sets out five 'Priorities for Care' for a person who is expected to die within the next few days or hours.

1 The possibility of imminent death is recognised and communicated clearly; decisions are made and actions taken in accordance with the person's needs and wishes; and these are regularly reviewed and revised accordingly.
2 Sensitive communication takes place between staff, the dying person, and those identified as important to them.
3 The dying person and those identified as important to them participate in decisions about treatment and care to the extent that the dying person wants.
4 The needs of families and others identified as important to the dying person are explored, respected, and met as far as possible.

5 An individual plan of care, which includes food and drink, symptom control and psychological, social, and spiritual support, is agreed upon, co-ordinated and delivered with compassion.

The goal is to move from the medical model to a more individualised, community-based experience, aiming to achieve a hospice level of care in all settings, including home, with privacy and dignity, optimal symptom control plus spiritual and psychological support. This requires good resources and excellent communication and coordination between patients and carers, primary and secondary care, social care, and the voluntary sector.

Recognising that patients are nearing the end of life enables us to plan for a 'good death' (see below). Older people tend to be philosophical about dying, but their families can sometimes have unrealistic expectations. Many middle-aged people have never experienced the death of a loved one or seen a dead person, so education is needed to ensure that patients and families understand what is happening and why.

Aspirations for a 'good death' might include:

- Being able to access information and expertise of whatever kind is necessary.
- Making sense of the universe within personal beliefs and value systems.
- Resolving personal conflicts and unfinished business (e.g. the funeral planned and paid for) and having time to say goodbye.
- Knowing that one's wishes will be respected.
- Confidence that life will not be prolonged unnecessarily when futile.
- Understanding that death is imminent and what is likely to happen.
- Dying at home or a place of choice.
- Being with family and friends.
- Feeling in control.
- Being free of pain and other unpleasant symptoms.
- Having appropriate spiritual and religious support.
- Having privacy, dignity, and compassionate care.

Statistics about UK deaths

The leading three causes of death in 2018 (before the COVID-19 pandemic) in men were IHD and dementia, followed by lung cancer. In females, dementia was followed by IHD and stroke.

- Between 2015 and 2019, the average number of annual deaths in the UK was 530,000.
- In 2020, this increased by 14.5% to 608,000 due to COVID.
- In the UK, 80% of deaths occur in people aged over 65.
- 65% of women die aged 75 years old or older.

Geriatric Medicine and Elderly Care: Lecture Notes, Ninth Edition. Claire G. Nicholl, K. Jane Wilson, and Shaun D'Souza.
© 2025 John Wiley & Sons Ltd. Published 2025 by John Wiley & Sons Ltd.
Companion website: www.wiley.com/go/lecturenotesgeriatricmedicine9e

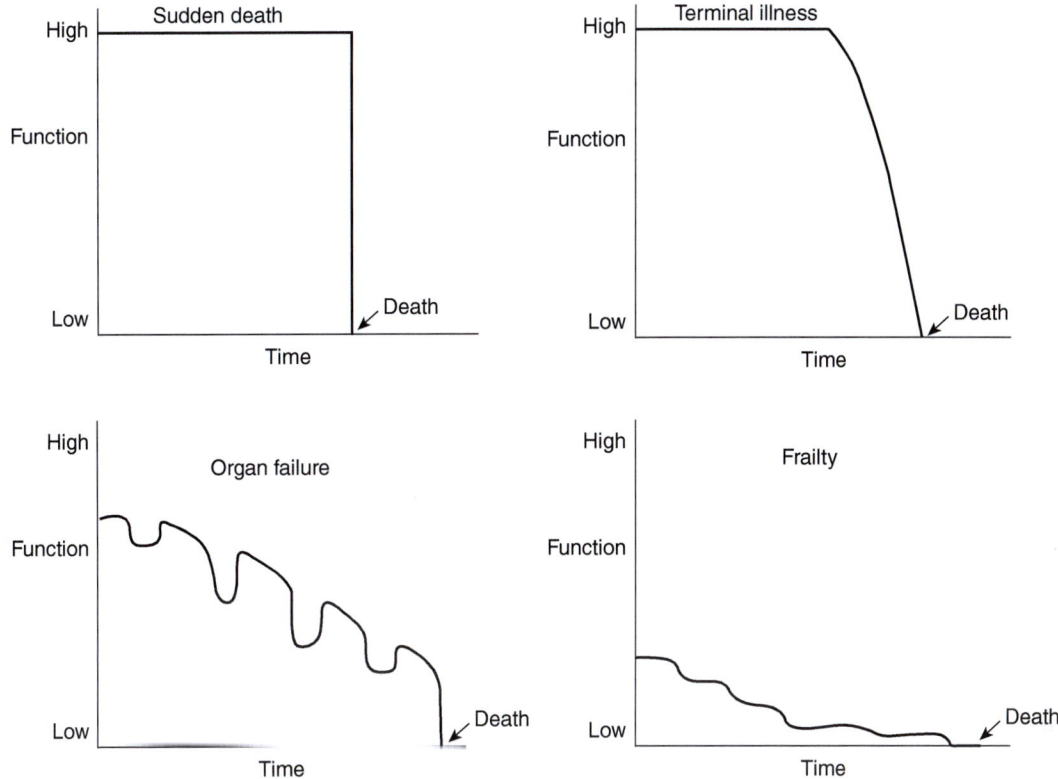

Figure 22.1 Trajectories of dying. *Source*: Lunney et al. (2002/John Wiley & Sons).

Table 22.1 Place of death of people aged 85 and above.

Location	Percentage of people in 2009 dying aged 85+	Percentage of people in 2020 dying aged 85+
NHS hospitals	55	37
Care homes	18	39
Own home	22	21
Hospice	5	2

Source: ONS data for 2009 and 2020.

- 70% of people would choose to die at home, but most deaths still occur in institutions (see Table 22.1).
- People over the age of 80 are more likely to die in nursing homes.
- People under the age of 65 are more likely to die at home.

Recognising the last year of life: the role of the Gold Standards Framework

People are living longer, often with multiple conditions, sometimes treated by several specialists. Therefore, it is important for generalists such as GPs and geriatricians to recognise when patients are becoming increasingly frail and deteriorating despite optimum treatment or when side effects are becoming too burdensome. In the UK, 95% of general practices now use the Gold Standards Framework (GSF). This aims to improve the early identification of patients who are deteriorating. Consider:

- Would you be surprised if this person were to die in the next 6–12 months?
- Do you think the person knows this?
- Can you talk to them about the likely trajectory?

When we identify such people, we can explain the significance of their condition to them and their family, provide information, reduce fear of the unknown, and offer better planning for supportive and palliative care. Futile and often unpleasant investigations and treatments can be cancelled.

Warning signs include:

- Recurrent hospital admissions.
- Weight loss >10% over 6 months, serum albumin <25 g/L.
- Exhaustion.
- Needing more help with activities of daily living.
- Already on maximal therapy.
- Cardiac cachexia, breathlessness at rest in heart failure.
- Oxygen dependency and right heart failure in COPD.
- Worsening renal failure with nausea, pruritus, and fluid overload.
- Deterioration of speech, swallowing, and recurrent aspiration in neurological conditions.

Breaking bad news

This might apply when a person is first diagnosed with a life-limiting illness or when they are likely to die soon. There are a few accepted guidelines:

- Suggest that the patient asks a family member or friend to be present at an agreed time: this warns them that the situation is serious and, if they consent to being accompanied, ensures that a trusted person knows the same information and can ask questions, provide support, etc.

- Pre-plan the discussion: check that you have all the relevant information, anticipate further questions, make sure that you have time (bleep-free), and ensure privacy.
- If possible, go to a quiet room away from the bedside and take another team member with you.
- Sit beside the patient, signalling that you are willing to spend time.
- Identify the relatives and introduce yourself and any colleagues.
- Start by checking what the patient already understands. Often, older patients will have insight that their dramatic weight loss must be due to cancer.
- Use a warning shot: 'I am afraid I have some bad news for you.'
- Avoid jargon. Explain in simple terms what the diagnosis is and what that is likely to mean.
- Break the news into small sections and check whether the patient understands what you have said.
- Do not be afraid of eye contact, physical contact, or silence.
- Try not to remove all hope or to give a precise prognosis.
- Offer a second opinion, if wanted.
- Do not be afraid to speak of dying, but only give as much information as they can cope with.
- Do not worry about being too detached – patients and relatives often appreciate it if they see that the doctor or nurse is affected emotionally.
- Offer to continue support and to emphasise good symptom control. Cancer nurse specialists are an excellent resource for patients with a new diagnosis of advanced cancer.
- If appropriate, explain how the palliative care team, Macmillan nurses, etc. will be involved.
- Ask if the patient or relative has questions. Some direct questions can be answered initially with, 'What makes you ask that?' It gives you a chance to think and may enable them to explain the worry behind the question, which will make your answer relevant.
- If you are asked something you do not know, say you will find out and tell them.
- Offer a further meeting if wanted.
- Record what was said and to whom in the notes.

Although patients have the right to know, they may not want to know, be in denial, or lack the mental capacity to understand. If a patient makes it clear that they do not wish to be burdened with diagnostic and prognostic information, do not force the issue. Offer a further meeting if they want to know more later. Remember your duty of confidentiality, and do not inform relatives without the explicit consent of a competent patient. The health care team is different because they are all bound by a similar ethical code, but this may not apply to the manager of a care home, so bear this in mind. The family may have insight into what the patient would have wanted, which is useful, particularly if the patient lacks capacity. However, if a patient has capacity, avoid being drawn into collusion.

Advance care planning

Advance care planning (ACP) has been defined as a process of discussion between the patient, their care providers, and often those close to them about their future care. This may be more challenging for frail older people with an uncertain prognosis, but this makes it more important. Although two-thirds of the public claim they are comfortable talking about death, less than a third have discussed their wishes with their families, and a tiny percentage have an advance statement.

ACP should be encouraged for everyone, as 'none of us has a crystal ball', but particularly for people:

- Identified as in the last year of life,
- With cancer on palliative treatment,

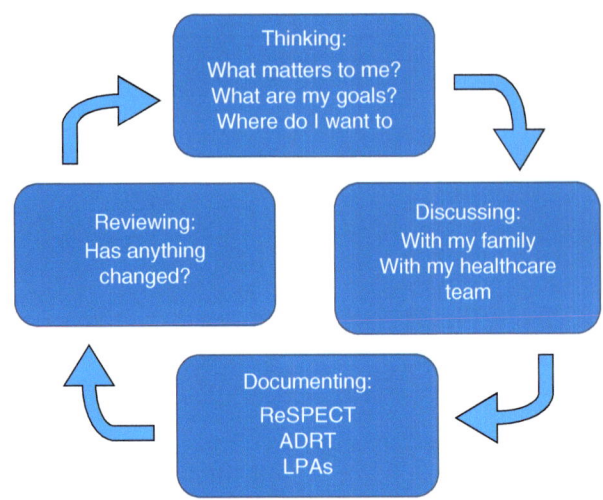

Figure 22.2 Advance care planning process. ReSPECT, recommended summary plan for emergency care and treatment; ADRT, advance decision to refuse treatment; LPA, lasting power of attorney.

- With long-term conditions, e.g. COPD, and especially where cognitive deterioration is likely, e.g. early dementia or PD.

A discussion can be triggered if there is a change in function or circumstances, such as after settling into a care home or the death of a spouse. A helpful approach is to acknowledge that the person is well now but ask whether they have views on what they would like to happen in the future. A general discussion may benefit the family and at least ensure that a will is made, and there is some discussion about funeral arrangements (Figure 22.2).

ACP is ongoing, evolves over time, and can take several forms.

Lasting power of attorney

A lasting power of attorney (LPA) allows a person to give someone they trust the legal power to make decisions for them in case they later lose capacity and cannot make decisions. There are two types of LPA:

1 An LPA for Health and Welfare covers decisions about health and care.
2 An LPA for Property and Financial Affairs covers decisions about money and property.

See Chapter 21 for the legal details.

Advance statement

A person can record their general wishes and care preferences, such as place of care, type of care and support. It is not legally binding.

Advance decision

Known more correctly as an advance decision to refuse treatment (ADRT) or colloquially as a 'living will', competent patients may choose to refuse life-sustaining treatments such as CPR, ventilation, PEG tubes, dialysis, and antibiotics. An ADRT needs to be:

- Written down.
- Signed.
- Signed by a witness.
- Clear that the person has understood that they might die as a result.
- Shared with their GP (who will scan it into the notes and code it).

If a person has both an LPA and an ADRT, the more recent document takes precedence.

Patients usually draw up a form with their family and GP. The decisions are legally binding in England, Wales, and Northern Ireland,

and doctors will respect them. In Scotland, the equivalent, an advance directive, is likely to be considered but is not recognised in law.

For a sample form with clear explanations, see the 'Compassion in Dying' website.

Euthanasia and assisted suicide currently remain illegal in the UK but there is ongoing debate in parliament.

Hospice care

This remains the gold standard provider of palliative and end-of-life care, but provision is limited and tends to focus on younger people with cancer.

- Offers short in-patient admissions to control difficult symptoms with a view to getting the patient home to die if that is their choice.
- Provides daycare facilities for symptom control, including diverse ways of managing pain such as relaxation and other psychological approaches.
- Provides opportunities to address emotional and spiritual needs with the family and group therapy for patients in similar situations.
- Enables outreach and co-ordination of care for a wider group of people dying at home.

Symptom control

Many hospitals have a palliative care team – do not hesitate to ask for advice, as it will improve your skills as well as care for your patient and reassurance for their family. The BNF has a section on prescribing in palliative care, and for detailed information, see *The Palliative Care Handbook* 2019.

Pain

Pain is multifactorial and exacerbated by fear, depression, and other factors. Ideally, identify the cause of the pain to target the most appropriate analgesia. Acute pain lasting 2–4 hours is treated with analgesia as needed; chronic pain, which is common in advanced disease, is better managed with longer-acting analgesics given in anticipation of pain. The dose will require titration for the individual. Most pain formularies are still based on the three-step WHO pain ladder.

1. Paracetamol, given regularly, can help moderate pain and be a co-analgesic in severe pain. Reduce the total dose for patients who weigh less than 50 kg or have hepatic failure. NSAIDs are usually avoided in old age (because of the risks of gastric erosion, renal impairment, and fluid retention), but they have a role in bone metastases.
2. The next step is a 'weak' opioid. High-dose codeine tends to cause disproportionately more nausea, constipation and confusion for the additional analgesia achieved. A synthetic opioid analogue is often used. Meptazinol may cause less confusion and constipation than the cheaper tramadol.
3. Strong opioids are usually given regularly, with additional doses as needed for breakthrough pain. Oral, rectal, transdermal, and injectable preparations are available. In the UK, the principal drug is morphine. In addition to analgesia, some gain benefit from the euphoriant effect of these drugs, but others find this distressing.

The main problems associated with strong opioids are:

- Drowsiness, which may be unacceptable, usually wears off within a few days.
- Constipation is universal. Prescribe a strong laxative such as macrogol, which combines lubricant and stimulant properties.
- Nausea. Co-prescribe regular anti-emetics initially, but again, nausea usually wears off (see Table 22.2).
- Respiratory depression, cough suppression, and hypotension rarely limit the use of these agents in end-of-life care.

Table 22.2 Causes and treatment of nausea and vomiting.

Symptom	Likely mechanism	Causes	Treatment
Persistent, severe nausea, little vomiting	Chemical/metabolic	Uraemia	Haloperidol
		Hypercalcaemia	
		Opioids	Ondansetron
		Chemotherapy	
Early satiety. Intermittent mild nausea, large volume vomiting	Gastric stasis/outflow obstruction	Drugs, including opioids and anticholinergics	Metoclopramide
		Local tumour	
		Hepatomegaly	
Dysphagia with little nausea relieved by vomiting	Regurgitation	Oesophageal or mediastinal disease	Dexamethasone
Intermittent nausea completely relieved by vomiting	Bowel obstruction	Malignant: tumour in the lumen, wall or pressing on the bowel wall	Metoclopramide only if there is no colic
Large-volume vomiting may be faeculent, sometimes with little warning		Benign: adhesions after surgery, enteritis from radiotherapy, oedema of the bowel wall due to inflammation	Hyoscine butyl bromide, if colic is present
			Cyclizine and/or haloperidol
May be associated with abdominal pain, distension, and constipation			Octreotide
		Faecal impaction	Enema, suppositories
Nausea and headaches worsen in the mornings	Intracranial disease	Intracranial tumour	Dexamethasone
		Cranial radiotherapy	Cyclizine
		Raised intracranial pressure	Levomepromazine
Mixed picture	Multiple causes	Combination of the above	Levomepromazine

- Tolerance and addiction. These are not issues in end-of-life care, but explain this to the patient so they do not ration themselves.

Causes of pain requiring specific treatment

- Neuropathic pain: responds better to tricyclic antidepressants, anticonvulsants (e.g. pregabalin, gabapentin or valproate) or transcutaneous electrical nerve stimulation (TENS) than conventional analgesics. Nerve blocks and other specialist interventions can be helpful.
- Bony metastases: NSAIDs with a proton pump inhibitor (PPI); avoid if there is serious risk of GI bleeding. Intravenous bisphosphonates are often helpful. Hormonal treatment usually relieves the pain of prostatic secondaries. A single bony deposit will respond well to a palliative dose of radiotherapy.
- Headache due to raised intracranial pressure: dexamethasone 16 mg in divided doses at breakfast and lunchtime (not at night as it increases alertness) is given for a week and then reduced by 2 mg a week to 4–6 mg daily, again with a PPI.
- Nerve compression: dexamethasone 8 mg orally a day can help; consider local anaesthetic infiltration.
- Pain from hepatic capsule stretch due to liver metastases: prednisolone 20 mg a day.
- Intestinal colic due to partial bowel obstruction: try loperamide and hyoscine *hydrobromide* as Kwells sublingually (see later for parenteral management).

Using opiates

- Start with immediate-release oral morphine sulphate solution or tablets, e.g. regular 2.5–5 mg every 4 hours. Oramorph solution contains 10 mg/5 mL.
- Titrate up until pain relief is adequate. Note the total dose needed over the last 24 hours.
- Convert to morphine sulphate modified-release tablets, capsules, or suspension using the same total amount of morphine in two equal doses. Prescribe immediate-release morphine as needed for breakthrough pain or before an activity that causes pain, e.g. wound dressing.
- To convert to morphine injections, use half the oral dose of morphine. The usual route is subcutaneous, by syringe driver if needed regularly.
- Fast-acting fentanyl lozenges, 'lollipops' provide a boost of analgesia to cover incident pain from dressing changes and personal care.
- Transdermal patches of fentanyl and buprenorphine have a wide dose range and duration, ranging from 72 hours to 7 days. Conversion tables from oral morphine are available. Patches are long-acting, so they are not suitable for titration, but they reduce the tablet burden.
- In renal failure, use low-dose tramadol or oxycodone orally and alfentanil subcutaneously.

Restlessness and confusion

Look for physical causes, e.g. a distended bladder or rectum, or a respiratory or urinary infection. Oxycodone may cause less confusion and agitation than morphine. If restlessness and agitation persist, try midazolam 2.5 mg subcutaneously or haloperidol 0.5 mg.

Nausea and vomiting

These are unpleasant symptoms, especially early in the dying process, and may prevent the patient from preparing food, eating with their family, or enjoying their daily routine. In hospital, boredom may make the symptoms seem even worse.

Identify any precipitating causes and treat those that are reversible.

- Always prescribe anti-emetics and laxatives when commencing opioids.
- Treat constipation.
- Treat hypercalcaemia; rehydrate with intravenous fluids; or give intravenous pamidronate.

If there are no reversible precipitants, identify the cause to choose the most appropriate anti-emetic. All causes of nausea and vomiting produce gastric stasis, so use parenteral preparations until symptoms are controlled. See Table 22.2.

- Metoclopramide is a pro-kinetic (muscarinic agonist) in gastric and small intestinal smooth muscle and a D2 blocker (and 5-HT$_3$ blocker in higher doses) at the chemoreceptor trigger zone (CTZ). Domperidone remains useful in palliative care; the cardiac cautions are not relevant, and it causes fewer extrapyramidal effects.
- Cyclizine is an antihistamine (H$_1$ blocker) and central anti-muscarinic. Avoid metoclopramide with cyclizine, which is anti-kinetic, as they counteract each other.
- Granisetron and ondansetron are 5-HT$_3$ receptor antagonists. Both cause constipation. Granisetron is longer-acting. They can be highly effective for vomiting due to chemotherapy.
- Haloperidol, a butyrophenone, is another option for chemically induced nausea as it blocks D2 and 5-HT$_3$ receptors in the CTZ.
- Levomepromazine, a phenothiazine D2 blocker with sedative properties, is used for a mixed picture of vomiting, severe pain, and distress.
- Octreotide, a somatostatin analogue given subcutaneously reduces intestinal secretions and vomiting in bowel obstruction.
- Dexamethasone reduces oedema.

Anorexia and malaise

Prednisolone 20 mg a day

Breathlessness

About 75% of all dying patients suffer from breathlessness, not just those with end-stage heart failure or lung disease. Where possible, identify and treat the cause in the usual way. The following types of dyspnoea require specific management:

- Superior vena cava obstruction. This is an oncological emergency presenting with increasing breathlessness and facial oedema. Treat with radiotherapy. Dexamethasone (16 mg a day) can be used if there is any delay.
- Lymphangitis carcinomatosis. When cancer cells infiltrate the lung lymphatic system, the prognosis is poor (usually months). Dexamethasone can reduce the associated breathlessness.
- Pleural effusions. Fluid usually reaccumulates after drainage. Consider pleurodesis.
- Intractable breathlessness of any cause can be treated using opioids, diazepam, and/or oxygen, whichever gives the best relief. Get input from the breathlessness intervention service (usually physios). A hand-held fan can reduce the associated claustrophobic fear.
- The 'death rattle' occurs as secretions are inadequately cleared by dying patients. The patient is usually unconscious by this stage, but it is upsetting for relatives who need reassurance that the patient is not distressed. Glycopyrronium 0.6–1.2 mg/24 hr subcutaneously will help dry up the secretions. Avoid suctioning, as this will not remove secretions in the lower respiratory tract but will agitate the patient and family.

Fungating tumours

Older women sometimes ignore breast tumours, and present when there has already been a breakdown of the overlying skin. Radiotherapy can reduce pain and bleeding. Topical metronidazole and charcoal dressings reduce odour and exudate.

Bowel obstruction

Depending on the prognosis, this might be best managed by palliative colostomy or stenting. If surgical intervention is no longer appropriate, try to avoid the 'drip and suck' regime. Allow the patient to take small sips and talk to their family without a nasogastric tube. The pain can be relieved by a morphine infusion. Colicky pain should be alleviated by subcutaneous hyoscine *butylbromide* (Buscopan) 60–240 mg over 24 hours. Vomiting is common; strong parenteral anti-emetics and octreotide (300–600 mcg subcutaneously) may be required. A phosphate enema may relieve the associated constipation. Offer patients who respond small quantities of food and fluid.

Other problems and possible solutions

- **Hiccup:** use metoclopramide or haloperidol.
- **Dysphagia:** consider stent or laser treatment for oesophageal carcinoma.
- **Dry or painful mouth:** good mouth care, artificial saliva such as Biotene Oral Balance, a quarter of a vitamin C tablet, and treating candidiasis with fluconazole.
- **Diarrhoea:** treat the cause. Do not forget overflow secondary to constipation.
- **Constipation:** treat the cause. If very severe, may need manual evacuation.
- **Cough:** oxygen, opioids, local anaesthetic lozenges, and hyoscine.
- **Insomnia:** treat the cause, e.g. pain, depression, fear.
- **Hypercalcaemia:** treat if symptomatic.
- **Ascites:** drain if causing discomfort.
- **Spinal-cord compression:** an oncological emergency – radiotherapy if diagnosed early.
- **Lymphoedema:** pressure device, support sleeves.
- **Pruritus:** treat the underlying cause where possible, e.g. switch morphine to oxycodone, practise careful hygiene, use soap substitutes and emollients.

Enabling people to die at home

In most cases, it is possible to achieve good symptom control. The pain service and community palliative care nurses can offer specialist expertise in difficult cases. Check that the patient is getting Attendance Allowance and apply under the special rules if not. If the patient is in hospital and the prognosis is short weeks, apply for 'fast-track' NHS continuing care. Depending on the prognosis, special equipment may be needed (hospital bed, pressure-relieving mattress, hoist, and commode). Usually, care for older people will comprise a care package from social services, plus support from the district nurse to manage syringe drivers, etc. In 90% of cases where dying patients are admitted to hospital, the reason is inadequate community support or the distress of the relatives.

Additional support may be available from the following:

- Marie Curie nurses provide hands-on care for cancer patients, including personal care, dressing changes and emotional support for the family. They can visit during the day or night to allow the family to rest.
- Macmillan nurses are trained to provide good symptom control. They also have an educational role, so they can answer questions. They work 9-5 and do not offer emergency support.

- An outreach team from the local hospice may provide advice and offer short-term admission if symptom control is not optimal.
- Patient support groups may provide practical advice and support.

Diagnosing dying

In a perfect world, doctors would recognise when death is imminent, but it can be surprisingly difficult. The trajectory of metastatic cancer is more predictable than that of heart failure, stroke, and respiratory failure. It can be very difficult to recognise the final dip in function of frail, older people, often with dementia, who may have had multiple admissions. A particular 'trap' is a post-ictal state after an unwitnessed fit when a patient may appear moribund only to recover 24 hours later. Often, the nurses, who have more hands-on time with the patients, are better at predicting imminent death.

Signs of impending death include:

- Becoming bedbound.
- Lack of interest in eating and drinking.
- Poor swallowing and not taking medicines.
- Agitation or distress.
- Drop in level of consciousness.
- Cheyne–Stokes breathing.

Recognising this point enables:

- Communication of this with the patient (if sufficiently alert), family and team.
- The family to gather and say goodbye.
- Ongoing support for the wishes of the patient and family regarding end-of-life care, place of death, spiritual and emotional support, etc. If the patient has been admitted to hospital it may be possible to expedite discharge if the patient wants to die at home. If this is feasible, it is essential to supply 'just in case' medication in anticipation of what may be needed and to phone the community team and GP.
- Focus on symptom control, especially mouth care, and stopping management that is no longer relevant, e.g. prophylactic dalteparin, blood tests, and cannulation. Reduce disruptive interruptions, e.g. routine observations. Check that a DNACPR order has not been overlooked.
- Pre-emptive prescribing for ongoing symptom control when oral medication can no longer be taken.
- Explanation and ongoing discussion with the family about aspects of care. If relatives understand that someone who is dying does not usually want to eat or drink, they are less likely to feel that the nurses are not making enough effort to feed them. Reassure about signs such as the 'death rattle' (see discussion above).

If the patient is dying in hospital, it can be useful to have something positive to offer, e.g. a side room if available referral to the palliative care team, the chaplain or to facilitate the family helping with mouth care if desired, etc.

How a patient is managed in their last few days of life influences satisfaction with medical and nursing care and affects the way their relatives think about their loved one's last days, which will have an impact on their grieving. Good symptom control and communication improve the reaction to bereavement. This benefits the team by reducing the desire to blame and, therefore, complaints.

Using a syringe driver

When patients are unable to take medications orally but are distressed, a subcutaneous syringe driver is an excellent method of providing symptom control. It is often possible to predict that a 'pump' will be needed soon. Ask the nurses to check that one is available. Drivers used in the NHS include the McKinley T34 and the Graseby pump. Your trust may have a syringe driver prescription proforma (online or paper). Get help from your team, the ward pharmacist, or palliative care about what to include, and make sure the drugs are available. Tell the patient, if alert and the family what you are doing and why. Use 'as needed' subcutaneous doses to gain control of symptoms and ensure that symptom control is maintained without interruption. Common options are:

- **Morphine:** for pain and severe distress.
- **Anti-emetic:** consider cyclizine (may cause site irritation and limited compatibility), haloperidol or levomepromazine.
- **Midazolam:** to control fits and for terminal restlessness.
- **Glycopyrronium:** to reduce respiratory secretions.

Water for injection is the commonest diluent, but some units prefer 0.9% saline (incompatible with cyclizine but essential for levomepromazine and dexamethasone).

Emotional support

Support the family and carers and encourage them to talk with and listen to the patient. Enable them to work through feelings of grief, loss, and fear. Explain that it is entirely normal for the patient to feel sad, angry, guilty, and depressed about their illness and impending death. The patient may be anxious and fearful about what will happen to their spouse or family. Talking things through and bringing them into the open will help the patient find some resolution of their emotional conflicts. Encourage discussions regarding the last few days and the patient's wishes for their funeral.

Spiritual and religious support

Spiritual care for a patient approaching the end of life is centred on their need to find a meaning for their life, their illness, and their impending death. It may include helping the patient find self-worth or just enabling them to express themselves. Spiritual support should be available for people of all faiths and none. Patients may find great comfort in religious support, prayer, and rites.

It may be difficult to assess the spiritual needs of patients. Earlier in their journey ask open questions such as 'How do you usually make sense of things?' and 'How do you cope?' This may reveal a specific religious need or a more nebulous desire to talk things through. All care professionals can provide some spiritual care but should avoid projecting their beliefs on the patient. The chaplaincy service and other faith leaders can deliver specialist spiritual help. Simply ask 'Would you like to see someone from the chaplaincy?'

The chaplaincy service is multi-faith and has adapted to a more secular society. Chaplains can offer counselling, help with ethical decisions, support for the family and ward team and education, as well as worship and liaison with the community and faith leaders. They are very willing to see people with no religion.

Considerations for people of different faiths dying in hospital

In England and Wales in the 2021 census 46% described themselves as Christian, 37% as having no religion, 6.5% as Muslim, 1.7% as Hindu, 0.9% as Sikh, 0.5% as Jewish and 0.5% as Buddhist. Religious adherence will vary with age and place; your ward team will be familiar with the local population.

Work with the ward team to be flexible – in traditions where many friends and relations wish to gather with the patient before and after death a side room makes this easier. If rapid cremation or burial is desired, expedite the death certificate. The following list gives some examples but ask the patient/family what they want, as people differ in their adherence to their faith.

Christianity includes many traditions and allows burial or cremation.

- Anglican patients may want a chaplain (or their parish priest) to visit, say prayers at the bedside, and offer Holy Communion.
- Roman Catholic patients derive comfort from the priest performing the Sacrament of the Anointing the Sick (the Last Rites) before death. The priest may offer Confession and Holy Communion.
- Free Church patients may wish for prayers around the time of death.

A Muslim patient's family will traditionally keep vigil.

- If able, the patient may continue to pray five times a day and may need help to wash before prayer.
- The family will take turns at reading from the Quran.
- An imam is not required but may provide support.
- When death is near, the closest family member encourages the patient to say the Islamic declaration of faith, the Shahada.
- After death, the head is turned towards the right shoulder to enable the body to be buried facing Mecca.
- Traditionally, the body is cared for and washed by Muslims of the same sex.
- The funeral and burial should be as soon as possible. Post-mortem is only allowed if required by law.

Hindu patients may wish to have religious items around them, as they believe a dying person's state of mind influences rebirth.

- Many relatives may wish to visit, and a Hindu priest may perform the last rites.
- Just before death, the sacred tulasi leaf and Ganges water may be administered to the dying person.
- The body is washed and dressed by the family.
- Cremation takes place as soon as possible after death.
- Be sensitive if a coroner's post-mortem is required, as this is felt to be disrespectful to the dead.

The family of Sikh patients or a priest from the local Gurdwara may read from Sri Guru Granth Sahib Ji.

- A few drops of holy water will be placed in the patient's mouth at the time of death.
- Usually, families choose to wash and dress the body, but if they are not present, do not remove the Five Ks (Kesh: hair kept under a turban for men; kangha: comb; kara: bracelet; kachera: undershorts; kirpan: short sword).
- Cremation takes place as soon as possible after death.
- There is no religious objection to a post-mortem.

Jewish beliefs depend on whether the patient is Orthodox, Reform, or Conservative.

- Patients may want their own rabbi to visit.
- When nearing the end, the patient may make the final confession, or Viddui.
- The body should not be left alone, and it should not be undressed until it is washed and prepared for burial.
- The funeral should be as soon as possible after death.
- The family will need support if a coroner's post-mortem is needed.

Buddhism includes many different traditions.

- Buddhists prefer to be mentally alert at the time of death, so avoid sedatives and discuss the use of painkillers that may decrease awareness.

- The teachings of Buddha, known as sutras, may be chanted by friends and family to reduce fear and distress.
- Buddhism teaches that a person is not fully dead until several hours after death to allow the being to continue its journey, so the body should be disturbed as little as possible.
- Most Buddhists choose to be cremated.
- Buddhists accept post-mortems but prefer a delay of several days to ensure the soul has had time to depart.

Care after death

See Chapter 21 for information regarding death certification and informing the coroner. Some trusts offer an opportunity for relatives to come back to the hospital to meet the consultant after every bereavement. At Addenbrooke's, this is handled by the chaplaincy and patient affairs. A letter of condolence and an offer to meet the consultant are sent to the next of kin 6 weeks after every death. If the family wants to accept the offer, the chaplaincy liaises to find out what the family wants to discuss and arranges the meeting. Most people who die in hospitals are older, so most of this work is done by geriatricians.

This feels like 'extra' work, but it is informative to find out what questions a family has, explanations can be given, and any misconceptions can be corrected. Families usually express great satisfaction for this opportunity, and although difficult to prove, it probably helps with their grieving and reduces formal complaints.

Bereavement

After the age of 75, 30% of men and 64% of women are widowed. Four (or five) main phases of grief have been described, but grief varies enormously between individuals, and few people progress steadily through each stage in a predictable way. Sometimes, e.g. when a loved one has dementia, part of the work of grieving may be undertaken before the death (anticipatory grieving).

1 **Shock and disbelief:** characterised by numbness and an inability to accept what has happened.
2 **Yearning:** may be characterised by acute pangs of severe loss and pining and a restless search for the dead person, who often appears in dreams and hallucinations. Periods of guilt and anger are directed at oneself, the dead person or other family members, friends, and hospital staff.
3 **Depression and apathy:** a time of hopeless despair with periods of joyless monotony. It is often associated with profound depression and a loss of self-confidence. Guilt and anger are again common features. This emotional turbulence may continue for a year or more.
4 **Acceptance:** of the reality that the loved person is dead and that life has changed. The bereaved person resumes a lifestyle that, to a greater or lesser extent, is adapted to his or her new status. This phase enables the bereaved person to let go of their dead loved one and to start a new sort of life.

The first of these phases may last for days, and the second for weeks. The third phase is likely to last for months, but most people adjust to a major bereavement within 1–2 years. Hallucinations, in which the dead person is vividly seen, may continue for a prolonged period. Mourning is associated with a number of 'tasks', which include acceptance of reality, experiencing the pain, adjusting to the unfamiliar environment, and redirecting energy towards new relationships and activities.

The inability to work through the phases of grief is sometimes called a pathological grief reaction and is particularly likely to occur following sudden or untimely deaths. There is a high incidence of ill health and death in the surviving spouse following bereavement. Most areas of the UK now have a branch of Cruse Bereavement Care, a charity that offers help to bereaved people ranging from talking to a trained volunteer to meeting other bereaved people to share their feelings. The website has practical advice on what to do after someone dies.

📖 REFERENCES AND FURTHER READING

Lunney JR, Lynn J, Hogan C (2002) Trajectories of dying. Profiles of older Medicare decedents. *J. Am. Geriatr. Soc.* 50:1108–12. https://doi.org/10.1046/j.1532-5415.2002.50268.x

Lancet Commission on the Value of Death bringing death back into life (2022): https://www.thelancet.com/commissions/value-of-death

Dying Matters https://www.hospiceuk.org/our-campaigns/dying-matters

Leadership Alliance for the Care of Dying People. *One Chance to get it Right* (2014) https://assets.publishing.service.gov.uk/government/uploads/system/uploads/attachment_data/file/323188/One_chance_to_get_it_right.pdf

ONS Leading causes of death in the UK 2001 to 2018 www.ons.gov.uk/peoplepopulationandcommunity/healthandsocialcare/causesofdeath/articles/leadingcausesofdeathuk/2001to2018

Gold Standards Framework www.goldstandardsframework.org.uk

NICE Guidelines *Advance care planning* www.nice.org.uk/about/nice-communities/social-care/quick-guides/advance-care-planning

Palliative care adult network guidelines http://book.pallcare.info/index.php

The Palliative Care Handbook (2019) https://www.ruh.nhs.uk/for_clinicians/departments_ruh/palliative_care/documents/palliative_care_handbook.pdf

Public Health England *Faith at the end of life.* (2016) https://assets.publishing.service.gov.uk/government/uploads/system/uploads/attachment_data/file/496231/Faith_at_end_of_life_-_a_resource.pdf

BGS *Guidance on End of Life Care in Frailty* (2020). Comprises a comprehensive suite of chapters: www.bgs.org.uk/resources/resource-series/end-of-life-care-in-frailty

INFORMATION FOR PATIENTS AND FAMILIES

Compassion in Dying website: Making a Living Will: https://beta.compassionindying.org.uk/living-will-advance-decision

Advance Care Plan England and Wales: http://advancecareplan.org.uk/advance-care-plan-journey

A short video describing the ReSPECT process and form: https://www.youtube.com/watch?v=qyNvBgo_VGI

Marie Curie Cancer Care: www.mariecurie.org.uk

Cruse bereavement support: www.cruse.org.uk

Kathryn Mannix With the End in Mind. Collins (2017), paperback (2022), ISBN-13 978-0008210915

All websites were accessed in September 2024.

Index

Geriatric Medicine and Elderly Care: Lecture Notes, Ninth Edition. Claire G. Nicholl, K. Jane Wilson, and Shaun D'Souza.
© 2025 John Wiley & Sons Ltd. Published 2025 by John Wiley & Sons Ltd.
Companion website: www.wiley.com/go/lecturenotesgeriatricmedicine9e